Small Animal Medical Diagnosis

Small Animal Medical Diagnosis

EDITED BY

Michael D. Lorenz, B.S., D.V.M.

Diplomate, American College of Veterinary Internal Medicine;
Professor of Small Animal Medicine and Associate Dean for Academic Affairs
College of Veterinary Medicine
The University of Georgia,
Athens, Georgia

Larry M. Cornelius, D.V.M., Ph.D.

Diplomate, American College of Veterinary Internal Medicine;
Professor of Small Animal Medicine
College of Veterinary Medicine
The University of Georgia
Athens, Georgia

WITH 11 CONTRIBUTORS

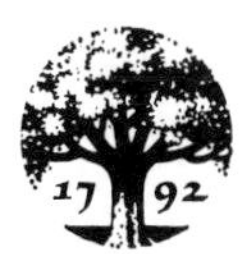

J. B. Lippincott Company

Philadelphia • London • Mexico City
New York • St. Louis • São Paulo • Sydney

Sponsoring Editor: Delois Patterson
Manuscript Editor/Production Coordinator: Lee Henderson
Indexer: Ann Cassar
Design Director: Tracy Baldwin
Design Coordinator: Don Shenkle
Designer: Patricia Pennington
Production Supervisor: Carol A. Florence
Compositor: Bi-Comp, Inc.
Printer/Binder: R. R. Donnelley & Sons Company
Cover Printer: Philips Offset

1 3 5 6 4 2

Library of Congress Cataloging-in-Publication Data

Small animal medical diagnosis.
Bibliography: p.
Includes index.
1. Veterinary medicine—Diagnosis. I. Lorenz, Michael D. II. Cornelius, Larry M.
SF771.S59 1987 636.089'6075 86-15358
ISBN-0-397-50555-8

The authors and publisher have exerted every effort to ensure that drug selection and dosage set forth in this text are in accord with current recommendations and practice at the time of publication. However, in view of ongoing research, changes in government regulations, and the constant flow of information relating to drug therapy and drug reactions, the reader is urged to check the package insert for each drug for any change in indications and dosage and for added warnings and precautions. This is particularly important when the recommended agent is a new or infrequently employed drug.

This book is dedicated to our colleagues
who have championed the problem-oriented method,
and to our many students
who have faithfully applied this method in their practice
of veterinary medicine.

Contributors

Dennis N. Aron, d.v.m.
Diplomate, American College of Veterinary Surgeons;
Assistant Professor of Small Animal Medicine
College of Veterinary Medicine
The University of Georgia
Athens, Georgia

Jeanne A. Barsanti, d.v.m., m.s.
Diplomate, American College of Veterinary Internal Medicine;
Professor of Small Animal Medicine
College of Veterinary Medicine
The University of Georgia
Athens, Georgia

Scott A. Brown, v.m.d.
Resident in Small Animal Internal Medicine
College of Veterinary Medicine
The University of Georgia
Athens, Georgia

Clay A. Calvert, d.v.m.
Diplomate, American College of Veterinary Internal Medicine;
Associate Professor of Small Animal Medicine
College of Veterinary Medicine
The University of Georgia
Athens, Georgia

JONATHAN N. CHAMBERS, D.V.M.
Diplomate, American College of Veterinary Surgeons;
Associate Professor of Small Animal Medicine
College of Veterinary Medicine
The University of Georgia
Athens, Georgia

LAINE A. COWAN, D.V.M.
Resident in Small Animal Internal Medicine
College of Veterinary Medicine
The University of Georgia
Athens, Georgia

CRAIG E. GREENE, D.V.M., M.S.
Diplomate, American College of Veterinary Internal Medicine;
Professor of Small Animal Medicine
College of Veterinary Medicine
The University of Georgia
Athens, Georgia

MICHAEL R. LAPPIN, D.V.M.
Resident in Small Animal Internal Medicine
College of Veterinary Medicine
The University of Georgia
Athens, Georgia

CHARLES L. MARTIN, D.V.M., M.S.
Diplomate, American College of Veterinary Ophthalmologists;
Professor and Director
Veterinary Medical Teaching Hospital
College of Veterinary Medicine
The University of Georgia
Athens, Georgia

JOHN E. OLIVER, D.V.M., M.S., Ph.D.
Diplomate, American College of Veterinary Internal Medicine—Neurology;
Professor and Head
Department of Small Animal Medicine
College of Veterinary Medicine
The University of Georgia
Athens, Georgia

JAMES P. TOOMBS, D.V.M., M.S.
Assistant Professor of Small Animal Medicine
College of Veterinary Medicine
The University of Georgia
Athens, Georgia

Preface

Veterinary medical education, like other scientific fields, must come to grips with a knowledge explosion unparalleled in medical history. It is very apparent that the development of factual knowledge is occurring at a rate that surpasses the capacity of human memory. In an attempt to deal with the knowledge explosion, specialization has developed. However, veterinary students and practitioners are usually generalists and are required to acquire a data base for many diseases and surgical procedures for several species of animals. Educators now recognize that a student cannot possibly remember all the facts that he encounters in 4 years of veterinary medical education; however, sufficient facts must be retained to provide a core data base that allows effective problem-solving.

Having observed veterinary students and practitioners solve problems for the past 16 years, we are convinced that problem-solving must occur early in the educational process. *Small Animal Medical Diagnosis* has been written for the veterinary student and the general small animal practitioner. It provides the core information necessary to effectively evaluate the major medical problems in dogs and cats. It does not replace the traditional textbooks that are disease oriented.

We are indebted to our colleagues for their contributions based on their many years of experience in veterinary education. Special thanks are extended to Kip Carter for the medical illustrations and to Patti Carter and Joan Hoffman for their typing assistance. We also extend our appreciation to the staff of J. B. Lippincott Company, especially Bill Burgower, Delois Patterson, and Sandy Reinhardt, for their patience and guidance in the development of *Small Animal Medical Diagnosis*.

MICHAEL D. LORENZ, B.S., D.V.M.

LARRY M. CORNELIUS, D.V.M., Ph.D.

Contents

PART SIX: CARDIOVASCULAR PROBLEMS

PART SEVEN: RESPIRATORY PROBLEMS

PART EIGHT: DIGESTIVE PROBLEMS

PART TWELVE: NEUROLOGIC PROBLEMS

PART THIRTEEN: SPECIAL SENSATION PROBLEMS

PART FOURTEEN: LABORATORY-DEFINED PROBLEMS

1

The Problem-Oriented Approach

MICHAEL D. LORENZ

In the 1960s, the problem-oriented medical record (POMR) was introduced in medical practice.[3,4] The POMR encourages the user to employ sound logic in thoughts about patients and provides a convenient display system for medical data and actions.[1] In 1971, the Department of Small Animal Medicine at The University of Georgia adopted the POMR for use in the Small Animal Teaching Hospital. Since that date, the concepts of the POMR have evolved into a problem-solving system based on identification and management of an animal's problems. These concepts have also been incorporated into lecture and laboratory courses.[2]

The basic tenet of the problem-oriented approach (POA), and thus the POMR, is that disease alters anatomy and function to cause clinical signs and symptoms. These changes in anatomy and function are called "problems." The focus in the POA is away from the classic method of diagnostic impressions and lists of differential diagnosis. Instead, emphasis is placed on critical identification of the patient's problems and a clear understanding of the mechanisms (pathophysiology) that create each problem. When the mechanisms are clearly understood, the diseases that cause each problem are more easily recalled. In the POA, the term *rule out* is used to describe the potential causes of any problem. The most appropriate diagnostic procedure for documentation of each rule out is then listed. Thus, possible causes of problems are always coupled with the most appropriate diagnostic procedures.

The clinical reasoning process utilized in the POA is based on four steps: (1) data base collection, (2) problem identification, (3) plan formulation, and (4) assessment and follow-up.

STEP 1: DATA BASE COLLECTION

The initial data base should contain the information necessary to allow identification of all problems in the patient. The size of the data base for any particular patient should be specified in advance. This is the guaranteed data base and it is collected for each animal. Although the size of the guaranteed data base is often debated, there is no disagreement that it must include a complete history and a complete physical examination. A strong argument for the inclusion of a complete blood count and urine analysis in the guaranteed data base can be made, since these procedures broadly screen many body systems. In this regard, these diagnostic procedures can be viewed as an extension of the physical examination. In this book, the problems described are largely those identified through the history and physical examination.

A problem-specific data base is the information necessary to properly evaluate the possible causes or rule outs for that problem. Each chapter of this book has a diagnostic plan that lists the data base for each problem.

History

Next to the physical examination, the history is the most important aspect of correct medical problem solving. One must resist the temptation to substitute diagnostic tests for a thorough history. The history alerts the clinician to the presence of potential problems and increases one's curiosity during physical examination of the patient. Begin by determining the chief complaint. Pursue this complaint in depth, noting any additional problems and their chronologic development. Be sure to list all medications given, since treatment often alters the normal progression of many diseases. Review each body system and question the owner about the presence of signs that would indicate organ or system dysfunction.

In taking the history, two different techniques are usually employed. The first technique, called the cross-examination or interrogation style, allows the clinician to ask questions in an organized and chronologic manner. Some owners are inhibited by this style, whereas others may answer questions falsely, particularly when the question is not understood. The second technique is the open-ended story style, in which the owner is asked to describe the pet's problems. This style may be disorganized and lack the chronologic specificity needed in a good history. The author prefers a combination of the two techniques, using just enough cross-examination to clarify problems and add good chronology to the history.

Physical Examination

The physical examination is the most important aspect of the data base. Problems not identified in the physical examination are usually also missed when more invasive or expensive diagnostic tests are performed. In addition, the proper interpretation of laboratory tests involves correlation with the history and physical examination findings. A complete physical examination should not require more than 5 to 8 minutes. Each body system should be examined. Particular attention should be given to those body systems in which dysfunction is suspected from the history. Ocular and neurologic evaluations (frequently slighted during the physical examination) must be included.

The author suggests that a physical examination form be followed that stresses a complete review of body systems (Fig. 1-1). Abnormalities are recorded for each system on the form. Special examination forms for the integumentary system, eye, and nervous system are very helpful and reduce writing time (Figs. 1-2, 1-3, and 1-4).

PRESENTING COMPLAINT OR REQUEST

REFERRING VETERINARIAN

ADDRESS

PHONE

ADMISSION HR. | PREVIOUS ADMISSION | DISCHARGE HR.

(1) GEN	☐ N ☐ ABN ☐ NE	(2) INTEG.	☐ N ☐ ABN ☐ NE	(3) M	☐ N ☐ ABN ☐ NE	(4) CIRC	☐ N ☐ ABN ☐ NE	(5) RESP	☐ N ☐ ABN ☐ NE	(6) DIG	☐ N ☐ ABN ☐ NE
(7) GU	☐ N ☐ ABN ☐ NE	(8) EYES	☐ N ☐ ABN ☐ NE	(9) EARS	☐ N ☐ ABN ☐ NE	(10) NS	☐ N ☐ ABN ☐ NE	(11) L	☐ N ☐ ABN ☐ NE	(12) MUCOSA	☐ N ☐ ABN ☐ NE

DESCRIBE ABNORMAL (USE NUMBERS ABOVE) T ______ P ______ R ______ WT ______

STUDENT SIGNATURE ______________ PHYSICAL EXAMINATION ADM. CLINICIAN SIGNATURE ______________

Fig. 1-1. System-oriented physical examination form.

DATE: ______

GRADE LESIONS:
1 if few or mild
2 if several or moderate
3 if many or severe

Primary Lesions

Papule___ Pustule___ Vesicle___ Bulla___
Plaque___ Nodule___ Tumor___ Cyst___
Macule___ Patch___ Wheal___ Abscess___

Secondary Lesions

Scale___ Epidermal Collarette___ Crust___
Alopecia___ Erythema___
Hyperpigmentation___ Lichenification___
Erosion___ Excoriation___ Ulcer___
Comedone___ Hyperkeratosis___ Callus___
Fissure___ Scar___ Hypopigmentation___

(Circle)
Pruritus: Int. Mod. Mild None
Thickness: Norm. Inc. Dec.
Elasticity: Norm. Inc. Dec.
Easy Epilation: Yes No
Hair Coat: Norm. Dry Dull Brittle Oily

INITIAL WORK-UP (Circle)

Scrape: Sarcoptes Demodex Neg.
Other ______
Parasites: Fleas Flea Dirt Ticks
Other ______
Woods Light: - + DTM submitted
Direct Smear: ______

DISTRIBUTION OF LESIONS

VENTRAL DORSAL

DIFFERENTIAL DIAGNOSIS

Teaching Hospital
College of Veterinary Medicine
University of Georgia
Athens, Georgia

9/85 (#615/3-N) **Dermatology Exam.**

Fig. 1-2. Dermatologic examination form for the integumentary system.

STEP 2: PROBLEM IDENTIFICATION

The second step in medical problem-solving is problem identification. In small animal veterinary medicine, a problem is defined as any abnormality requiring medical or surgical management or one that interferes with the quality of life. It is important for problems to be stated at their current level of understanding. An overstated problem may cause expensive, invasive, and needless diagnostic tests

OPHTHALMIC CONSULTATION REQUEST

DATE REQUESTED	TIME AM ☐ PM ☐	LOCATION OF ANIMAL	SPECIES	ADDRESSOGRAPH
REQUESTING CLINICIAN		STUDENT		
Hx/PROBLEMS				
PRIOR OCULAR AND SYSTEMIC THERAPY				

OD	OPHTHALMIC EXAMINATION	OS
	ORBIT/GLOBE	
	LIDS Palpebral Reflex	
	CONJUNCTIVA & MEMBRANA NICTITANS	
	NASOLACRIMAL SYSTEM	
	CORNEA Sensation	
	IRIS Direct Reflex Consensual Reflex	
	ANTERIOR CHAMBER, ANGLE, & IOP	
	LENS	
	FUNDUS	
	VITREOUS	
	VISUAL ACUITY Menace Reflex	
	OCULAR MOTILITY & VESTIBULAR REFLEXES	

PROBLEMS		OS-Left Eye OU-Both Eyes NE-Not OD-Right Eye N-Normal Examined
		DATE AND TIME COMPLETED / / AM ☐ PM ☐
		BY

Fig. 1-3. Ophthalmic examination form.

to be performed. Many times problems identified in the history need to be documented, since the owner's observations may be erroneous. Problems are numbered consecutively and dated chronologically on a separate sheet of paper called the master problem list (MPL). As additional problems are identified, they are dated and assigned the next number.

The POMR couples all notations in the medical record to numbered problems on the MPL (Fig. 1-5). The MPL should be placed in the front of the

Neurologic Examination
University of Georgia

I. Subjective

II. Objective (circle or describe)

A. Observation: Mental Status: Alert Stupor Depressed Coma ____________

Posture: Normal, Head Tilt, Tremor, Falling L-R ____________

Gait: Normal, Post Paresis, Tetraparesis Ataxia, Dysmetria, Circling ____________

B. Palpation: Muscle or Skeletal Abnormality

C. Postural Reactions

L	Reaction	R
	Hopping, Front	
	Hopping, Rear	
	Proprioception Front	
	Rear	
	Placing, Tactile Front	
	Rear	
	Placing, Visual Front	
	Rear	

D. Cranial Nerves

L	Nerve + Function	R
	II vision menace	
	II + III pupil size	
	Stim. L. eye	
	Stim. R. eye	
	II Fundus	
	III, IV, VI Strabismus	
	Nystagmus	
	V Sensation	
	V Mastication	
	VII Facial Muscles	
	Palpebral	
	IX, X Swallowing	
	XII Tongue	

E. Spinal Reflexes

L	Reflex Spinal Segment	R
	Triceps C-7–T-1	
	Ext. Carpi Rad. C-7–T-1	
	Quadriceps L-4–6	
	Flexion, Fore C-6–T-1	
	Flexion, Hind L-5–S-1	
	Perineal S-1–2	

F. Sensation: Location

Hyperesthesia ____________
Superficial Pain ____________
Deep Pain ____________

G. Assessment:

Note significant findings and localize lesion.

H. Plan: Dx

Sig: ____________ DVM

Fig. 1-4. Neurologic examination form.

medical record. It serves as a table of contents that directs the medical care of each patient.

Problems are subject to several "fates" (see section on assessment and follow-up). Problems can be redefined to a higher level of understanding or they may be combined. The clinical reasoning process has problem resolution as its primary goal. Problems may be resolved or combined to a diagnosis or only resolved therapeutically. Problems can be inactivated when no further diagnostic or therapeutic action is warranted but resolution has not occurred.

DATE ACTIVE	NO.	**MASTER PROBLEM LIST** CONTINUED	DATE RESOLVED

Fig. 1-5. Master problem list form (the "table of contents" or "index" to the medical record) (this page, front; page 8, back).

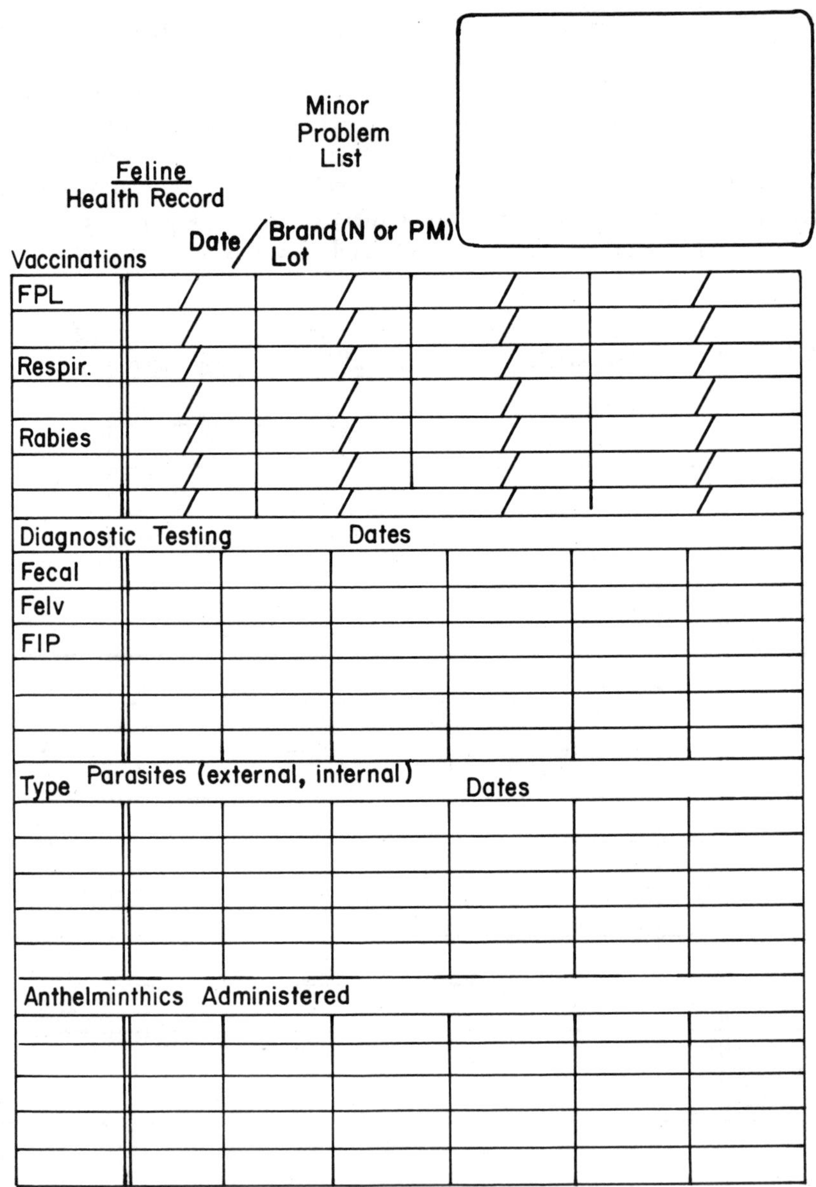

Minor Problem List

Feline Health Record

Vaccinations	Date/Brand (N or PM) Lot				
FPL	/	/	/	/	
	/	/	/	/	
Respir.	/	/	/	/	
	/	/	/	/	
Rabies	/	/	/	/	
	/	/	/	/	
	/	/	/	/	

Diagnostic Testing	Dates					
Fecal						
Felv						
FIP						

Type Parasites (external, internal)	Dates					

Anthelminthics Administered						

Fig. 1-5. (*Continued*)

STEP 3: PLAN FORMULATION

Once the problems are identified and the MPL formulated, attention is given to development of an initial plan (Fig. 1-6). This is a critical step in the clinical reasoning process, since it will dictate medical action for the first 24 to 48 hours.

Temporary Problem List
Initial Plan

Problem	Dx:	Rule outs, Procedures	Rx:	CE·

Student Signature

Clinician Signature

Fig. 1-6. Form for construction of the initial plan.

Each plan has three components: (1) a diagnostic section, (2) a therapeutic section, and (3) a client/owner education section. The initial plan emphasizes components 1 and 2. Plans are also a component of the assessment and follow-up step described below.

The Diagnostic Plan

A diagnostic plan is formulated and written for each problem. The plan should be organized with the most important or serious problems listed first. Rule outs (causes) are listed under each problem, with priority given to the most likely causes. Diagnostic procedures are coupled with each rule out. In this manner, logical clinical reasoning can be displayed and audited. The clinician in effect has stated the thought process, that is, "Here are the problems I've identified," "These are the most likely causes in my opinion," and "I will perform these diagnostic procedures to test my hypothesis." When displayed in the POMR, the clinical reasoning process can be evaluated by any knowledgeable individual.

Developing a well-founded diagnostic plan is based on the logic and information contained in each chapter of this book. As stated earlier, the POA emphasizes the management of problems through knowledge of their mechanisms and causes. By listing the problems, interrelationships can be more easily elucidated. Certainly, a disease or condition that appears as a major rule out for more than one problem should be highly suspected as the primary target for clinical diagnostic efforts.

The management of certain problems involves the collection of data beyond that contained in the guaranteed data base. This information constitutes the problem-specific data base. It includes tests or procedures that help establish the cause and the metabolic or biochemical consequences of the problem. Clinical algorithms are sequential steps in clinical reasoning based on the results of the problem-specific data base. Clinical algorithms are used in this book to display a logical progression of problem management. Realize that "perfect" algorithms do not exist. Therefore, understanding the reasons for each decision is important. Algorithms are very useful in medical management since it is impossible to remember all the causes of many problems.

The Therapeutic Plan

Therapy must be coupled with the problem that it is intended to resolve or help. When this is not done, the logic of therapeutic decisions cannot be audited. During formulation of the initial plan, a clinician must weigh the possible benefits of symptomatic therapy against the alterations that therapy may produce in laboratory tests results. In many cases, serum should be saved prior to therapy for future biochemical or immunologic tests. In medicine, as much time is spent diagnosing what was done to an animal as is spent in diagnosing the underlying disease.

A therapeutic plan is also part of the assessment and follow-up step.

Client/Owner Education

This section of the initial plan describes the information given to clients about their animals' problems, general condition, and prognosis.

STEP 4: ASSESSMENT AND FOLLOW-UP

The fourth step in medical problem solving is the assessment of data collected from the initial plan (or the problem-specific data base). These results must be correlated with the history and physical findings. The clinician is actually assessing hypotheses stated in the initial plan. The assessment should be written in the medical record in relationship to each problem and should accurately interpret the results of diagnostic tests or procedures. It reflects the logic for changes in the MPL.

Follow-up represents actions to be taken based on the results of the initial plan or daily plans. In the POMR, follow-up is maintained in the daily progress notes. Progress notes contain three sections and are written in a problem-oriented manner, that is, information is grouped according to the problem it affects. Section 1 is for new or additional data, section 2 is the assessment, and section 3 is the plan (remember that plans always have three components). Orienting follow-up information by problems allows the display of the clinical reasoning process so that audit of this process can be efficient and effective.

SUMMARY

The problem-oriented approach to medical management is based on logical concepts. Disease creates clinical signs or problems. When problems are logically pursued, the underlying disease(s) can be discovered. When the diagnosis still escapes identification, proper problem management improves the quality of life. The POA is not a new system: it follows the logic that clinicians have used for many years. The POMR is new: it provides a structured format for display of an old system of medical management. The POA is no panacea for the "ills" of medical management. It will not correct the problems created by superficial data collection. Poor histories, poorly performed physical examinations, poorly understood pathophysiologic processes, and deficiencies in basic concepts of therapy are not corrected by this system. It is a system that functions well when all steps are meticulously followed.

This book is about problems: how they are identified, why they occur, what diseases are ultimately responsible, how they are logically pursued, and how they are symptomatically managed. There is little or no discussion of particular diseases. Other books are available that describe disease in detail. When the knowledge of disease is coupled with the knowledge of problems, the clinical reasoning process operates at its highest level. The author sincerely believes that the clinical reasoning process is greatly improved when knowledge of problems is understood first, followed by the knowledge of disease.

The POA is a logical way to think about diagnosis and patient management. A POMR is not necessarily needed for the clinician to think in terms of "problem solving." However, when the POMR is used, it reflects a problem-oriented approach to case management.

REFERENCES

1. Hurst JW: Ten reasons why Lawrence Weed is right. N Engl J Med 284:51, 1971
2. Lorenz MD: Problem directed instruction in small animal clinical endocrinology. J Vet Med Ed 12:6, 1985
3. Weed LL: Medical records, patient care, and medical education. Ir J Med Surg 6:271, 1964
4. Weed LL: Medical records that guide and teach. N Engl J Med 278:593, 1968

Part One

GENERAL (POLYSYSTEMIC) PROBLEMS

2

Pyrexia (Fever)

MICHAEL D. LORENZ

PROBLEM DEFINITION AND RECOGNITION

Pyrexia is an elevation of body temperature caused by disease. It is only a clinical sign and occurs in a wide variety of pathologic conditions. Fever is synonymous with pyrexia. Hyperpyrexia relates to a fever in excess of 105°F. Intermittent fever is one in which the temperature falls to normal and rises again each day. A remittent fever is characterized by marked variation in temperature level each day; however, the low point is still above normal. A relapsing fever has short periods of increased temperature interspersed by periods of one or more days of normal temperature. A septic fever has large daily oscillations in body temperature.

To understand the significance of fever, it is necessary to present some background information concerning the regulation of body temperature and the pathogenesis of fever.

REGULATION OF BODY TEMPERATURE

Mammals are endothermic vertebrates that are capable of generating sufficient heat to regulate their body temperature by altering heat production and heat loss. Temperature regulation is a complicated reflex integrated by a thermoregulatory center in the hypothalamus. Thermal sensors are located throughout the body but are most abundant in the skin, spinal cord, abdomen, and hypothalamus.[4] The effectors of the reflex are those structures actually involved in raising or lowering body temperature. Examples of these effectors include skeletal muscle, skin, and the respiratory system.

Body heat is generated largely by the liver's oxidation of nutrients. During physical activity, much heat is generated by the muscles. The muscular system is very important to thermal regulation since its heat production can be rapidly increased or decreased according to need. Heat can be eliminated from the body in three ways: radiation, vaporization, and convection. In dogs and cats, the primary mechanism for heat loss is radiation and vaporization. Since small animals are covered with hair and have few sweat glands, heat is not rapidly dissipated through the skin. Panting is the primary means of dissipating excessive heat.

The central thermoregulator is set at 101°F to 102°F. It responds to changes of less than 0.2°C[3] and heat production is greatly augmented when skin temperatures are below 33°C. As the animal senses falling body temperature, two important effectors are stimulated. Peripheral vasoconstriction helps decrease heat loss, and increased muscular activity (shivering) generates additional heat. If body temperature increases in the normal animal, peripheral vasodilation, panting, and decreased muscular activity are used to dissipate heat. In general, the mechanisms for raising body temperature are sympathetic controlled whereas depression of temperature is largely parasympathetic regulated.

In summary, body temperature is controlled by a thermoregulator that receives information from a variety of thermal sensors. Small changes in body temperature elicit marked sympathetic or parasympathetic responses that alter heat production and heat loss.

Pathophysiology of Fever

Diseases or substances that induce fever (are pyrogenic) do not affect the effector side of the thermoregulatory reflex. Pyrogenic conditions affect the sensory and/or integrating parts of the reflex.[4] Fever represents the ability of an animal to regulate its body temperature at a higher level. Fever occurs when the thermoregulatory set point is raised above normal. Body temperature may or may not be raised to the same level.

Activators of Fever

Fever-inducing substances are called pyrogens. Bacterial endotoxins, gram-positive bacteria, viruses, hypersensitivity reactions, and tumors are sources of so-called *exogenous pyrogen*. It is unlikely that these substances directly affect the thermoregulatory center because the size and molecular complexity of most exogenous pyrogens preclude their entrance into the hypothalamus.[2]

All the activators of fever probably induce the formation of protein mediators called *endogenous pyrogen*. Endogenous pyrogen is the actual fever-inducing compound. It is released from neutrophils, monocytes, and eosinophils. Lymphocytes do not release endogenous pyrogens; however, sensitized lymphocytes reacting with antigen release a soluble lymphokine that stimulates production of endogenous pyrogen in neutrophils and macrophages.[1] Endogenous pyrogen is also released from fixed phagocytes such as Kupffer cells, splenic sinusoidal cells, alveolar macrophages, and peritoneal cells. Endogenous pyrogen does not exist as a preformed compound in the cells. Rather, its synthesis is stimulated when leukocytes or macrophages become activated by an exogenous source.

There is considerable evidence that endogenous pyrogen either directly or indirectly elevates the thermoregulatory set point in the hypothalamus. The exact mechanism is unknown but probably involves monoamines, prostaglandins, and cyclic AMP. Once the temperature set point is elevated, the body temperature is perceived as too low. Heat conservation (vasoconstriction) and increased heat production (chills, shivering) occur. These processes elevate the body temperature. When the fever stimulus is removed, the hypothalamic thermostat resets at normal and body temperature is lowered by peripheral vasodilation, sweating, and panting.

FUNCTION OF FEVER

There is no conclusive proof that fever is either harmful or beneficial. The majority of clinicians approach fever as a nonbeneficial sign that should be suppressed to make the patient feel better. Based on experiments in animals, fever may have the following beneficial effects. Fever may directly inhibit the growth of microorganisms, both bacteria and viruses. For instance, neonatal puppies have lower body temperatures than adult dogs and are much more susceptible to herpes viral infection. The suppressive effects of fever on the growth of microorganisms may be coupled with host defense mechanisms. For instance, serum iron levels decrease in animals with infection. The reaction is most likely due to endogenous pyrogen and makes an essential nutrient less available for bacterial metabolism. In addition, fever decreases the ability of bacteria to trap or chelate iron.

Several immune responses may be affected by fever. Lysosomes are more easily broken down during fever, and proteolytic enzymes that are destructive to viral agents are released. Fever may also increase the production of interferon that infers with the growth of viruses. There is some evidence that leukocyte mobility and phagocytic activity are enhanced by fever. The bactericidal activities of leukocytes may be increased by fever. Lastly, fever may enhance lymphocyte transformation.

The fever that accompanies noninfectious conditions apparently has little useful purpose and may aggravate the other clinical signs. However, fevers below 106°F in dogs and cats are potentially beneficial. Fevers above 106°F are potentially harmful to cellular metabolism and should be suppressed.

DIAGNOSTIC PLAN

Fever that results from acute inflammatory processes is usually easy to explain, and the cause is often found in the physical examination. Obscure or unexplained fevers are usually caused by chronic inflammatory processes that are difficult to define with routine physical or laboratory procedures. These fevers have been defined as fever of unknown origin. These fevers have three characteristics: (1) duration of at least 2 weeks, (2) temperature must exceed normal by 1.5° on several occasions, and (3) the etiology is obscure. There are four major

(Text continues on p 20)

Table 2-1. Causes of Obscure Fever in Dogs

DISEASE	SUGGESTIVE CLINICAL SIGNS	DIAGNOSTIC CLUES	SPECIAL TESTS
GENERALIZED INFECTIONS			
Bacterial endocarditis	Shifting leg lameness, joint effusion, heart murmur, cardiac arrhythmia, limb edema, history of recent surgical or medical illness	Changing cardiac murmur, splenomegaly, neutrophilic leukocytosis, microscopic hematuria, suppurative joint effusions, cardiac arrhythmia	Aerobic and anaerobic blood cultures, urine culture, joint fluid culture, ECG
Systemic mycoses	Chronic cough, chronic diarrhea, lymphadenopathy, suppurative skin nodules, history of endemic exposure	Evidence of diffuse granulomatous pneumonia on thoracic radiographs. Granulomatous skin lesions. Chorioretinitis, anterior uveitis, occasional neurologic signs	Demonstrate organism in bronchial secretions, exudate, lymph node aspirates, or tissue biopsies. Culture organisms from tissue or exudates. Occasionally serology is needed to confirm diagnosis.
Ehrlichosis	Epistaxis, petechiation, pallor, chronic weight loss, anorexia, serous ocular and nasal discharges	Thrombocytopenia, leukopenia, anemia (nonregenerative). Presence of brown dog ticks on patient or in its environment.	Demonstrate intracytoplasmic morula in mononuclear cells from peripheral blood or bone marrow Indirect fluorescent antibody test for *Ehrlicha canis* antibody
Rocky Mountain spotted fever (*Rickettsia rickettsia*)	Chronic anorexia, weight loss, peripheral limb and scrotal edema	Thrombocytopenia, mild anemia; chronic renal failure may develop	Serology for *R. rickettsia*; FA test on skin biopsy
Toxoplasmosis	Variety of clinical syndromes, including diarrhea, icterus, chronic cough, muscle pain and weakness, neurologic signs, chorioretinitis	The presence of myositis, chronic liver failure, chronic pneumonia, chronic CNS signs, or chorioretinitis are suggestive.	Serologic examination for toxoplasma antibodies and identification of organisms in affected tissue (muscle, liver, brain)
LOCALIZED INFECTIONS			
Pyothorax	Chronic cough, dyspnea, muffled lung sounds	Pleural effusion on thoracic radiographs	Thorocentesis for fluid analysis and bacterial and fungal cultures

Chronic hepatic disease	Chronic weight loss, vomiting and anorexia. Icterus may or may not be present. Vague neurologic signs.	Persistent increased concentrations of SGPT, hypoalbuminemia, low BUN. Radiographic evidence of small liver.	BSP and ammonia tolerance test; hepatic biopsy
Chronic pyelonephritis	Absent unless disease progresses to chronic renal failure. Anterior abdominal pain may be present.	Persistent hematuria, pyuria, and bacteria on cystocentesis urine specimens	Excretory urogram; renal biopsy
Chronic prostatitis or abscess	Dysuria, hematuria, tenesmus	Enlarged or painful prostate found on rectal palpation	Prostatic ejaculate, prostatic biopsy, double contrast cystography
IMMUNE-MEDIATED DISORDERS			
Systemic lupus erythematosus	Shifting leg lameness, muscle pain or weakness, joint effusion and pain, anemia	Nonerosive, nonseptic, suppurative polyarthritis; autoimmune hemolytic anemia; idiopathic thrombocytopenia; polymyositis; glomerulonephritis	ANA titer, LE prep, Coomb's test, antiplatelet antibody, renal biopsy
Rheumatoid arthritis	Progressive lameness, joint pain, joint enlargement	Progressive erosive polyarthritis	Arthrocentesis, rheumatoid factor titer
Polymyositis	Progressive lameness, muscle weakness, atrophy	Diffuse muscle pain	Muscle enzymes (CPK, LDH), muscle biopsy for histopathology and immunofluorescence, EMG
Lymphosarcoma	Signs largely depend upon tissue or organ involved. Enlarged peripheral or abdominal nodes are very suggestive.	Nonregenerative anemia, pancytopenia, neutropenia	Lymph node aspiration or biopsy, organ biopsy, bone marrow examination
Leukemia and other myeloproliferative disorders	No specific clinical signs	Evidence of leukemia in blood smear. May be associated with anemia and thrombocytopenia.	Bone marrow examination
DRUG-INDUCED			
Tetracycline	None	Associated with antibiotic therapy	Response to withdrawal of medication

ECG, electrocardiogram; FA, fluorescent antibody; CNS, central nervous system; SGPT, serum glutamic-pyruvic transaminase; BUN, blood urea nitrogen; ANA, antinuclear antibody; LE, lupus erythematosus; CPK, creatine phosphokinase; LDH, lactic dehydrogenase

disease categories to consider when seeking the etiology of an obscure fever: (1) infections (bacterial, viral, fungal, rickettsial), (2) immune-mediated, (3) neoplastic, and (4) drug-induced. The diagnostic plan should be formulated to explore each of these potential causes. In the dog, bacterial endocarditis, systemic lupus erythematosus, and lymphoreticular neoplasia are the most common causes of obscure fever. The data base should include a complete blood count (CBC), biochemical profile, urine analysis, aerobic and anaerobic blood cultures, antinuclear antibody (ANA) test, and thorough palpation of the abdomen and peripheral lymph nodes. Any abnormality detected in these procedures is followed up, since it may be a clue to the location of the fever-inducing disease.

The most common causes of obscure fever in cats are the systemic viral infections: feline infectious peritonitis and feline leukemia-related diseases. The data base for a cat with obscure fever should include a CBC, biochemical profile, urine analysis, feline leukemia test, and feline infectious peritonitis titer. The eye grounds should be carefully examined since these viral infections may produce chorioretinitis. If these procedures are negative, blood cultures, ANA tests, and determination of toxoplasmosis titers are indicated.

Tables 2-1 and 2-2 list the diagnostic criteria for the major diseases that produce obscure fevers in dogs and cats, respectively. The tables do not list every possible cause of obscure fever; rather, the most common causes are described. Localized organ involvement (*e.g.*, hepatic abscess) may cause obscure fever. The initial data base must be carefully examined to identify clues that suggest disease in a particular organ. Chest radiographs are useful for evaluation of the lungs and pleural space.

SYMPTOMATIC THERAPY

It is usually unnecessary to suppress fever unless the body temperature exceeds 105°F. Fevers above this level may be harmful to body metabolism and may need to be suppressed. Hyperpyrexia (body temperature above 106°F) should be treated with cool water baths, ice packs, alcohol rubdowns, or cool water enemas. Cooling procedures should continue until the body temperature is down to 103°F.

Several drugs have antipyretic effects and do not lower body temperature unless fever is present. Aspirin and other salicylate-like antipyretics do not affect the production of endogenous pyrogen. Rather, the antipyretic effect may be related to the antiprostaglandin properties of these compounds. Although controversial, prostaglandins may play a role in the mechanisms that allow endogenous pyrogen to induce fever. Aspirin and dipyrone are the drugs most commonly used in small animals. The dosage must be carefully monitored since these drugs have side effects such as gastrointestinal irritation and ulceration and, with dipyrone only, bone marrow suppression.

Glucocorticoids have potent antipyretic effects. These drugs reduce the amount of endogenous pyrogen released from leukocytes in response to endo-

Table 2-2. Causes of Obscure Fever in Cats

DISEASE	SUGGESTIVE CLINICAL SIGNS	DIAGNOSTIC CLUES	SPECIAL TESTS
SYSTEMIC INFECTIONS			
FeLV-related disease	Chronic infections, abortion, anemia, vomiting, diarrhea, dyspnea, anorexia, and weight loss	Nonregenerative anemia, immature blood cells in peripheral circulation Pleural effusion, organ enlargement, abdominal masses	FeLV tests, bone marrow examination, organ biopsy
Feline infectious peritonitis	Depends on form of disease present. Effusive form causes abdominal and pleural effusion. Noneffusive form may cause nonspecific neurologic signs, anterior uveitis, and renal and liver failure.	Hyperglobinemia, nonregenerative anemia, suppurative modified transudate in thorax or abdomen	FIP titer, liver or renal biopsy, examination of body cavity effusion, CSF examination
Toxoplasmosis	Dyspnea, icterus, enlarged abdominal lymph nodes, neurologic signs, iritis, retinitis, abortion	Bilirubinemia, diffuse pneumonia, leukopenia, anemia	Serology, demonstration of organism in tissue
IMMUNE-MEDIATED DISORDERS			
Systemic lupus erythematosus	See Table 2-1.	See Table 2-1.	See Table 2-1.
Polyarthritis	Progressive lameness, pain and enlargement of carpal and tarsal joints	Soft tissue swelling, degenerative joint disease, and erosion of carpal or tarsal joints	FeLV test

FeLV, feline leukemia virus; FIP, feline infectious peritonitis; CSF, cerebrospinal fluid

toxin and sepsis. Thus, glucocorticoids may actually mask the fever of a serious disease. Fever monitoring is important in assessing response to therapy for septic conditions. Corticosteroids suppress leukocyte migration, local inflammatory responses, and immunologically mediated processes that may stimulate endogenous pyrogen release. Glucocorticoids may also inhibit prostaglandin release and, through this mechanism, centrally inhibit fever production. In general, it is very risky to use glucocorticoids to suppress fever since they actually potentiate and mask the progression of serious infections. Glucocorticoids, as antipyretic agents, may be useful in immune-mediated and neoplastic conditions.

Certain phenothiazine compounds generally inhibit prostaglandin synthesis, interfere with central regulation of body temperature, and increase peripheral vasodilation. These effects may dramatically decrease fever. The drug most commonly used in veterinary medicine is dipyrone. It may cause bone marrow suppression in cats if used repeatedly.

Obviously, the decision to suppress fever must be weighed against its potential benefits. In the treatment of infection, fever suppression is seldom justified since this removes one method for monitoring the effectiveness of other drugs.

REFERENCES

1. Chao P, Francis L, Atkins E: The release of an endogenous pyrogen from guinea pig leukocytes in vitro: A new model for investigating the role of lymphocytes in fevers induced by antigen in hosts with delayed hypersensitivity. J Exp Med 145:1288–1298, 1977
2. Dinarello CA, Wolff SM: Pathogenesis of fever in man. N Engl J Med 298:607–612, 1978
3. Kluger MJ: Temperature regulation, fever, and disease. Int Rev Physiol 20:209, 1979
4. Pickering G: Regulation of body temperature in health and disease. Lancet 1(1):59, 1958

3

Disturbances of Food Intake: Anorexia and Polyphagia

MICHAEL D. LORENZ

Disturbances of food intake are frequently the first clinical signs observed by owners when an animal is ill. Owners tend to be very observant of their animals at meal time, since most people associate a good appetite with good health. Many systemic and even localized disease processes affect food intake. Unfortunately, a disturbance of food intake is not definitive of a specific disease process; rather, it represents a clinical finding common to many diseases. To meaningfully approach this problem, one should understand how food intake is regulated in the normal animal.

REGULATION OF FOOD INTAKE

Definitions

Hunger

Hunger means a craving or a desire to ingest food. In humans, hunger is often associated with intense rhythmic contractions of the stomach. In animals with the stomach removed, the apparent psychic sensations of hunger still occur and the animal still searches for an adequate food supply.

Appetite

In animals, appetite and hunger are often used as synonymous terms; however, appetite actually implies hunger for specific foods. Thus, appetite reflects the quality of food intake, whereas hunger reflects the quantity of food intake.

Satiety

Satiety is the opposite of hunger and results from a filling meal, particularly when the energy and nutritional requirements of the animal are fulfilled.

Neural Regulatory Mechanisms

Hypothalamic Centers for Hunger and Satiety

The hunger or feeding center is located in the lateral hypothalamus. Stimulation of this area causes an animal to eat voraciously. The feeding center directly stimulates the psychic drive to search for and ingest food. Stimulation of the ventromedial nuclei of the hypothalamus causes complete satiety even in the presence of stimuli that would normally incite hunger. It is believed that the satiety center primarily inhibits the feeding (hunger) center. Neuronal lesions that destroy the ventromedial hypothalamic nuclei cause voracious eating; lesions that destroy the lateral hypothalamic nuclei cause complete disinterest in food and progressive weight loss. The function of the hypothalamic center is to control the quantity of food intake by exciting activity of lower centers.

Other Mechanisms for Neuronal Control of Feeding

Centers higher than the hypothalamus also affect feeding, presumably via their influence on the feeding and satiety centers. These higher centers include the amygdala and the cortical areas of the cortex. They are closely coupled with the hypothalamus. The amygdala is one of the major parts of the olfactory nervous system and probably couples appealing odors with the desire to eat. Although the amygdala may both stimulate and inhibit feeding, its major function appears to be in the area of food discrimination (appetite). The cortical regions of the limbic system function in much the same manner as the amygdala, except that they play a major role in the animal's drive to search for food when hungry.

Nutritional and Alimentary Regulation of Food Intake

Nutritional Regulation

Nutritional regulation is concerned primarily with maintenance of normal quantities of nutrient stores in the body. The feeding center in the hypothalamus is influenced by the nutritional status of the body. In general, inadequate nutritional stores cause feeding, whereas abundant nutritional stores favor satiety.

Effects of Glucose and Amino Acid Concentrations

The concentration of blood glucose has important effects on feeding. An increased blood glucose concentration increases activity of the satiety center and secondarily decreases activity of the hunger center. The satiety center concentrates glucose, whereas other areas of the hypothalamus do not. Thus, it is assumed that glucose acts to regulate feeding by increasing the degree of satiety. Increased blood amino acid concentrations also reduce feeding, although the effect is less dramatic than that of glucose.

Effects of Fat Metabolites

The degree of adipose tissue in the body inversely affects feeding. As the degree of adipose tissue increases, the rate of feeding decreases. The quantity of free fatty acids and fat metabolites in the blood is directly proportional to the quantity of adipose stores in the body. It is likely that free fatty acids and other fat metabolites have a negative feedback regulatory effect on feeding. This lipostatic mechanism may be a major factor in long-term feeding regulation.

Alimentary Regulation

Several short-term physiologic stimuli affect feeding. Although habits related to eating are important, factors related to the alimentary tract also play important roles.

Gastrointestinal Distention

Distention of the stomach and intestinal tract inhibits feeding. Nervous impulses arising from mechanoreceptors in the wall of the distended tract stimulate the satiety center and inhibit the feeding center. The inhibitory effects of stomach distention are not completely removed by denervating the stomach wall. Therefore, overstretching the abdominal cavity and nutritional signals from the liver may also be involved. These mechanisms are especially important considerations since diseases of the liver, stomach, small intestine, and abdominal cavity are frequently associated with anorexia.

Cephalic Regulation

Various factors related to feeding, such as chewing, salivation, swallowing, and tasting, may also inhibit the feeding center after a certain amount of food has passed through the mouth. These cephalic factors decrease feeding in animals with esophageal fistulas that prevent food from entering the stomach.

ANOREXIA

Anorexia is the lack of or disinterest in the ingestion of food. In clinical terms, total anorexia is the pathologic absence of hunger. Its presence is associated with many disease processes that either directly inhibit or suppress activity in the hunger center or stimulate or increase activity in the satiety center. Anorexia may be partial or complete, pathologic, physiologic, or psychologic. The major task confronting the veterinary clinician is to determine whether anorexia is pathologic or physiologic/psychologic in origin.

Pathophysiology

Many diseases or disorders produce anorexia because they disturb the normal neurologic, endocrinologic, and mechanical mechanisms that control hunger and feeding. In certain disorders such as cancer, the underlying mechanisms are not totally understood. The basic causes of anorexia have been identified (see Classification for the Causes of Anorexia). This classification scheme may be somewhat artificial since most diseases produce a combination of factors leading to anorexia. The classification scheme does provide a logical method for finding the cause of anorexia, particularly when other manifestations of the disease are obscure.

Classification for the Causes of Anorexia

- I. Primary Anorexia
  - A. Neurologic dysfunction
    - 1. Increased intracranial pressure
      - a. Cerebral edema
      - b. Hydrocephalus
    - 2. Intracranial pain
    - 3. Hypothalamic disorders
      - a. Neoplasia
      - b. Infection
      - c. Trauma
  - B. Psychologic disorders
    - 1. Anorexia nervosa (humans)
    - 2. Unpalatable diets
    - 3. Stress
    - 4. Altered daily routine or environment
  - C. Loss of smell
- II. Secondary Anorexia
  - A. Pain
    - 1. Abdominal
    - 2. Thoracic
    - 3. Musculoskeletal
    - 4. Urogenital
  - B. Abdominal organ disorders
    - 1. Enlargement or serosa distention
    - 2. Inflammation
    - 3. Neoplasia
  - C. Toxic agents
    - 1. Exogenous
      - a. Drugs
      - b. Poisons
    - 2. Endogenous
      - a. From organ failure (*e.g.*, metabolic wastes)
      - b. Endotoxin
      - c. Pyrogens?—Fever
  - D. Endocrine
    - 1. Adrenal insufficiency
    - 2. Hypercalcemia

- E. Neoplasia of any site
- F. Infectious disease
- G. Miscellaneous
  1. Cardiac failure
  2. Malnutrition with ketosis
  3. Motion sickness
  4. High environmental temperature
  5. Autoimmune disease

III. Pseudoanorexia
- A. Disorders of the oral cavity
  1. Abscessed or broken teeth
  2. Foreign bodies
  3. Stomatitis, pharyngitis, tonsillitis
- B. Hypoglossal paralysis
- C. Mandibular paralysis
- D. Maxillary or mandibular fractures or dislocations
- E. Retrobulbar disease
  1. Abscess
  2. Inflammation
  3. Neoplasia
- F. Blindness
- G. Esophagitis
- H. Tetanus
- I. Temporo-mandibular myositis

Primary Anorexia

For the purpose of diagnosis, it is convenient to initially think of anorexia in three general categories: primary, secondary, or pseudo. Primary anorexia results from direct disease processes involving the appetite centers of the hypothalamus or from psychologic disorders that impact directly on neural control of feeding.

Diseases or disorders that destroy or structurally inhibit the appetite centers are listed in the Classification for the Causes of Anorexia. Destruction of the appetite center results in complete anorexia. Other neurologic signs related to hypothalamic dysfunction may be present if the lesion is of sufficient size to disrupt other neuronal centers in the brain stem. A thorough neurologic examination may detect these abnormalities. This form of anorexia is relatively uncommon in dogs and cats.

Psychologic disorders, although more easily defined in humans, are extremely difficult to differentiate from other causes of anorexia in animals. The causes listed in this chapter are probably quite common except for anorexia nervosa, a disease not documented in small animals. Conditions that evoke fear, anxiety, and depression may result in anorexia. Changes of environment that disrupt normal daily activities may cause anorexia in animals, especially cats. Anorexia nervosa is a neuropsychiatric abnormality of young girls, which results in severe weight loss and pituitary dysfunction. It is likely that the endocrinologic abnormalities (low serum T3 levels, increased half-life of cortisol, altered estrogen metabolism, and abnormal gonadotropin secretion) are the result of this disease and not an inherent cause.[2]

Severe pain arising from any part of the body may cause anorexia since these neural signs may inhibit the appetite center. Intracranial pain, that is, headache, is probably most important; however, this type of pain is nearly impossible to document in animals. The administration of analgesics may greatly improve appetite when musculoskeletal diseases are present.

Secondary Anorexia

The diseases that produce secondary anorexia occur in areas outside the brain and affect the neural and endocrine control of hunger. In many diseases, compounds may be produced that inhibit activity of the appetite center. This category is the major cause of anorexia in animals. It must be recognized that anorexia is commonly associated with nausea or vomiting. This is not surprising since these centers are probably neuronally interconnected. The type of stimuli for anorexia, nausea, and vomiting may be identical, the only difference being the magnitude of the stimulation.

Pain may cause anorexia by inhibiting neuronal stimulation of the appetite center. Pain also produces psychologic abnormalities that inhibit hunger.

Intra-abdominal disorders such as distention of the serosa or capsule of various abdominal organs cause anorexia via neuronal pathways or mechanisms that also produce vomiting. Distention of the stomach and small intestine (most significantly the duodenum) from obstruction are common causes of anorexia. Splanchnic sympathectomy will eliminate vomiting from intestinal obstruction; however, vagotomy is required to eliminate the associated anorexia.[4]

Inflammatory involvement of virtually any abdominal organ, pelvic organ, or visceral peritoneum may produce anorexia via neural pathways to the brainstem that inhibit appetite. Inflammatory diseases of the liver, pancreas, stomach, small intestine, and kidneys are the most commonly encountered causes of anorexia in small animals. These conditions may be associated with severe intra-abdominal pain. Inflammation of the liver may be associated with more severe anorexia than vomiting.[4] Severe uterine enlargement, as occurs in pyometra or late pregnancy, may also cause anorexia through stimulation of neuronal pathways that eventually inhibit the appetite center. In pyometra, toxic compounds from the uterus may also inhibit the appetite center.

Toxic agents, either endogenous or exogenous, are common causes of anorexia and nausea. Toxins produce anorexia by two primary mechanisms: directly by affecting the appetite centers and indirectly through involvement of intra-abdominal organs, creating inflammation, necrosis, and organ failure. Many drugs and toxins apparently stimulate the chemoreceptor trigger zone in the medulla, producing vomiting, nausea, and anorexia. Digitalis works through this mechanism, whereas amphetamines directly inhibit the appetite center.

Endogenously produced metabolic wastes that result from organ failure (such as uremia from renal failure, hyperammoninemia from liver failure, and ketosis from insulin deficiency) are serious causes of anorexia and its closely related problems of nausea and vomiting. Microgram quantities of bacterial enterotoxin are capable of inducing anorexia and may partially explain the anorexia common to a variety of febrile diseases.[4] One must wonder if endogenous pyrogen also has the property of inhibiting the appetite center, since anorexia is so commonly associated with fever from bacterial, viral, mycotic, and autoimmune diseases.

Endocrine disorders (deficiency of glucocorticoid hormones from adrenal gland failure) commonly result in anorexia. The exact mechanism is unknown. In classic Addison's disease, azotemia and hyperkalemia contribute to the anorexia of glucocorticoid deficiency. Hypercalcemia from any cause produces anorexia by an unknown mechanism.

Neoplastic disease is a serious cause of anorexia in animals. In many patients, anorexia is the primary complaint and may not be associated with other clinical signs. Cancer in animals produces peptides or nucleotides that inhibit feeding regulators.[5] Hyperphagic rats (produced by destruction of the satiety center) develop anorexia within 2 weeks of neoplastic transformation.[1] Liberation of heat from cancer cells and altered taste sensation also appear to promote anorexia in cancer patients.[3] Cancer of intra-abdominal organs may produce anorexia by any of the previously described mechanisms.

Cancer is a prime rule out for all patients with chronic anorexia. Other clinical signs may be lacking, which makes diagnosis extremely difficult in some cases.

Miscellaneous causes, including cardiac failure, prolonged malnutrition with ketosis, motion sickness, and inner ear disease, are causes of anorexia, nausea, and sometimes vomiting. Loss of smell, although rare, should not be overlooked as an obscure cause of anorexia.

Pseudoanorexia

Diseases in this category do not directly suppress the desire to eat. Rather, they result in the ability to pick up, masticate, or swallow food. These conditions are frequently so painful that animals will not eat even though they are hungry. The causes of pseudoanorexia listed in the Classification for Causes of Anorexia are usually identified by a thorough physical examination.

Diagnostic Plan

Since anorexia is a common sign of many diseases, the approach to its diagnosis is the identification of the underlying cause. In this regard, the physical examination is extremely important since most causes of pseudoanorexia can be identified by observation of the animal when presented with food and careful examination of the head, mouth, and throat. These animals may try to eat but experience pain or discomfort that prevents normal eating. Examination of the head may reveal pain when the jaws are opened or the masticatory muscles are palpated. Oral examination can reveal foreign bodies, tooth disease, stomatitis, or hypoglossal paralysis. Dysphagia and regurgitation are common problems associated with pharyngeal and esophageal disorders.

When no abnormalities of the head or oral cavity are detected, the next diagnostic step is to uncover causes of secondary anorexia. Thorough abdominal palpation is critical and may reveal abnormalities that dictate future diagnostic plans. When the physical examination is unrevealing, a complete blood count (CBC), biochemical profile, and urine analysis should be performed to rule out a variety of systemic, metabolic, and endocrinologic diseases. Abnormalities detected in these procedures may dictate future courses of action.

When no abnormalities are detected in the laboratory procedures just described, consideration is given to the causes of primary anorexia. A thorough neurologic examination is given, with attention being given to subtle abnormalities. If the neurologic examination is normal, one then considers the possibility of a psychologic disorder. The owner's history may provide clues as to the cause.

The diagnostic plan for anorexia is schematically represented in Figure 3-1.

Symptomatic Therapy

The definitive treatment of anorexia is to find the underlying problem and resolve it. In certain disorders, anorexia is treated by improving the odor and palatability of the diet. Nonspecific treatment with B complex vitamins and androgenic steroids may improve appetites. Glucocorticoid hormones may also stimulate eating in some cases. In many cases, forced oral alimentation may be needed to prevent negative nitrogen and caloric balance. Diazepam and related compounds may stimulate eating in cats.

POLYPHAGIA

Polyphagia (ravenous appetite) is the consumption of food in excess of normal estimated or calculated intake. It must be differentiated from pica, the craving for abnormal substances (for example, soil or plants). As with anorexia, polyphagia may be physiologic, pathologic, or psychologic in origin. Overfeeding that results in obesity may be a form of psychologically acquired polyphagia.

Pathophysiology

In small animals, polyphagia usually results secondarily from diseases that create a negative caloric balance or an increased metabolic rate. These diseases cause inhibition of the satiety center and stimulation of the appetite center. Primary examples include hyperadrenocorticism, hyperthyroidism, diabetes mellitus, pancreatic exocrine insufficiency, and primary intestinal malabsorption. These diseases result in muscle wasting as well as polyphagia. Certain drugs such as glucocorticoid hormones and the anticonvulsants phenobarbital, primidone, and phenytoin may directly stimulate the appetite center.

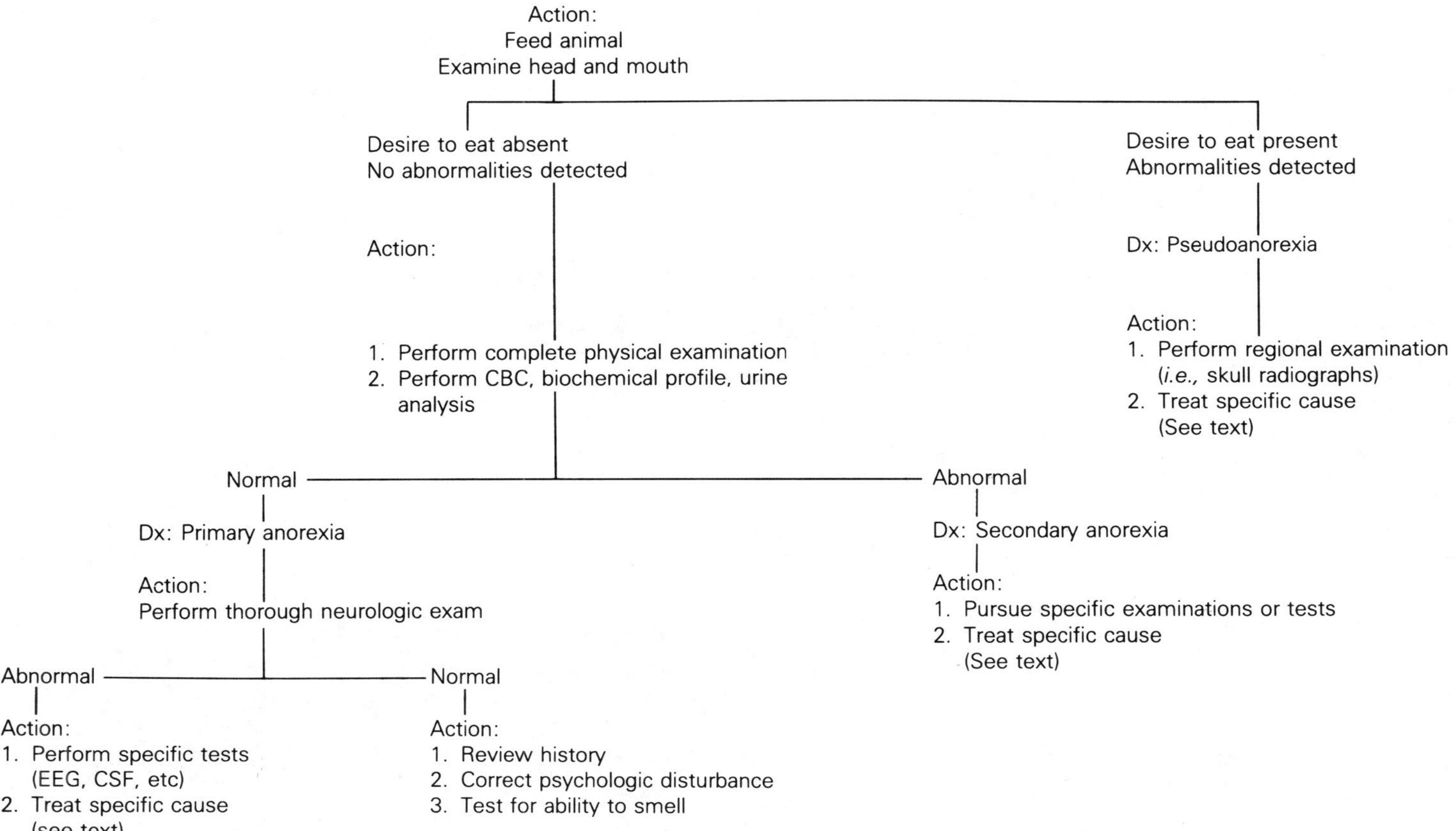

Fig. 3-1. Algorithm for the diagnosis of anorexia.

Primary polyphagias are disorders that directly destroy the satiety center in the brainstem and result in severe obesity. These conditions are rarely encountered. Overfeeding that leads to obesity is another form of primary polyphagia. This condition is probably acquired through feeding habits, although a genetic basis may also be responsible in certain breeds. The obese animal appears to lose one part of the feeding regulatory mechanism. In the normal animal, the accumulation of fat stores in the body tends to decrease feeding, whereas in the obese animal, feeding continues despite the obvious accumulation of adipose tissue.

Diagnostic Plan

The causes of polyphagia are classified as primary or secondary (see Classification and Causes of Polyphagia). The secondary causes of polyphagia are most common. All of the causes of polyphagia result in weight gain, except those that develop secondary to an increased metabolic rate or a catabolic disorder. The initial diagnostic step is to determine if the animal's weight has decreased, increased, or remained the same. If weight loss has occurred, the clinician should then search for evidence of caloric deficiency diseases or disorders that result in an increased metabolic rate. The history and physical examination usually provide evidence of associated problems such as polydipsia, polyuria, diarrhea,

Classification and Causes of Polyphagia

I. Primary Polyphagia
   A. Destruction of satiety center (rare)
      1. Neoplasia
      2. Trauma
      3. Infection
   B. Psychologic
      1. Overfeeding
II. Secondary Polyphagia
   A. Increased metabolic rate
      1. Hyperthyroidism
      2. Low environmental temperature
   B. Catabolic disorders
      1. Hyperadrenocorticism
      2. Diabetes mellitus
      3. Pancreatic exocrine insufficiency
      4. Malabsorption syndrome
      5. Hypoglycemia
      6. Low calorie diet
   C. Drug-induced
      1. Glucocorticoid hormones
      2. Anticonvulsants

nervousness, and accelerated heart rate. A CBC, urine analysis, and biochemical profile can establish a confirmed diagnosis of diabetes mellitus and hypoglycemia. Specialized tests such as serum thyroxine determinations and plasma cortisol assay are usually needed to confirm a diagnosis of hyperthyroidism and hyperadrenocorticism, respectively.

Animals with digestive disorders that produce polyphagia usually have diarrhea or bulky, malformed stools. Fecal digestion tests and oral fat or D-xylose absorption tests are required to differentiate pancreatic exocrine insufficiency from primary intestinal malabsorption.

If weight has increased, attention should be given to the causes of primary polyphagia or the administration of appetite-stimulating drugs. The most common cause in this category is overeating or overfeeding. The history may be helpful, although most owners deny that they overfeed their pets.

Symptomatic Therapy

The treatment of primary polyphagia is to restrict the diet in quantity and caloric density. If weight loss is desired, a good exercise program must be followed. The treatment of secondary polyphagia is removal of the primary cause.

REFERENCES

1. Anand B: Nervous regulation of food intake. Physiol Rev 41:667–708, 1961
2. Boyar RM: Endocrine changes in anorexia nervosa. Med Clin North Am 62:297, 1978
3. Crow SE, Oliver J: Cancer cachexia. Comp Cont Ed 3:682, 1981
4. McGuigan JE: Anorexia, nausea, and vomiting. In MacBryde CM, Blacklow RS (eds): Signs and Symptoms, 5th ed. Philadelphia, JB Lippincott, 1970
5. Theologides A: Anorexia-producing intermediary metabolites. Am J Clin Nutr 29:552–558, 1976

4

Episodic Weakness

MICHAEL D. LORENZ

PROBLEM DEFINITION AND RECOGNITION

Weakness that occurs with exercise and dissipates with rest is termed *episodic.* It is recognized as early fatigue with mild exercise, although in some cases, more vigorous exercise may be needed to induce the problem. Signs of weakness include an ataxic or paretic gait, severe panting, reluctance to walk or run, lying down, and collapse. The animal may be alert or depressed. Following rest, muscle strength improves greatly.

PATHOPHYSIOLOGY

The correct approach to diagnosis of this problem is based on the normal physiology of muscle function during exercise and at rest. In addition, the function of other organs that support muscle metabolism (*i.e.*, by supplying oxygen, calories) during exercise must be considered. The wise clinician is able to quickly and accurately recall the neuromuscular events that control muscle contraction and relate these to cardiopulmonary support.

Muscle and nerves are tissues that generate electrical activity, called action potentials, along the cell membranes. Action potentials are generated by the movement of sodium and potassium ions through the cell membrane. The movement of these ions is controlled by calcium. Disorders that cause electrolyte imbalances may produce episodic weakness as the primary clinical manifestation. Table 4-1 describes the effects of various electrolyte disturbances on the production of action potentials and the resultant clinical signs or problems.

In the normal animal, skeletal muscle fibers are stimulated to contract by the lower motor neurons. The muscle fibers are connected to the nervous system via neuromuscular junctions (also called motor endplates). The motor endplate transmits electrical activity (action potentials) from the axon to the muscle fiber. Acetylcholine is the neurotransmitting agent released in the motor endplate that stimulates action potential production on the muscle fiber membrane. The re-

Table 4-1. Effects of Electrolyte Imbalance on the Production of Action Potentials, Motor Endplate Function, and Muscle Function

DISORDER	EFFECT ON ACTION POTENTIAL PRODUCTION	EFFECT ON MOTOR ENDPLATE FUNCTION	EFFECT ON MUSCLE CONTRACTION	PRIMARY CLINICAL SIGNS OR PROBLEMS
Hyperkalemia	Decreased intensity due to hypopolarization of membrane Decreased membrane potential		Decreased strength of contraction Block conduction of cardiac impulse	Muscle weakness, bradycardia, sinoatrial arrest
Hypokalemia	Membrane hyperpolarization		Decreased strength of contraction	Muscle weakness
Hypocalcemia	Increased membrane excitability Spontaneous impulses	Decreased release of acetylcholine	Decreased strength of contraction	Tetany
Hypercalcemia	Decreased membrane excitability	Increased release of acetylcholine	Spontaneous contractions may occur. Muscle strength may decrease.	Muscle fasciculations and muscle weakness

lease of acetylcholine is modulated by calcium ion (see Table 4-1) and is inactivated by acetylcholine esterase enzyme. Thus, disturbances of calcium homeostasis or disorders that affect the activity of acetylcholine esterase may adversely affect neuromuscular transmission and can produce episodic weakness.

Special receptors on the muscle fiber membrane bind the acetylcholine released by the axonal foot process. Although this binding occurs for only a few milliseconds, it creates an action potential on the muscle fiber. Normally, three to four times more electrical activity is generated than needed to stimulate muscle contraction. This is the so-called "safety factor" of the neuromuscular junction; "fatigue" of this synapse almost never occurs under normal exercise conditions. Myasthenia gravis is an autoimmune disease affecting the acetylcholine receptors. In myasthenia gravis, the number of effective acetylcholine receptors is reduced so that normal muscle contractions may occur at rest but, during work or exercise, the fibers easily fatigue since sufficient electrical stimulation cannot be sustained.

An action potential, generated on the surface of muscle fibers, is conducted into the cell, where it stimulates the release of calcium ions stored within the sarcoplasmic reticulum. Calcium ions then stimulate contraction of the myofibrils. A physiologic pump within the muscle cell effectively stores calcium ions in the sarcoplasmic reticulum, and this mechanism keeps the concentration of calcium ions in the myofibrils at an extremely low level except during periods of excitation. Therefore, the concentration of calcium ions within the body is critical for normal muscle contraction. Disturbances of calcium homeostasis at this level may result in episodic weakness.

During muscle contraction, much energy is required. The primary initial source of energy is muscle glycogen, which is utilized by the process of aerobic glycolysis. Muscle glycogen can be rapidly expended during exercise; blood glucose then becomes the primary source of energy. In hypoglycemic conditions, this source of energy is not available; therefore, episodic weakness is a common problem associated with hypoglycemia.

Aerobic glycolysis is the most efficient means of generating energy within skeletal muscle. In conditions of reduced oxygen tension (*e.g.*, reduced oxygen in the blood, reduced hemoglobin concentration) or with vigorous exercise, insufficient oxygen is present to maintain aerobic glycosis. Anaerobic glycolysis, although less effective, generates some energy for muscle function. High levels of lactic acid are produced, which may cause disturbances within the muscle cell. Therefore, conditions of decreased oxygen concentration in the blood may result in episodic weakness, since, during exercise, the increased metabolic demands in muscle tissue cannot be met.

Primary muscle disease such as early degenerative disorders (myopathies) or inflammation (myositis) may cause episodic weakness via damage to any of the steps necessary for normal muscle contraction. These diseases may asymmetrically affect muscle fibers within a muscle or a group of muscles. Thus, sufficient function may be maintained to sustain mild work; however, the increased demands of exercise cannot be sustained since insufficient numbers of healthy fibers are present for recruitment.

Table 4-2. Causes of Episodic Weakness

CATEGORY	CONDITION	DOCUMENTATION	UNDERLYING DISEASE	SPECIFIC DIAGNOSTIC TEST
Metabolic	Hyperkalemia	Serum K^+	Adrenal insufficiency	Plasma cortisol profile
			Severe acidosis	Blood gases and *p*H
			Severe renal failure	Blood urea nitrogen
				Urine analysis
				Complete blood count
	Hypokalemia	Serum K^+	Severe vomiting	See chapter 32.
			Diuretic therapy	
	Hypocalcemia	Serum Ca^{++}	Hypoparathyroidism	Urine, calcium, and phosphorus
				Serum phosphorus
				PTH assay
	Hypercalcemia	Serum Ca^{++}	Pseudohyperparathyroidism (Lymphosarcoma)	Complete blood count
				Lymph node aspirate or biopsy
			Primary hyperparathyroidism (Parathyroid tumor)	Serum PTH assay
				Presence of parathyroid mass
				Urine calcium and phosphorus
				Serum phosphorus
	Hypoglycemia	Fasting blood glucose	Functional beta cell carcinoma	Insulin–glucose ratio
				Glucagon response test
			Adrenal insufficiency	Plasma cortisol profile
				Serum electrolytes
			Glycogen storage disease	Glucagon response test
				Tissue biopsy (liver, muscle)
Cardiovascular	Arrhythmias	ECG	See chapter 21.	See chapter 21.
	Conduction failure	ECG	See chapter 21.	See chapter 21.
	Congestive heart failure	Thoracic radiographs	*Dirofilaria*	Knott's test
				Occult heartworm test
				ECG
Neuromuscular	Myasthenia gravis	Repetitive nerve stimulation	Thymoma	Tensilon response test
			Autoimmune disease	
	Polymyositis	Serum muscle enzyme levels	Eosinophilic myositis	Biopsy
			Autoimmune disease (systemic lupus)	Antinuclear antibody
		Muscle biopsy		Direct FA of muscle
			Toxoplasmosis	Biopsy, serology

PTH, parathyroid hormone; ECG, electrocardiogram; FA, fluorescent antibody

DIAGNOSTIC PLAN

The diseases or disorders that cause episodic weakness are listed in Table 4-2. The diagnostic plan is based on the mechanisms that cause this problem plus knowledge of their relative frequency in dogs and cats.

The history and physical examination may provide clues to the underlying mechanism or disease. In this regard, the history and physical examination usually provide clues of cardiopulmonary disease (*e.g.*, coughing, cyanosis, edema, ascites, pale muscle membranes, abnormal pulse, heart murmurs [see related chapters]). A neurologic examination is valuable, since organic disease of the nervous system usually creates constant signs of weakness (see chapter 47), and signs may be localizing to a segment or region of the nervous system. Except for depression or, rarely, seizures, the neurologic examination is usually normal with the diseases listed in Table 4-2. Muscle palpation is very important since primary muscle diseases may cause pain (see chapter 46) and/or atrophy. The presence of polysystemic signs, vomiting, polydipsia-polyuria, anorexia, or weight loss may indicate the presence of a metabolic disorder. A minimum data base (see Minimum Data Base for Episodic Weakness) should be collected to evaluate this problem.

Several of the diseases that cause episodic weakness may create problems suggestive of other diseases. For instance, polymyositis may cause acquired megaesophagus and thus regurgitation (see chapter 32). The regurgitation may cause aspiration pneumonia and clinical signs of severe pulmonary disease. The pulmonary disease may be assumed to be the cause of the episodic weakness and, thus, the primary disease can be easily overlooked.

SYMPTOMATIC THERAPY

There is no reliable symptomatic therapy for this problem. Therapy is predicated on establishing the correct diagnosis.

Minimum Data Base for Episodic Weakness

1. History
2. Physical examination; include neurologic examination
3. Laboratory
   a. Complete blood count
   b. Urine analysis
   c. Complete biochemical profile
   d. Knott's test
4. Electrocardiogram
5. Thoracic radiographs

5

Polydipsia and Polyuria

MICHAEL D. LORENZ

Polydipsia and polyuria (P&P) are associated clinical signs that commonly occur in small animals as the result of several different polysystemic disorders. In most cases, these signs suggest a disorder in water homeostasis that has disturbed normal plasma and cellular osmolality. Polyuria is the increased production of urine usually of low specific gravity. Polydipsia is increased thirst. In many instances, polydipsia is a compensatory mechanism for polyuria; however, in rare instances, polydipsia may be primary and polyuria is a compensatory mechanism for excretion of the excess water load. This chapter provides a concise review of P&P and outlines a diagnostic plan for animals with these problems.

Normal regulation of body fluid volume and osmolality depends upon a balance between water loss and water intake. Drinking and urine loss are the most important mechanisms for regulation of body water. If increased drinking is not compensated by increased urine loss, body water must increase, with resulting cellular overhydration. Conversely, if urine loss is not compensated by increased drinking, body water decreases, with resulting cellular dehydration. Water and sodium regulation are closely interrelated since extracellular fluid osmolality is almost totally determined by sodium concentration. Fluid osmolality and, ultimately, body fluid volume are controlled by neuroendocrinologic and renal mechanisms. To logically pursue the problems of P&P, clinicians should understand these basic mechanisms.

THE THIRST MECHANISM

Thirst is the conscious desire for water. The stimulus to drink is generated in the thirst center in the hypothalamus. The involved neurons lie in close proximity to the antidiuretic hormone (ADH) control centers and are controlled by extracellular fluid osmolality. A 2% increase in osmolality is sufficient for stimulation of thirst. The basic stimulus for exciting the thirst center is intracellular dehydration; this mechanism has been termed *primary thirst.* A second stimulus for the thirst center arises from volume and pressure receptors located in the left atrium and large vessels. A reduction in blood volume by 8% to 10% can induce thirst by neural stimulation of the thirst center from these pressure receptors. Although the role of primary thirst mechanisms is well understood, primary thirst is not the primary mechanism that determines water intake in normal animals. Secondary thirst is a poorly understood mechanism that anticipates water needs before actual deficiencies occur. The stimulus for drinking is from oropharyngeal cues or is related to the circadian rhythm of eating. It is well established that animals will drink nearly the exact amount of water in 5 minutes required to relieve anticipated or existing dehydration even though it may take hours for this fluid load to be distributed within the body. Evidence that supports the concept of secondary thirst includes thirst despite lack of dehydration or maximally concentrated urine.

Other mechanisms may also stimulate the thirst center. For example, both renin and angiotensin stimulate thirst by direct action on neurons in the thirst center. Compounds with this capacity are termed *dipsinogenic.* This mechanism may be important in certain diseases in which these substances accumulate in large amounts.

Pathologic Thirst

Primary polydipsia is increased drinking not explained as a compensatory mechanism for excessive fluid loss. Among the causes of pathologic thirst (see Causes of Pathologic Thirst), compulsive water drinking (pseudopsychogenic polydipsia) is probably most important in animals. Although the cause is not known, psychogenic factors such as boredom may be involved. Water intake exceeds body needs and a compensatory polyuria results. Unlike in humans, osmoregulation is still present in affected animals. When deprived of water, urine is concentrated and thirst decreases when ADH is administered. The condition is treated by controlling water intake and eliminating predisposing environmental factors.

Causes of Pathologic Thirst

- Neuronal irritation (hypothalamic)
    - Tumor
    - Trauma
    - Inflammation
- Compulsive water drinking (pseudopsychogenic polydipsia)
- Increased plasma renin
- Other
    - Hypercalcemia
    - Thoracic caval constriction

RENAL CONCENTRATING MECHANISMS

The structure of the kidney enables animals to excrete a large solute load and still conserve most of the water that appears in glomerular filtrate. In water excess, urine is diluted and urine volume increases. In water deficit, the opposite process occurs. In a 25-pound (10.5-kg) dog, 68 liters of fluid is filtered by the glomeruli each day; however, less than 500 ml is excreted as urine. Urine volume control is primary regulated by the ADH and countercurrent systems.

The ADH–Osmoreceptor Control System

Water homeostasis is largely dependent upon extracellular fluid sodium concentration: sodium concentration is inversely related to water content but directly related to fluid osmolality. Osmolality of extracellular fluid is regulated by thirst and the ADH feedback control mechanisms. ADH is produced by specialized neurons in the hypothalamus and is stored in nerve endings in the neurohypophosis. Large amounts of ADH are normally stored in these nerve endings, called pituicytes. Increased extracellular fluid osmolality stimulates the osmoreceptors in the hypothalamus to release ADH from the pituicytes. Under the influence of ADH, the permeability of the collecting tubules to water is greatly enhanced. Water is then reabsorbed along concentration gradients established in the renal medulla by the countercurrent system. The increased absorption of water conserves fluid while allowing the excretion of solute waste in the urine. The retention of water in relationship to sodium decreases the osmolality, lowering the output of ADH. When the extracellular fluid becomes hypoosmotic, less ADH is released. Excess water is lost in the urine, increasing the osmolality back to normal. A 2% change in osmolality will increase or decrease ADH secretion. An 8% decrease in blood pressure or volume will also stimulate ADH secretion. Volume receptors in the left atrium and the carotid sinus pressure receptors are responsible for these effects on ADH secretion.

The mechanism of ADH action to increase tubular permeability to water is not known. In addition to increasing water reabsorption, ADH also increases the reabsorption of urea. This is an important step in the renal urea cycle that influences renal medullary hypertonicity.

The Countercurrent System

Water reabsorption from glomerular filtrate is dependent upon a high osmotic gradient in the renal medulla. Two solutes, sodium chloride and urea, are primarily responsible for maintaining this osmotic gradient. Large concentrations of sodium chloride remain in the renal medulla for two reasons: (1) sluggish blood flow in the peritubular capillaries (vasa recta) and (2) a countercurrent multisystem at work in the loop of Henle (LH) and vasa recta. Urea also becomes highly concentrated in the renal medulla and may contribute nearly half of the hypertonicity of the inner medulla.

Renal Tubular Functions

Glomerular filtrate is isothenuric, meaning it has a specific gravity equal to that of plasma (1.008 to 1.012). Tubular functions (passive and active reabsorption) dilute or concentrate this filtrate depending upon body needs. In most cases, the final product, urine, is more concentrated than glomerular filtrate.

Nearly 75% of glomerular filtrate is reabsorbed in the proximal tubule regardless of need. In a 25-pound (10.5-kg) dog filtering 68 liters a day, 51 liters of fluid is reabsorbed in the proximal tubule and 17 liters passes on to the remainder of the renal tubule. Filtered water is passively reabsorbed in the proximal tubule following osmotic gradients produced by the active transport of solutes such as glucose, sodium, and amino acids. Diseases that affect the proximal tubule (primary renal disease, renal glycosuria, Fanconi syndrome) or those that result in solute loads that overwhelm proximal tubule absorptive capacity (diabetes mellitus) create an osmotic diuresis by overloading absorptive functions in the LH and distal tubules. An obligatory water loss accompanies this increased solute excretion.

Fluid entering the LH has a volume of 17 liters and is nearly isotonic (specific gravity, 1.008 to 1.012). The LH generates a high concentration gradient within the renal medulla, which is necessary for water conservation and urine concentration. The ascending limb of LH generates solute-free water. The thick portion of LH actively reabsorbs chloride and sodium but is impermeable to water. Fluid leaving the LH has a volume of 12 liters and a specific gravity of 1.003 (hyposthenuric). Thus, the LH dilutes tubular fluid to maintain renal medullary hypertonicity and while absorbing approximately 7% of the glomerular filtrate. Urine specific gravities less than 1.008 suggest normal tubular function through the LH since urine is diluted below isothenuria at this level. Abnormal LH function results in polyuria because of decreased renal medullary hypertonicity. Disorders that affect LH function include primary renal disease and diuretics such as furosemide

The final steps in water conservation occur in the distal tubule and collecting ducts. In the distal tubule, sodium and water are reabsorbed while potassium is actively secreted. This process is strongly enhanced by aldosterone. Fluid leaving the distal tubules has a specific gravity of 1.003 to 1.010 and a volume of 8 liters. Approximately 6% of the tubular fluid is reabsorbed in the distal tubule. Epithelial cells in the collecting ducts are relatively impermeable to water unless stimulated by ADH. In the absence of ADH, tubular fluid becomes somewhat more dilute because of sodium and other solute reabsorption. In the presence of ADH, water is reabsorbed; this process is responsible for water homeostasis in normal animals. The collecting ducts in our 25-pound example dog can reabsorb nearly 8 liters of fluid depending upon body needs.

Table 5-1 illustrates the effects of ADH relative to urine volume and specific gravity. As urine specific gravity doubles, urine volume is halved. Thus, when urine is hyposthenuric, small changes in specific gravity have profound effects on urine volume. However, as urine becomes hyperosmotic, large changes in

Table 5-1. Urine Specific Gravity Versus Urine Volume in ADH Deficiency

SPECIFIC GRAVITY	VOLUME	SPECIFIC GRAVITY	VOLUME
1.001	5 liters	1.010	500 ml
1.002	2.5 liters	1.020	250 ml
1.003	1.7 liters	1.040	125 ml
1.004	1.25 liters	1.050	100 ml
1.005	1.0 liter		

specific gravity have smaller effects on urine volume. With ADH deficiency, profound polyuria occurs because the urine has a very low specific gravity.

Several disorders produce P&P by disturbing distal and collecting tubular function. These include primary renal disease, diabetes insipidus, pyometra, hyperadrenocorticism, hypoadrenocorticism, liver failure, and hypercalcemia. Glucocorticoid and spironolactone therapy also has these effects.

Medullary Washout

Certain diseases produce polyuria by decreasing renal medullary osmotic gradients. Failure of the sodium chloride pump in the LH is a primary mechanism for this abnormality. Failure of the urea cycle or urea depletion, as occurs in chronic liver failure, may also decrease renal medullary hypertonicity. Prolonged P&P produces medullary washout by increasing the rate of fluid flow through the LH and vasa recta. This decreases the effectiveness of the countercurrent mechanism and results in the production of isotonic urine. The importance of medullary washout is discussed more thoroughly later in this chapter in regard to its effect on urine concentration tests.

APPLIED PATHOPHYSIOLOGY

As stated previously, many diseases produce polyuria because they affect renal concentrating mechanisms or stimulate primary polydipsia. Table 5-2 lists the various diseases that produce P&P and summarizes the altered physiology that actually produces these signs.

DIAGNOSTIC PLAN

The evaluation of an animal that may have P&P proceeds in four steps: (1) documentation that the problem exists; (2) inspection of the data base for clues to diagnosis; (3) performance of urine concentration tests; and (4) performance

Table 5-2. Pathogenesis of Polydipsia and Polyuria in Various Diseases and Iatrogenic Disorders

	MAJOR ABNORMALITY	MECHANISM OF P&P
Spontaneous disease or abnormality		
Diabetes insipidus		
Neurogenic	Hypothalamic or posterior pituitary injury	Deficiency of ADH
Nephrogenic	Tubular enzyme deficiency or receptor unresponsiveness	Tubule unresponsive to ADH
Diabetes mellitus	Insulin deficiency → hyperglycemia	Glycosuria: excessive absorbable solute in proximal tubule
Hyperadrenocorticism	Excessive endogenous production of glucocorticoids. Adrenal cortical hyperplasia or neoplasia	ADH inhibition at collecting duct. May inhibit ADH release.
Hypercalcemia (hypercalcemic nephropathy)	Parathyroid tumor: excessive parathormone Lymphosarcoma: osteoclast stimulating factor	Early: inhibition of ADH Stimulation of thirst Late: mineralization of kidney; chronic renal failure
Hyperthyroidism	Autonomously functioning thyroid tumor → Excessive thyroid hormones	
Liver failure	Liver insufficiency ↓ Urea synthesis and ↓ Renin catabolism	↓ Renal medullary hypertonicity Dipsinogenic activity of renin
Medullary washout	Loss of countercurrent multipler system (various disorders)	↓ Renal medullary hypertonicity
Pyometra	Endometrial hyperplasia Bacterial endotoxins??	Tubule unresponsive to ADH
Pseudopsychogenic polydipsia (compulsive water drinking)	Primary polydipsia	Compensatory polyuria Medullary washout??
Renal disease	Renal tubular dysfunction Renal medullary dysfunction	Alteration of many renal concentrating mechanisms
Iatrogenic disorders (drug therapy)		
Alcohol		Inhibition of ADH release
Glucocorticoids		ADH inhibition
Mannitol	Nonabsorbable solute	Osmotic diuresis
Dextrose	Excessive absorbable solute	Osmotic diuresis
Furosemide	Inhibition of active chloride transport in loop of Henle	Osmotic diuresis Medullary washout
Phenytoin		Inhibition of ADH release
Vitamin D intoxication	Excessive vitamin D absorption → Hypercalcemia	Early ↑ ADH inhibition Late ↑ renal mineralization

ADH, antidiuretic hormone

of special diagnostic tests or procedures. These procedures will also allow the clinician to decide which is the primary versus the compensatory event. In most small animals, polyuria is the primary problem and polydipsia is the compensatory disorder.

Documentation

Many owners may complain that their pets are urinating or drinking excessively. However, it is difficult for owners to quantitate water intake or urine output unless the problem is severe. As related earlier, a 25-pound (10.5-kg) dog with a urine specific gravity of 1.010 produces roughly 500 ml of urine. Only very astute owners are able to detect polyuria of this magnitude. The signs of lower urinary tract disease, dysuria and pollakiuria, are often confused by owners with polyuria. Because of false information related by owners, it is important to quanitate the problem of P&P. Initial evaluation includes a complete physical examination, accurate determination of the animal's weight and hydration status, determination of packed cell volume (PCV) and plasma proteins, and assessment of urine specific gravity. Animals with urine specific gravities above 1:035 are probably not polyuric (Table 5-1). The animal's water consumption should be measured accurately. For many patients, the owner can perform the procedure at home. With hospitalized patients, water consumption, urine output, and urine specific gravities are measured. In marginal P&P, 48- to 72-hour determinations are necessary, whereas in severe P&P, 24-hour determinations usually are sufficient. Normal daily water intake and urine output for dogs and cats are listed in Table 5-3.

Inspection of Data Base

The completed initial data base (history, physical examination, hematology, biochemical profile, and urine analysis) is carefully searched for clues to the cause of P&P. For instance, the presence of glucosuria would imply the possible presence of diabetes mellitus or renal proximal tubular defects. In this case, further tests to document P&P would be withheld until the glucosuria problem is resolved. Table 5-4 lists the various diseases that produce P&P as a major sign and describes the most important clues indicative of that disorder.

Table 5-3. Water Intake, Urine Output, and Urine Specific Gravities in Normal Dogs and Cats

SPECIES	WATER INTAKE (ml/kg/Day)	URINE OUTPUT (ml/kg/Day)	URINE SPECIFIC GRAVITY (EXPECTED RANGE)	URINE SPECIFIC GRAVITY (MAXIMUM)
Dog	20–90	20–45	1.018–1.045	1.065
Cat	0–45	20–40	1.030–1.050	1.085

(Text continues on p 48.)

Table 5-4. Differential Diagnosis of Diseases That Produce Primary Polydipsia and Polyuria: Diagnostic Clues and Special Tests

RULE OUT	PREDOMINANT CLINICAL SIGNS (OTHER THAN P&P)	HEMATOLOGY	BIOCHEMISTRY	URINE ANALYSIS (OTHER THAN SPECIFIC GRAVITY)	SPECIAL TESTS
Pseudopsychogenic polydipsia (compulsive water drinking)	No consistent clues Search for predisposing environmental or emotional problems.	No consistent clues	No consistent clues	No consistent clues	None Response to control of water intake
Hyperadrenocorticism (also see diabetes mellitus)	Alopecia Thin skin, elasticity ↓ Calcinosis cutis Muscle weakness Polyphagia Hepatomegaly	Lymphopenia Eosinopenia	BUN N or ↓ SGPT N or ± ↑ Alk Phos ↑ ↑ Cholesterol ↑ Glucose N or ↑	WBC ↑ or N Bacteria N or ↑ Glucose N or ↑	Plasma cortisol Dexamethasone suppression tests
Hypercalcemia	(Depends on precipitating disease) 1. Weakness, depression 2. Muscle tremors 3. Anorexia	Usually normal unless associated with lymphosarcoma PCV ↓ WBC N	BUN N or ↑ Creatinine N or ↑ Calcium ↑ Phosphorus N, ↓, or ↑ (depends on stage of disease)	Calcium crystals	Lymph node aspirate or biopsy Bone marrow aspirate PTH assay
Hyperthyroidism	Polyphagia Voluminous stools Weight loss Nervousness, hyperactivity	Usually normal	Cholesterol ↓ Glucose N or ↑	Rarely glucosuria	Serum T4 test
Diabetes insipidus	Marginal dehydration	PCV N or ↑ TS N or ↑	BUN N or ↑ Na N or ↑ Cl N or ↑		ADH response test Water deprivation test
Diabetes mellitus (also see hyperadrenocorticism)	Weight loss Polyphagia Vomiting Lethargy Hepatomegaly	Lipemia PCV N or ↑ WBC N or ↑ Lymphopenia Eosinopenia	BUN N or ↑ SGPT N or ↑ Alk Phos ↑ Glucose ↑ ↑ TCO_2 ↓	Glucosuria Ketonuria	Glycogenated hemoglobin Glucose tolerance Serum amylase, lipase Blood gases

Liver failure	Vomiting Diarrhea Weight loss Neurological signs Icterus	PCV N or ↓ TS ↓	BUN N or ↓ T Prot ↓ Alb ↓ SGPT ↑ Alk Phos ↑	Ammonium biurate crystals	Serum ammonia BSP Coagulogram Liver radiographs Biopsy
Early renal failure	No consistent clues	Normal	If not azotemic, no consistent clues	Protein N or ↑	PSP Creatinine clearance Assess renal size Palpation Radiographically
Renal failure	Weight loss Vomiting Anorexia	Nonregenerative anemia Lymphopenia	↑ BUN ↑ Creatinine ↑ Phosphorus ↓ TCO_2	Protein N or ↑ Casts +	Renal biopsy Renal size
Pyelonephritis	Fever Vomiting Mild abdominal pain Weight loss	WBC N or ↑	Normal or ↑ BUN etc	WBC ↑ Bacteria + Protein ↑	Urine culture Excretory urogram
Pyometra	Anorexia Vomiting Depression ↑ Uterus History of estrus Vaginal discharge	WBC ↑ (may be normal if early or open)	BUN N or ↑	WBC ↑ Protein ↑	Abdominal radiography Exploratory laparotomy
Hypoadrenocorticism	Anorexia Vomiting Depression Diarrhea Weakness Hypotension	Lymphocytosis Eosinophilia PCV N, ↑, ↓	BUN ↑ Na N or ↓ K N or ↑ Cl N or ↓	No consistent clues	Plasma cortisol

BUN, blood urea nitrogen; N, normal; ↓, decreased; ↑, increased; SGPT, serum glutamic-pyruvic transaminase; Alk Phos, alkaline phosphatase; PCV, packed cell volume; WBC, white blood cells; PTH, parathormone; ADH, antidiuretic hormone; TS, total solids; TCO_2, total carbon dioxide; T Prot, total protein; BSP, Bromsulphalein; PSP, phenolsulfonphthalein

During the initial evaluation of animals with suspected P&P, approximately 50% are found to not have the problem, suggesting that owner observations were probably in error. A significant number of cases have sufficient clues in the data base to suggest a primary cause for the P&P; however, in many documented P&P animals, no cause for the P&P can be identified. Diabetes insipidus, nonazotemic renal failure, certain cases of hyperadrenocorticism, and psychogenic polydipsia are examples of disorders that are not easily differentiated in the initial data base. Patients with unexplained P&P at this point are evaluated with urine concentration procedures.

Urine Concentration Tests

These tests are indicated for patients with P&P not explained by steps 1 and 2 in the diagnostic plan. In small animals, two procedures are used: the water deprivation test and the ADH (pitressin) response test. In certain cases, the animal may be fluid deficient (dehydrated) during the evaluation of steps 1 and 2. Obviously, a documented dehydrated patient with low urine specific gravity is not a candidate for water deprivation since it is already apparent that either renal disease or a deficiency in the action or presence of ADH is likely present. It is more logical and safer to perform an ADH response test in these animals. Therefore, before beginning urine concentration tests, the hydration status of the patient must be accurately assessed. This is done clinically by measuring the PCV, total plasma proteins, and, if possible, plasma osmolality. If little evidence of dehydration is present and no other contraindications exist, one should proceed with water deprivation.

Water Deprivation Test

The abrupt test is indicated when poorly controlled water deprivation results in either negative or equivocal findings. The contraindications for this test are azotemia, dehydration, and hypercalcemia.

The test is conducted as follows:

1. Following a 12-hour fast, obtain a blood sample for serum osmolality.
2. Obtain urine for specific gravity and save a small quantity for osmolality.
3. Store serum and urine in a refrigerator.
4. Allow patients to urinate and defecate before recording accurate body weight.
5. Place animal in metabolism cage and withhold food and water.
6. Evaluate animals every 3 to 4 hours by assessing body weight, urine specific gravity, dehydration, and general well-being.

The water deprivation test is terminated when one of three criteria is achieved: (1) production of concentrated urine, (2) weight loss of 7%, or (3) demonstration of hemoconcentration (increased plasma protein concentration or osmolality). At termination of the test, urine produced during the last half hour is collected and the specific gravity is determined. A small amount of urine should be saved for osmolality determination.

Normal dogs, when water deprived, can maximally concentrate urine to a specific gravity of 1.065. Cats produce even more concentrated urine under similar conditions. It appears that most normal dogs and cats will achieve urine specific gravities of 1.045 or greater. Values of 1.035 to 1.045 are considered a grey zone, and values below 1.035 are abnormal. Failure to concentrate urine following water deprivation indicates one of the following possibilities: (1) deficiency of ADH, (2) renal unresponsiveness to ADH, (3) primary renal disease, or (4) renal medullary washout. Failure to concentrate urine following this procedure usually eliminates primary polydipsia unless medullary washout is present.

A gradual water deprivation test is indicated when medullary washout is suspected or for severely polyuric animals that are at increased risk of severe hemoconcentration if suddenly deprived of all water. In this procedure, water intake is measured for 2 days and then gradually decreased over 3 to 4 days. The patient is closely monitored as described for the abrupt procedure. As stated earlier, normal renal medullary hypertonicity is reestablished within 1 to 3 days. Failure to concentrate urine during this procedure eliminates medullary washout as the cause of polyuria. The results of water deprivation tests in various diseases are summarized in Table 5-5.

ADH (Vasopressin) Response Test

This test is indicated for animals that fail to concentrate urine after water deprivation or for animals for which water deprivation is viewed as a risky procedure. In most cases, ADH response tests can be performed immediately following water deprivation tests. A urine specific gravity is obtained prior to starting the test. Water and food are given *ad libitum*. Vasopressin tannate in oil

Table 5-5. Response to Urine Concentration Tests in Certain Diseases That Produce Polydipsia and Polyuria

DISEASE	USUAL RANGE OF URINE SPECIFIC GRAVITY (NONCHALLENGED)	RESPONSE TO WATER DEPRIVATION	RESPONSE TO ADH ADMINISTRATION
Diabetes insipidus (neurogenic)	1.001–1.017	Negative	Positive
Diabetes insipidus (nephrogenic)	1.001–1.017	Negative	Negative
Primary renal disease (nonazotemic)	1.008–1.030	Negative	Negative
Hyperadrenocorticism	1.001–1.035	Positive	Positive
Renal medullary washout	1.008–1.012	Negative–abrupt Positive–gradual	Negative
Pseudopsychogenic polydipsia	1.001–1.030	Positive	Positive

is given intramuscularly and urine specific gravities are obtained every 4 to 6 hours during the subsequent 24 hours. The dosage of ADH is 5 units for dogs weighing more than 6.5kg and 2.5 units for dogs less than this weight. Adult cats are given 2.5 units. The vial of vasopressin must be vigorously agitated to suspend the precipitated vasopressin. Failure to suspend the vasopressin in the oil vehicle will give false-negative results. Most animals with normal kidneys achieve urine specific gravities of 1.030 or greater. Failure to respond to ADH suggests the presence of primary renal disease, nephrogenic diabetes insipidus, or medullary washout. If questionable results are obtained, the ADH response test should be repeated. The results of urine concentration tests in various diseases are summarized in Table 5-5.

Special Diagnostic Tests

The final step in evaluation of animals with P&P is the selection and performance of specialized tests. These tests vary according to the diseases under investigation. They are listed by the appropriate disease in Table 5-4.

Part Two

BEHAVIORAL PROBLEMS

6

Misdirected Aggression

JOHN E. OLIVER

PROBLEM DEFINITION AND RECOGNITION

Aggression is difficult to define, even by authorities in the field. A comprehensive definition is "an overt act the goal of which is either to eliminate, consume or cause the escape of, an opponent by inflicting organic damage upon the latter, or to induce the opponent to escape by noncontactual means; that is, via a ritualized attack or threat."[10] What is meant by aggression is more clear when the various forms are listed (Table 6-1).[7,9] Many forms of aggression are normal behaviors in a species and are only a problem when they are misdirected in terms of our environment. Misdirected aggression is the most frequent problem presented to behavioral specialists.[2,7,8,15]

PATHOPHYSIOLOGY

Aggressive behavior may be caused or modified by organic brain lesions, genetic predisposition, learning or conditioning, early socialization, and gender. Although organic brain disease has been considered an infrequent cause of aggression, there is little documentation that it is not important.[2,3,7,9]

The limbic system is considered the anatomic substrate for most behavior. It is a complex interconnection of nuclei in the more primitive parts of the cerebrum with areas in the thalamus, hypothalamus, and midbrain.[4] Stimulation or destruction of some of these structures will enhance or reduce aggressive behavior. A summary of some of these findings is included in Table 6-1.[13] Focal lesions of one of these structures could cause aggression in the clinical patient, but few documented cases have been reported. Most of the reported cases of aggression with brain lesions involved diffuse or multifocal lesions, generally a nonsuppurative encephalitis.[3,4]

Psychomotor seizures may have an aggressive component.[2,4,7,12] Animals may run blindly, bite at anything in their path, and bite at themselves or inani-

Table 6-1. Forms of Aggression

	ANATOMIC SUBSTRATE	
TYPE	Activators	Suppressors
Predatory	Lateral hypothalamus	Ventromedial hypothalamus Basolateral amygdala
Competitive and intermale	Centromedial amygdala Ventrolateral posterior thalamus Central gray matter	Olfactory bulbs Septal nuclei Head of caudate nucleus
Fear-related	Centromedial amygdala Fimbria of the fornix	Ventromedial hypothalamus Septal nuclei Dorsal hippocampus
Territorial	Lateral hypothalamus	Basolateral amygdala
Maternal	Hypothalamus Ventral hippocampus	Septal nuclei Basolateral amygdala
Sex-related	Hypothalamus Ventral hippocampus Centromedial amygdala	Septal nuclei Basolateral amygdala Cingulate gyrus
Irritative	Dorsomedial hypothalamus Posterior hypothalamus Anterior cingulate gyrus	Ventromedial hypothalamus Basolateral amygdala Head of caudate nucleus Posterior cingulate gyrus
Learned	Cerebral cortex(?)	Unknown
Pain-related	Unknown	Unknown
Seizures	Limbic system	
Idiopathic	Unknown	Unknown

mate objects; finally, they may have a generalized seizure. Some animals exhibit this behavior when fed, attacking themselves or the food dish. The behavior is stereotyped: the animal is not aware of its surroundings. Anticonvulsants may reduce the episodes (see chapter 50).

Early socialization can have a major effect on aggressive tendencies. Most of the information is on dogs, but it probably applies to other species as well. If the dog has little contact with people in early life, especially from 3 to 12 weeks of age, it is likely to be fearful of human contact and may be a fear biter. Removal of the dog from the litter at 3 to 4 weeks of age prevents normal socialization with other dogs, and it may be aggressive toward dogs as an adult. Social dominance in the household is also important. Early obedience training is useful to establish the owner's dominance at an early age. This is especially important in breeds that tend to be aggressive by nature. Hart has rated dogs on reactivity (affection, excitability, excessive barking, snapping, and activity), aggressiveness (territorial defense, watchdog barking, aggression to dogs, and dominance over owner), and trainability (obedience training and housebreaking).[6] The aggressive tendencies are summarized in Table 6-2. It is clear that genetic factors are important in the level of aggression. In addition, there are a few breeds that are reported to have "idiopathic aggression." These include the Saint Bernard,[7] Doberman pin-

Table 6-2. Levels of Aggressive Tendencies in Dogs

VERY LOW	LOW	MEDIUM	HIGH	VERY HIGH
Basset hound	Australian shepherd	Beagle	Afghan hound	Airedale terrier
Bloodhound	Brittany spaniel	Bichon frise	Alaskan malamute	Akita
English bulldog	Chesapeake Bay retriever	Boston terrier	Boxer	Cairn terrier
Norwegian elkhound	Collie	Cocker spaniel	Chow Chow	Chihuahua
	German shorthaired pointer	English springer spaniel	Dalmatian	Dachshund
	Golden retriever	Irish setter	Great Dane	Doberman pinscher
	Keeshond	Lhasa apso	Saint Bernard	Fox terrier
	Labrador retriever	Maltese	Samoyed	German shepherd
	Newfoundland	Pekingese	Siberian husky	Rottweiler
	Vizsla	Pomeranian		Schnauzer (miniature)
		Poodle (all sizes)		Scottish terrier
		Pug		Silky terrier
		Shetland sheepdog		West Highland white terrier
		Shih Tzu		
		Weimaraner		
		Welsh corgi		
		Yorkshire terrier		

(Data from Hart BL, Hart LA: Selecting pet dogs on the basis of cluster analysis of breed profiles and gender. J Am Vet Med Assoc 186:1181–1185, 1985)

scher,[7] German shepherd,[7] English springer spaniel,[5,10] English cocker spaniel,[11] and Bernese mountain dog.[7,10]

Male animals are more aggressive than females.[7] Prepubertal castration has little effect on this difference, but castration, either prepubertal or postpubertal, reduces intermale aggression in about half of dogs.[7]

Dogs can be taught to be aggressive. Aggressive tendencies can also be shaped by positive feedback (*e.g.*, the fear biter may be reinforced by successfully driving people away). Early training is critical in the development of social behavior, especially in animals that are normally most aggressive.[7]

DIAGNOSTIC PLAN

Aggressive animals are dangerous, so all procedures should be conducted with the objective of avoiding injury to the examiner, support personnel, and the client. The history is usually the most important part of the evaluation of behavioral disorders. Adequate time should be allowed to extract all of the necessary information. Items to be analyzed are the usual medical information (see chapter 50) and specific data on the animal's behavior, including early socialization, times of normal and abnormal behavior and events surrounding each, owner–animal interaction, training, and environment. If the behavior is sudden in onset, events occurring at the time should be explored carefully.

The physical, neurologic, and laboratory examination should rule out systemic and neurologic disease in most cases (see chapter 50). If the animal is normal except for the behavioral problem, then the type of aggression should be determined (see Table 6-1). Factors likely to relate to the type of aggression are also listed in Table 6-1. This information should lead to the source of the problem. The causes of each type of aggression are so numerous that they defy cataloguing. For more details, see one of the references.[1–3,7–9,11,14,15]

SYMPTOMATIC THERAPY

Gender-related aggression, including intermale, maternal, and sex-related, are the simplest to recognize. Intermale aggression is normal in most species. It becomes a problem when it is inappropriate for our environment. If the animals are in the same household, the problem is usually owner intervention in the dominance structure. Allowing the animals to set the structure will often establish a normal relationship. If the actions are toward strange dogs, the problem may be territorial or true intermale aggression. Castration is effective in about half of dogs in this type of aggression.[7] Progestins (medroxyprogesterone by injection, 5 mg/kg; megestrol acetate, 0.5 mg/kg daily) may be effective in about 75% of castrated males.[7] Another solution is behavioral therapy, such as counterconditioning. Maternal and sex-related forms of aggression are also normal behavior that can be managed best by avoidance of the stimulus. Conditioning of the female can usually overcome maternal aggression.

Dominance-related aggression is usually a function of the owner's behavior. Early obedience training, especially in dogs with strong aggressive tendencies (see Table 6-2), will usually prevent the problem. It is less likely to help once the dog has gained dominance. One approach is for the owner to regain dominance through force. The dog must be punished at every instance of aggressive behavior. Shaking by the scruff of the neck and use of a choke chain are methods of asserting dominance. The owner must be convinced of the necessity for physical punishment. The alternative is to withhold all affection and feeding from the dog except when the dog responds appropriately to a command.

Fear-related aggression is treated by a combination of desensitization and counterconditioning. Desensitization involves gradual presentation of the fear-inducing stimulus in small steps. Counterconditioning is a reward in association with the stimulus. The two are employed together and may be enhanced by the use of tranquilizers.[5]

Dogs with idiopathic aggression directed toward people are usually unresponsive to treatment. These animals are dangerous, especially in large breeds, and should be euthanized.[7]

Management of aggressive behavior is difficult and time consuming and requires a thorough understanding of normal and abnormal behavior. Referral to a specialist is recommended when possible.

REFERENCES

1. Beaver B: Veterinary Aspects of Feline Behavior. St. Louis, CV Mosby, 1980
2. Borchelt PL, Voith VL: Aggressive behavior in dogs and cats. Comp Cont Ed Pract Vet &:949–960, 1985
3. Caldwell DS, Little PB: Aggression in dogs and associated neuropathology. Can Vet J 21:152–154, 1980
4. De Lahunta A: Veterinary Neuroanatomy and Clinical Neurology, 2nd ed. Philadelphia, WB Saunders, 1983
5. Hart BL: Behavioral indications for phenothiazine and benzodiazepine tranquilizers in dogs. J Am Vet Med Assoc 186:1192–1194, 1985
6. Hart BL, Hart LA: Selecting pet dogs on the basis of cluster analysis of breed profiles and gender. J Am Vet Med Assoc 196:1181–1185, 1985
7. Hart BL, Hart LA: Canine and Feline Behavioral Therapy. Philadelphia, Lea & Febiger, 1985
8. Houpt KA: Aggression in dogs. Comp Cont Ed Pract Vet 1:123–128, 1979
9. Houpt KA Wolski TR: Domestic Animal Behavior for Veterinarians and Animal Scientists. Ames, IA, Iowa State University Press, 1982
10. Karczmar AG, Richardson DL, Kindel G: Neuropharmacological and related aspects of animal aggression. Prog Neuropsychopharmacol 2:611–631, 1978
11. Mugford RA: Aggressive behavior in the English cocker spaniel. Vet Ann 25:310–314, 1984
12. Oliver JE, Jr, Lorenz M: Handbook of Veterinary Neurologic Diagnosis. Philadelphia, WB Saunders, 1983
13. Valzelli L: Human and animal studies on the neurophysiology of aggression. Prog Neuropsychopharmacol 2:591–610, 1978
14. Voith VL: Applied animal behavior for the veterinary practitioner. Proceedings AAHA 47th Annual Meeting, 1980, pp 15–33
15. Voith VL: Diagnosis and treatment of aggressive behavior problems in dogs. Proceedings AAHA 47th Annual Meeting, 1980, pp 35–38

7

Self-Mutilation

MICHAEL D. LORENZ

PROBLEM DEFINITION AND RECOGNITION

Self-mutilation is the destruction of any body part through the voluntional acts of an animal. It is usually recognized by the injuries induced through biting, chewing, or rubbing of the limbs, feet, tail, or head. Autoamputation of a foot or tail is the result of many severe self-mutilation syndromes. This chapter describes those syndromes that cause self-induced destruction of a body part other than primary dermatologic conditions (see chapter 15).

PATHOPHYSIOLOGY

The pathophysiology of self-mutilation syndromes is poorly understood in dogs and cats, since these animals are incapable of expressing their feelings regarding pain, pruritis, or abnormal behavior. In veterinary medicine, the assumption has been that self-mutilation is the animal's response to the perception of altered sensation. More recently, attention has focused on a psychologic basis for self-mutilation.

Basically, self-mutilation can be classified into the following etiologic categories: (1) primary sensory neuropathy or neutritis, (2) psychogenic, (3) psychomotor epilepsy, (4) encephalitis, and (5) intractable severe pruritis or pain secondary to soft tissue or bone inflammation (see Diseases That Cause Self-Mutilation in Dogs and Cats). Category 5 may overlap with category 1.

Primary sensory neuropathies or neuritis may be congenital or acquired. Damage to sensory nerves from trauma, compression, neoplasia (neuroma), or viral infection (herpes virus, pseudorabies virus) may cause pain or paresthesia (morbid or perverted sensation). Paresthesia is described by humans as a burning, searing, or prickling sensation. Causalagia is a burning pain caused by injury or scar tissue in the sympathetic nerves innervating the skin. It is assumed that damage to peripheral nerves or sensory nerve roots in dogs and cats results in

Diseases That Cause Self-Mutilation in Dogs and Cats

- Neuropathies
  - Traumatic
    - Neoplasia
    - Neuroma
    - Neurofibroma
  - Compression
    - Skeletal fractures
    - Skeletal subluxation
    - Lumbar spinal stenosis
  - Inflammation
    - Trigeminal neuritis
    - Pseudorabies virus
    - Canine distemper virus
  - Congenital sensory neuropathy
    - English pointer
    - Dachshunds
- Behavioral
  - Acral pruritic nodule
  - Feline hyperesthesia syndrome/neurodermatitis
- Psychomotor epilepsy
- Encephalitis
  - Pseudorabies virus
  - Canine distemper virus
- Soft tissue or bone inflammation

similar sensations. The altered sensation may be referred to that area of the skin or limb (tail) innervated by the affected sensory nerve. The animal's response to this sensation is severe chewing, biting, and licking. Autoamputation is common.

Psychogenic causes of self-mutilation cannot be conclusively proven in the dog or cat. However, self-mutilation may be worsened or initiated by changes in the environment that could be viewed as "stressful." These syndromes may be alleviated by mood-altering drugs (see chapter 15). Acral pruritic nodule, feline hyperesthesia syndrome, and feline lick granuloma are dermatoses commonly attributed to a psychogenic abnormality. Autoamputation is rare and the neurologic exam is normal.

Psychomotor epilepsy is a seizure disorder characterized by episodes of abnormal behavior such as hysteria, rage, salivation, and hallucinations. During the seizures, especially if rage is a component, self-mutilation of a body part may occur. Frequently when food is the apparent stimulus, dogs will violently attack their pelvic limbs and tail, causing severe lacerations. Autoamputation is rare. Unlike the preceding causes, psychomotor seizures are preceded by an aura and the animal is usually completely unresponsive to commands during the ictus.

Loss of consciousness is not a feature of this syndrome. Psychomotor seizures result from functional abnormalities in the limbic system of the brain.

Viral encephalitis may cause self-mutilation through involvement of the brain stem and/or cranial and peripheral nerves (neuritis). Pseudorabies is the outstanding example of those viral diseases that cause intense pruritis and severe self-mutilation. In pseudorabies, self-mutilation is most severe on the head, face, neck, and shoulders. Other signs of viral encephalitis are usually present and include abnormal behavior, fever, hypersalivation, and generalized convulsions. Pets are usually infected by eating contaminated pork.

Viral encephalitis that causes severe behavioral changes from brain stem disease may cause self-mutilation through changes in the function of sensory neurons. Canine distemper encephalitis is one example. In most cases, other clinical signs of neurologic disease are present. There is no evidence that herpes viruses other than pseudorabies virus are associated with self-mutilation syndromes in dogs and cats. Herpes zoster infection in humans frequently causes intense pruritis and burning via inflammation of cranial or peripheral neurons.

Severe inflammation of soft tissue and underlying bone may cause chronic irritation of sensory receptors. This may be perceived as severe pruritis, pain, or burning. Severe excoriations or self-mutilation may result from the animal's intense chewing or licking.

DIAGNOSTIC PLAN

A diagnostic plan for the problem of self-mutilation is presented in Figure 7-1. The initial step is to identify any neurologic signs or deficits that may be present. A thorough neurologic examination is required. If neurologic signs are present, the lesion should be localized to the central or peripheral nervous system (see chapter 47). The presence of seizures associated with self-mutilation is strong evidence of central nervous system disease. A thorough seizure workup is indicated (see chapter 50).

Peripheral nerve lesions causing a sensory neuropathy are extremely difficult to diagnose. In some cases, pain perception may be decreased from the affected area; other sensory or motor deficits may be present. In most cases, there are few, if any, signs of neurologic disease. In these animals, one must consider the presence of a sensory neuropathy due to trauma, neoplasia, entrapment, or compression. Radiographs of the affected body part and that region of the vertebral column from which the affected nerves originate should be closely examined for bony or soft tissue changes that might cause a neuropathy. Measurement of sensory nerve conduction times and evoked potentials may be helpful in the identification of a sensory neuropathy. Unfortunately, only a few large referral centers are equipped to perform these electrodiagnostic procedures.

Biopsy of affected skin for histopathology and possible bacterial and fungal culture should be performed, especially when the lesions are swollen, nodular, or infected.

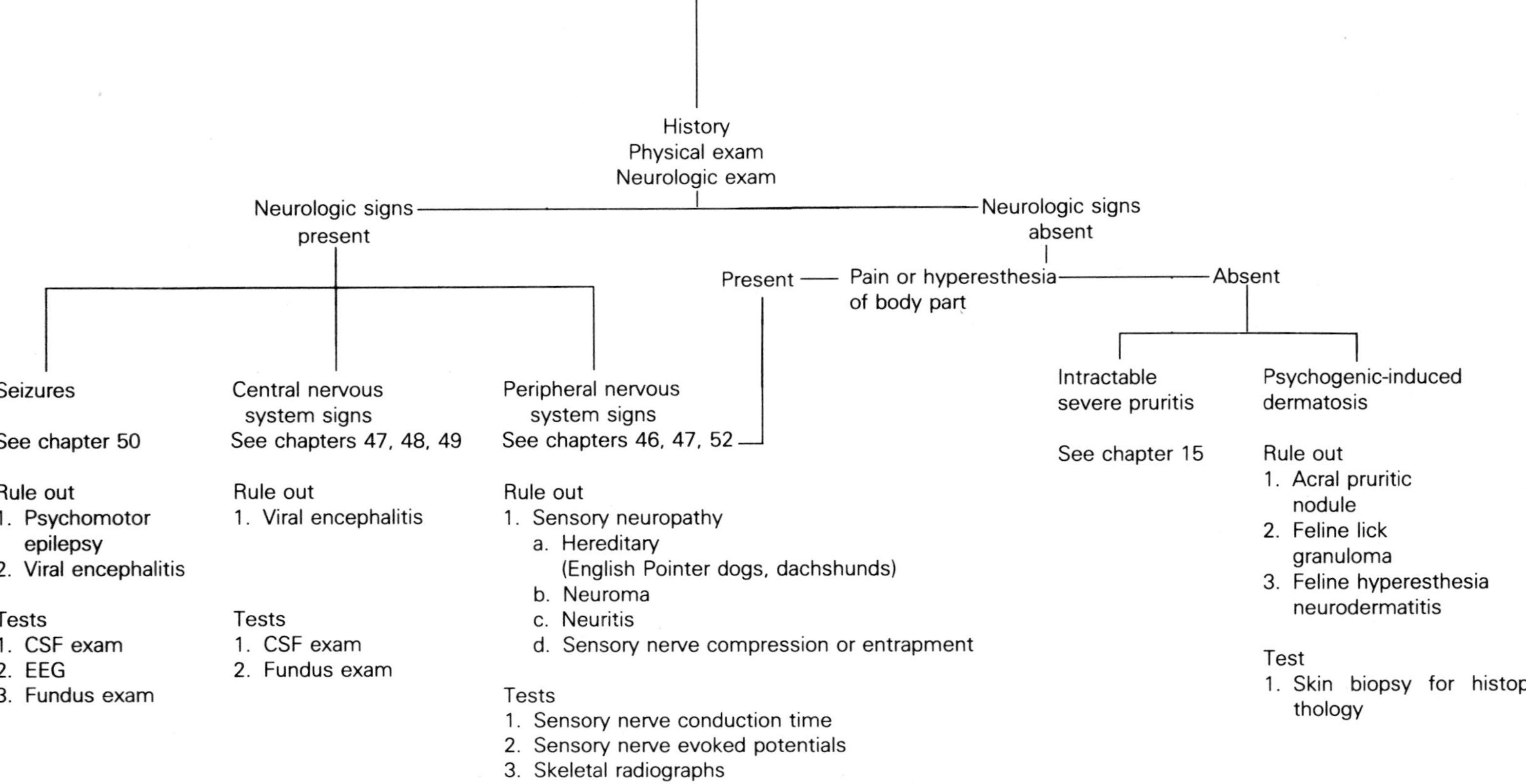

Fig. 7-1. Diagnostic plan.

Behavioral studies should be undertaken when there is no evidence of organic disease to explain the self-mutilation. Changes in an animal's "normal" daily routine may be associated with self-mutilation. Introduction of a new animal or person in the environment or moving the animal to new surroundings may initiate excessive chewing and licking. Animals placed under unusual stress such as heavy obedience work from a demanding trainer may also initiate self-mutilation.

SYMPTOMATIC THERAPY

Definitive therapy is obviously dependent on discovery of the underlying cause. Excessive chewing or licking of a body part can be prevented with the use of Elizabethan collars or side braces. These procedures are most helpful in the treatment of tail or foot chewers.

So-called psychogenic dermatoses can be treated with drugs such as diazepam, phenobarbital, hydroxyzine, and the progesterone compounds such as megesterol acetate. Megesterol acetate is more beneficial in cats. Destruction of sensory receptors in the skin has been advocated; however, these procedures are currently not indicated since they are seldom effective.

Self-mutilation of the feet or tail may be so severe that amputation may be warranted. In the author's experience, the animal usually mutilates another area or continues to mutilate the body part proximal to the site of amputation.

8

Coprophagy and Pica

MICHAEL D. LORENZ

PROBLEM DEFINITION AND RECOGNITION

Coprophagy is the ingestion of feces. It is not uncommon in dogs, but it is rare in cats. Coprophagic dogs usually ingest dog or cat feces, although other animal feces may be eaten if available. In certain situations, coprophagy is considered normal animal behavior. For instance, lactating bitches normally ingest the feces of their puppies from birth to 3 weeks of age.

Pica is a craving for and the ingestion of unnatural articles. Dogs may eat dirt (geophagy), rocks, sticks, or cat litter or lick concrete. Cats may crave wool yarn. Both dogs and cats may ingest green grass, which is most commonly observed in the spring. Coprophagy is a pica for feces.

PATHOPHYSIOLOGY

Although many causes for pica and coprophagy have been proposed, the underlying cause for this behavior is unknown. Except for the coprophagy of lactating bitches, most forms of pica should be considered an abnormality of behavior.

Veterinarians and laypeople have assumed that coprophagy results from certain dietary deficiencies. One theory proposes a deficiency of amylase perpetuated by a high-carbohydrate diet. Other theories propose that coprophagy results from a deficiency of proteolytic enzymes.[1] None of these theories has any scientific merit. Coprophagy may occur in well-nourished dogs with no evidence of digestive system disease.

Animals with pancreatic exocrine insufficiency may become severely coprophagic, apparently in an attempt to ingest sufficient calories to prevent starvation. Any disease that causes polyphagia may also cause coprophagy (see chapter 3). Coprophagy has been associated with hyperadrenocorticism, glucocorticoid therapy, diabetes mellitus, intestinal malabsorption syndromes, intestinal parasitism, hyperthyroidism, and nonspecific dietary deficiencies.

There are usually few deleterious consequences associated with coprophagy. Severe halitosis is a common complaint of owners. Dogs that ingest large quantities of horse manure may develop acute gastroenteritis. The ingestion of dog feces may cause repeated infection with gastrointestinal parasites. The ingestion of foreign matter may cause gastrointestinal obstruction. Some dogs with acquired megacolon may impact the colon with sand, rocks, or garbage material. Geophagic dogs may develop excessive wear of the teeth. In humans, geophagia (ingestion of clay soil) may cause hypokalemia, iron deficiency, and zinc deficiency; this has not been reported in dogs or cats.

DIAGNOSTIC PLAN

Since many animals with coprophagy or pica are thought to have behavioral problems, a thorough history regarding the environment and handling of the pet is indicated. Stressful conditions or abrupt changes in the animal's normal routine should be identified and eliminated. The diet should be carefully analyzed for any deficiencies, especially of trace minerals.

Gastrointestinal disease, pancreatic exocrine insufficiency, hyperthyroidism, hyperadrenocorticism, and diabetes mellitus should be considered as possible etiologies. A urine analysis and biochemical profile should be performed to evaluate the possible presence of these disorders. A complete blood count (CBC) may detect iron deficiency. Fecal flotations are indicated since chronic intestinal parasitism may be associated with coprophagy.

SYMPTOMATIC THERAPY

Avoidance of the offending substance is the most effective therapy. Feces should be cleaned up each day and litter pans should be placed in areas or containers unavailable to dogs. Empirically, the feeding of digestive enzymes or foods that contain large quantities of proteolytic enzymes (for example, pineapple, figs, and squash) may decrease coprophagic tendencies in some dogs.[1,2] Commercial meat tenderizers, lightly sprinkled on the dog's food, may add some digestive enzymes to the diet. Pancreatic enzymes added to the diet may be helpful but are modestly expensive.

The addition of small quantities of sulfur to the diet may make the feces less attractive to the dog. A mineral-iron supplement can also be tried in dogs with geophagy.

REFERENCES

1. McCuistion WR: Prevention of coprophagy. In Kirk RW (ed): Current Veterinary Therapy III. Philadelphia, WB Saunders, 1968
2. Morris ML: Index of diatetic management. In Kirk RW (ed): Current Veterinary Therapy VI. Philadelphia, WB Saunders, 1977

9

Urine Spraying in Cats

JEANNE A. BARSANTI

DEFINITION AND RECOGNITION

Urine spraying in cats is a method of marking territory. The cat will typically smell the target area, turn around, and forcibly express uring while standing with its tail upright. The urine is sprayed horizontally onto a vertical object. Another form of urine marking in cats is voiding a small amount of urine while squatting. Cats may also void outside of litterboxes because of factors related to the litterbox itself as well as urinary tract diseases. Spraying becomes a form of inappropriate urination (voluntary urination in the wrong place or at the wrong time) when the target is in the owner's house. Inappropriate urination must always be distinguished from urinary incontinence (see chapter 40). This chapter will deal with inappropriate urination in cats in general as well as spraying in particular, since some clients do not understand the specific terminology and since many identify the problem by finding urine but do not actually observe the act of urination.

PATHOPHYSIOLOGY

Inappropriate urination is the most common behavioral problem in cats. The incidence of spraying is highest in intact males, but spraying also occurs in intact females, especially during estrus. Even in cats neutered younger than 10 months of age, 10% of males and 5% of females sprayed urine more than once a month. This high incidence of a "behavioral problem" is related to continuation of a normal feline behavior during indoor confinement with people who obviously find it objectionable.

Normal Behavioral Considerations

Cats spray urine or squat to void a small amount of urine to establish their territory and to communicate their presence to other cats. Cats by choice prefer a low population density, where each can establish its own territory. They adhere to regular schedules of movement to avoid confrontations with other cats except during breeding season. The frequency of spraying is increased by the sight, odor, and sounds of other cats. Androgens also increase the frequency of spraying, while progestogens decrease it. The problem of spraying arises when cats become house pets, particularly when confined with other cats. The incidence of spraying is directly proportional to the number of cats in the household, particularly with male cats. In households of ten or more cats, a spraying problem is inevitably present in at least one cat. In contrast to popular opinion, one survey found that neutered male cats were more likely to spray if in a household including female cats as opposed to a household containing only other males.

Other Considerations

Cats may void urine outside of a litterbox because of aversion to the box. Most cats are easily litter trained because of their natural tendency to urinate in sand or loose dirt. However, cats possess this tendency to varying degrees. Some cats avoid certain types of litter (especially that containing deodorants such as chlorophyll), dirty litter, litter being used by another cat, and litter in certain types of containers (such as those with lids or with or without high sides). Cats may also learn to avoid litterboxes if the box is associated with punishment, injury, or pain whether inflicted from without or associated with cystitis.

Cats may become attracted to an alternate area for voiding urine, because of house soiling by another pet or because of discovery of a surface or material that they individually prefer to litter.

Environmental changes may also cause a cat to begin to urinate outside the litterbox. These can include moving to a new house, redecorating an existing dwelling, adding a new person or pet to the household, or longer-than-accustomed absences of the owner.

Urinary tract problems that cause dysuria or polyuria may also result in urination outside of the litterbox (see appropriate chapters).

Once a cat begins to urinate outside a litterbox, it may continue to do so for reasons different from that which initiated the problem. For example, the cat may object to a new litter, but after the litter is changed it continues to urinate outside the box because it has learned to prefer the new location whether because of odor, material, or the location itself.

DIAGNOSTIC PLAN

Primary rule outs for a cat urinating outside the litterbox are (1) problems related to disease such as dysuria (voiding urgency), polyuria (requiring more frequent trips to the litterbox or increased soiling of the box), and musculoskeletal problems (which inhibit access to the litterbox), (2) urine marking, and (3) a change in urination area preference (see Rule Outs for Inapproprate Urination in Cats).

Rule Outs for Inappropriate Urination in Cats

Diseases

- Those that cause dysuria
  - Feline urologic syndrome (idiopathic hematuria)
  - Bacterial cystitis/urethritis
  - Cystic or urethral calculi
  - Lower urinary tract neoplasia
- Those that cause polyuria
  - Renal failure
  - Diabetes mellitus
  - Hepatic failure
  - Hyperthyroidism
  - Others (see chapter 5)
- Musculoskeletal problems inhibiting mobility

Urine Marking

- Spraying
- Squatting to void small urine volumes without dysuria

Urination Preference

- Aversion to litter or litterbox
- Preference for a new material or location
- Environmental change

History

A thorough history is essential; however, owners seldom know what terms such as spraying, incontinence, polyuria, and dysuria mean. Some owners consider any urination outside the litterbox as spraying, while others have never heard the term. An exact description of the cat's position during urination or whether the urine is found on a horizontal or vertical surface will help determine if spraying urine has occurred. The owner should be questioned regarding the presence of dysuria, hematuria, and polyuria (see chapters on dysuria, abnormal urine color, and polyuria) since disease in the urinary tract may cause inappropriate urination. Urinary incontinence must be distinguished from inappropriate urination (see chapter on incontinence). Any changes in the household or management of the cat are important as are any other behavioral changes, medical problems, or drug usage. Androgen therapy in cats may induce urine marking.

Sometimes owners of more than one cat do not know which cat is inappropriately urinating. One proposed method to determine the culprit is to inject 0.3 ml of sodium fluorescein subcutaneously, (Fluorescite Injectable, 10%, Alcon Laboratories) or give 0.5 ml orally to the most likely suspect. The urine should fluoresce with a Wood's light for the next 24 hours. Each cat in the household can be checked by evaluating one every other day.

Physical Examination and Diagnostic Tests

A complete physical examination should be performed on the affected cat. Urine collected by cystocentesis should be analyzed. If abnormalities suggestive of urinary tract infection are present (pyuria, bacteriuria, hematuria), a culture of urine collected by cystocentesis is indicated. A fraction of the sample for urine analysis can be refrigerated so that a culture can be performed without a second cystocentesis. Urine analysis and urine culture should be performed on the *same* day as collection. Survey and contrast radiographs may also be indicated to determine whether calculi or neoplasia is the cause of the abnormal urine analysis. If the urine is marginally concentrated (urine specific gravity less than 1.040), blood urea nitrogen and/or serum creatinine should also be assessed. A blood chemistry profile and complete blood count may also be indicated to rule out other causes of polyuria (see chapter on polyuria).

TREATMENT

Any medical problems should be treated appropriately. If no medical problems are identified, the problem is one of urine marking or change in urination area preference. If possible, these problems should be differentiated. Spraying indicates urine marking. It can be difficult to determine whether squatting to urinate is due to marking or change in preference. Small volumes suggest marking and larger volumes suggest a change in preference.

Neutering is highly effective therapy for urine marking in intact male cats. Immediate improvement in approximately 80% of male cats and gradual improvement over 2 to 3 months in another 10% has been reported. Neutering may also help intact female cats, although this is less well proven. If the cat is already neutered, the most effective therapy is to reduce the number of contact cats. If this is not possible, behavioral modification efforts, progestogen therapy, or, as a last resort, olfactory tractotomy can be tried.

Behavioral modification can be attempted for both urine marking and urination area preference changes and can be both positive and negative. Positive methods suggested have included increasing attention to the cat and praise for litterbox use. Negative methods include a loud noise from an inanimate object such as a horn or slapping a table or spraying with water. The problem with these methods is that they require observation of the act of urination and they must be consistently and immediately applied. Most clients do not have the time to carry out these techniques. Cats also quickly learn to urinate out of the owner's presence. One mistake clients may make is to take the cat to the litterbox when urination outside the box occurs or urine is found. If the owner is angry and tries to correct the cat this way, the cat will associate the litterbox with punishment and the problem may worsen.

For both urine marking and urination area preference problems, attention should be payed to the litterbox, although the emphasis may be different. The box should be cleaned daily; the litter should be completely changed at least once a week. One litterbox should be provided per cat. The location of the box can be changed to one that is less busy or to the area where the cat is urinating. The box could then be gradually moved to a more appropriate location.

If the cat repeatedly urinates in the same inappropriate place, that area should be established for feeding or playing. This may discourage the urination. Access to the area can be prohibited or the area covered with a surface the cat does not like such as plastic or aluminium foil.

For the problem of litter avoidance, the owner must determine the type of material the cat likes and associate this with the litterbox. This may be as simple as returning to a previously acceptable litter. In other cases, the owner will have to determine what the cat likes to scratch in, since scratching in any material is correlated with urinating in it. Pieces of rug, paper, cloth, sand, earth, or other materials may have to be considered.

Areas where the cat has urinated should be thoroughly cleaned to avoid repeated odor attraction to that location. A 50 : 50 solution of white vinegar and water or club soda has been recommended. Ammonia should be avoided because it may be an attractive odor to some cats.

For cats that do not respond to the above methods, progesterone therapy is indicated. Approximately 30% of cats will respond to medroxyprogesterone acetate (MPA) or megestrol acetate (MA). The response rate is better in neutered males (50%) than females (10%) and better in cats from single cat households (50%) than in those from multiple cat households (20%). The best response was in neutered males in single cat households (80%) and the worst in neutered females in multicat households (0%). The dosage of MPA is 10 to 20 mg/kg subcutaneously or intramuscularly. If there is no response in a few weeks, the dosage may be repeated. Repeat doses may be required every 3 to 6 months. The recommended dosage of MA is 5 mg/day for 7 to 10 days, then 5 mg every other day for 2 weeks, then 5 mg twice a week for 2 weeks, then 5 mg once a week for 8 weeks, then 2.5 mg once a week for 4 weeks, and so forth until the minimum dose and frequency of administration is determined. If improvement is not seen at 5 mg/day after 7 days, treatment with MA should be stopped. These doses were initially randomly determined; lower doses need to be evaluated for efficacy since progesterone therapy in cats has potential side effects. These include polyphagia, depression, mammary gland hyperplasia, mammary gland neoplasia, diabetes mellitus, pyometra, and decreased sperm production. Because of potential uterine disease and because the potential for mammary neoplasia may be higher, these drugs should not be used in intact females. Changes in pigmentation at the injection site have been reported with use of MPA. Since systemic side effects of MPA were less than those of MA in one study, MPA should be tried first. MA may be effective if MPA fails.

Diazepam has been occasionally recommended for urine marking and for emotional problems related to environmental changes to reduce anxiety. The dosage is 1.25 to 2.5 mg. This drug may produce behavioral changes in cats. It should be reserved for short-term use.

As a last resort, olfactory tractotomy can be tried. This was effective in 6 of 12 neutered male cats and 4 of 4 neutered female cats with few side effects.[1]

CLIENT EDUCATION

The attitude of the owner regarding the cat is extremely important. Owners often consider euthanasia for a cat with this problem even though they are attached to the animal. Since the cat is otherwise healthy, this decision may be difficult and associated with guilt. The owner may be willing to accept potential side effects of therapy when the alternative is euthanasia. In any case, sympathy with the owner's plight and efforts on his behalf with counseling in regard to environmental changes, drug therapy, and surgery are indicated. Some form of treatment will correct the problem in most cats. In those that do not respond, emotional support of the owner may be required if euthanasia is elected.

REFERENCE

1. Hart BL: Olfactory tractotomy for control of objectionable urine spraying and urine marking in cats. J Am Vet Med Assoc 179:231–234, 1981

SUGGESTED READING

Borchelt PL, Voith VL: Elimination behavior problems in cats. Compend Cont Ed Pract Vet 3:730–738, 1981

Hart BL: Objectionable urine spraying and urine marking in cats: Evaluation of progestin treatment in gonadectomized males and females. J Am Vet Med Assoc 177:529–533, 1980

Hart BL: Olfactory tractotomy for control of objectionable urine spraying and urine marking in cats. J Am Vet Med Assoc 179:231–234, 1981

Hart BL, Barrett RE: Effects of castration on fighting, roaming, and urine spraying in adult male cats. J Am Vet Med Assoc 163:290–292, 1973

Hart BL, Cooper L: Factors relating to uring spraying and fighting in prepubertally gonadectomized cats. J Am Vet Med Assoc 184:1255–1258, 1984

Hart BL, Leedy M: Identification of source of urine stains in multi-cat households. J Am Vet Med Assoc 180:77–78, 1982

Part Three

CONFORMATIONAL PROBLEMS

10

Abdominal Distention

LARRY M. CORNELIUS

Abdominal distention may be defined as a sudden or gradual increase in the size of the abdomen. Distention may be intermittent or persistent and asymptomatic or painful. Abdominal distention may be due to either fluid or nonfluid causes (Table 10-1). Ascites is an abnormal accumulation of fluid transudate or modified transudate in the peritoneal cavity. Since exudates must also be ruled out whenever abdominal fluid is present, they will be included in this discussion of ascites. Associated signs such as vomiting, diarrhea, abdominal pain, polydipsia, polyuria, polyphagia, and edema, if present, may be clues to the etiology of abdominal distention and ascites.

PATHOPHYSIOLOGY

Pathophysiologic mechanisms of ascites are similar to those of expansion of extracellular fluid elsewhere in the body (edema). There appear to be two general groups: (1) those in which the primary event is escape of plasma into tissue spaces with resultant hypovolemia and secondary renal retention of water and electrolytes and (2) other types in which the primary disturbance is excessive renal retention of electrolytes and water, leading to extracellular fluid expansion and transudation of fluid from plasma into tissue spaces.[2] General mechanisms of ascites formation include increased capillary hydrostatic pressure, increased capillary permeability, decreased colloid osmotic pressure of plasma (hypoalbuminemia), obstruction of lymph flow, and excessive renal retention of sodium and water. More than one of these causes are often present in clinical cases of ascites.

Abdominal venous obstruction results in increased capillary hydrostatic pressure and may cause ascites. Protein content of ascitic fluid varies depending upon the anatomic site of venous obstruction and thus may be helpful in establishing the cause of ascites (Table 10-1).[1] Obstruction of blood flow draining hepatic sinusoids (postsinusoidal obstruction) causes production of high protein

Table 10-1. Causes of Abdominal Effusion

HIGH-PROTEIN (>2.5 g/dl) ASCITES		LOW-PROTEIN (<2.5 g/dl) ASCITES
Exudate	**Modified Transudate**	**Transudate**
Protein (g/dl) > 3.5	2.5–6.0	<2.5
Cells/cmm > 30,000	250–20,000	<1000
Inflammatory	Cardiac	Hypoalbuminemia (<0.8 g/dl)
Bacterial (septic)	Right-sided congestive heart failure	Glomerular disease
Bowel rupture	Intracardiac tumors	Hepatic insufficiency
Penetrating wounds	Cardiomyopathy (dog)	Gastrointestinal loss (diarrhea)
Ruptured abscess	Neoplasia in abdomen	Chronic starvation
Chemical	Obstruction of hepatic vein or thoracic caudal vena cava	Sustained portal hypertension
Intraperitoneal drug	Thrombosis	Cirrhosis
Pancreatitis	Stricture	Chronic active hepatitis
Leakage of	Vascular anomaly	Chronic cholangiohepatitis
Bile	Thrombosis of hepatic vein or thoracic caudal vena cava	Abdominal or hepatic neoplasia with sustained portal hypertension and/or hypoalbuminemia
Urine	Chyle	
Circulatory compromise	Lymphadenitis	
Thrombosis	Ruptured lymphatic	
Torsion	Inflammatory	
Intussusception	Feline infectious peritonitis	
Physical injury		
Postsurgical manipulation		
Trauma		

(>2.5 g/dl) ascites derived from hepatic lymph. Protein content is high because hepatic sinusoidal capillaries are much more porous and "leaky" than capillaries elsewhere in the body. Extrahepatic portal venous pressure is normal or only slightly increased.

Experimentally produced *transient* portal venous obstruction alone does not cause ascites. Lymph flow from the bowel markedly increases and probably compensates for obstructed portal venous drainage. *Sustained* portal hypertension causes ascites. Persistently increased capillary hydrostatic pressure causes dilation of intestinal lacteals and increased fluid transudation into the bowel lumen and from the serosa into the peritoneal cavity. Intestinal lymph is relatively low in protein; therefore, ascites caused by chronic portal hypertension is generally low in protein (<2.5 g/dl).[1]

Abdominal masses (neoplasms, granulomas, "walled-off" abscesses) may cause vascular damage and leakage of blood or plasma, resulting in high protein ascites. If the mass restricts portal blood flow (presinusoidal), resulting in sustained portal hypertension, low protein intestinal lymph contributes to the formation of the ascitic fluid. Low protein ascites (with normal serum albumin) in the presence of an abdominal mass signifies that portal venous obstruction is present.[1]

Hypoalbuminemia, in the absence of other causes of ascites, must be severe (<0.8 g/dl) to sufficiently lower plasma oncotic pressure to cause ascites; however, lesser degrees of hypoalbuminemia facilitate formation of ascitic fluid whenever other mechanisms such as increased capillary permeability are also present.

The pathophysiologic events of intra-abdominal exudate formation vary with the particular exudate. Rapid accumulation of blood in the abdomen, such as may occur following trauma or rupture of a splenic hemangiosarcoma, may be associated with signs of hypovolemic shock. A rent in the urinary system with accumulation of urine in the peritoneal or retroperitoneal spaces will result in signs of uremia. Leakage of bile into the peritoneal cavity causes signs of chemical peritonitis. A ruptured bowel usually leads to septic peritonitis with signs of endotoxemia and septic shock.

For the nonfluid causes of abdominal distention, the pathophysiologic mechanisms also vary depending on the cause. For example, ileus may be secondary to peritonitis or an obstructed bowel. Lack of normal bowel motility may allow proliferation of pathogenic intestinal bacteria and subsequent absorption of endotoxins. Intra-abdominal masses may impinge on normal abdominal organs and cause disruption of function, resulting in signs such as anorexia, vomiting, diarrhea, and icterus. With gastric volvulus, abdominal venous return is severely restricted and signs of hypovolemic shock may occur.

DIAGNOSTIC PLAN

History and Physical Examination

The history may be helpful in narrowing the possible causes of abdominal distention. An example would be a history of polydipsia, polyuria, and polyphagia in a dog with a distended, pendulous abdomen suggesting hyperadrenocorticism. The physical examination should be complete. Detection of associated findings such as dyspnea, tachycardia, heart murmurs, and peripheral edema usually help in determining the etiology of abdominal distention and the appropriate diagnostic plan. Ballottement of the abdomen should be done carefully to determine if a fluid wave is present. With experience, false-positive results are minimal, but small amounts of abdominal fluid usually cannot be detected by this method.

Other Diagnostic Procedures

Whenever an abdominal fluid wave is easily observed, paracentesis and fluid analysis prior to other diagnostic procedures are appropriate. This is accomplished by using a 20- to 22-gauge, 1-inch needle and a 6-ml syringe. If the animal is fractious, it is safer to use a butterfly needle unit. Although the risks of this procedure are minimal, it is probably better to tap the right cranial quadrant to avoid the spleen. Appropriate clipping and skin preparation should be done. Fluid analysis, including protein content, cell count and differential, sediment examination, and culture/sensitivity if indicated, should be performed. Only a

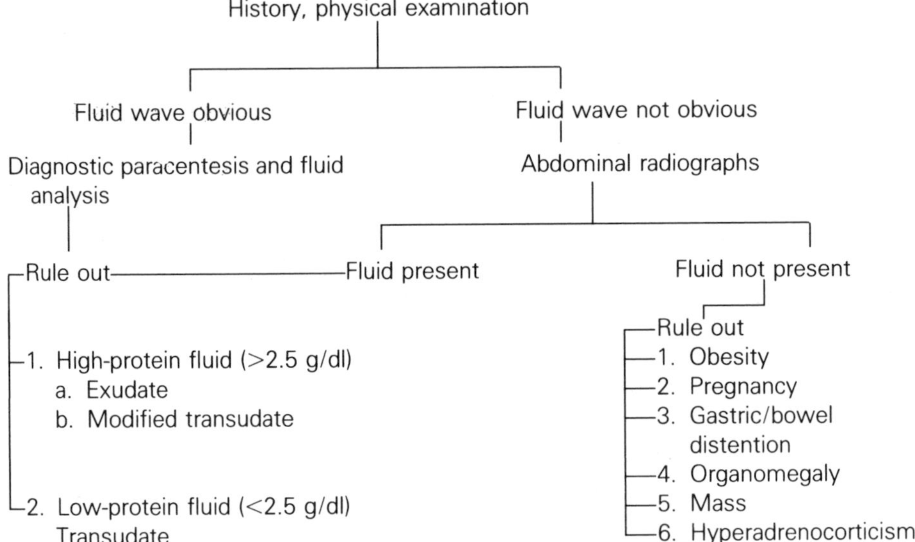

Fig. 10-1. Initial plan for diagnosing abdominal distention.

small amount of fluid (<1 ml) is required. Removal of large amounts of ascitic fluid should be avoided unless fluid distention is causing respiratory distress (see symptomatic therapy).

Abdominal and thoracic radiographs are often needed to evaluate an animal with abdominal distention. Although smaller quantities of fluid are best detected radiographically, large amounts of abdominal fluid often obscure detail. A suggested initial diagnostic plan for abdominal distention is shown in Figure 10-1.

SYMPTOMATIC THERAPY

Treatment of abdominal transudates and exudates depends upon the cause. Therapy of ascites is often unsatisfactory unless the primary cause is successfully managed within a reasonably short time. Symptomatic treatment of ascites is best done by using diuretics such as furosemide (Hoechst-Roussel Pharmaceuticals, Somerville, NJ) and restricting dietary sodium. Diuretics are more efficient in mobilizing edema than ascites but are helpful nonetheless. Side-effects include dehydration, reduced glomerular filtration resulting in increased blood urea nitrogen, and potassium depletion. Intermittent (every 2 or 3 days) use of diuretics and potassium supplementation (potassium gluconate [Adria Labs, Columbus, OH]) in the diet (1 to 3 mEq K^+/kg/day) lessens the severity of these complications.

Paracentesis is usually reserved for patients that do not respond to diuretics and sodium restriction within 48 hours. The exception is the animal with dyspnea in which ascites is restricting lung expansion and causing difficult breathing. Paracentesis should be done without delay in such cases. Ascitic fluid may be rapidly withdrawn without causing signs of cardiovascular collapse, but hypoalbuminemia and hyponatremia often worsen due to subsequent fluid retention and reformation of ascites. Dietary sodium restriction markedly slows the rate at which ascitic fluid is reformed and lessens the severity of hypoalbuminemia and hyponatremia.[1]

Symptomatic treatment of intra-abdominal distention caused by exudates depends upon the cause. Restoration of circulating blood volume with intravenous fluids and whole blood may be necessary.

REFERENCES

1. Greene CE: Ascites: Diagnostic and therapeutic considerations. Comp Cont Ed Small Animal Practice, 1979
2. Schroeder HA: Edema. In MacBryde CM, Blacklow RS (eds): Signs and Symptoms, pp 804–833. Philadelphia, JB Lippincott, 1970

11

Edema

CRAIG E. GREENE

PROBLEM DEFINITION

Edema results from expansion of the interstitial fluid volume. This increase in the extravascular components of the extracellular fluid can occur in a localized or generalized distribution depending on the primary cause. Determining the cause of edema formation is usually of utmost importance; however, increased tissue fluid pressure may require immediate treatment because it directly interferes with physiologic functions such as proper tissue nutrition.

PATHOPHYSIOLOGY

The interstitial fluid space is highly structured: it consists of collagen fibers embedded in a gel matrix. Fluid within this network, although relatively immobile, is in dynamic equilibrium with the blood capillary network.

Most intravascular fluid that enters the interstitial space as a result of hydrostatic pressure on the arteriolar network is reabsorbed by the local venous circulation so that minimal amounts of fluid exist. The narrow pores in the capillary endothelium normally restrict the migration of large plasma proteins into the interstitial space while allowing free passage of water and small solute molecules. Since the interstitial fluid protein concentration is normally much lower than that of plasma, the colloidal osmotic pressure from intravascular protein facilitates fluid retention in the vascular space. Excess fluid filtered into the interstitial space does not accumulate under normal circumstances but is returned to the blood via lymphatic vessels. Fluid return via lymphatic circulation is also somewhat dependent upon the interstitial compartment compliance. Under normal circumstances, the entry of fluid into the interstitial space causes marked increases in tissue pressure, which further restricts movement of fluid out of the vascular space.

Increased capillary permeability from endothelial damage can result in increased interstitial fluid accumulation. Hypoproteinemia will also result in expansion of the interstitial compartment, as will decreased flow or obstruction of the lymphatic or venous circulation.

Albumin, the smallest plasma protein, is the primary source of plasma colloidal oncotic pressure. Edema usually becomes evident when the serum albumin concentration falls below 2.0 g/dl. Extensive generalized edema associated with decreased plasma volume and increased extracellular fluid space is associated with decreased renal excretion of sodium and by presumed hormonal mechanisms. This continued retention of fluid exacerbates edema formation.

An increase in free fluid volume accounts for the pitting phenomenon that is seen in edematous states. Pressure applied to an edematous area forces the mobile fluid out of the region, resulting in a permanent indentation. The mobility of fluid also explains the continuous weeping of wounds in edematous tissues and the mobility of edema to the lowest portions of the body. Generalized edema is greatest in the dependent parts of the body due to increased venous pressure in these areas.

RULE OUTS AND DIAGNOSTIC PLAN

A thorough history and physical examination will help determine if an inflammatory process is the cause of edema (see Rule Outs for Edema). Fever, warm swelling, and enlarged or painful lymph nodes are associated with inflammatory conditions. Enlarged peripheral lymph nodes may also occur with lymphoreticular neoplasia that may cause edema. Arteriovenous fistulas may be detected by the presence of a continuous murmur auscultated in the affected extremity. Cardiovascular disorders may be detected on physical examination on the basis of pulse, respiratory rate, and cardiac auscultation. Suspicious findings can be followed-up with electrocardiography and thoracic radiography. Measurement of central venous pressure using a catheter and manometer is useful in determining the presence of venous obstruction. Venous occlusion can also be detected by contrast radiography.

The presence of ascites should be determined in any edematous patient since its presence may help determine the cause of both disorders. Ascitic fluid formation occurs by itself or prior to subcutaneous edema with cardiac disorders but also can occur in conjunction with edema in hypoproteinemic states. Analysis of the ascitic fluid to determine cell and protein content (see chapter 10) will also contribute to understanding the cause of edema formation.

Essential laboratory screening should include a complete blood count with a leukocyte differential and, most importantly, the measurement of plasma and urine protein concentrations. A refractometer can be used for initial screening of plasma protein concentration; albumin and total protein measurements should also be determined. If hypoproteinemia is found, other causes of this problem should be considered (see chapter 63). Electrolyte concentrations in plasma and urine can be examined to determine if extracellular fluids are being retained in

Rule Outs for Edema

- Decreased capillary integrity (increased permeability)
    - Inflammation
    - Vasculitis
        - Infectious
        - Immune-mediated
    - Allergy
    - Trauma
    - Burns
- Change in tissue gel
    - Myxedema
    - Serous atrophy of subcutaneous fat from cachexia
- Noninflammatory increase in tissue fluid
    - Decreased plasma oncotic pressure
        - Hypoproteinemia (albumin)
        - Increased loss
            - Renal
            - Gastrointestinal
            - Body cavities
            - Wounds
            - Vasculitis
            - Nephrotic syndrome
            - Protein-losing enteropathy
            - Protein malabsorption
        - Decreased production
            - Hepatic insufficiency from any cause
    - Lymphatic hypertension or obstruction
        - Surgical or traumatic injury
        - Neoplasia
        - Lymphatic or lymph node inflammation
        - Congenital lymphedema
    - Increased capillary hydrostatic pressure
        - Venous hypertension
            - Venous obstruction
            - Right heart failure or obstruction
            - Arteriovenous fistula
            - Overhydration
        - Arteriolar hypertension
            - Hyperaldosteronism
            - Inappropriate secretion of antidiuretic hormone
            - Acute renal failure

excess of or equal to electrolytes; this may help determine whether the process is primary or secondary to renal or adrenal dysfunction. Suspected immune or infectious disorders, based on clinical or laboratory findings, have to be confirmed using additional serologic tests. Enlarged lymph nodes should be aspirated or biopsied for cytologic evaluation. Edema may originate from a variety of disturbances; therefore, multiple abnormalities in laboratory tests may be apparent.

SYMPTOMATIC THERAPY

A rational approach to therapy of edema depends upon an understanding of the underlying disease process that produces it. Many factors, either alone or in combination, can contribute to edema formation, so the actual cause is not often apparent. Antimicrobial therapy should be instituted when multisystemic signs suggest an infectious disorder, such as rickettsial disease or bacteremia, to be the cause of generalized edema. Until this can be determined, the use of glucocorticoids should be restricted.

Hyproproteinemic disorders can be managed temporarily by plasma transfusions; however, the administration of exogenous plasma can lead to systemic hypertension and ascites formation. When hypoproteinemia is caused by renal proteinuria, treatment of the primary renal disease is desired. The two major causes of proteinuria, amyloidosis and glomerulonephritis, have vastly different therapies: dimethyl sulfoxide (DMSO) and glucocorticoids, respectively. The primary renal disease should be confirmed by renal biopsy before treatment is instituted.

Cardiac disease initially should be treated with low salt diet and diuretics as needed to control edema formation. The use of cardiac glycosides is warranted only under certain conditions.

While diuretics are the mainstay of therapy for edema of any cause, they must be used with caution. Depending on the cause of edema, intravascular volume is reduced and the addition of a potent diuretic may contribute to the development of hypotension and shock. In many edematous animals with hypoproteinemia, repletion of serum albumin by transfusion followed by the judicious use of diuretics would be more desirable than the use of diuretics alone. Plasma transfusion provides temporary improvement when protein loss is continual. In hypoproteinemic states, a high quality/low quantity protein diet will meet caloric protein needs without excess sodium intake and will reduce the excess nonprotein nitrogen load on reduced hepatic or renal function.

Orthostatic edema, which develops in the dependent portions of the body of many edematous animals, occurs because gravity impairs venous return. Any procedure that facilitates venous return (such as elevation of the affected extremity, use of support bandages, increased muscle activity, use of cage padding, or preventing the animal from lying on the extremity for extended periods) will decrease the edema.

12

Retarded Growth

MICHAEL D. LORENZ

PROBLEM DEFINITION AND RECOGNITION

Retarded growth is failure to attain the weight and/or height standards characteristic of a given breed of dog or cat. The problem is more difficult to define in mongrels, since absolute standards are not available to guide one's judgment. Standards for the various breeds of dogs are available from the American Kennel Club. Canine and feline growth charts have been published elsewhere.[7]

Dwarfism is marked underdevelopment of the body. It is one cause of retarded growth; however, not all small-sized animals are truly dwarfs.

PATHOPHYSIOLOGY

To understand why this problem occurs, it is necessary to know the mechanisms that control growth in normal animals. Normal growth is a critical balance of proper nutrition, oxygen, hormonal interactions, and genetic influences that control cell division and growth.[1]

Genetic Control

The genetic information that ultimately controls cell division and growth is primarily contained in the sex chromosomes, although the autosomes probably contribute to growth regulation. In humans, it is known that the genes that allow normal growth are contained in the X chromosome. In addition, the Y chromosome also contains growth-promoting genes.[1] The greater size of male animals is probably explained by the positive influence of the Y chromosome. If the amount of Y chromosomes is increased, as in XYY individuals, greater-than-normal stature is encountered, whereas retarded growth occurs in XO individuals.

Prenatal Growth

Growth of the fetus is dependent on maternal health and nutrition and the ability of the placenta to transfer necessary nutrients to the developing fetus. Placental size and function may be directly related to the size and weight of newborns. So-called runts may never achieve normal size, since no makeup growth occurs after birth.

Hormonal abnormalities during fetal life appear to exert relatively little influence on somatic growth. Fetal growth is not appreciably impaired by failure of the fetal thyroid, and animals with congenital hormone deficiencies are usually of normal size at birth.

Postnatal Growth

Normal growth is dependent on the secretion and interaction of several key hormones. In addition, adequate nutrition, including calories, protein, essential fatty acids, minerals (especially zinc and calcium), and vitamins (especially vitamin A) are necessary for maximum growth. Deficiency of growth-promoting hormones, malnutrition, and metabolic diseases are the most common causes of retarded growth.

Hormonal Regulation of Growth

The most commonly recognized hormonal regulator of growth is growth hormone (GH), or somatotropin. This polypeptide hormone of pituitary origin has both catabolic and anabolic effects. The catabolic effects (lipolysis, restricted glucose transport) are directly induced by the hormone, whereas the growth-promoting effects are mediated by insulinlike growth factors (IGFs), or somatomedins.[2]

Recent studies in German shepherd dwarf dogs have shown that both GH and IGF levels are extremely low compared to those in normal dogs.[5] In addition, the IGF levels in these dogs appear to be subject to the control by GH.[5] In dogs there is a parallel relationship between body size and plasma IGF levels.[4] Larger dog breeds have the highest IGF levels, which progressively decrease in smaller breeds.[4] Surprisingly, there is little difference in plasma GH levels across the various breeds, regardless of size. In a study of the poodle breed, the small stature of the toy poodle was clearly associated with lower concentrations of IGF and the larger stature of the standard poodle with higher concentrations of IGF, even though GH levels were remarkably similar.[3]

Although GH deficiency results in retarded growth, a deficiency of IGF may also cause this problem. Since IGF is largely made in the liver, any serious liver problem during growth may result in small stature.

Thyroxine is a general stimulator of cellular metabolism and has a strong positive effect on growth. Hypothyroidism that occurs in the neonatal or juvenile animal results in severe growth suppression and slow cerebral development. Congenital hypothyroidism is rare in dogs and cats.

Insulin may be necessary at the cellular level for GH to exert its effects. Small stature (retarded growth) is common in dogs with congenital diabetes mellitus (keeshond, golden retriever).

Malnutrition

Probably the most common cause of retarded growth is malnutrition resulting from dietary deficiency or severe gastrointestinal parasitism. When these problems are severe or prolonged, reduced growth may never be totally made up during the catch-up growth phase that occurs once normal nutrition is established. Deficiencies of vitamin A almost always cause growth retardation. Initially, deficiency of vitamin D does not slow growth; however, the resulting abnormalities in bone metabolism and bone growth may cause severe growth suppression. The mechanism by which zinc deficiency causes growth suppression is unknown.

Animals with congenital heart defects or chronic progressive lung disease grow slowly and often fail to develop normal size. A deficiency of oxygen in the tissues is the primary mechanism.

Disease of the digestive system that results in maldigestion or malabsorption of nutrients may cause severe growth retardation. Pancreatic insufficiency in dogs may occur prior to puberty and result in severe growth retardation. The syndrome known as *juvenile pancreatic atrophy* occurs in large breeds such as the German shepherd and great dane. Congenital megaesophagus may also cause retarded growth.

Metabolic Diseases

The most common metabolic causes of retarded growth are liver disease and kidney failure. Severe liver disease due to portosystemic shunts, copper intoxication (Wilson's syndrome), or infection such as feline infectious peritonitis virus is a common cause of retarded growth. Congenital renal diseases such as polycystic kidneys and progressive renal failure of Lhaso Apso and Norwegian elkhounds cause severe growth reduction.

Although growth reduction occurs in these diseases, more specific signs are likely to be present.

DIAGNOSTIC PLAN

The classification and causes of retarded growth are listed in the accompanying box. Table 12-1 lists the differentiating features of the most important causes of growth retardation.

The initial steps in the diagnosis of growth retardation is to determine the presence or absence of signs suggestive of metabolic or polysystemic disease. The degree of retarded growth and the symmetry of the reduced size should be determined. For example, endocrine disorders usually cause severe but propor-

(*Text continues on p 89.*)

*Classification and Causes of Retarded Growth**

Abnormal Endocrine Regulation

- Growth hormone deficiency
  - Pituitary dwarfism—German shepherd
- Congenital hypothyroidism
- Diabetes mellitus
  - Rottweiler
  - Golden retriever
  - Keeshond

Genetic Disorders of Bone and Cartilage

- Chondrodysplasia
  - Alaskan malamutes—chondrodysplastic dwarfs
- Mucopolysaccharidiosis—Siamese cats
- Achondroplasia
  - Basset hound
  - Collie
  - Miniature poodle
  - Scottish terrier

Nutritional Deficiencies

- Major nutrients
  - Protein (essential amino acids)
  - Fat
  - Carbohydrates
- Minerals
  - Zinc
  - Calcium
- Vitamins
  - A
  - D
- Oxygen
  - Congenital heart disease (developmental defect)
  - Chronic lung disease (as in "swimmer puppies")

Congenital (Inherited) Disorders of Cell Metabolism

- Lysosomal storage diseases
- Glycogen storage diseases

Chronic Inflammation, Infection, and Parasitism

- Immunodeficiency diseases
- Intestinal parasitism

Congenital or Acquired Major Organ Failure

- Congenital heart failure due to developmental defects
- Hepatic failure
  - Portosystemic shunts
- Renal failure
  - Familial progressive renal insufficiency
    - Lhaso Apso
    - Shih Tzu
    - Norwegian elkhounds
  - Canine Fanconi syndrome
  - Congenital polycystic kidneys
- Digestive tract disease

* Note: The diseases listed above are major examples of the causes of retarded growth. The lists are not inclusive of every breed or disease.

Table 12-1. Differential Diagnosis of Retarded Growth

DISEASE	MAJOR ASSOCIATED SIGN(S)	SUGGESTIVE LABORATORY FINDING(S)	RADIOGRAPHIC CHANGE(S)
Abnormal endocrine regulation			
Growth hormone deficiency	Hyperpigmentation Severe alopecia Absence of primary hair Delay in permanent dentition	Suppression of growth hormone and insulinlike growth factors	Delayed closure of growth plates
Congenital hypothyroidism	Sparse hair coat Dull, depressed attitude	Low serum T-4 Inadequate response to thyroid-stimulating hormone	None
Diabetes mellitus	Polydipsia, polyuria	Glycosuria Elevated blood glucose	None
Genetic disorders of bone and cartilage			
Chondrodysplasia (Alaskan malamutes)	Shortening of the radius and ulna Carpal enlargement Lateral bowing of the forelimbs	Complete blood count—regenerative anemia due to hemolysis Bone marrow—normoblastic erythroid hyperplasia	Evidence of chrondrodysplasia at 8–12 weeks of age
Mucopolysaccharidosis (Siamese cats, etc.)	Dwarfism Severe skeletal deformities Neurologic deficits Retinal atrophy	Metachromatic inclusion bodies in circulating leukocytes Increased levels of dermatan sulfate in urine	Bony proliferation and fusion of cervical vertebrae Entire spine may be evolved Broad, irregular epiphyses and ankylosis of joints
Achondroplasia (collie, basset hound, miniature poodle, Scottish terrier)	Abnormally short limbs May be associated with muscle weakness	None	Disturbance of epiphyseal, chondroblastic growth Impaired ossification of long-bone cartilage
Nutritional Deficiencies			
Zinc	Infection Poor wound healing Dry, scaly skin Hyperkeratotic foot pads	None	None

Calcium	Lameness Bone pain Pathologic fractures Neurologic signs	Serum calcium and phosphorous in low-normal range Alkaline phosphatase may be increased.	Generalized skeletal demineralization Evidence of fractures (healed, etc.)
Vitamin A	Thick cranial bones Delayed growth of nervous tissue Zerophthalmia Hydrocephalus Suppurative skin lesions	None	Shortening and thickening of the long bones Thick cranial bones
Vitamin D	Muscle pain Bending and distortion of long bones Nodular enlargements on bones	Low-normal serum calcium	Flattening and mushrooming of the growth plates Bending of the long bones
Oxygen	Cyanosis Rapid breathing Syncope Ascites etc.	Increased packed cell volume Decreased arterial PO_2	Depends on condition
Congenital (inherited) disorders of cell metabolism			
Lipid storage diseases	Various neurologic signs suggesting cortical, cerebellar, or brainstem disease	None	None
Glycogen storage diseases	Muscle weakness Hepatomegaly Seizures	Blood glucose decreased or normal	Hepatomegaly
Congenital or acquired major organ failure or insufficiency			
Cardiopulmonary failure Congenital heart or great vessel defect Chronic pulmonary disease	Dyspnea Cyanosis Exercise intolerance Syncope Ascites Cough Tachycardia	Packed cell volume may be increased. Abdominal transudate Decreased blood PO_2	Depends on cause: cardiomegaly, pulmonary edema, pleural effusion, pulmonary infiltrates, or fibrosis

(*Continued*)

Table 12-1. Differential Diagnosis of Retarded Growth *(Continued)*

DISEASE	MAJOR ASSOCIATED SIGN(S)	SUGGESTIVE LABORATORY FINDING(S)	RADIOGRAPHIC CHANGE(S)
Hepatic failure	Seizures Neurologic signs Vomiting Anorexia Hemostatic problems Ascites	Decreased serum albumin Increased serum ammonia	Small liver Angiography may reveal portosystemic shunt.
Renal failure	Polyuria Polydipsia Vomiting Anorexia Renal rickets Dehydration	Decreased packed cell volume Increased blood urea nitrogen, creatinine, phosphorus Decreased calcium in some cases Isosthenuria	Small kidneys Bone demineralization
Digestive Tract			
Megaesophagus	Regurgitation	None	Decreased esophageal motility and esophageal dilatation Aspiration pneumonia
Pancreatic atrophy	Diarrhea	Negative fecal trypsin Suppressed BT-PABA test	None

tional dwarfism. In contrast, chondroplastic dwarfism that occurs in Alaskan malamutes is characterized by bilateral stunting of the forelimbs with carpal enlargement.[6,7] Careful examination of the long bones may provide additional clues. For instance, enlargement of the diaphyseal region of the long bones may suggest vitamin D deficiency and rickets.

The data base must include radiographs of a long bone, a complete blood count, urine analysis, and biochemical profile. See Table 12-1 for abnormalities of the tests associated with the various disorders. Radiographs can be very useful, since various forms of dwarfism have characteristic changes (see Table 12-1).

When endocrinopathies are suspected as the cause of dwarfism, specific hormonal assays are warranted. Thyroxine concentrations measured pre- and post-TSH (thyroid-stimulating hormone) stimulation plus a TRH (thyrotropin-releasing hormone) response test should be performed. If thyroxine levels are normal, GH concentrations before and after intravenous clonidine (10 μg/kg) stimulation should be measured.[2] Blood samples are collected at 0, 15, 30, 45, 60, and 90 minutes after clonidine stimulation. Measurement of insulinlike growth factor I may also be useful.[2] In clinical practice it is difficult to find a reliable laboratory for the assay of GH and IGF.

SYMPTOMATIC THERAPY

Once the epiphyses have closed, correction of the underlying cause will not correct the retarded growth. Administration of growth hormone to pituitary dwarfs may increase the growth rate; however, the epiphyses may close before normal size is achieved. The availability of growth hormone for veterinary use is severely restricted at this time.

REFERENCES

1. Daughaday WH: Growth and sex development. In MacBryde CM, Blacklow RS (eds): Signs and Symptoms, 5th ed, p 32. Philadelphia, JB Lippincott, 1970
2. Eigenmann JE: Growth hormone and insulin-like growth factor in the dog: Clinical and experimental investigations. Domestic Anim Endiocrinol 2:1–16, 1985
3. Eigenmann JE, Patterson DF, Froesch ER: Body size parallels insulin-like growth factor I levels but not growth hormone secretory capacity. Acta Endocrinol (Copenh) 106:448–453, 1984
4. Eigenmann JE, Patterson DF, Zapf J, Froesch ER: Insulin-like growth factor I in the dog: A study in different dog breeds and in dogs with growth hormone elevation. Acta Endocrinol (Copenh) 105:294–301, 1984
5. Eigenmann JE, Zanesco S, Arnold U, Froesch ER: Growth hormone and insulin-like growth factor I in German shepherd dwarf dogs. Acta Endocrinol (Copenh) 105:289–293, 1984
6. Fletch SM, Pinkerton PH, Brueckner PJ: The Alaskan Malamute chondrodysplasia (dwarfism–anemia) syndrome: In review. J Am Anim Hosp Assoc 11:353–361, 1975
7. Kirk RW, Bistner SI: Normal physiologic data. In Handbook of Veterinary Procedures and Emergency Treatment, 4th ed, pp 885, 888. Philadelphia, WB Saunders, 1985
8. Tarpin T, Roach MR: Chondrodysplasia in the Alaskan Malamute: Involvement of arteries, as well as bone and blood. Am J Vet Res 42:1865–1873, 1981

13

Weight Loss

MICHAEL D. LORENZ

PROBLEM DEFINITION AND RECOGNITION

Weight loss is a physical condition that results from a negative caloric balance such as when metabolic utilization plus excretion of essential nutrients exceed the supply. Weight loss does not necessarily imply malnutrition; however, in many disease states this is actually what occurs. When the nutritive deficiency is restricted to calories, stored fats may be lost, which may be desirable as in obesity. Weight loss may result from the loss of body fluids as in dehydration or from the elimination of ascites or edema. In this chapter, only weight loss due to undernutrition (calorie deficiency, protein deficiency, or both) will be discussed. The reader is referred to other chapters dealing with the problems of dehydration, edema, and ascites.

Weight loss is considered significant when a 10% decrease in normal body weight occurs unassociated with loss of body fluids. Certainly, undernutrition is present when the small reserves of body protein are gone and body tissue protein is utilized for calories. Growth and weight charts should be consulted when one considers the significance of any weight loss. In addition, body conformation, muscle mass, and bone structure characteristics of the different breeds should be considered.

Emaciation is extreme weight loss due to severe undernutrition and is characterized by prominence of the skeleton due to catabolism of body fat and protein. Cachexia is a state of extreme ill health associated with weight loss, anorexia, weakness and mental depression.

PATHOPHYSIOLOGY

When any of the many etiologic factors discussed in subsequent sections becomes of sufficient magnitude or persists for a sufficient time, the deficient nutrient is withdrawn from body stores or tissues that contain it. The first stage is a negative balance of the nutrient factor, causing abnormalities in growth, repair, or maintenance. Subsequent changes in approximate order are tissue depletion, biochemical changes, functional alterations, and anatomic defects.

In caloric undernutrition (negative caloric balance), balance must be achieved by reducing activity or by utilizing body tissues for energy. During the stage of tissue depletion, body stores of fat and limited stores of protein are used first. Because of body reserves, tissue depletion may be advanced before signs develop.

Several biochemical disturbances may occur in the undernourished animal. When tissue protein has been greatly depleted, total serum proteins may decrease, largely due to a decrease in serum albumin. Other biochemical changes likely to occur include an increase in extracellular fluid; vitamin deficiencies; calcium/phosphorus imbalance, affecting bone metabolism, with an increase in serum alkaline phosphatase activity; low serum iron concentration and microcytic anemia; and decreased concentrations of thyroid hormones.

The functional changes associated with undernutrition occur because of decreased metabolism and tissue depletion. Fatigue, lack of energy, and mental depression are common signs. The body temperature decreases in response to the decreased metabolic rate. Decreased thermiogenesis obviously saves calories. Bradycardia and hypotension are common. Nonregenerative anemias, in addition to iron deficiency anemia, may occur since less hemoglobin is required to carry a reduced concentration of oxygen that supports the lower metabolic rate.

Extreme undernutrition results in anatomic lesions that are easily recognized. The fat padding is lost first, and muscles are catabolized later for energy. Pallor; skin hemorrhages; edema; dry, wrinkled skin that is inelastic; dry, brittle hair; reproductive failure or failure to cycle; gonadal atrophy; and peridontal disease are the most common anatomic lesions.

Once all adipose tissue is exhausted, severe depression, hypotension, and death will occur.

CAUSES OF WEIGHT LOSS

In general, there is but a single cause of weight loss: insufficient calories are present to meet the metabolic needs. However, caloric deficiency may be divided into three major categories (see Causes of Weight Loss): (1) inadequate food intake, (2) failure to assimilate calorigenic nutrients, and (3) excessive caloric expenditure. All categories may be in effect, but there is always a negative caloric balance.

The degree of appetite may be an important clue to the diagnosis of certain diseases since weight loss in the face of a normal or increased appetite suggests an inadequate diet, maldigestion syndrome, or excessive caloric expenditure as occurs in hyperthyroidism or diabetes mellitus. However, serious undernutrition may cause anorexia in a patient that initially had a normal appetite. Many diseases may cause anorexia late in their courses (see chapter 3).

Causes of Weight Loss

- Inadequate food intake
  - Dietary deficiency
    - Inadequate amount
    - Poor digestibility
    - Protein–calorie imbalance
  - Oropharyngeal disease (dysphagia, prehension, and mastication problems)
  - Vomiting and regurgitation
  - Anorexia (numerous causes; see chapter 3)
- Malassimilation of calorigenic nutrients
  - Maldigestion
    - Pancreatic exocrine insufficiency
    - Bile salt deficiency
  - Malabsorption syndromes
    - Villous atrophy
    - Infiltrative diseases
      - Inflammatory bowel disease
      - Lymphosarcoma
      - Histoplasmosis
  - Diarrhea
- Excessive caloric expenditure
  - Increased metabolic rate
    - Hyperthyroidism
    - Fever
    - Infection/sepsis
    - Malignancy
    - Heart failure
    - Trauma
  - Loss of caloric nutrients
    - Diabetes mellitus (glucosuria)
    - Renal disease (proteinuria)
    - Burns (serum protein)
    - Severe pyoderma (serum protein)
    - Protein-losing enteropathy (albumin and globulin)
    - Intestinal parasites
    - Chronic blood loss
  - Physiologic
    - Pregnancy
    - Lactation
    - Extreme exercise
    - Increased thermogensis (decreased environmental temperature)

Effects of Disease on Nutrition and Weight Loss

Various types of illness may affect the absorption, intake, utilization, or excretion of various nutrients. The reader is referred to the list of the clinical manifestations of undernutrition. Two important causes of weight loss will be discussed.

Infection, Pyrexia, and Weight Loss

One of the earliest consequences of infection is anorexia and a tendency to drink only liquids. Antimicrobial therapy may interfere with the intestinal synthesis of certain nutrients such as vitamins. Fever, by increased metabolic rate, causes catabolism of body tissue.

Infection and fever cause a stress reaction qualitatively similar to that of pain and fear. Cortisol released in response to stress mobilizes aminoacids from skeletal muscle for glyconeogenesis in the liver. This process causes a depletion of body protein and a negative nitrogen balance because the mobilized aminoacids are deaminated to make glucose and the nitrogen is excreted as urea in the urine. In certain infections, especially those associated with diarrhea, deficiences of vitamin A and the B vitamins may develop. This is especially of great concern in cats, in which gastrointestinal synthesis of B vitamins is limited.

The malnutrition and weight loss associated with infectious disease result in several adverse effects. The outcome of infection is frequently worsened by the malnutrition since malnutrition may decrease antibody formation, inhibit or delay phagocytic reactions, lower tissue resistance to infection, decrease the rate of wound healing and collagen formation, and delay the destruction of bacterial toxins.

Clinical Manifestations of Undernutrition

- Weight loss
- Failure to grow
- Fatigue, muscle weakness
- Nervous irritability
- Delayed convalescence
- Poor wound healing
- Dehydration
- Anorexia
- Impaired liver function
- Protein deficiency
- Mineral, trace element deficiency
- Vitamin deficiency
- Anemia
- Edema, ascites (hypoalbuminemia)

Effects of Neoplastic Disease That Cause Weight Loss

- Anorexia (see chapter 3)
  - Suppression of appetite center
  - Pain
  - Disease of abdominal organs
- Maldigestion syndromes
  - Deficiency of pancreatic enzymes
    - Pancreatic cancer
    - Diffuse infiltration of duodenum (obstruction of pancreatic ducts)
    - Bile salt deficiency
    - Obstruction of bile duct (bile duct carcinoma)
- Malabsorption syndromes
  - Diffuse small intestinal neoplasia (*e.g.*, lymphosarcoma)
  - Gastric hypersecretion (apudomas)
- Protein-losing enteropathies
  - Diffuse small intestinal neoplasia with lymphatic obstruction (*e.g.*, lymphosarcoma)
  - Carcinoma (gastric, small intestinal, colonic)
- Electrolyte and fluid imbalances
  - Vomiting
  - Diarrhea
  - Hypercalcemia (ectopic production of parathormonelike compounds)
- Increased metabolic rate
  - Adrenal cortical neoplasia (*e.g.*, increased gluconeogenesis due to hypercortisolemia)
  - Thyroid neoplasia
  - Pheochromocytoma
- Cancer therapy
  - Surgical resection
    - Chewing or swallowing difficulties
    - Malabsorption (gastric or intestinal resection)
    - Pancreas
      - Maldigestion
      - Diabetes mellitus
- Radiation treatment
  - Anorexia
  - Regurgitation
  - Diarrhea
  - Malabsorption
- Chemotherapy
  - Anorexia
  - Vomiting
  - Diarrhea
  - Abdominal pain
  - Intestinal ulceration

Cancer Cachexia

Malignant disease frequently results in severe weight loss and malnutrition. In fact, weight loss may occur as a very early finding in cancer even prior to the development of other clinical signs. Thus, cancer, especially of the liver, pancreas, or intestinal tract, should be considered in the initial diagnostic plan for unexplained weight loss. In the cat, feline-leukemia-virus-associated disease or malignancy should receive priority in the diagnosis of weight loss.

As discussed in chapter 3, cancer has an unexplained effect in causing anorexia and wasting. This may occur when obvious intestinal obstruction, sepsis, and endocrine disorders are not present.[1] The weight loss observed in animals with cancer is usually associated with anorexia, vomiting, diarrhea, or severe dysfunction of the liver or pancreas (see Effects of Neoplastic Disease That Cause Weight Loss). It is possible that certain types of cancer cause direct suppression of the appetite center through unexplained mechanisms. Human cancer patients may have alterations in taste, although this is usually not the primary factor responsible for anorexia.[1]

Cancer may alter energy metabolism so that requirements are increased beyond those of normal animals.[1] Some cancer patients experience increased resting metabolic expenditure during a time of decreased caloric intake. A number of metabolic changes that change energy requirements may occur in cancer patients. Fever, infection, and stress-induced glucocorticoid release are not uncommon, and these cause increased gluconeogenesis and protein catabolism. In addition, the direct metabolic activity of certain tumors may be large enough to cause a significant drain on host tissues.

DIAGNOSTIC PLAN

A scheme for the diagnosis of weight loss is presented in Figure 13-1. It is based on the diseases listed under Causes of Weight Loss. A review of chapter 3, Anorexia, may also be useful in the diagnosis of weight loss.

SYMPTOMATIC THERAPY

Therapy for weight loss is directed at correcting the underlying cause and providing an immediate positive caloric-nitrogen balance. The method of achieving a positive caloric balance depends on the underlying cause. Oral alimentation is negated in animals with vomiting or diarrhea. Parenteral hyperalimentation may be the only way of securing calories for the patient when the gastrointestinal tract is not available for digestion and absorption of nutrients.

Anorectic animals can be given appetite stimulants such as diazepam and tube-fed gruels containing sufficient quantities of calories and protein. Pharyngostomy tubes or naso-oral tubes can be used. Vitamin, mineral, and iron supplementation should be considered. B vitamin therapy is essential in anorectic cats since gut synthesis of B vitamins is limited in this species.

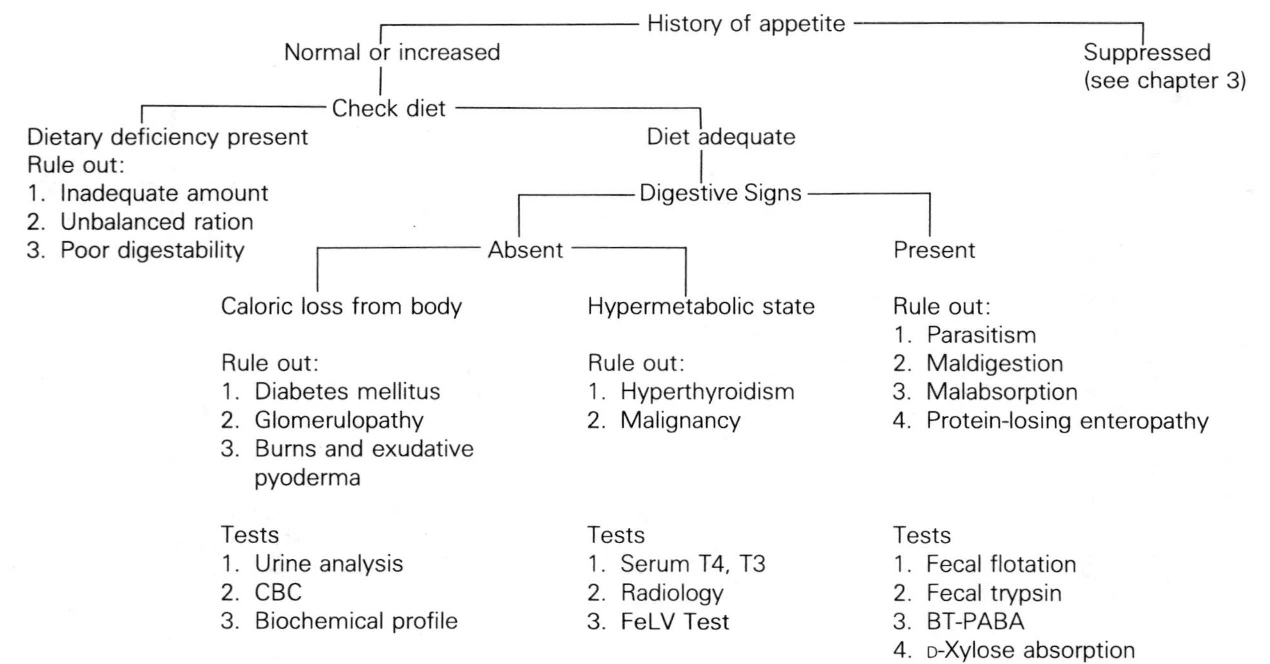

Fig. 13-1. **Diagnostic plan for weight loss.**

It is extremely important to anticipate the undernutrition that may accompany any disease or surgical procedure prior to the actual detection of weight loss. Certainly the restricted intake of oral nutrients that is used in the symptomatic treatment of vomiting, gastroenteritis, acute pancreatitis, or surgery preparation may result in acute weight loss and must be considered when animals can have "nothing per os." It is far easier to prevent weight loss than to correct the problem after it is well established.

REFERENCE

1. Shils ME: Nutritional problems induced by cancer. Med Clin North Am 63:1009, 1979

14

Obesity

SCOTT A. BROWN

PROBLEM DEFINITION AND RECOGNITION

Obesity is a condition of excess body fat. It is the most common nutritional disorder in veterinary medicine, with reported prevalences of 25% to 44% in dogs[4,5] and 6% to 12% in cats.[5] It should not be considered synonymous with excess body weight, although the two conditions often occur simultaneously in an animal. The term *common or simple obesity* refers to adipose tissue that occurs in a normal body distribution. Dystrophic obesity, with a pathologic alteration in body fat distribution pattern, has not been reported in veterinary medicine. However, canine patients with hypercortisolism often have fatty deposits over the dorsum and intrabdominally, which may be a form of dystrophic obesity. Common obesity is divided into two types: Hyperplastic obesity, due to excessive numbers of adipocytes, may have a genetic component and is associated with overeating early in life. Hypertrophic obesity is due to increased fat cell size; it usually occurs in adult life and is believed to be more prevalent in veterinary medicine.

Variable conformation and body size make it difficult to determine "normal" body weight limit tables in veterinary medicine. Ultrasound, girth measurements, and water displacement have been utilized to quantitate canine body fat content. Identification of clinically significant obesity in veterinary patients is dependent upon subjective evaluation of body fat stores. This can be accomplished by palpation over the rib cage. The outline of the ribs should be readily palpable. Ribs obscured by subcutaneous fat are indicative of obesity. Ribs readily visible without palpation suggest the animal is too thin. Excess fat may be deposited over the iliac crests in older, obese dogs. Ventral abdominal subcutaneous fat may be helpful in assessing feline obesity, although fat in this area is frequently confused with mammary gland development. Recognition is subjective, but obesity is often marked and apparent to the veterinarian. Obesity causing a 15% excess in body weight is generally considered clinically significant and injurious to the patient and should be treated.[5]

Conditions that may be confused with obesity include generalized subcutaneous edema (anasarca) or abdominal distention due to any cause. Differentiation is generally possible on physical examination. Edematous subcutaneous tissue will generally "pit" upon compression, in contrast to the loose feel of subcutaneous fat. Abdominal distention due to obesity is accompanied by excess subcutaneous fat. Occasional cases of abdominal distention may be difficult to distinguish on physical examination; differentiation may require radiographs and/or abdominocentesis. The radiographic density of fat is intermediate to air and soft tissue (fluid); excess fat offers excellent radiographic contrast.

PATHOPHYSIOLOGY: DEVELOPMENT OF OBESITY

Obesity is always caused by prolonged caloric intake in excess of body needs. It may be due to overeating, reduced physical activity, or both. Genetic, endocrine, and social factors play contributory roles.

Obesity develops in two stages. In the first stage (the dynamic stage), body fat accumulates due to excess caloric intake. The pet's diet contains an excess number of calories during this stage. In the second, or static, stage, food intake is balanced by energy expenditure. In this stage, the obese sedentary dog may consume relatively few calories. Owners of pets in this stage of obesity will be correct when they claim that their dog eats only a small quantity of food daily.

Food intake is under control of the feeding and satiety centers of the hypothalmus, which determine a "set point" for body weight.[5,9] This set point is not as tightly controlled as that for body temperature (see chapter 2). It may be affected by psychologic factors (forebrain input), nutrient type, metabolic/endocrine diseases, food availability and palatability, and social factors (competition with other household pets and owner encouragement of food intake).[5,9] Boredom, idleness, and nervousness increase food intake in humans and may have a similar effect in animals. Highly palatable fatty or sweet foods are likely to be consumed more readily and will increase the animal's set point for body weight. The use of predigested animal tissue ("digest") in commercial cat food has contributed to the rise in prevalence of obesity in cats.[5] High fat or high carbohydrate nutrients are utilized more efficiently by the pet's body and will lead to the development of obesity.[2,5]

Although an underlying disease condition predisposing the animal to obesity is not usually present, it is important to determine if such a condition exists and institute specific therapy where indicated. Commonly identified predisposing pathologic conditions (Table 14-1) include hypothyroidism and hyperglucocorticoidism (endogenous or exogenous). Other conditions that have been incriminated include cerebral/hypothalamic brain lesions and insulinoma. Even when a predisposing condition is identified, the condition of obesity is still dependent upon caloric intake in excess of needs and can be managed symptomatically, as outlined below.

There appears to be a genetic predisposition to obesity, with cocker spaniels; Labrador retrievers; Cairn, West Highland, and Scottish terriers; and collies hav-

Table 14-1. Clinical Diseases Predisposing to the Development of Obesity

DISEASE	SUGGESTIVE CLINICAL SIGNS	LABORATORY FINDINGS	SPECIAL TESTS
Hypothyroidism	Lethargy, thick skin alopecia, bradycardia, thermophilia, somnolence, hypothermia	Nonregenerative anemia	TSH response test
Hypercortisolism	Polyuria/polydipsia, pot belly appearance, thin skin, alopecia, hepatomegaly	Stress leukogram, hyperglycemia, elevated alkaline phosphatase, urinary tract infections	ACTH response test Dexamethasone suppression test
Cortical/hypothalmic lesion	Neurologic deficits		Neurologic exam, CSF tap, EEG
Insulinoma	Weakness, seizures	Hypoglycemia	Amended glucose-insulin ratio

TSH, thyroid-stimulating hormone; ACTH, adrenocorticotropic hormone; CSF, cerebrospinal fluid; EEG, electroencephalogram

ing an increased incidence. Boxers, fox terriers, and Sealyham terriers are reported to have a low incidence of obesity.[4,5] Obese-prone animals may have a body weight set point disturbance due to heightened responsiveness to food palatibility.[7] There is an increased incidence with advancing age of the pet, probably due to a reduction in basal metabolic rate and physical activity. Females are more commonly obese than males. Neutering has been associated with an increase in body weight in both sexes. In males, castration frequently reduces activity levels and also removes the androgenic hormone, testosterone, which normally diverts energy and amino acids into muscle protein production.[2] The result may be increased fat production. In females, ovariohysterectomy does not usually result in marked obesity. However, in occasional cases, spayed female dogs will become severely obese. Reduced activity levels and increased food intake are believed to be contributory. Hormonal imbalance[2] (including high follicle-stimulating hormone levels, which stimulate feed intake, and low serum estrogen levels, which normally inhibit food intake) may also play a role. Prevalence of obesity in pets is higher when the pet is owned by middle-aged, elderly, or overweight individuals.[4] This may be due to reduced exercise and/or increased caloric intake due to treats and table scraps.

The prevalence of obesity appears to be on the rise in veterinary medicine. The increased confinement of pets during the working day in suburban/urban environments plays a role through reduction in physical activity. The highly palatable/energy dense pet foods on the grocery shelf are a product of a highly competitive industry where palatability is at a premium. Obesity in veterinary patients is principally attributed to the use of these diets, which are offered in large amounts on a frequent or easily accessible basis. Reduction in energy expenditure due to low levels of physical activity, reduced metabolic rate, and genetic/endocrine factors further exacerbate this condition.

EFFECTS OF OBESITY

A list of health problems linked to obesity in dogs and cats is presented in Table 14-2.[2,4,5,7,9] Obese pets are frequently fed a diet consisting predominantly of table scraps.[4] Such unbalanced, fatty foods present significant health risks beyond obesity and may predispose the animal to nutritional deficiencies, pancreatitis, diabetes mellitus, and other systemic diseases.

DIAGNOSTIC PLAN

Every attempt should be made to diagnose the predisposing pathologic conditions for obesity. A thorough history, physical examination, and basic laboratory tests are very useful in the differential diagnosis of these conditions. Table 14-1 lists the predisposing causes of obesity with their suggestive clinical signs, laboratory findings, and special diagnostic tests.

SYMPTOMATIC THERAPY

As with all medical problems, not all overweight pets should be treated in the same manner. If the pet is not markedly obese, a few minutes spent warning the client about the complications of obesity and reviewing the feeding regimen/food type used will be adequate. In other cases, more stringent measures will be necessary. Careful nutritional counseling is critical in cases involving overweight young, growing pets, since development of hyperplastic obesity refractory to therapy may occur. In general, any pet estimated to be more than 15% above optimum weight should be placed on a weight reduction program. A complete program for the obese dog involves client education, increased physical activity, and reduced caloric intake.

Table 14-2. Deleterious Effects of Obesity

ORGAN/SYSTEM	EFFECT OF OBESITY
General	Lethargy, irritability, fatigability, heat intolerance, inactivity, increased risks with anesthesia and surgery, technical difficulty with many diagnostic and therapeutic procedures
Musculoskeletal	Arthropathies, metabolic bone disease
Cardiovascular	Increased cardiac workload, myocardial fatty deposits, myocardial hypoxia, and arrhythmias
Gastrointestinal	Increased risk of pancreatitis and hepatic lipidosis
Endocrine	Glucose intolerance, increased risk of diabetes mellitus
Respiratory	Dyspnea, alveolar hypoventilation ("pickwickian syndrome"), exacerbation of any respiratory disease (especially tracheal collapse)
Immune	Increased susceptibility to infection, delayed healing
Reproductive	Dystocia, infrequent cycling, reduced reproductive efficiency

(Data from references 1 through 5)

The first and most critical component is client education. Failure to concentrate on this aspect of the weight reduction program invariably results in failure. Education includes emphasizing the negative effects of obesity; setting a reasonable goal; designing a program for recording daily exercise, food intake, and daily weights at home; and setting a reexamination schedule. Simply pointing out that the pet is overweight often does not result in any significant long-term weight reduction. First, many owners (31% in one study[4]) deny that obesity is present, even in pets that are severely obese. Second, once willing to accept that their pet is obese, owners must be convinced that this problem presents a significant health risk to their pet. There are several client education aids that may help the veterinarian.[1,3,6] Other owners will deny their pet's obesity because of guilt feelings or the presence of obesity in the owner. The latter situation presents the veterinarian with a particularly difficult problem. The veterinarian must utilize special tact in this situation.

Frequently, owners are obsessed with care of the obese pet and may not act in an apparently rational manner. The decision to enter into a weight control program ultimately rests with the owner and should be respected. It is not the veterinarian's role to become angry or attempt to force the owner to follow the prescribed path, since this will only alienate the client.

A weight control chart should be kept by the owner at home, with daily notation of weight, exercise, and feed. This involves the client and is the best assurance of compliance with the weight reduction program. The home record should be reviewed at each reexamination. Thoracic girth measurement at the level of the xiphoid process is an alternative to daily weight recording for large dogs or frail clients.[7] This measurement should not serve as the sole assessment of progress, since it tends to lag behind weight reduction and is subject to mechanical errors.

It is important to encourage the client to break their pet of the habit of begging for food. Many obese pets have dominant personalities, making frequent demands for treats. Absolutely no table scraps or treats should be allowed, since an occasional treat serves as intermittent reinforcement, which is a stronger stimulus for begging than is regular reward. At the outset of the weight control program, the pet will try every means available to maintain its caloric intake. The owner will need to be encouraged not to revert to previous bad feeding habits.

Prior to instituting dietary therapy or increasing physical activity, it is important to examine the pet thoroughly to determine if other medical problems are present. A thorough history, physical examination, complete blood count, biochemical profile, and urine analysis are indicated at this point. It is important to determine if there are other contributory diseases or if an unrelated disease is present that will be adversely affected by an exercise/calorie restriction program.

Increased Physical Activity

Total energy utilized by an animal's body represents the sum of basal metabolic rate (BMR), physical activity, calorie utilization from meal intake/digestion (specific dynamic action), and heat production. Ideally, increasing all of these factors would be achieved. The use of a feeding regimen involving small, frequent meals may increase calorie usage for digestion and reduce efficiency of food utilization. Besides maintaining the pet outdoors in cold weather, little can be done to increase calorie loss due to heat production. Recent evidence indicates that reduction of dietary intake will cause a compensatory decrease in BMR as the body attempts to preserve its energy stores (fat). Benefit can be derived from increasing energy utilization through exercise. Increasing physical activity will blunt this reduction in BMR, consume calories, reduce the pet's set point, and mobilize body lipid stores. Obese dogs should be placed on an exercise program. Daily leash walks, object retrieval, and other forms of physical activity should be encouraged. The owner should be instructed as to exactly how much activity would be appropriate. Some severely obese dogs will not tolerate any more than 100 yards at a slow walk, while others can be very active. As with other parts of the weight reduction program, specific goals must be outlined and the owner encouraged to record daily exercise as part of the home record.

A program to increase physical activity is difficult to implement in obese feline patients. Obese cats should not be locked outside simply to encourage physical activity, since they may be unable to adequately defend themselves from attack by other cats or dogs. Any injuries incurred will heal poorly in such patients.

Reduced Caloric Intake

The basic diet may consist of a commercial weight reduction diet or a homemade diet (Table 14-3). This is often a matter of personal preference of the veterinarian and owner. Commercial diets have the advantages of being balanced diets of reduced caloric density and providing dietary bulk that may reduce the pet's hunger. However, feeding special reducing diets may cause some owners to believe that quantity of intake is unimportant or that snacks are needed or justified. Simply dispensing a diet does not usually constitute an adequate weight reduction program.

Table 14-4 provides recommendations for total caloric intake for weight loss. Small frequent feedings are recommended. The table is based upon feeding 60% of maintenance caloric requirements for the veterinarian's estimate of the ideal weight for the pet. An alternative is to feed 50% of maintenance for the dog's current obese weight. Utilizing the diets from Table 14-3 and the following chart, weight reduction can generally be achieved within 8 to 12 weeks. If the pet does not lose weight as documented during weekly weigh-ins and if tactful questions do not indicate an alternate source of caloric intake, further reduction in food intake of 25% should be instituted.

To prepare the owner, it is best to estimate the rate of weight loss and time expected to completion. In general, it will require 8 to 12 weeks with a weight loss of 0.5 to 2 pounds (2% to 4% of the body weight) per week.

An alternative to the above program is hospitalization for caloric intake restriction. Although this is an expensive alternative, it should be considered

Table 14-3. Reducing Diets

DIET	CALORIC DENSITY (kcal METABOLIZABLE ENERGY)
Canine R/D*	330/can, 186/cup dry
Canine Cycle 3†	355/can, 257/cup dry
Fit n Trim‡	270/cup
Canine low-fat diet[2]	
¼ lb cooked lean ground beef	
½ cup uncreamed cottage cheese	
2 cups carrots	250/pound
2 cups green beans	
1.5 tsp dicalcium phosphate	
Vitamin–mineral supplement	
Feline R/D*	350/can
Feline low-fat diet[2]	
1.5 lb cooked liver, ground	
1 cup cooked rice	587/pound
1 tsp vegetable oil	
1 tsp calcium carbonate	
Vitamin–mineral supplement	

* Hill's Pet Products
† Gaines Foods, Inc.
‡ Ralston Purina Co.

when it is apparent the owner is frustrated or when progress in weight reduction is considered inadequate.

If the above methods are ineffective, consideration of a plan for hospitalization and total caloric restriction is acceptable if the owner is willing, although many will consider this inhumane. Care must be taken to supply a balanced vitamin/mineral supplement, ascertain that the dog has no preexisting medical illnesses, and regularly evaluate the dog's clinical condition. With starvation there is an initial rapid weight loss principally due to fluid and electrolyte loss, with an overall weight loss of 25% in 6 weeks.[2] Research indicates that total

Table 14-4. Caloric Requirements (kcal/lb/Day)[2]

OPTIMUM WEIGHT (lb)	MAINTENANCE	REDUCTION
Dog		
5	50	30
10	40	24
20	35	21
30	30	18
75	25	15
200	20	12
Cat		
8–12	30	20

Outline of the Weight Reduction Plan

1. Obtain client cooperation.
2. Supply written instructions and a home record chart for precisely recording daily weights, exercise, and food intake.
3. Caution the owner to feed no table scraps, snacks, or sweets. A change in basic diet is best (Table 14-3).
4. Initial weekly appointments to discuss problems and weigh the pet should be instituted. If 2 consecutive weeks without weight loss occur, the owner should be carefully questioned about alternate sources of food, such as a family member, garbage can, or neighbor. If no alternate explanation is found, decrease the amount fed by 25%.
5. Once the ideal weight is reached, maintenance of this weight is the final, yet critical, part of the weight reduction program. Ideally, reduction of body weight set point would be achieved by increased physical activity, reduction in palatability of diet, and reduction in boredom and "emotional stress." It is usually desirable to maintain the dog on some modification of the weight reduction program. This usually means routine leash walks, measured portions of a "reducing diet," and maintenance of a modified home record. The pet's record should be flagged so that weight will be carefully checked and recorded on each subsequent visit to allow the veterinarian to follow trends and note weight gain before it becomes a severe problem again.

fasting for 6 weeks does not result in serious clinical problems in otherwise *healthy* dogs.[2] Opponents argue that rebound weight gain is likely since there is no organized weight reduction program instituted in the home prior to the pet's return. The total restriction also poses a health risk to the obese animal who frequently has subclinical/clinical medical illnesses. Proponents argue that their experience has been favorable, with less hunger exhibited by dogs on this program and more control by the veterinarian since pets are hospitalized.[2] This type of restriction should never be instituted in obese cats, since hepatic lipidosis and hepatic encephalopathy represent only two of several possible ill effects in this species.

Other Treatments

Drugs and hormones have an effect of food intake and energy balance. Corticosteroids increase food intake. Thyroid hormone will increase BMR and promote weight loss. Its use should be reserved only for those patients with proven hypothyroidism on the basis of a thyroid-stimulating hormone test result. Nearly 75% of the weight loss while being treated with thyroid hormone will be at the expense of body protein rather than fat, and excess levels of thyroid hormone may lead to the development of cardiac and skeletal myopathy and other complications.

There are several other categories of drugs that have been utilized in weight reduction programs. Appetite suppressants constitute the major category, and include the central acting amphetamine derivatives, peripheral acting hormones and prostaglandins.[8] Amphetamine and fenfluramine are two centrally acting compounds that have been used for weight reduction in dogs without effect.[2,5] The citric acid analog, threochlorocitric acid, is a peripherally acting appetite suppressant that induces satiety by slowing gastric emptying time.[8] It has shown some effectiveness experimentally in dogs and may hold promise for the future. Other drugs reduce the availability of dietary nutrients. Fenfluramine and cholestyramine inhibit fat absorption, but there is no evidence for their effectiveness in dogs or cats. Amylase inhibitors to block carbohydrate digestion and absorption have been tried in dogs with little effect.[5,8] Endogenous opioids are believed to increase food intake in people under stress[8] and may play a similar role in animals. Sucrose polyester may be used in the future as an indigestible food additive with the taste of fat to increase palatability.[5] At this time, drug therapy has little place in the weight reduction program, with the exception of thyroid hormone replacement in the hypothyroid animal.

In obese human patients, jaw wiring, gastrointestinal bypass procedures, surgical lipectomy, and vagotomy have been used as surgical therapy with mixed results. These procedures are associated with a high morbidity rate and are not recommended for veterinary patients.

REFERENCES

1. McKinley JH (ed): ANCOM (A-V System). Lincoln, NE, Hill's Riviana Foods
2. Anderson GL, Lewis LD: Obesity. In Kirk RW (ed): Current Veterinary Therapy VII. Philadelphia, WB Saunders, 1980
3. Care of the Overweight Dog. Canine Practice 10:445–448, 1983
4. Mason E: Obesity in pet dogs. Vet Rec 86:612, 1970
5. Morris ML, Lewis LD: Obesity. In Small Animal Clinical Nutrition. Topeka, KS, Mark Morris Associates, 1984
6. Obesity, Pet Health Information Series. Topeka, KS, Hill's Pet Products Inc.
7. Sibley KW: Diagnosis and management of the overweight dog. Br Vet J 140:124–131, 1984
8. Sullivan AC, Nauss-Karol C, Cheng L: Pharmacological treatment I. In Greenwood MRC (ed): Obesity. New York, Churchill Livingstone, 1983
9. Ward A: The fat-dog problem: How to solve it. Vet Med 79:781–786, 1984

Part Four

DERMATOLOGIC PROBLEMS

15

Pruritus

MICHAEL D. LORENZ

PROBLEM DEFINITION AND RECOGNITION

Pruritus is defined as an unpleasant sensation that provokes the desire to scratch. In veterinary medicine, this sensation is impossible to differentiate from other stimuli such as burning, since the animal's responses to these stimuli are similar. Self-mutilation (see chapter 7) is a common sequala to offensive stimuli in the skin of small animals. The presence of excoriations is evidence of a pruritogenic disorder.

PATHOPHYSIOLOGY

Pruritus should be regarded as one of five primary cutaneous sensations; heat, cold, pain and touch are the other four forms of sensation. Pruritus is an epidermal sensation, whereas pain can also be perceived from denuded skin. The sensory receptors are naked nerve endings located in the epidermis. The axons that carry pruritic sensation are small unmyelinated C fibers. They ascend in the ventrolateral spinothalamic tracts via the thalamus to the cerebral cortex. Certain areas of the skin may have increased numbers of "itch" receptors or are more sensitive to pruritic stimuli. Although fewer nerve endings are present in chronic dermatitic skin, those present have a lower threshold for pruritic sensation.

Mediators of Pruritus

For many years, histamine was believed to be the major pruritogenic substance. It is now believed that proteolytic enzymes are the major mediators of pruritus. These enzymes may be released from bacteria, fungi, mast cells, epidermal cells (cathepsin), leukocytes (leukopeptidases), and capillary dilatation (plasmin). Although pruritus is a common feature of allergic skin disease, many other diseases cause pruritus through the release of proteolytic enzymes (see Factors That May Initiate Pruritus).

Factors Affecting Pruritus

Certain conditions may actually potentiate the pruritic sensation. Boredom may increase the cerebral response to physiologic itch stimuli and actually convert the sensation to a pathologic state. This mechanism may play a role in the etiology of acral pruritic nodules, feline lick granuloma, feline hyperesthesia syndrome, and idiopathic acute moist dermatitis ("hot spots"). Chronically diseased skin has limited perception because of decreased pruritic receptors; however, stimuli applied to this skin are perceived as either a burning sensation or itch. Thus, stimuli not usually considered noxious may be converted to pruritus (conversion itch). In addition, the remaining nerve endings may have a lower threshold for pruritic sensation. Chronic inflammation and secondary bacterial infections potentiate pruritus by aiding the accessibility of proteases to the nerve endings.

Scratching is the primary physiologic response for the control or temporary relief of pruritus. Temporary relief occurs because other stimuli (heat, cold, touch, pain) suppress the sensation of itch by competing for neuronal circuits within the internuncial sensory neuronal pool in the spinal cord. To be effective, the competing stimulus must be applied to the same dermatome from which the pruritic sensation originated. Scratching may actually potentiate pruritus since the induced epidermal damage may increase the release of proteolytic enzymes. This is the basis for the itch-scratch-itch cycle common to many skin diseases.

Factors That May Initiate Pruritus

- Physical factors
  - Heat
  - Cold
  - Light
  - Electrical stimuli
- Vasodilation
- Anoxia
- Proteolytic enzymes
- Histamine
- Serotonin
- Bile acids
- Calcium salts and uremia
- Asteatosis (dry skin)

DIAGNOSTIC PLAN

Pruritus is frequently associated with several primary skin lesions. These include papules, pustules, vesicles, and hyperemia. Secondary skin lesions observed with pruritus include excoriations, scales, crusts, lichenification, and hyperpigmentation. The nature of these lesions, their distribution pattern, and the degree of pruritus are very important factors to consider in the differential diagnosis of dermatologic conditions.

The desire to stop pruritus and its associated self-mutilation must be tempered by the desire to establish a correct diagnosis. Unfortunately, glucocorticoid drugs are frequently given to control pruritus with little regard for finding the underlying cause. The dermatologic history and physical examination should answer at least these five basic questions: (1) is it pruritic?, (2) what are the basic skin lesions?, (3) what is the distribution pattern?, (4) is it contagious?, and (5) are other body systems involved?

A problem-specific data base should include a complete history, a description of the dermatologic lesions and their pattern, analysis of multiple skin scrapings, and results of Wood's light examination. This data base should be expanded to include a variety of other procedures based on the dermatologic findings (see Expanded Data Base for the Pruritic Animal).

The diseases characterized by pruritus and their differentiating features are listed in Table 15-1.

SYMPTOMATIC THERAPY

Both local and systemic medications may be used to decrease pruritus.

(*Text continues on p 115.*)

Expanded Data Base for the Pruritic Animal

- Microbiologic tests
  - Fungal culture
  - Bacterial culture
- Immunologic procedures
  - Intradermal skin tests
  - Direct fluorescent antibody
- Histopathology
- Provocative exposure
  - Environment
  - Diet
  - Drugs

Table 15-1. Classification of Skin Diseases on the Degree of Pruritus Usually Observed

DISEASE	HISTORY	LESION(S)	DISTRIBUTION	SPECIAL TEST(S)
VERY PRURITIC CONDITIONS				
Sarcoptic mange	May be contagious Dogs of all ages affected Nonseasonal	Papules, excoriations	Elbows, ear margins, ventral abdomen	Skin scraping, response to therapy
Atopy	Age: 1–5 years Breeds: terriers, poodles, Irish setters Seasonal and nonseasonal	Many cases only pruritus—later papules, excoriations	Face, ear pinna, axilla, abdomen	Intradermal skin test
Flea allergy dermatitis	Dogs and cats usually older than 1 yr Seasonal except in subtropical climates	Papules, excoriations Cat: miliary crusty or papular lesions	Dog: Tail head, inner thighs Cat: Neck, back	Response to flea control
Superficial staphylococcal dermatitis	Usually young dogs—more common during warm months Can be chronic Tendency to relapse	Papules, superficial pustules, erythematous collarettes with scales	Abdomen—may generalize	Response to antibiotic therapy
Feline hyperesthesia syndrome	Usually house cats Any age Psychologic episodes	Pulling of hair	Usually back—limbs	None
Feline miliary dermatitis (see feline flea allergy)				
Rhabditic dermatitis	Animals on wet straw	Papular	Ventral—Abdomen and legs	Skin scraping
Notoedric mange	Cats: contagious	Papules, excoriations, crusts	Head	Skin scraping

Subcorneal pustular dermatitis (SPD)	Recurrent vesiculopapular eruptions Nonresponsive to antibiotics and corticosteroids	Papules—vesicles, erosions, crusts	Body and face (nose and ears)	Histopathology—subcorneal pustules—response to dapsone
Pemphigus (foliaceous and erythematous)	Dogs and cats of any age Recurrent lesions	Vesiculopustular eruptions—erosions, scales, and crusts	Face, body, and feet Mucocutaneous lesions are rare	Histopathology—subcorneal acantholysis Positive direct FA
Dermatitis herpetiformis	See SPD	Vesiculopustular eruptions	Body	Histopathology—subcorneal pustules Response to dapsone
Bacterial folliculitis	Younger short-haired dogs	Papules, small pustules	Body	Skin biopsy
Acral pruritic nodule (lick granuloma)	Usually solitary dogs Constant licking of limb	Nodule with eroded surface	Forelimb	Skin biopsy Radiography of limb
Drug eruption	Recent drug therapy	Papulomacular eruption	No specific distribution	Response to drug withdrawal
Food allergy dermatitis	Dogs and cats of any age Nonseasonal occurrence Acute and chronic signs common	Papules, erythematous plaques, excoriations Lesions may be severe Cats: may cause miliary dermatitis	Dogs: no specific distribution Cats: facial, may generalize	Response to hypoallergenic diet Skin biopsy
Allergic contact dermatitis	Nonseasonal occurrence Signs may wax and wane	Papuloeruptive to erythematous plaques	Ventral: feet, legs, abdomen, chest, axilla, neck	Provocative exposure to potential allergens
MILD TO MODERATELY PRURITIC CONDITIONS				
Pediculous	Young animals	Scales—small papules	Generalized	None
Cheletellia Dermatitis	Young animals	Scales—small papules	Generalized	None
Demodectic mange	Usually dogs less than 3 years of age	Alopecia, scales, erythema, pustules	Localized—face, legs Generalized—face, body, ear canals, feet	Skin scraping

(*Continued*)

Table 15-1. Classification of Skin Diseases on the Degree of Pruritus Usually Observed *(Continued)*

DISEASE	HISTORY	LESION(S)	DISTRIBUTION	SPECIAL TEST(S)
Pyoderma	No significant clues	Pustules Fistulous tracts	Depends on type	Bacterial culture
Dermatomycosis	Young animals	Circular scaling or asymmetric patches of alopecia	Head and legs usually Body in some severe cases	Fungal culture
Seborrhea	No significant clues	Asymmetric patches of scales	Body, face, ears	None
Nodular panniculitis	Recurrent painful or pruritic nodules	Nodules with necrotic centers	Body	Histopathology—necrosis and inflammation of fat
Sporotrichosis	Often develops following skin injury	Nodules—suppurative lymph nodes	Limbs—may follow lymphatics	Fungal culture Histopathology—PAS and methenoamine silver stains

FA, fluorescent antibody; PAS, periodic acid–Schiff

Local Therapy

The application of heat may increase pruritus; however, cool water baths are usually beneficial. The effect may last for 30 minutes to 1 hour. Cooling and drying agents such as camphor or alcohol are of transient benefit. Weak acid solutions (salicylic, tannic, or acetic acid) are astringents that may temporarily deaden irritated nerve endings in localized excoriations. One must be careful that the irritated skin is not aggravated by the medication. Radiation therapy may also relieve pruritus in localized lesions.

Systemic Therapy

Glucocorticoids

Glucocorticoids are very effective antipruritic agents because they affect the pathophysiology in several places. They are anti-inflammatory membrane stabilizers that decrease the effect of proteolytic enzymes. Glucocorticoids must be used with discretion because of their potential adverse effects. The short-acting oral preparations are preferred.

Antihistamines

Antihistamines, unless given in sedation doses, are poor antipruritic agents in dogs and cats.

Centrally Acting Antipruritic Agents

Trimeprazine is a phenothiazine tranquilizer that may decrease the awareness of pruritus. Hydroxyzine hydrochloride may act in a similar fashion. Both drugs are usually given as adjuncts to glucocorticoids.

Serotonin Antagonists

Cyproheptadine is a serotonin antagonist with marginal antipruritic properties in dogs and cats.

Megesterol Acetate

This progesterone-type drug has anti-inflammatory and subsequently antipruritic activity in cats. Because of severe adverse reactions in long-term use, it is a poor substitute for glucocorticoid therapy.

16

Diagnostic Significance of Various Skin Lesions

MICHAEL D. LORENZ

The morphology of skin lesions is extremely important in the diagnosis of dermatologic conditions. This chapter describes the morphology and diagnostic significance of the primary and secondary lesions. All lesions must be carefully examined so that the primary lesions are differentiated from the secondary changes.

PRIMARY SKIN LESIONS

Papule

Morphology

Papules are small, solid ruptions in the epidermis and are approximately 1 cm in diameter or smaller. Most papules are erythematous, reddened swellings produced by tissue infiltration of inflammatory cells, epidermal edema, or epidermal hypertrophy. Papules, when present as a group, may form erythematous plaques or rashes. The elevation may not be visible but can usually be felt with the fingertips. The surface epithelium of true papules remains intact unless secondarily traumatized.

Diagnostic Significance

Papules are the basic lesions in many allergic and parasitic skin diseases (*e.g.*, flea allergy dermatitis and sarcoptic mange). Papules are also the earliest stage in pustule formation and may be confused with the initial stages of small vesicular eruptions. Therefore, papules may be observed in pustular diseases such as bacterial folliculitis, pemphigus foliaceous, subcorneal pustular dermatoses, and dermatitis herpetiformis. It is very important to examine the stratum corneum covering the eruption. With pustules and vesicles, the stratum corneum is usually separated from the underlying epidermal layers and the resulting cleft may be filled with various amounts of fluid or inflammatory exudates. Most diseases with papular eruptions are pruritic. Since scratching may dramatically alter the appearance of the skin, lesions should be characterized in nontraumatized areas.

Pustule

Morphology

Pustules are small circumscribed or larger asymmetric eruptions in the skin. The cavity of the pustule is filled with inflammatory (suppurative) exudate. Pustules may be superficial (just under the stratum corneum, *i.e.*, subcorneal) or deep (extending down to the hypodermis). Pustules may be yellow, erythematous, or hemorrhagic in appearance. Rupture of the pustule may leave a superficial erosion or, with deep pustules, a necrotic fistulating tract.

Diagnostic Significance

Subcorneal pustules are associated with superficial bacterial infection (superficial staphylococcal dermatitis, folliculitis), pemphigus foliaceous, subcorneal pustular dermatoses, and dermatitis herpetiformis. Deep pustules are frequently seen with deep pyodermas and certain fungal diseases such as sporotrichosis. In the differential diagnosis of pustular eruptions, the contents of an intact pustule should be microscopically examined for bacteria and acantholytic epithelial cells and aseptically cultured for bacteria. Pemphigus foliaceous, subcorneal pustular dermatitis, and dermatitis herpetiformis form pustules that are sterile.

Vesicle

Morphology

Vesicles are circumscribed eruptions in the epidermis filled with clear fluid. Bulla are large vesicular eruptions. The "dome" covering the vesicle or bulla in dog and cat skin is very fragile and easily ruptured. Therefore, vesicular eruptions in dog and cat skin are short-lived and can be easily missed. Ruptured vesicles expose the underlying epithelium, creating erosions. Early vesicles may appear as papules and the term *vesiculopustular eruptions* is used when papules and vesicles coexist in the skin.

Diagnostic Significance

Vesicles may be associated with contact irritants or burns. Bulla are the basic lesions in pemphigus vulgaris and bullous pemphigoid, which are autoimmune skin diseases that produce clefts within the epidermis. Vesiculopustular or vesiculopapular eruptions are also associated with subcorneal pustular dermatoses, dermatitis herpetiformis, pemphigus foliaceous, pemphigus erythematosis, and drug eruptions.

Wheals

Morphology

Wheals are circumscribed, raised lesions, usually with a flat surface. They are usually erythematous and consist of localized edema.

Diagnostic Significance

Wheals may be associated with cutaneous anaphylactoid reactions such as insect bites, drug allergy, food allergy, or contact irritation. The classic wheal in dogs is the positive reaction to intradermal skin test antigens. Wheals are uncommon lesions in most allergic dermatoses of dogs and cats.

Macule

Morphology

Macules are circumscribed to slightly asymmetric spots in the skin characterized by hyperpigmentation, depigmentation, or erythema.

Diagnostic Significance

Hyperpigmented macules are occasionally associated with endocrine disorders such as hyperadrenocorticism, Sertoli cell tumor, and hypothyroidism. Hyperpigmented macules frequently occur as the final stage in the healing of circumscribed superficial erosion (*e.g.*, superficial staphylococcal dermatitis). Erythematous macules are observed with many acute dermatoses and probably represent erythematous plaques. Depigmented macules are usually large and are called patches. They are associated with vitiligo and, rarely, hypothyroidism. Hyperpigmented macules are characteristic of many dog breeds and may be more apparent in puppies. In some breeds, these juvenile macules disappear near puberty and may reappear in later life.

Nodule

Morphology

Nodules are solid, usually round elevations in the skin that may extend into the deeper layers. The surface may be intact or ulcerated. Nodules are caused by cellular accumulations in the skin.

Diagnostic Significance

Nodules may be granulomatous (inflammatory) or neoplastic. Neoplastic nodules are called tumors. Biopsy of the nodule and histopathologic examination of the tissue are indicated to identify the underlying reaction. Callus, lick granuloma, nodular panniculitis, and histiocytoma are examples of nodular disorders.

SECONDARY SKIN LESIONS

Ulcer

Morphology

Ulcers represent denuded epithelium that exposes the dermis. Hair is usually devoid in such lesions.

Diagnostic Significance

Severe necrotizing or inflammatory diseases produce ulcers. Ulcers generally heal, with scar formation. Neoplastic conditions such as squamous cell carcinoma, burns, toxic epidermal necrolysis, and severe autoimmune diseases will produce ulcers. Ulcerated skin provides a break in the barrier to bacterial infection and must be properly managed to prevent infection.

Erosion

Morphology

Erosions represent denuded epithelium that leaves the basement membrane intact. Hair is usually present in the erosive lesions.

Diagnostic Significance

Erosions are the common lesions that remain when pustules, vesicles, or bulla rupture. Because the basement membrane is intact, erosions heal without scar tissue formation.

Excoriation

Morphology

Excoriations are symmetric or asymmetric superficial erosions caused by scratching, biting, or rubbing. The surface of the lesion is usually moist and contains hair.

Diagnostic Significance

Excoriations reflect the presence of a pruritic skin disease. The term *hot spot* is used by laypeople to describe this lesion.

Scale

Morphology

Scales are loose fragments of keratin debris that accumulate in the coat or on the skin. Most scales in the dog are dry, powdery, or flaky. Occasionally, waxy or greasy scales are found.

Diagnostic Significance

Scales represent a disorder of the keratinization process. Scales often represent a lack of hydration in the stratum corneum. Waxy scales or scaley plaques are the basic lesions observed in primary seborrhea. Scales are nonspecific lesions that result from a variety of inflammatory and endocrine disorders.

Crust

Morphology

Crusts are dried blood, serum, pus, scales, or topical medications that cover the surface of ulcers or erosions.

Diagnostic Significance

See pustules, erosions, and ulcers.

Scar

Morphology

Scars are fibrous tissue that has replaced normal epithelium in the healing of an ulcer. Scars are depigmented and hairless.

Diagnostic Significance

Scars may follow severe burns and deep pyodermas. Irregular scars occur on the face and limbs of dogs and cats with the cutaneous manifestations of systemic lupus erythematosus. Canine solar dermatitis frequently heals with scar tissue formation.

Lichenification

Morphology

Lichenification is thickening of the skin with exaggeration of the superficial skin markings. Histologically, the skin is characterized by marked acanthosis (thickening of the prickle cell layer). Lichenified skin is usually hyperpigmented.

Diagnostic Significance

Lichenification is most commonly observed in chronically inflammed skin and may result from constant scratching or rubbing. It is also observed in acanthosis nigricans and the male feminizing syndrome. In many parts of the United States, the most common cause is chronic flea allergy dermatitis.

Hyperkeratosis

Morphology

Hyperkeratosis is an increased thickness of the stratum corneum. It may occur on the body, planum nasale, and digital pads. Scales are frequently associated with hyperkeratotic reactions.

Diagnostic Significance

See scales. In addition, hyperkeratotic reactions are associated with dermatophyte infections.

17

Alopecia

MICHAEL D. LORENZ

Alopecia is the loss or lack of hair in any amount or distribution up to complete baldness. Alopecia may be a primary event; however, it most commonly occurs secondary to an acquired disorder.

PATHOPHYSIOLOGY

The basic mechanisms that produce alopecia include (1) abnormalities in follicular structure; (2) abnormalities in follicular function (alteration of hair growth cycle); (3) structural abnormalities of the hair shaft; and (4) traumatic removal of hair.

Abnormalities in Follicular Structure

Primary alopecia is caused by inherited abnormalities of follicular structure. These may range from complete absence of hair follicles to absence of hair follicles that produce hair of a particular color.

Secondary (acquired) alopecias may be caused by diseases that disturb the follicular environment, prompting the disruption of hair growth and the dislodgement of hair from the follicles. Bacterial folliculitis, demodectic mange, severe necrotizing processes, and follicular hyperkeratosis are examples of acquired diseases that adversely affect follicular structure.

Abnormalities in Follicular Function

Diseases in this category do not destroy follicular structure *per se*, but they adversely affect the normal cyclic phases of the hair follicle. The phases of follicular activity are anagen (growth phase), catagen (transitional phase), and telogen (resting phase). The normal follicular cycles in the dog and cat have seasonal variations; however, hair growth is not synchronized but follows a mosaic pattern. The majority of follicles are in anagen, yet a few neighboring follicles may be in catagen or telogen. Certain conditions or diseases cause alopecia by promoting the development of telogen follicles. Estrogens, testosterone, and adrenocortical hormones delay the initiation of anagen. Thyroid hormone accelerates follicular activity. Conditions such as severe illness, fever, pregnancy, and lactation may cause the simultaneous precipitation of many follicles into catagen and telogen. The resulting alopecia is called "telogen effluvium." Certain drugs may also arrest mitotic activity of the follicle, causing alopecia.

The endocrine disorders may also produce follicular hyperkeratosis that results in follicular plugging. Follicular plugging disturbs normal hair growth.

Structural Abnormalities of the Hair Shaft

Certain diseases may weaken the hair shaft so that normal tension on the hair causes it to break. This is a primary mechanism for the alopecia that results from dermatophyte infections. Weakened, brittle hair shafts may be found in certain endocrine disorders such as hypothyroidism.

Traumatic Removal of Hair

This is a common mechanism for the alopecias associated with pruritic dermatosis. Constant self-mutilation mechanically removes or breaks the hair. The underlying inflammatory process may delay the initiation of anagen.

CLASSIFICATION

Alopecia may be classified as to onset (primary *vs.* secondary) or by its distribution.

The distribution pattern of the alopecia may be characteristic of the specific underlying disease. By distribution, alopecias may be classified as diffuse, regional, multifocal, or focal.

Diffuse Alopecia

The generalized or diffuse alopecias are primarily trunkal and tend to spare the head and limbs. Endocrine disorders are the most important cause of nonpruritic diffuse alopecias. Their differentiating features are listed in Table 17-1. Occasionally, allergic, bacterial, fungal, or immune-mediated diseases cause generalized alopecia. Telogen effluvium has been previously described as a cause of diffuse alopecia.

Regional Alopecia

Regional alopecias occur in a variety of dermatoses that have a predisposition for certain areas of the body. These distribution patterns are useful in formulating a

Table 17-1. Differential Features of Endocrine Alopecias

DISEASE	DERMATOLOGIC SIGNS	MAJOR SYSTEMIC SIGN(S)	PROFILE FINDINGS	SPECIAL TEST(S)
Hypothyroidism	Intense hyperpigmentation Thickened skin Dry, brittle coat	Lethargy Cold intolerance Weight gain Myxedema Anestrus	↑ Serum lipids Rarely, nonregenerative anemia	T4 before and after TSH stimulation
Canine Cushing's syndrome	Thin skin, lack of skin elasticity Calcinosis cutis Pigmented macules	Polyuria/polydipsia Muscle weakness Abdominal enlargement Hepatomegaly Polyphagia Anestrus	Lymphopenia ↑ Alk phos ↑ Serum lipids ↑ Glucose ↓ Urine specific gravity	Plasma cortisol before and after ACTH stimulation Dexamethasone suppression tests
Sertoli cell tumor	Gynecomastia Thin skin Pigmented macules	Pendulous prepuce Cryptorchidism Enlarged retained testicle	Rarely, anemia and thrombocytopenia	None
Male feminizing syndrome	Hyperpigmentation and lichenification of the caudal abdomen and flanks Gynecomastia	Attraction to male dogs	No consistent clues	None
Adult-onset growth hormone deficiency	Variable degrees of alopecia and hyperpigmentation of rump, flanks, and body	None	No consistent clues	Growth hormone assay before and after xyalazine stimulation
Estrogen deficiency	Patchy alopecia of flanks and back Very soft skin Very soft and fine hair	Occasionally urinary incontinence	No consistent clues	Response to estrogen therapy
Feline endocrine alopecia	Alopecia of caudal abdomen, rear legs Occasionally diffuse trunkal alopecia	None	No consistent clues	None
Hypotestosteronism	Diffuse trunkal alopecia Mild hyperpigmentation	Castrated Testicular atrophy	No consistent clues	Serum testosterone Response to testosterone therapy

↑, increased; TSH, thyroid-stimulating hormone; Alk phos, alkaline phosphatase; ACTH, adrenocorticotropic hormone

differential diagnosis. The conditions likely to involve the face, ears, feet, mucocutaneous junctions, and caudal body are given in the accompanying lists.

Multifocal Alopecia

Multifocal alopecia is probably the most common distribution pattern. It may begin with a focal pattern, but multiple lesions develop as the disease progresses. See Diseases Producing Multifocal Alopecia.

Diseases With Marked Facial Alopecia

- Demodectic mange
- Dermatophytosis
- Canine and feline acne
- Feline food allergy dermatitis
- Systemic lupus erythematosus
- Discoid lupus
- Pemphigus erythematosus
- Pemphigus foliaceus
- Canine solar dermatitis
- Atopy
- Epidermolysis bullosa simplex/dermatomyositis
- Juvenile pyoderma
- Lipfold pyoderma
- Subcorneal pustular dermatosis
- Notedric mange
- Drug eruption

Diseases With Ear Alopecia

- Dermatophytosis
- Demodectic mange
- Sarcoptic mange
- Pemphigus foliaceus
- Pemphigus erythematosus
- Seborrhea
- Marginal ear pinna alopecia and seborrhea
- Periodic ear pinna alopecia of miniature poodles
- Subcorneal pustular dermatitis
- Solar dermatitis (cats)
- Cold agglutinin disease
- Fly bite dermatitis
- Bacterial otitis externa
- Otodectic otitis externa
- Atopy

Diseases With Alopecia of the Feet

- Contact dermatitis
- Discoid lupus
- Demodectic mange
- The pemphigus group
- Bullous pemphigoid
- Interdigital pyoderma
- Thallium poisoning

Diseases With Mucocutaneous Involvement and Alopecia at Mucocutaneous Junctions

- Pemphigus vulgaris
- Bullous pemphigoid
- Candidiasis
- Thallium poisoning
- Drug eruption
- Toxic epidermal necrolysis

Diseases With Alopecia of Caudal Trunk and Abdomen

- Flea allergy dermatitis
- Feline endocrine alopecia
- Male feminizing syndrome
- Hypoestrogenism
- Adult-onset growth hormone deficiency

Focal Alopecia

This form of alopecia may initiate a multifocal distribution pattern and is caused by many of the diseases that produce multifocal alopecia. Diseases such as demodectic mange, acral pruritic nodule, dermatophytosis, and solitary neoplasms may remain as a focal pattern throughout the course of the disease.

DIAGNOSTIC PLAN

Although the distribution pattern of alopecia may provide clues to the diagnosis, characterization of the primary and secondary lesions is also very important. The diagnostic significance of the various skin lesions is described in chapter 16.

In certain cases, direct examination of the hair shaft and root may provide some clues as to the underlying etiology. Club hairs have a tiny white ball at the

Diseases Producing Multifocal Alopecia

- Demodectic mange
- Dermatophytosis
- Pyoderma
- Superficial staphylococcal dermatitis
- Cutaneous neoplasia
- Autoimmune skin diseases
  - The pemphigus group
  - Bullous pemphigoid
  - Systemic lupus
  - Discoid lupus
- Dermatitis herpetiformis
- Subcorneal pustular dermatosis
- The deep mycoses
- Seborrhea
- Nodular panniculitis
- Cutaneous candidiasis
- Zinc-responsive dermatosis

root end, and root sheaths are absent. Club hairs indicate a telogen hair follicle; however, the removal of club hair may initiate anagen. Anagen hairs plucked from the follicle have a larger expanded root surrounded by a root sheath. Hair can be carefully plucked from the coat so that the anagen-telogen ratio can be determined. When telogen hairs predominate, endocrine disorders, normal shedding, and telogen effluvium should be considered. Diseases that attack the hair shaft such as dermatophytes cause the hair to break; the root end may appear like a spear. Traumatic alopecias are characterized by hair broken midway up the shaft. These hairs may be more difficult to pluck from the follicle.

SYMPTOMATIC THERAPY

Definitive therapy of alopecia requires correction of the underlying disease process. In certain cases of persistent idiopathic alopecia (as occurs following surgical clipping), empirical thyroid hormone supplementation may stimulate anagen.

PROGNOSIS

The reversibility of alopecia depends on two factors: (1) the presence of viable hair follicles and (2) the correction of the underlying pathology. Alopecia is permanent when hair follicles are congenitally absent or reduced in number (hypotrichosis) or when lesions heal with scar tissue formation. Scar tissue is devoid of hair follicles since it is derived from connective tissue.

18

Abnormalities of Skin, Hair, and Mucous Membrane Pigmentation

MICHAEL D. LORENZ

Abnormalities of skin or coat color are of great concern to pet owners, especially when the abnormality is an obvious fault in a show animal. Of greater importance to veterinarians is the realization that these disorders may reflect a serious underlying disease. An understanding of normal pigmenting processes is necessary in order to correctly diagnose these disorders.

NORMAL SKIN AND HAIR PIGMENTATION

Three basic pigments and the optical effect called scattering are responsible for normal skin color. Scattering is the rearrangement of light as it passes through a turbid medium (*e.g.*, skin, hair, mucosa). The degree of pigment plus the density of the medium containing the pigment combine to give the various colors.

Skin and Hair Pigments

Melanin

Melanin is formed by specialized cells (melanocytes) in the basal cell layer of the epidermis, hair follicle, and mucous membranes. Melanogenesis involves the oxidation of tyrosine to melanin. This reaction is catalyzed by a copper-containing enzyme called tyrosinase. Melanin is injected through dendritic processes from the melanocytes into epithelial cells. Some free melanin pigment is engulfed by dermal cells called melanophages. Melanogenesis is increased by ultraviolet light, increased temperature, and friction. Sulfhydryl compounds inhibit tyrosinase activity and thus decrease melanin production.

The intensity of melanin pigment is not determined by the number of melanocytes but by the size and number of melanin granules contained in epithelial cells. Dark-skinned animals have larger, more numerous melanin granules in several layers of epithelial cells. Albino individuals have sufficient melanocytes but cannot form melanin because of a defect in tyrosinase activity.

The colors produced by melanin range from brown when diluted to yellow, orange, or orange-red when concentrated. Melanin is a strong pigment and usually obscures the other pigments in dark-skinned animals.

Melanin is the primary black-brown pigment of hair and pheomelanin is the yellow-red pigment. Pigmentation may be uniform throughout the shaft or have alternating bands of varying degrees of pigment. White hair is largely devoid of melanin. Pigment cells within the hair root (bulb) deposit the pigment in or between the cortical and medullary hair cells. The amount of pigment placed in the hair is genetically determined and creates the optical effects characteristic of particular breeds. The distribution of melanocytes within hair follicles is also genetically determined. This accounts for spotting, ticking, and other color patterns.

Hemoglobin

Blood vessels of the mucous membranes, sparsely pigmented skin, and white nails are penetrated by light and thus contribute to the color of these tissues. The primary pigment is hemoglobin. Oxyhemoglobin is more red, and reduced hemoglobin is more blue. Thus, the overall hue is determined by the ratio of oxyhemoglobin to reduced hemoglobin. Rapid changes in skin, mucous membrane, or nail color result from changes in vessel diameter, blood flow, and degree of hemoglobin oxidation. Increased reddening of the skin, mucous membranes, and nails is caused by vasodilation, whereas vasoconstriction or hypotension has the opposite effect. Cyanosis is apparent when reduced hemoglobin is present in concentrations of 5 g or more per deciliter of blood. Extreme cold may also cause increased skin redness because the lower temperature may decrease oxygen utilization in local tissue. Thus, more oxyhemoglobin is present to give the red color.

Carotene

Carotene and its related pigments impart a yellowish color to the skin. It is relatively unimportant in small animals.

INCREASED SKIN PIGMENTATION

This process may involve melanin, hemoglobin, carotene, and pigments of endogenous (bilirubin) or exogenous origin. Melanin and bilirubin are the most clinically important pigments.

Melanosis

Melanosis is hyperpigmentation due to increased amount of melanin. Several factors may potentiate excessive melanin production. It is more common in canine skin (see Causes of Melanosis in Dogs) and occurs infrequently in cats.

Causes of Melanosis in Dogs

- Chronic eczematous dermatoses
  - Flea allergy dermatitis
  - Atopy (chronic)
  - Allergic contact dermatitis
  - Food allergy dermatitis
- Focal superficial dermatoses
  - Superficial staphylococcal dermatitis
  - Dermatomycosis
- Hormonal conditions
  - Hypothyroidism
  - Hyperadrenocorticism
  - Sertoli cell tumor
  - Male feminizing syndrome
- Miscellaneous conditions
  - Acanthosis nigricans
  - Friction
  - Tanning (only in areas of alopecia exposed to light)

External Causes

Melanosis resulting from ultraviolet light exposure is called tanning. It is of little clinical significance in animals since the hair coat tends to prevent light exposure to the skin. The planum nasale and ear tips of white cats may actually suffer sunburn because of insufficient melanin protection.

Heat, radiation therapy, and mechanical irritation (as from a collar or harness) may cause localized melanosis.

Chronic Inflammation

Melanosis is a common finding in chronic inflammatory dermatoses. The pattern may be focal, multifocal, or regional. The underlying mechanism is not completely known but may be related to mechanical irritation (scratching, rubbing). The inflammatory process may also directly stimulate melanin production. Melanosis is most common in lichenified skin that results from chronic allergic conditions (*e.g.*, chronic flea allergy dermatitis).

Hormonal Control

The pituitary gland plays the dominant role in controlling melanin metabolism. Melanocyte-stimulating hormone (MSH) is secreted by the pituitary gland and increases melanin production in the skin. It is structurally similar to adrenocorticotropic hormone (ACTH), which also may stimulate melanosis in humans. Apparently ACTH has little, if any, MSH activity in dogs or cats that is clinically important.

Melatonin is a hormone found in the pineal gland of mammals. It decreases melanin production and may be useful in treating acanthosis nigricans. Melatonin has little effect in humans.

Glucocorticoids have an antimelanin effect. Since ACTH apparently has little MSH activity in dogs, it is difficult to rationalize the diffuse melanosis observed in hypercortisol states such as canine Cushing's syndrome. Unlike the disease in humans, melanosis is not a feature of canine adrenal insufficiency.

Estrogens tend to stimulate melanosis, whereas testosterone has little or no effect. Thus, the melanosis of hyperestrogenism can be explained; however, the hyperpigmentation observed in male feminizing syndrome is difficult to rationalize if the etiology is actually hypoandrogenism.

Thyrotropin (TSH) has a melatonin-like effect, whereas increased levels of thyroid hormones stimulate melanosis in humans. Hypothyroid dogs frequently develop generalized melanosis. This reaction is difficult to rationalize since the hormonal changes should reduce melanin production. Obviously, other unknown factors must be present in hypothyroid dogs.

Melanoplakia

Melanoplakia is focal melanosis of the mucous membranes. It has been observed in certain breeds of dogs and orange tabby cats. Melanoplakia has little clinical significance other than cosmetic. It should be differentiated from malignant melanoma.

Yellow Pigmentation

Jaundice (Icterus)

The serum bilirubin must reach 2 mg to 4 mg/dl before jaundice is clinically detectable. Tissue staining lags plasma staining, whereas the reverse is true when icterus is subsiding. Biliverdin imparts a greenish hue to the yellow color and usually occurs with biliary obstruction. Elastic tissue has a great affinity for bilirubin, which may explain the accentuation of icterus in the sclerae, conjunctiva, and mucous membranes. Icterus cannot be detected in edematous skin.

Medication

Quinacrine hydrochloride (Atabrine) is a drug utilized in the treatment of *Giardia* infection, solar dermatitis, and discoid lupus. It may produce a diffuse yellow color of the skin. Unlike bilirubin, the pigmentation is less intense in the sclerae.

Hemoglobin Pigmentation

Blood diffused through the skin and subcutaneous tissue at first has a purplish blue or blackish blue color. As the blood breaks down, bilirubin and biliverdin are formed. These pigments produce localized yellowish or yellowish-green discoloration.

Polycythemia produces an erythematous to purplish-red discoloration of the skin and mucous membrane. The vessels of the mucous membranes are very congested and appear slightly cyanotic. This condition, erythremia, represents the effects of red oxyhemoglobin tinted blue by an increased amount of reduced hemoglobin due to sluggish blood flow through the microcirculation.

Carbon monoxide poisoning produces a cherry-red color of the skin and mucous membranes because of the formation of carboxyhemoglobinemia. Cyanohemoglobinema due to cyanide poisoning produces a similar effect. If death occurs, the bright red color persists. Methemoglobinema produces a brownish-blue discoloration.

DECREASED SKIN PIGMENTATION

Abnormal skin, hair, or mucous membrane color may result from the loss of one or more normal pigments or modification of their appearance by some anatomic or physiologic factor.

Anemia

Pallor is the effect of decreased hemoglobin in blood vessels. Hemolytic anemia produces a combination of pallor and icterus. The yellow pallor of intravascular hemolysis may be modified by the presence of hemoglobinemia.

Decreased Melanin Production

Albinism

Albinism is a genetically controlled defect in the conversion of tyrosine to melanin. There is no deficiency of melanocytes or the substrate tyrosine. The entire skin, eyes, and hair are devoid of pigment. All white small animals are not true albinos in that some melanin pigment is present in the eyes and skin. Albino animals are predisposed to sunburn of the ears and nose or of the skin when the hair is clipped or lost from disease.

Vitiligo (Leukoderma)

Vitiligo is an acquired loss of melanin pigmentation in focal areas of the hair and mucous membranes. It has a patchy distribution of white hair or depigmentation of the gums, mucous membranes, eyelids, and nose. Vitiligo has been recognized in the Belgian truverian, Doberman pinscher, Appaloosa horse, and other dark-coated breeds of dogs.

Several potential causes of vitiligo have been recognized. It may result from anatomic destruction of melanocytes (freezing, severe necrosis, scar tissue), inhibition of melanin formation (copper deficiency), nervous influences, and autoimmune antibody formation. The underlying cause in dogs has not been determined. Affected animals are healthy in all other respects, and the disease is usually slowly progressive. In humans, vitiligo may be caused by Addison's disease, hyperthyroidism, diabetes mellitus, and pernicious anemia.

A localized form of vitiligo involving the planum nasale has been observed in dogs eating from rubber food dishes that contain *p*-benzylhydroquinone. Apparently this chemical is absorbed through the skin and inhibits melanin synthesis. The condition is reversible.

Depigmentation of the nose is a feature of canine solar dermatitis and discoid lupus erythematosus. Apparently, sunlight activates an autoimmune response directed at the melanocytes or melanin pigment. Severe ulceration of the planum nasale results from continual licking or rubbing and the inflammatory reaction.

SYMPTOMATIC THERAPY

Melanosis

In many cases, correction of the underlying problem obviates the use of topical therapy. In certain conditions such as acanthosis nigricans or chronic exzematous dermatoses with melanosis, topical therapy may be beneficial. Topical corticosteroids, salicylic acid, and coal tar preparations are useful for the conditions mentioned. These drugs are applied three times a day and rubbed in well. They help melanosis by decreasing the skin thickness, thus decreasing the layers of skin containing melanin. Pigmented spots may be bleached with 2% stabilized hydroquinone applied topically.

Melatonin, given parenterally, may be beneficial in acanthosis nigricans.

Depigmentation

There is no satisfactory treatment for vitiligo. Depigmentation of the planum nasale may be treated with sun screens and tatoo procedures.

Part Five

HEMATOLYMPHATIC PROBLEMS

19

Prolonged Bleeding

CRAIG E. GREENE

PROBLEM DEFINITION AND RECOGNITION

Bleeding disorders can involve deficiencies in platelets, in the extrinsic or intrinsic coagulation systems, or in vascular integrity, alone or in combination. An outline of extrinsic and intrinsic coagulation sequences is presented in Figure 19-1. The character of the hemorrhagic tendency may aid the clinician in arriving at a diagnosis. Capillary bleeding is commonly associated with defects in microvascular integrity or in platelet function and number. This "purpuric" or primary bleeding tendency is caused by microscopic lesions in the blood vessel wall, resulting from impaired formation of platelet plugs at sites of microvascular injury. Animals with such defects show multifocal pinpoint petechial or ecchymotic hemorrhages most commonly on the skin and mucosal surfaces. Epistaxis, melena, and hematemesis may be seen in severe cases. In contrast, secondary bleeding associated with abnormalities in the extrinsic and intrinsic clotting systems is usually characterized by large spreading subcutaneous hematomas and rebleeding following venipuncture and surgical dissection. In general, animals with clotting defects in the latter stages of the intrinsic pathway show greater incoagulability than those with abnormalities in early intrinsic stages or in the extrinsic pathway.

Because of the differences in clinical presentation, hemorrhagic disorders, regardless of cause, have also been classified as hereditary or acquired. *Hereditary* clotting disorders are being recognized with increasing frequency in domestic animals, most notably the dog and cat. Frequently, affected animals have a history of recurrent hemorrhagic episodes. The severity of clinical signs is dependent upon several factors, including the type of defect, the degree of the deficiency, and individual variation. Moderately to severely affected animals with hereditary bleeding disorders are commonly young at presentation. Tail docking, ear cropping, dew claw removal, and neutering may initiate the problem. However, with the absence of surgical or traumatic insult or of stress, overt clinical signs may not be evident. *Acquired* clotting disorders arise in animals of any age

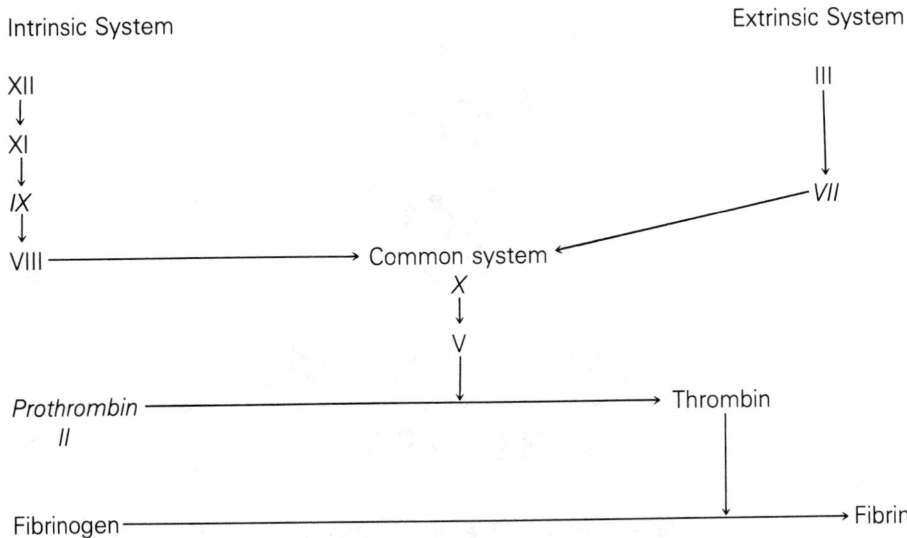

Fig. 19-1. Coagulation cascade. Vitamin K–dependent factors are in italics.

as a pathophysiologic response to preexisting disease. The hemorrhagic diathesis is often only one part of the clinical spectrum associated with the underlying disease.

PATHOPHYSIOLOGY

Hereditary coagulation defects (see Hereditary Platelet Disorders) arise as genetic mutations and have increased in prevalence because of the high degree of inbreeding of domestic dog and cat populations. A defect usually results in a malfunctioning coagulation protein and generally involves one coagulation factor (Table 19-1). Undoubtedly, there is some heterogeneity with respect to the severity and underlying cause of the coagulation defect even within the same disease. Von Willebrand's disease is caused by a deficit in a coagulation protein that is responsible for both platelet and coagulation factor dysfunctions.

Acquired bleeding disorders can involve abnormalities in platelets, clotting factors, or both (see Acquired Platelet Disorders and Acquired Clotting Factor Disorders). In contrast to hereditary disorders, clotting disorders that arise as pathophysiologic responses to preexisting disease frequently are associated with a wide variety of hemostatic alterations. Rather than a single defect, multiple factor deficiencies can compound the bleeding tendency in a single patient.

RULE OUTS AND DIAGNOSTIC PLAN

Diagnostic laboratories can screen for coagulation disorders using a number of tests, including the prothrombin time (PT), partial thromboplastin time, thrombin time (TT), coagulation factor assays, and fibrin(ogen) degradation products

Hereditary Platelet Disorders

Thrombocytopenia

- Decreased platelet production
  - Neonatal virus disease
  - X-linked trait (Wiskott-Aldrich syndrome)
  - Autosomal traits (various diseases such as Bernard-Soulier syndrome)

Platelet Dysfunction

- Thrombasthenia
  - Glanzmann's disease
- Thrombopathia
  - Bernard-Soulier syndrome
  - Storage pool disease
  - Albinism
  - Ehlers-Danlos syndrome
  - Wiskott-Aldrich syndrome
  - Osteogenesis imperfecta
  - Others

Susceptible breeds: Otterhounds, basset hounds, isolated in other breeds, Simmenthal cattle, cats, fawn hooded rats

Acquired Platelet Disorders

Thrombocytopenia

- Decreased or ineffective thrombopoiesis
  - Irradiation, myelophthistic diseases, hypothyroidism, drugs (estrogens, cytotoxic agents)
- Increased destruction, consumption, or sequestration
  - Immunologic: idiopathic, isoantibodies, hypersplenism, infectious agents, vaccination, ehrlichiosis, drug-induced, autoimmune disease
  - Coagulatory: mechanical (extracorporeal circulation), vascular disease (hemangiosarcoma, vasculitis) disseminated intravascular coagulation
  - Sequestration: splenomegaly (splenic neoplasia, portal hypertension)
- Dilutional by transfusion of platelet-free fluids such as stored blood products, crystalloids, or colloids

Thrombocytosis

- Increased production: hemorrhage, hemolysis, iron deficiency, rebound, cirrhosis
- Decreased storage: exercise, stress, epinephrine, vincristine

Platelet Dysfunction

- Disease-associated: hyperfibrinolysis, uremia, hepatic dysfunction, paraproteinemias, scurvy, polycythemia
- Drug-induced: aspirin, phenylbutazone, heparin, estrogen, phenothiazines, local anesthetics, plasma expanders, warfarin, sulfonamides

Table 19-1. Hereditary Clotting Factor Deficiencies

FACTOR	DISEASE	SPECIES OR BREED	TYPE OF DEFICIT	CLINICAL SIGNS
I	Afibrinogenemia Hypofibrinogenemia	Saanen goats	AID	HD; severe
II	Hypoprothrombinemia	Boxers	AID	Neonatal HD; epistaxis, mild
VII	Hypoproconvertinemia	Beagles Alaskan Malamutes	AID	Mild; bruising, demodicosis
VIII	Hemophilia A (classic hemophilia)	Most dog breeds, mongrels, cats, horses	X-linked	HD; severe, moderate, or mild
IX	Hemophilia B (Christmas disease)	Cairn terriers, St. Bernards, coonhounds, French bulldogs, particolored Cocker spaniels, Alaskan Malamutes, British shorthair cats	X-linked	HD; usually severe
von Willebrand factor + platelets + epithelium	von Willebrand's disease	German shepherds, miniature Schnauzers, Golden retrievers, Doberman pinschers, Scottish terriers, Pembroke Welsh corgis, Manchester terriers, Chesapeake Bay retrievers, other breeds of less frequency, Poland-China swine, rabbits	AID	HD; usually moderate or mild; severe postsurgical bleeding; otitis externa; panosteitis; epistaxis; melena; stress-induced bleeding; often lethal in homozygotes
X	Stuart factor deficiency	Cocker spaniels	AID	Neonatal HD; lethal in homozygotes
XI	Plasma thromboplastin antecedent (PTA) deficiency	Springer spaniels, Great Pyrenees, Kerry Blue terriers, Holstein cattle	AID	HD; mild; hematuria; severe or lethal bleeding 12–24 hr after surgery
XII	Hageman trait Hageman factor deficiency	Cats, marine mammals, reptiles, birds	AR in cats	None

AID, autosomal, incomplete dominance; HD, hemorrhagic diathesis; AR, autosomal recessive

Acquired Clotting Factor Disorders

- Primary hyperfibrinolysis
- Disseminated intravascular coagulation (DIC)
  - Vitamin K deficiency
  - Rodenticide ingestion
  - Complete biliary obstruction
  - Prolonged enteric antimicrobial therapy
- Circulating anticoagulants
  - Heparin administration
  - Plasma expander therapy
  - Antifactor antibodies
- Liver disease
  - DIC
  - Vitamin K deficiency
  - Factor dysfunction
  - Decreased factor synthesis

(FDPs) test. Tables 19-2 and 19-3 summarize the tests used to distinguish the most common hereditary and acquired bleeding disorders seen in small animals.

A platelet count and an activated coagulation time (ACT) can be used as rough screening tests to separate the various bleeding disorders and to aid in the initial decision regarding appropriate therapy. These two tests have the advan-

Table 19-2. Summary of Coagulation Screening Test Results in Most Common Hereditary Bleeding Disorders

	FACTORS XII, XI, IX, AND VIII AND VON WILLEBRAND	FACTORS III, VII	FACTORS I (FIBRINOGEN), II, V, X	THROMBO-CYTOPATHY
SCREENING TESTS				
Platelet count	N	N	N	N
ACT	P	N	P	N*
LABORATORY TESTS				
PT (extrinsic)	N	P	P	N
PTT (intrinsic)	P	N	P	N
Fibrinogen	N	N	N†	N
FDPs (clot lysis)	–	–	+	–
Decreased factors	As above	As above	As above	–

N, normal; ACT, activated coagulation time; PT, prothrombin time; PTT, partial thromboplastin time; P, prolonged; –, absent; +, present; FDPs, fibrinogen degradation products

* May be slightly prolonged in some cases, only by 20 seconds or less when counts are less than 20,000

† Decreased in Factor I (fibrinogen) deficiency

Table 19-3. Summary of Coagulation Screening Test Results in the Most Common Acquired Bleeding Disorders

	THROMBO-CYTOPENIA	HEPATIC DYSFUNCTION	DISSEMINATED INTRAVASCULAR COAGULATION			VITAMIN K DEFICIENCY	HYPERFIBRINOLYSIS
			Low-grade	Acute	End-stage		
SCREENING TESTS							
Platelet count	D	N	D	DD	D	N	N
ACT	N*	P	N	P	PP	P	P
LABORATORY TESTS							
PT (extrinsic)	N	P	N	P	PP	P	P
PTT (intrinsic)	N	P	N	P	PP	P	P
Fibrinogen	N	D	N	D	DD	N	D
FDPs (clot lysis)	−	±	−	+	+ +	−†	+
Decreased factors	−	I, II, V, VII IX, X	I, II, V, VII, VIII, X, XIII			II, VII, IX, X	I, V, VIII

D, decreased; N, normal; DD, very decreased; ACT, activated coagulation time; P, prolonged; PP, very prolonged; PT, prothrombin time; PTT, partial thromboplastin time; FDPs, fibrinogen degradation products; −, absent; ±, variable; +, present

* May be slightly prolonged in some cases but only by 20 seconds or less when counts are less than 20,000

† Increased FDPs are seen in some cases with extensive extravascular hemorrhage.

tages of being simple to perform and readily available to most veterinary practitioners. Enumeration of platelets is performed indirectly by estimating platelet numbers relative to leukocytes on stained blood films or directly by counting using a hemacytometer and a commercially available diluting-lysing solution (Unopette Microcollection System No. 5855, Becton Dickinson Co, Rutherford, NJ). On blood films, there are normally three to five platelets per oil immersion field. Platelet morphology can also be evaluated at this time since large forms appear in consumptive states. The ACT is a relatively reproducible measure of the intrinsic and common coagulation pathways. Commercially supplied tubes (activated coagulation time tubes No. 6522, Becton Dickinson Co, Rutherford, NJ) are available for this procedure. Blood taken by clean venipuncture is injected directly into the prewarmed (37°C) vacuum tube or transferred by syringe. The time interval from injection of the blood into the ACT tube until the first evidence of a visible clot is determined to be the ACT.

SYMPTOMATIC THERAPY

The initial management of bleeding disorders requires that the type of disorder be determined. The guidelines listed above will aid in this determination.

Hereditary Factor Deficiencies

There is no specific therapy for hereditary bleeding disorders. If one is suspected based upon clinical or familial history or on the basis of factor analysis, then precautions should be taken prior to surgical procedures. Therapeutic administration of fresh or frozen plasma to arrest or prevent hemorrhage is preferable to the use of whole blood, because the need for repeated transfusions in some animals will lead to sensitization to erythrocyte antigens if whole blood is used.

Thrombocytopenia

The most common causes of thrombocytopenia are related to immune-mediated (idiopathic thrombocytopenic purpura [ITP]), infectious diseases, or disseminated intravascular coagulation (DIC). Animals with immune-mediated diseases such as ITP present only with clinical signs of bleeding. Therefore, patients with few other signs of systemic illness should be given prednisone or prednisolone (1 mg/lb) daily. The platelet count should be checked within 1 week since it usually increases during this interval, although it may take up to 10 days. If no improvement is evident, then dexamethasone should be used at 0.1 to 0.2 mg/lb daily. A lack of response within 3 to 5 days warrants the use of vincristine at approximately 0.01 mg/lb once weekly. If there is no improvement after 1 week, these regimens can be combined. Splenectomy may have to be considered as a last resort. It is possible that animals with rickettsial disease or low-grade DIC could have very similar coagulatory abnormalities, although, in contrast to ITP, they usually have multisystemic signs in addition to bleeding. When these disorders are suspected, therapy with either tetracycline or heparin may be considered for 24 to 48 hours before starting the glucocorticoids.

Vitamin K Deficiency

Administration of Vitamin K_1 (phytonadione) provides the most rapid response to vitamin K deficiency. The daily subcutaneous or oral dosage is 0.22 mg/kg (for warfarin intoxication) to 5 mg/kg (for newer, more potent rodenticides). Therapy may have to be continued for up to 3 weeks to avoid relapse, which may be caused by many of these newer compounds. Blood or plasma transfusions may be required if bleeding is excessive and the ACT is greater than 4 minutes or the hematocrit is decreasing rapidly.

Disseminated Intravascular Coagulation

Correction of the underlying disease process is the most effective means of removing the procoagulatory stimulus. This includes correction of hypotension and volume deficits with fluid therapy, of hypoxemia with ventilatory assistance and oxygen, of sepsis with appropriate antimicrobial drugs, and of acidosis with alkalinizing agents. Supportive care is essential for organ systems that are compromised by the coagulation process. Adequate diuresis is needed to prevent renal shutdown.

The most controversial aspect of DIC concerns the recommendation of restoring the hemostatic balance. A rational therapeutic approach depends upon the stage at which DIC is identified. Prophylactic therapy or mild anticoagulation using aspirin (5 mg/kg daily for dogs; 25 mg/kg twice weekly for cats) or low-dose subcutaneous heparin (100 to 200 U/kg for dogs; 50–100 U/kg for cats) given three times daily should be used in low-grade or early DIC, which is characterized by thrombocytopenia and normal ACT. Twice these dosages should be used in acute DIC (thrombocytopenia and moderately prolonged ACT) when the predisposing disease cannot be readily eliminated or effectively treated. Anticoagulation is not the only therapeutic measure in endstage DIC when thrombocytopenia is evident and ACTs are very prolonged (>200 seconds for dogs; >120 seconds for cats) and the animal is bleeding profusely. In this situation, heparinization must be accompanied by immediate replacement therapy with fresh blood or plasma transfusions. The danger of accelerating the clotting process is outweighed by the immediate (within 15 minutes) and continued administration of low or prophylactic dosages of subcutaneous heparin as outlined for early DIC therapy.

20

Lymphadenopathy

CRAIG E. GREENE

PROBLEM DEFINITION AND RECOGNITION

There are hundreds of lymph nodes and lymphoid aggregates of varying size in the dog and the cat but only a few are palpable on routine physical examination. Palpable superficial nodes include the mandibular, superficial cervical, popliteal, and inguinal lymph nodes. Determining what constitutes mild enlargement is somewhat subjective since the size of lymph nodes vary according to body weight, breed, amount of body weight, and hydration status. Clinical experience is the best judge of the amount of enlargement. If lymph nodes are exceptionally enlarged, thorough clinical and laboratory testing should be performed based on the location and number of lymph nodes involved.

PATHOPHYSIOLOGY

Lymph nodes are the sites of lymphocyte production and formation of antibodies in response to an antigenic stimulus. In certain diseases involving extramedullary hematopoiesis or myeloid metaplasia, the lymph nodes may produce erythrocytes, platelets, and neutrophils. The causes of lymphadenopathy can be classified by cytomorphologic findings (see Causes of Lymphadenopathy). Enlargement of lymph nodes, which can be localized or generalized, usually reflects the extent of the pathologic process. Acute enlargement from inflammatory processes generally is accompanied by warmth, tenderness, and reddening of the overlying skin. The enlargement may be discrete or, if it extends into surrounding tissues, the node may be adherent and immobile. This latter process is a common finding with severe localized granulomatous conditions. Necrosis and rupture with drainage are common sequelae to chronic lymph node suppuration associated with infection caused by certain bacteria, such as *Pasteurella, Actinomyces, Nocardia,* and *Yersinia.* Marked lymph node enlargement in the absence of signs of local inflammation frequently reflects lymphatic neoplasia.

Causes of Lymphadenopathy

- Granulomatous
  - Fungus
  - Bacteria
    - Persistent intracellular forms
- Reactive hyperplasia
  - Infectious
    - Protozoa
    - Metazoa
    - Virus
    - Rickettsiae
  - Immune-mediated
    - Allergic
    - Immunologic
    - Autoimmune
- Suppurative
  - Bacteria
    - Extracellular types
  - Streptococci, staphylococci, *Pasteurella*
- Neoplasia
  - Primary or metastatic
    - Lymphosarcoma
    - Plasma cell neoplasia
    - Metastatic neoplasia
  - Cellular proliferation
    - Extramedullary hematopoiesis

Noninflamed enlarged lymph nodes usually do not cause physical discomfort. An animal with this type of enlargement is not presented for examination unless the owner observes the swelling or unless blood vessels, lymphatics, or airways are sufficiently occluded to cause additional problems such as edema.

Localized infections usually induce lymphadenopathy, which is limited to the area of regional drainage. If the infection becomes systemic or if there is spread of infection, generalized lymph node enlargement occurs.

RULE OUTS AND DIAGNOSTIC PLAN

A summary of diagnostic laboratory testing for lymphadenopathy is listed under Ordered Diagnostic Plan for Lymphadenopathy. Laboratory testing should always be preceded by a detailed physical examination. The location of lymphadenopathy may suggest the site of origin of the disease causing it. In metastatic neoplasia, the site of primary tumor must be sought carefully since the secondary lymphadenopathy may be more prominent than the primary lesion. Rectal,

Ordered Diagnostic Plan for Lymphadenopathy

1. Lymph node aspirate
2. Complete blood count, including platelets
3. Biochemistry, including albumin/globulin ratio
4. Urine analysis
5. Bone marrow analysis
6. Serum or immunoelectrophoresis
7. Specific infectious disease testing
   a. Persistent bacteria (*e.g., Brucella, Mycobacterium*)
   b. Persistent viruses (*e.g.*, feline leukemia virus, feline infectious peritonitis virus)
   c. Rickettsiae
   d. Fungi
   e. Protozoa (*e.g., Toxoplasma*)
8. Chest or abdominal radiography to document additional involvement
9. Lymph node biopsy with special staining for microorganisms, if indicated
10. Culture of lymph node or tissue biopsy

deep cervical, and abdominal palpations and thoracic and abdominal radiography may be needed when routine physical examination fails to reveal the lesion site. To complete oral and nasopharyngeal examinations, sedation and general anesthesia may be necessary.

The most direct and important, but often overlooked, clinical diagnostic procedure for lymphadenopathy is lymph node aspiration. The area over the enlarged node is clipped free of hair and surgically prepared. The operator immobilizes the node securely between the thumb and forefinger of one hand and percutaneously pierces the node using a sterile 20- to 22-gauge needle and 6- to 10-ml syringe held in the other hand. The tissue is aspirated rapidly to a minimum volume of 6 ml and then the needle is withdrawn. Smears of the aspirated tissue are made by gently dispensing the contents of the syringe onto a clean glass slide to avoid cellular disruption. The slide can be initially stained with new methylene blue to determine if the collection of cells has been satisfactory and to be used for preliminary examination. Subsequently, the smear should be stained with Wright's stain for a permanent slide and a more accurate cytomorphologic assessment. Gram staining for bacteria should be done when suppurative cytology is present. Lymph node aspirates are most helpful in differentiating hyperplastic and neoplastic conditions.

Excisional biopsy of an enlarged node should be performed if the findings on needle aspiration are nonspecific. Selection of the site is usually made on the basis of the largest palpable node. Surgical biopsy provides greater amounts of tissue that are needed for special staining and cultural procedures and gives information as to the overall architecture of the diseased lymph node. Impression smears should always be made from the excised nodes prior to fixation.

Impression smears of biopsied tissue give more detailed information as to the morphology of individual cells than does histologic examination.

The results of cytologic and histologic examination of enlarged lymph nodes can usually be divided into several categories (see Causes of Lymphadenopathy). Neoplasia, either primary or secondary metastatic forms, can be detected on the basis of abnormal cellular morphology. Specific infectious agents such as *Mycobacterium*, some rickettsiae, *Leishmania*, *Toxoplasma*, and deep mycotic agents may be detected on direct examination of the node. Other bacterial and fungal agents usually produce suppurative or granulomatous reactions, but organisms are seldom seen. Reactive hyperplasia has the cytologic appearance of a normal node in that small lymphocytes are the predominant cell, while there are lesser numbers of larger, variably sized lymphocytes, macrophages, and plasma cells. Since normal lymph nodes have a similar cytologic appearance, the fact that the lymph node is enlarged indicates hyperplasia, which is usually seen as a reaction to viral, rickettsial, or noninfectious antigens. Because the cytologic appearance of granulomatous lymph node enlargement also can be similar to reactive hyperplasia, histologic examination may be needed to differentiate these two syndromes.

Abnormal findings of routine hematologic and biochemical tests and urinalysis done prior to surgical lymph node biopsy may suggest the presence of a systemic disorder. Additional diagnostic testing may be performed on the basis of the cytologic or histologic findings of the node. If an infectious disease is suspected on the basis of lymph node cytomorphology, then specific serologic testing or cultural procedures should be employed. Bone marrow examination may be indicated if neoplasia is suspected based on the presence of abnormal cell types.

SYMPTOMATIC THERAPY

The mode of treatment of lymphadenopathy usually involves specific therapy for the cause. Complications of lymphadenopathy, such as edema from lymphatic obstruction, may be controlled by symptomatic physical therapy, diuretics, and anti-inflammatory agents (See chapter 11). Indiscriminate use of glucocorticoids should be avoided until the possibility of an infectious disorder has been eliminated. Presumed bacterial infections should be treated with broad-spectrum antimicrobial therapy until the results of a culture and sensitivity analysis of the aspirated or biopsied tissue or blood culture have been returned. If a rickettsial infection is suspected, the animal should respond to tetracycline.

Part Six

CARDIOVASCULAR PROBLEMS

21

Disturbances of the Heart: Rate, Rhythm, and Pulse

CLAY A. CALVERT

PROBLEM DEFINITION AND RECOGNITION

Disturbances of the cardiac rate and rhythm with associated pulse characteristics are among the most common clinical signs of underlying cardiac or extracardiac disorders. The heart rate and rhythm are determined by either cardiac auscultation or palpation of the arterial pulse. Pulse deficits occur when successive contractions occur so rapidly that left-ventricular diastolic filling is insufficient to generate a normal pulse pressure.

CLASSIFICATION

Disturbances of the heart rate can be broadly classified as being bradycardias or tachycardias (Table 21-1). Disturbances of the heart rate are termed *arrhythmias* and are abnormalities of the rate, regularity, site of origin of the cardiac impulse, or conduction of the electrical impulse generated by a pacemaker. The mechanism of cardiac arrhythmias involves disturbances of impulse formation or impulse conduction. Arrhythmias arise from abnormalities of automaticity, conduction, or both.

Sinus tachycardia and sinus bradycardia are probably the most common cardiac rhythm disturbances. These arrhythmias are often physiologic in origin and are frequently not associated with organic heart disease.

Ventricular premature contractions, atrial premature contractions, atrial fibrillation, first and second degree atrioventricular block, and ventricular tachycardia were the most commonly diagnosed arrhythmias in dogs in one clinical study.[11] In another study, atrial arrhythmias occurred in approximately 10% of 2000 dogs evaluated during routine examinations because of suspected arrhythmias or for the evaluation of antiarrhythmic drug therapy. Ventricular arrhythmias occurred in approximately 6% of the dogs. Atrial premature beats, ventricular premature beats, atrial fibrillation, first and second degree atrioventricular

Table 21-1. Classification of Heart Rate Abnormalities and Common Associated Conditions

CLASSIFICATION	COMMON ASSOCIATION(S)
Tachycardia	
Sinus tachycardia	Physiologic
	Congestive heart failure
	Systemic disorders
	Hypoxemia
	Drug administration
Atrial tachycardia	Atrial enlargement
	Pulmonary disease
	Drug administration
Atrial fibrillation	Cardiomyopathy
	Mitral insufficiency
Ventricular tachycardia	Cardiomyopathy
	Mitral insufficiency
	Myocarditis
	Contusion
	Toxemia
	Bacteremia
	Ischemia
	Drugs
Bradycardia	
Sinus	Physiologic
	Systemic disorders
	Hypoxemia
	Drugs
Sinoatrial block or arrest	Physiologic
	Drugs
	Sick sinus syndrome
Sinoventricular conduction	Hyperkalemia
Advanced second-degree and complete atrioventricular heart block	Idiopathic myocardial fibrosis
	Feline cardiomyopathy
	Hyperkalemia

block, and ventricular tachycardia were, in that order, the most common arrhythmias.[13]

PATHOPHYSIOLOGY

The inherent heart rate and rhythm are constantly modified by numerous physiologic mechanisms, primarily chemical and neurologic in nature. Electrocardiographic analysis is required for the definitive diagnosis of disturbances of cardiac rate and rhythm.

Chemical control is exerted by certain ions and endocrine hormones. Sodium and potassium are the predominant electrolytes important in the control of the cardiac rate and rhythm. The adrenal gland, when stimulated by its sympathetic nerve supply, secretes a mixture of epinephrine and norepinephrine, hormones having a profound effect on heart rate and contractility. The autonomic nervous system is responsible for the innervation of the heart (Fig. 21-1). The autonomic nervous system regulates the rate of intrinsic impulse formation, controls the conduction of impulses, and influences the state of myocardial contractility.[1,3,6,9]

The nerve impulses of the autonomic nervous system are transmitted by a chemical mediator. The neurotransmitter of both the sympathetic and parasympathetic preganglionic neurons as well as the postganglionic parasympathetic neurons is acetylcholine. They are cholinergic neurons. The neurotransmitter of the postganglionic sympathetic neurons is norepinephrine.[2] They are adrenergic neurons.

The sympathetic preganglion neurons originate in the first four or five thoracic segments of the spinal cord and extend to the sympathetic chains.[2] The cardiac sympathetic nerves arise from the anterior thoracic sympathetic ganglion. Sympathetic stimulation of the heart increases both the rate and force of myocardial contraction.

The cardiac parasympathetic nerves originate in the medulla oblongata, specifically in the parasympathetic nuclei of the vagus nerve. The efferent fibers terminate primarily in the sinoatrial node, atria, and atrioventricular node.[8] The right vagus nerve innervates primarily the atrioventricular node.[5] Vagal stimulation results in a slowing of the sinoatrial rate and a decrease in the rate of

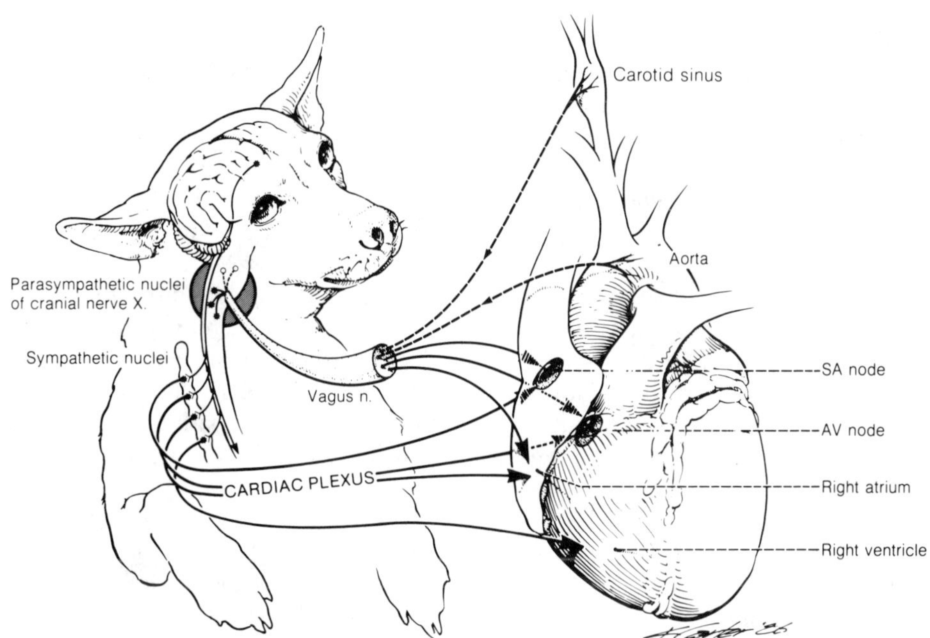

Fig. 21-1. Schematic representation of the cardiac conduction system of the dog.

impulse conduction through the atrioventricular node.[5] The vagus nerve is the efferent limb of a reflex arc with the vagal center in the medulla. Generally speaking, the potential afferent pathways capable of affecting the vagal center include all of the afferent nerves of the body. The more important afferent impulses for controlling the heart arise in portions of the circulatory system, especially those regions from which it receives and into which it discharges the blood: the right atrium and aorta, respectively. On the venous, or receiving, end the Bainbridge reflex causes acceleration of the heart when venous return is excessive to the point of overdistending the right atrium. The sensory endings are in the right atrium and adjacent vena cava and are stimulated by increased tension. The resultant nerve impulses are transmitted by the afferent fibers of the vagus nerve and inhibit the vagal center, thus increasing the heart rate.

On the arterial side is a depressor reflex, whose afferent fibers arise from the root and the arch of the aorta and course to the medulla within the vagus nerve. Increased tension within the aorta results in vagal stimulation and a slowing of the heart rate. The reverse occurs if the intra-aortic pressure becomes subnormal. A similar depressor reflex, dependent on the carotid artery pressure, has its afferent nerve endings in the carotid sinus. The afferent fibers from the carotid sinus reach the medulla via the glossopharyngeal and vagus nerves and the sympathetic trunk. The carotid sinus is a specially innervated part of the arteries and adjacent tissues located at the carotid artery bifurcation. Highly developed nerve endings in the carotid body, in the same location, are chemoreceptors sensitive to hypoxemia and hypercarbia, the response to which is cardiac acceleration.

The higher centers of the brain also may be a source for initiating afferent impulses to the medulla. Increased intracranial pressure usually is associated with slowing of the heart, brought about by overstimulation of the vagal center. This effect may be directly mechanical and due to ischemia resulting from increased pressure upon the blood supply of the medulla. Ischemia stimulates all of the medullary centers, including the vasomotor center, resulting in peripheral vasoconstriction and hypertension. Hypertension, in turn, acts on the aorta and carotid sinus to stimulate depressor reflexes that contribute to bradycardia.

The sympathetic and vagal centers in the medulla form a functional unit referred to as the cardiac center. The quantity and quality of blood reaching this center affect the heart rate. Slight hypoxia of the cardiac center results in an increased heart rate, as does slight hypercarbia. Severe hypoxia results in bradycardia; severe hypercarbia may produce a heart block. Such effects occur by means of efferent impulses coursing along the vagus or sympathetic nerves or both. Increased temperature of the blood perfusing the cardiac center accelerates the heart rate.

The sympathetic control of the heart is subordinate to vagal control. The afferent pathways of the sympathetic system are identical to those of the vagus nerve. The cardiovascular sensory areas of the right atrium, aortic root, and carotid sinus have an analogously intimate relationship with sympathetic control. Consequently, cardiac acceleration from an overdistended atrium, although predominantly brought about by inhibition of the vagus center, is partially produced by sympathetic nerve stimulation. Slowing of the heart by the vagus in the depressor reflex is enhanced by a concomitant decrease in sympathetic tone.

CONDUCTION SYSTEM ANATOMY

The cardiac conduction system consists of the sinoatrial node, the internodal tracts, the atrioventricular node, the bundle of His, the right and left bundle branches, and the Purkinje fibers (Fig. 21-2).[4,7,10,14,15] The sinoatrial node, situated in the upper right atrium, is the primary pacemaker. The internodal pathways conduct the electrical impulse generated by the sinoatrial node to the atrioventricular node. The atrioventricular node is on the right side of the lower portion of the interatrial septum and is continuous with the bundle of His.

The bundle of His establishes an electrical link between the atria and ventricles as it penetrates the atrioventricular ring. The bundle of His continues along the interventricular septum and bifurcates near the aortic valve. The right bundle branch courses down the right side of the interventricular septum to the anterior papillary muscle. Branching fibers then radiate over the right ventricular free wall. The left bundle branch courses along the left side of the interventricular septum and arborizes into two largely interconnected fascicles that course to the two papillary muscles. All diversions of the bundle branches divide into the Purkinje fiber network, which penetrates the ventricular myocardium.

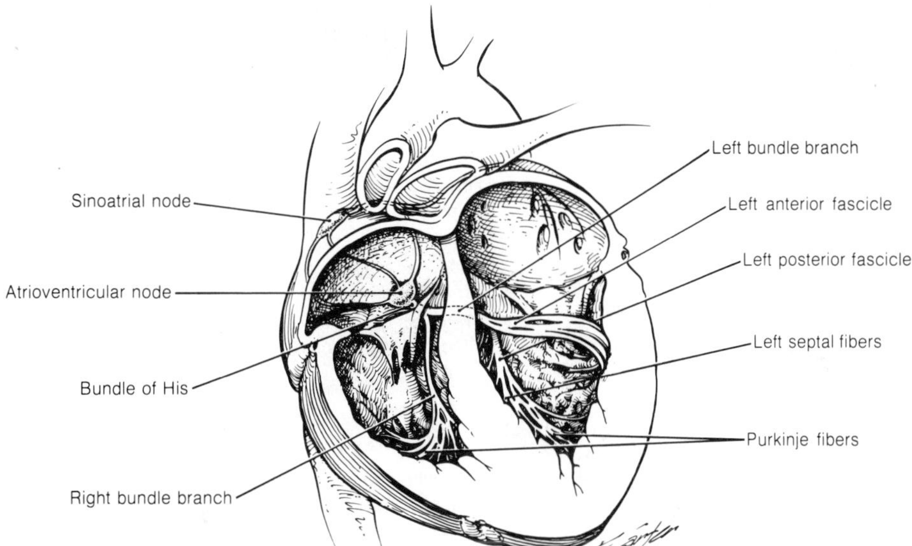

Fig. 21-2. Schematic representation of the autonomic innervation of the canine heart.

TACHYCARDIA

The most common type of tachycardia is referred to as sinoatrial or, usually, sinus tachycardia. In dogs and cats, the normal sinus rate is between 70 and 120 beats per minute. Most small dogs and cats have a resting sinus rate of 90 to 120 per minute. The causes of sinus tachycardia are numerous (Table 21-2) and are usually the result of extracardiac physiologic or pathologic stimuli. Transient tachycardia is a daily occurrence as a physiologic response to exertion, pain, and heat. Sinus tachycardia is usually the result of altered activity of the autonomic nervous system, rather than a primary disorder in the function of the sinus node. Physiologic sinus tachycardia occurs during and after stimuli resulting in anxiety and is an integral part of the "fight-or-flight" adaptive responses mediated through the sympathetic nervous system.

The heart rate in congestive failure may accelerate to maintain normal tissue perfusion. Extrinsic mechanisms, nervous or chemical, such as the Bainbridge and carotid sinus and aortic reflexes, are involved in the production of compensatory tachycardia in heart failure.

Sinus tachycardia tends to be persistent as long as its etiology persists. It is usually not paroxysmal unless the stimulus is also short lived. As a general rule, the rate of sinus tachycardia is usually between 120 and 180 beats per minute, although rates up to 210 to 220 per minute may occur. In puppies, kittens, and cats, rates may reach 240 to 260 per minute.

Table 21-2. Common Causes of Sinus Tachycardia

CATEGORY	CAUSES
Physiologic	Exercise
	Pain
	Excitement
Pathologic	Fever
	Shock
	Hemorrhage
	Hypotension
	Feline hyperthyroidism
	Anemia
	Hypoxia
	Drugs
	Atropine
	Catecholamines
	Hydralazine
	Congestive heart failure
	Toxicity
	Hexachlorophene
	Endotoxins
	Infections

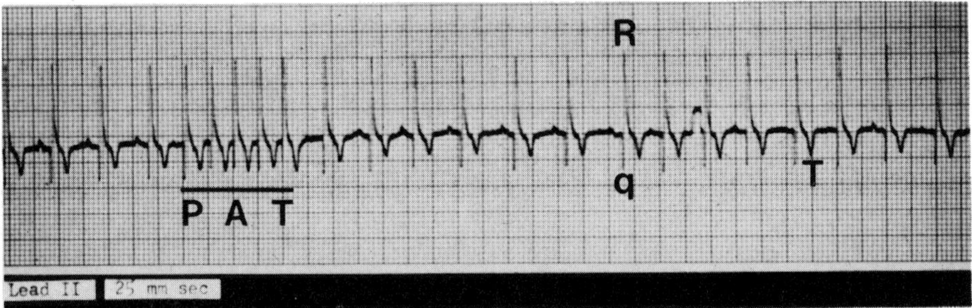

Fig. 21-3. Paroxysmal atrial tachycardia (*PAT*) in a 12-year-old miniature poodle with mitral valvular insufficiency and radiographic evidence of left atrial enlargement.

Atrial Tachycardia

Unlike sinus tachycardia, atrial tachycardia is usually paroxysmal, that is, persists for a few beats, to seconds, to minutes but seldom longer (Fig. 21-3). The rate associated with paroxysmal atrial tachycardia is usually in excess of 200 beats per minute and is typically in the range of 240 to 280 beats per minute. The exceedingly rapid rate and paroxysmal nature of atrial tachycardia are the most useful clues to the differential diagnosis (Table 21-3). An electrocardiogram is necessary for proof of the correct diagnosis. The exact character of the P wave and PR interval during normal sinus rhythm must be recorded to confirm the diagnosis. Since paroxysmal atrial tachycardia is usually of short duration, the P

Table 21-3. Differential Diagnosis of Sinus and Atrial Tachycardia

TACHYCARDIA	CRITERIA
Sinus	Sustained
	Vagal maneuvers unsuccessful*
	P-wave morphology unchanged†
	PR interval unchanged†
	RR interval slightly irregular‡
Atrial	Paroxysmal
	Vagal maneuvers successful§
	P-wave morphology different†
	RR interval regular‡

* Vagal maneuvers result in deceleration but tachycardia recurs after vagal maneuvers unless the etiology has abated.
† Compared with P-wave morphology and PR interval during normal sinus rhythm.
‡ Inconsistent finding
§ Vagal maneuvers break the tachycardia and normal sinus rhythms persist for minutes, hours, or indefinitely.

wave configuration and PR interval during normal sinus rhythm can usually be assessed and compared with those associated with the tachycardia.

Atrial tachycardia in dogs and cats is usually associated with chronic cardiac disease; severe left atrial enlargement is usually present. In the dog, these changes are most often the result of chronic mitral valve insufficiency (Table 21-4). In the cat, hypertrophic cardiomyopathy is the most common etiology. Chronic pulmonary disease in middle-aged and old, small breed dogs is often coexistent with mitral valve disease and may contribute to the genesis of the arrhythmia. The "sick sinus syndrome" of middle-aged and old female miniature Schnauzers is sometimes associated with paroxysmal atrial tachycardia. Following the tachycardia, periods of prolonged sinus arrest occur interspersed with junctional or, less frequently, ventricular escape beats and sinus arrhythmia (Fig. 21-3). Prolonged sinus arrest results in varying degrees of episodic weakness and syncope. Not all dogs manifesting the sick sinus syndrome experience paroxysmal atrial tachycardia.

Some degree of myocardial fibrosis, myocytolysis, edema, and inflammation are associated with most instances of atrial enlargement severe enough to result in paroxysmal atrial tachycardia. Atrial tachycardia may result from automaticity or re-entry. Most instances associated with severe left atrial disease probably result from re-entry. Digitalis glycosides can produce abnormal impulse formation, that is, ectopic atrial tachycardia. Paroxysmal atrial tachycardia with concomitant atrioventricular block (first-degree, second-degree, or both) or junctional tachycardia is usually the result of digoxin intoxication. Multifocal atrial tachycardia (also called "chaotic" atrial tachycardia) is also of ectopic origin and, although it may complicate severe cardiac disease, is usually the result of chronic lung disease.[12]

Although atrial tachycardia is unlikely to result in heart failure in younger animals and in those lacking severe cardiac disease, patients with cardiomy-

Table 21-4. Causes of Paroxysmal Atrial Tachycardia

CAUSE	ASSOCIATION(S)
Atrial enlargement	Mitral valve insufficiency (regurgitation)
	Chronic, acquired
	Congenital
	Cardiomyopathy
	Canine dilated congestive
	Feline hypertrophic
Hypoxemia	Congestive heart failure*
	Pulmonary disease*
Neoplasia	Hemangiosarcoma of the right auricle
Drugs	Digitalis glycosides
	Anesthesia
Hypokalemia	Diuretics
	Other

* Often coexistent.

opathy or advanced mitral valve disease may experience a significant decrease in cardiac output. Congestive heart failure (pulmonary edema) or shock may occur unless the tachycardia is short lived.

Atrial Flutter

Atrial flutter is an unusual tachycardia in dogs and cats and it results from a circus movement and re-entry. In most cases, the ventricular rate is considerably less than the atrial rate due to a variable and often high degree of atrioventricular block. The atrial flutter rate, although usually exceeding 180 beats per minute, is variable. In dogs, this arrhythmia is most often associated with atrial neoplasia or cardiac catheterization. It may occur rarely with severe left-atrial enlargement due to chronic mitral valve insufficiency or cardiomyopathy.

Atrial Fibrillation

Atrial fibrillation is a common arrhythmia in dogs but is uncommon in cats (Fig. 21-4). It is usually associated with severe organic heart disease (Table 21-5). Cardiomyopathies are the most common group of disorders associated with atrial fibrillation in the dog (dilated congestive) and cat (hypertrophic). Atrial

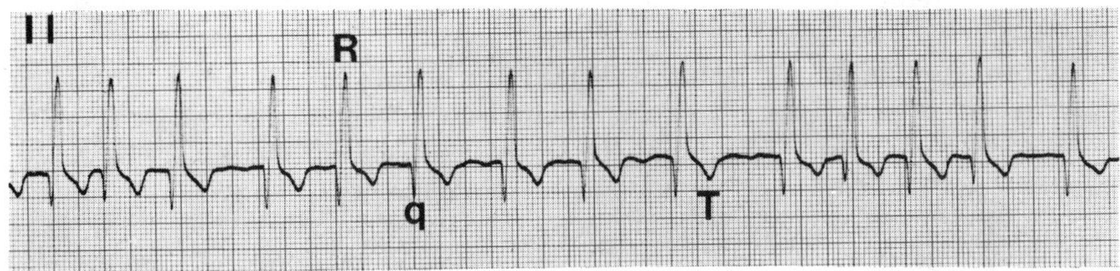

A

II
R
f

B

Fig. 21-4. (*A*) Atrial fibrillation in a 5-year-old Old English sheepdog with dilated congestive cardiomyopathy and bilateral congestive heart failure. The heart rhythm is rapid (200–220/min) and irregular. No P waves are visible. (*B*) Atrial fibrillation in a 7-year-old male Persian cat with radiographically confirmed severe left atrial enlargement and pulmonary edema. P waves are absent and f waves dominate the baseline.

Table 21-5. Causes of Atrial Fibrillation

CAUSE	ASSOCIATION(S)
Left atrial enlargement	Canine dilated congestive cardiomyopathy Feline hypertrophic cardiomyopathy Mitral insufficiency
Hyperkalemia	Hypoadrenocorticism*
Hypothermia*	

* Usually associated with ventricular rates of less than 180 beats per minute

fibrillation occurs occasionally in small dogs with acquired mitral valve insufficiency and severe left-atrial enlargement. Since mitral valve disease is very common in small breed dogs, atrial fibrillation, although uncommon on a percentage basis, is relatively common on an absolute basis.

Atrial fibrillation exacts two hemodynamic penalties: the ineffective writhing of atrial muscle deprives the heart of its atrial transport function and the incessant and irregular bombardment of the atrioventricular junction (with the latter's variable physiologic block) excites a rapid but irregular ventricular response. These hemodynamic consequences may precipitate congestive heart failure in dogs with advanced mitral valve disease or in dogs and cats with cardiomyopathy.

Atrial fibrillation may be paroxysmal at the onset, converting spontaneously to sinus rhythm. However, in association with organic heart disease, paroxysmal atrial fibrillation portends subsequent sustained atrial fibrillation. Initially, digoxin or digoxin plus propranolol therapy may result in conversion to sinus rhythm, but relapse usually occurs. Atrial fibrillation is occasionally found in overtly normal Irish wolfhounds, a condition analogous to "lone fibrillation" in humans, but the arrhythmia should be treated if the rate exceeds 170 beats per minute.

The diagnosis of atrial fibrillation should be suspected based on the physical examination. The heart rhythm is rapid and chaotic (irregularly irregular) and pulse deficits are frequent. Clinical signs consistent with advanced cardiac disease and heart failure are usually present. Auscultation of this chaotic sounding

---

Fig. 21-5. (*A*) Paroxysmal ventricular tachycardia in a 12-year-old Yorkshire terrier with chronic mitral valvular insufficiency and pulmonary edema. Capture beats (*c*) represent normal sinus beats that interrupt the tachycardia (25 mm/sec, 1/2 sensitivity). (*B*) Ventricular tachycardia (180/min) in a 7-year-old male Doberman Pinscher with dilated congestive cardiomyopathy and severe pulmonary edema. (*C*) Ventricular tachycardia (440/min) in a 5-year-old overtly healthy Doberman Pinscher that collapsed suddenly. Ventricular fibrillation and death occurred shortly following this ECG. (*D*) Paroxysmal ventricular tachycardia (480/min) in a 12-year-old Siamese cat with dilated congestive cardiomyopathy. Severe weakness, hypothermia, and pleural effusion were present. ▶

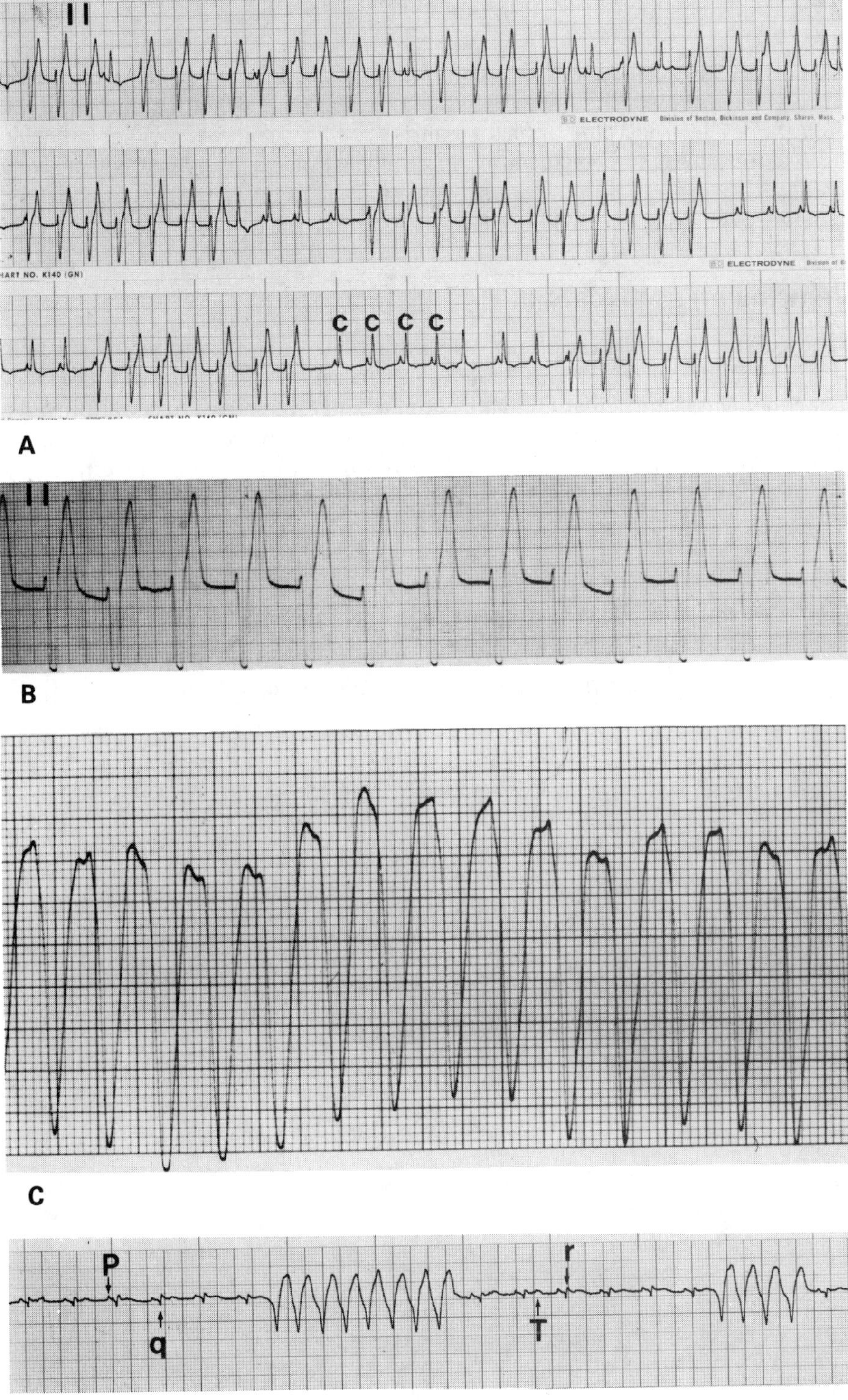
II
ELECTRODYNE Division of Becton, Dickinson and Company, Sharon, Mass.
ELECTRODYNE
CHART NO. K140 (GN)
C C C C
A
II
B
C
P
q
r
T
D

tachycardia in a giant breed dog exhibiting weight loss, dyspnea, ascites, pale mucous membranes, and exercise intolerance should leave little doubt as to the clinical and electrocardiographic diagnosis.

The physiologic mechanism of atrial fibrillation has not been conclusively established. Experimental evidence suggests that re-entry phenomena are the basis for sustaining this arrhythmia.

Ventricular Tachycardia

Ventricular tachycardia is a life-threatening arrhythmia and is strongly indicative of a diseased heart (Fig. 21-5; Table 21-6). In general, older, small breed dogs that experience ventricular tachyarrhythmias often have advanced mitral valve disease, chronic obstructive pulmonary disease, or both. Middle-aged, large breed dogs exhibiting ventricular tachyarrhythmias may have congestive cardiomyopathy; the differential diagnosis depends on associated clinical signs,

Table 21-6. Common Diseases and Disorders Associated With Ventricular Tachycardia

GENERAL ETIOLOGY	SPECIFIC DISORDERS
Myocardial disease or disorder	Cardiomyopathy
	Contusion
	Myocarditis
	Neoplasia (infiltrative cardiomyopathy)
Myocarditis	Parvovirus infection
	Bacteremia
Idiopathic cardiomyopathy	Doberman pinscher cardiomyopathy
	Boxer cardiomyopathy
	Canine dilated congestive
	Feline cardiomyopathies
Congestive heart failure	Cardiomyopathies
	Mitral valve disease (advanced)
Toxemia	Post-gastric torsion
	Bacteremia
	Pancreatitis
	Peritonitis
Hypoxemia	Congestive heart failure
	Anemia
	Pulmonary disease
Drug treatment	Digitalis glycoside
	Doxorubicin
	Anesthetics
	Ketamine
	Antiarrhythmic drugs
Metabolic disturbances	Uremia
	Hypokalemia
	Feline hyperthyroidism

laboratory findings, and radiographic abnormalities. Ventricular tachycardia occurring in middle-aged and especially old cats is usually the result of cardiomyopathy, particularly dilated congestive cardiomyopathy. The rapid and accurate diagnosis of this arrhythmia is essential and vital to the survival of the patient.

The mechanisms of ventricular tachycardia are numerous and include automaticity, triggered activity, micro–re-entry circuits in the ventricle, and macro–re-entry circuits confined to the specialized conduction system. Even in the same disease, the mechanism of the arrhythmia may vary.

BRADYCARDIAS

Bradyarrhythmias may result from disturbances of impulse formation or impulse conduction (see Classification of Bradyarrhythmias and Their Common Associations). The mechanism of such disturbances is often physiologic but may be pathologic.

Sinus Bradycardia

Sinus bradycardia is probably the most common bradyarrhythmia and is most often the result of increased vagal tone in brachiocephalic breeds (with concomitant sinus arrhythmia) and a normal variant in large breed dogs. Sinus bradycardia is usually the result of a disturbance of impulse formation. It is common in large breed dogs at rest and during sleep periods. Sinus bradycardia is a part of the normal reaction to vagal stimuli. Pharmacologic sinus bradycardia may result from digitalis glycosides, narcotics, beta-adrenergic blocking agents (propranolol), quinidine, quinidine-like antiarrhythmic drugs, xylazine, and anesthetics.

Pathologic sinus bradycardia may accompany the vagal stimulation produced by vomiting. It is also seen in association with obstructive jaundice, increased intracranial pressure, severe hypoxemia, and depressed mental status. Sinus bradycardia may portend cardiac arrest. Intrathoracic masses may produce a reflex sinus bradycardia due to irritation of the vagus nerve. Cervical masses such as thyroid gland neoplasia and carotid body tumors may produce sinus bradycardia through autonomic reflex arcs.

Vagal tone may be increased during surgical manipulation of abdominal organs, producing a marked sinus bradycardia. Hypothermia is associated with a number of cardiac rhythm disturbances, including sinus bradycardia.

Sinoventricular Conduction

Sinoventricular conduction is pathognomonic for hyperkalemia, most often resulting from hypoadrenocorticism. In this condition, the response of the sinoatrial node is slowed but conduction via the specialized internodal pathways continues. However, due to the atrial myocardium's increased susceptibility to

Classification of Bradyarrhythmias and Their Common Associations

Disturbances of Impulse Formation

- Sinus bradycardia
  - Physiologic
    - Increased vagal tone
      - Endogenous
      - Exogenous
        - Vagal maneuvers
        - Surgery
        - Drugs
    - Normal variant in large dogs
  - Pathologic
    - Systemic disease
      - Uremia
      - Toxemia
      - Peritonitis
    - Cardiac arrest
    - Hypoxemia
    - Hypothermia
    - Increase CSF pressure
    - Hyperkalemia
  - Drug Induced
    - Narcotics
    - Tranquilizers
    - Anesthetics
    - Antiarrhythmics
    - Beta-adrenergic blocking drugs

Disturbances of Impulse Conduction

- Sinoventricular conduction
  - Hyperkalemia
    - Hypoadrenocorticism
    - Oliguric renal failure
- Advanced atrioventricular heart blocks
  - Acquired
    - Idiopathic myocardial fibrosis
    - Cardiomyopathy
      - Feline dilated congestive
      - Feline hypertrophic
      - Canine hypertrophic
    - Infiltrative cardiomyopathy (neoplasia)
    - Hereditary stenosis of bundle of His
    - Bacterial endocarditis
    - Hyperkalemia
  - Drug Induced
    - Digoxin
    - Xylazine
    - Beta-adrenergic blocking drugs
    - Narcotics
    - Tranquilizers
    - Doxorubicin
    - Antiarrhythmic drugs

the resting membrane potential effects of hyperkalemia, an exit block occurs at the sinoatrial junction (junction between the sinoatrial node and perinodal-myocardial tissue). Thus, as the serum potassium concentration increases, a gradual decrease in the sinoatrial rate occurs (associated with gradual prolongation of the PR interval and decreasing P wave amptitude). The P wave eventually disappears (atrial standstill). Tall, spiked, T waves are typically present when this bradycardia develops. The ventricle is activated by the antegrade sinoatrial impulse being conducted via the specialized conducting fibers (internodal pathways, atrioventricular node, bundle of His), which are somewhat resistant to the depressant effect of hyperkalemia.

Sick Sinus Syndrome

The sick sinus syndrome causes episodic weakness and is characterized by sinus node depression, including sinus bradycardia and prolonged sinus (sinoatrial) arrest (Fig. 21-6). Prolonged sinus arrest is followed by delayed junctional (and occasional ventricular) escape beats and rhythms, alternating with sinus arrhythmia, sinus bradycardia, and prolonged sinus arrest. In some dogs, paroxysmal atrial tachycardia alternates with prolonged periods of sinus nodal inertia and often atrioventricular junctional inertia as well. This syndrome is common in middle-aged and older miniature Schnauzers (particularly females), but a similar pattern may be seen in the dachshund and other small breed dogs. Mitral valve disease and chronic pulmonary disease are often coexistent. Congestive heart failure due to mitral insufficiency eventually complicates the management of this syndrome.

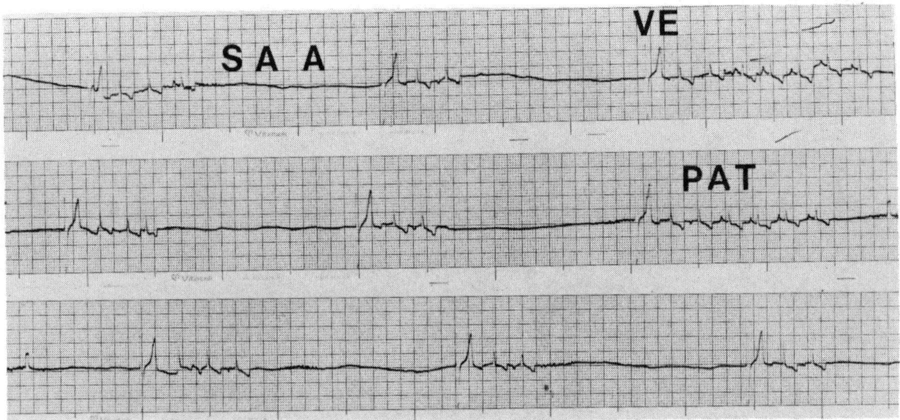

Fig. 21-6. Sinoatrial arrests (*SA A*) followed by ventricular escape beats (*VE*) and paroxysmal atrial tachycardia (*PAT*) in a 7-year-old female miniature schnauzer that was suffering from syncopal episodes.

Persistent Atrial Standstill

Persistent atrial standstill is a rare condition seen mostly in English springer spaniels.[1] Atrial hypoplasia is present to varying degrees, and sinoatrial node impulse conduction is absent. A junctional or ventricular escape rhythm maintains the ventricular rate at 40 to 60 beats per minute. P waves are persistently absent from the electrocardiogram.

HEART BLOCK

A variety of factors may affect propagation of cardiac impulses, particularly in depressed tissues. Thus, decremental conduction is likely to develop in the presence of a lower level of membrane potential and a slower rate of rise of phase 0 depolarization. These conditions can occur in any fibers showing incomplete repolarization or partial depolarization caused by various pathophysiologic factors. Fibers of the atrioventricular node (and possibly of the bundle of His) show the above characteristics even under physiologic conditions; therefore, decremental conduction is common in these tissues. Cardiac glycosides, hypokalemia, and ischemia enhance the degree of decremental conduction and thus may impair atrioventricular conduction, leading to heart block.

Advanced Heart Blocks

Advanced second-degree (Fig. 21-7) and complete (third-degree) (Fig. 21-8) atrioventricular heart block results in bradycardia. The ventricular rate of advanced second-degree heart block depends on the severity of the block (*i.e.*, 2 : 1, 3 : 1, 4 : 1, etc.) and the inherent sinoatrial rate. Thus, a 2 : 1 second-degree block associated with a sinus rate of 120 beats per minute results in a ventricular

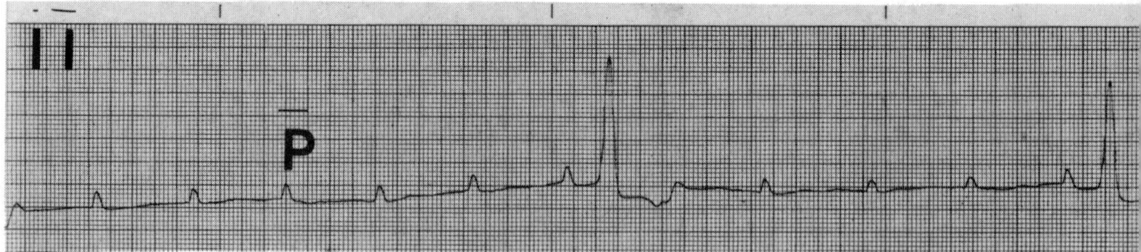

Fig. 21-7. Advanced second-degree atrioventricular (AV) heart block in a 10-year-old male cocker spaniel that was weak and lethargic. The sinus rate is 160/minute, while that of the ventricles is 40/minute. Notice that there is a consistent and normal PR interval preceding each R wave. Thus, the diagnosis of second-degree AV block is made. The R wave is of excessive duration, indicating that the block is below the AV node (type B block). This specific type of second-degree AV block often does not respond to atropine and may progress to complete heart block, as was the case in this dog.

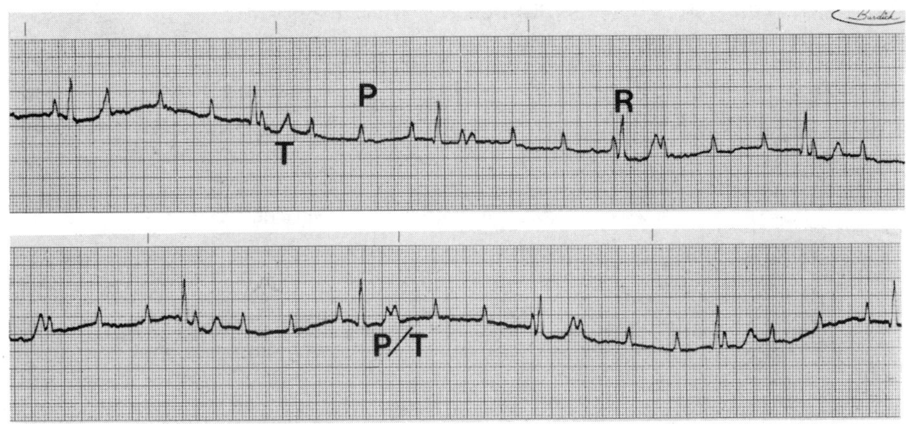

Fig. 21-8. Complete (third-degree) AV block in a 7-year-old English bulldog that was lethargic. Mitral and tricuspid valve endocardiosis and extensive ventricular fibrosis were present. There are no PR relationships; thus, the diagnosis of complete heart block was made. The sinus rate is 200/minute, while the ventricular rate is 60/minute.

rate of 60 beats per minute. A 3 : 1 block with a sinus rate of 180 beats per minute also produces a ventricular rate of 60 beats per minute.

Advanced (high-degree) second-degree atrioventricular heart blocks in dogs are most often associated with idiopathic myocardial fibrosis and mitral valve insufficiency in older, small, brachycephalic breeds. Such conduction disturbances are often precipitated or complicated by digoxin therapy. In the cat, advanced second-degree heart block is usually associated with hypertrophic cardiomyopathy. Electrolyte disturbances (hyperkalemia), hypoxemia, and hypercarbia from any cause can produce heart blocks.

Complete heart block results in a ventricular rate of 40 to 65 beats per minute. Complete heart block is usually associated with idiopathic myocardial fibrosis and mitral valve insufficiency in brachycephalic dog breeds and Cocker spaniels. In cats, complete heart block is usually the result of hypertrophic cardiomyopathy. Hyperkalemia may result in complete heart block.

ARRHYTHMIAS NOT PRODUCING ABNORMAL RATES

Some cardiac arrhythmias can result in rhythm disturbances without producing either a tachycardia or a bradycardia (Table 21-7). The physiologic, pathologic, and drug associations of these arrhythmias parallel those of more advanced arrhythmias of similar etiologies. Pulse deficits are common with premature contractions, while pauses are associated with ventricular premature contractions, sinoatrial arrest (or block), and simple second-degree heart block (one block of the antegrade sinoatrial impulse at the atrioventricular node and bundle of His occurs sporadically).

Table 21-7. Cardiac Rhythm Disturbances, Which May or May Not Be Associated With Tachycardia or Bradycardia, and Common Associations

ARRHYTHMIA	ASSOCIATION(S)
Sinus arrhythmia	Normal variation Inherent vagal tone Bradycardia possible Brachycephalic breeds
Supraventricular premature contractions	See Tables 21-1, 21-4, and 21-5.
Ventricular premature contractions	See Tables 21-1 and 21-6.
Sinoatrial block or arrest	Normal variation Exaggerated vagal tone Bradycardia possible See Table 21-1 and Classification of Bradycardia
Simple second-degree AV block	See Table 21-1 and Classification of Bradycardia

ABNORMALITIES OF THE PULSE

The arterial pressure pulse is produced by ejection of blood from the left ventricle into the great arteries at a rate faster than its runoff into the peripheral circulation. Although the peak rate of ejection of blood occurs prior to the peak pressure in the left ventricle or aorta, the pressure continues to rise in the aorta as long as blood is ejected into the aorta faster than it runs off into the peripheral arteries.

The form of the venous pressure pulse is determined by the rate of the blood return from the peripheral tissues into the venous segment, the pressure-volume characteristics of the segment of vein, the nature of the resistance to flow, the distensibility of the right atrium and ventricle, and the tissue overlying the veins at the point of observation. Although the venous pressure pulse wave travels peripherally away from the heart, there is at the same time a venous blood flow in the opposite direction toward the heart.

Arterial Pulse

The arterial pulse wave at any site is influenced by many factors, including the left ventricular stroke volume, the rate of ejection, the compliance of the aorta and large arteries, the peripheral vascular resistance, the heart rate, the systolic and diastolic blood pressures, the distance from the heart, the blood viscosity, and the size and pressure-volume characteristics of the artery.

The arterial pressure pulse enters the proximal aorta and travels distally at a velocity many times faster than maximum blood flow. The pressure wave is accompanied by a traveling wave distending the arterial wall; the pulse wave velocity increases as arterial wall distensibility diminishes. This increased velocity normally occurs distally as the arteries branch into smaller channels and their walls become stiffer.

The usual technique for palpating the arterial pulse is to press with the examining finger until the maximum pulse is sensed. The pulse is felt as changing displacement superimposed on the "baseline" displacement produced by compressing the artery.

The arterial pressure is divided into two phases: systole and diastole. Arterial pressure begins with the opening of the aortic valve and rapid ejection of blood into the aorta. This is followed by runoff of blood from the proximal aorta to the peripheral arteries. The arterial pressure waveform is characterized by a sharp rise in pressure followed by a decline in pressure. Diastole follows closure of the aortic valve and continues to the next systole. During this time, runoff to the peripheral arteries occurs without further flow from the left ventricle. The lowest point of diastole (end-diastole) is referred to as the arterial diastolic pressure. The systolic arterial pressure rise occurs immediately after ventricular depolarization, that is, after the QRS complex of the electrocardiogram (Fig. 21-9).

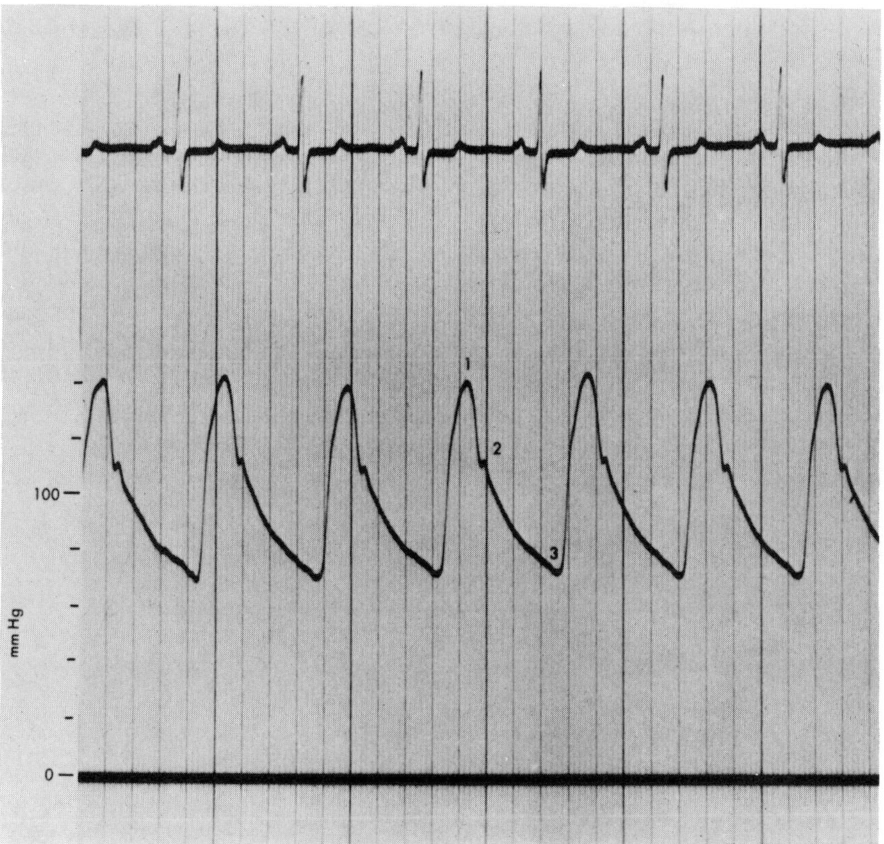

Fig. 21-9. Normal arterial pressure waveform. *1*, arterial systolic pressure (140 mm Hg); *2*, dicrotic notch; *3*, arterial end-diastolic pressure (72 mm Hg). The dicrotic notch coincides with aortic valve closure as the blood flow in the aorta temporarily reverses direction and blood pressure decreases.

Hyperkinetic Pulse

Large, bounding (hyperkinetic) arterial pulses usually indicate the rapid ejection of an increased volume of blood from the left ventricle. Commonly, the arterial pulse pressure is increased and the peripheral arterial resistance is diminished. The hyperdynamic arterial pulse is sometimes referred to in terms that describe a particular component of the pulse wave. Thus, the "water-hammer pulse," named after a Victorian toy, refers to an extremely rapid, forceful ascending limb of the arterial pulse wave. By contrast, "collapsing pulse" refers to a quick, marked decrease in the arterial pulse wave following its peak.

Hyperkinetic arterial pulses occur during exercise, fever, cardiac diseases associated with increased stroke volume, and marked bradycardia with increased stroke volume. A hyperdynamic pulse also occurs when abnormally rapid runoff of blood from the arterial system occurs (Table 21-8).

A hypokinetic (small, weak) arterial pulse may be present in patients with diminished left ventricular stroke volume (Table 21-9). Hypokinetic pulses are commonly associated with advanced mitral valve disease and left-sided congestive heart failure in the dog and congestive cardiomyopathy in the dog and cat.

Pulsus Alternans

Pulsus alternans is a characteristic pulse pattern in which the beats occur at regular intervals but in which there is a regular attenuation of the pulse pressure. Pulsus alternans is seen in association with ventricular bigeminy and myocardial failure. In congestive cardiomyopathy, it is postulated that alteration of the contractile state of at least part of the myocardium, which may be caused by the failure of electrochemical coupling in some cells during weaker contractions, can produce sustained pulsus alternans. Echocardiographic examination reveals alternating greater and lesser left ventricular shortening fractions. Pulsus alternans may be better appreciated on a peripheral rather than a carotid artery. The patient's respirations should be held since changes in arterial pressure may be produced by respiration.

Table 21-8. Causes and Associations of Hyperdynamic (Hyperkinetic) Pulses

CAUSE	ASSOCIATION(S)
Physiologic	Exercise Fever
Increased stroke volume	Hyperthyroidism Aortic regurgitation (insufficiency)
Bradycardia	Sinus bradycardia Advanced and complete heart blocks
Rapid runoff	Patent ductus arteriosus Peripheral arteriovenous fistulas Aortic regurgitation (insufficiency)

Table 21-9. Pulse Abnormalities and Associated Conditions

PULSE TYPE	ASSOCIATION(S)
Pulsus bisferiens	Aortic regurgitation (insufficiency)
	Aortic valve bacterial endocarditis
	Aortic stenosis with aortic regurgitation
	Patent ductus arteriosus
	Feline hypertrophic obstructed cardiomyopathy
Hypokinetic	Congestive cardiomyopathy
	Mitral valve insufficiency
	Aortic valve stenosis
	Hypovolemia
	Shock
Pulsus alternans	Ventricular bigeminy
	Dilated congestive cardiomyopathy
Pulsus paradoxus	Pericardial tamponade

Pulse Deficit

Pulse deficits can occur with various types of cardiac rhythm disturbances. Supraventricular or ventricular premature contractions (extrasystoles) may be associated with no pulse, a small amplitude pulse, or a normal pulse depending upon the timing and whether the left-ventricular pressure generated is able to open the aortic valve. The arterial pulse following a ventricular premature contraction may be enhanced because of decreased aortic impedence, increase left ventricular filling (compensatory pause), and augmented contractility (post-extrasystolic augmentation). Pulse deficits are commonly associated with ventricular tachycardia and atrial fibrillation.

Venous Pulse

The evaluation of the venous pulse is an integral part of the physical examination since the venous pulse reflects both the right atrial pressure and the hemodynamic events in the right atrium. Factors influencing the right atrial and central venous pressure include the total blood volume, the distribution of blood volume, and right atrial contraction. The two main objectives of examining the jugular veins are the estimation of the central venous pressure and the inspection of the wave form. Clipping of the hair, wetting the jugular furrow, and shining a light across the skin overlying the jugular vein enhance the detection of the jugular pulse. The patient should be relaxed and placed in recumbancy with the trunk inclined to various degrees.

The difference between venous distention and venous pressure must be considered. Veins may be markedly dilated with minimal increase in pressure or may not be visibly distended despite a very high venous pressure. Increased venous pressure may be detected with the patient in lateral recumbancy. The saphenous vein is visualized and the extremity is slowly and passively elevated

Table 21-10. Causes of Elevation of Jugular Vein Pressure and Jugular Pulses

CAUSE	ASSOCIATIONS

Right-sided congestive heart failure	Pulmonic stenosis (congenital)
	Tricuspid insufficiency
	  Congenital
	  Acquired
	Cardiomyopathies
	Cor pulmonale
	  Chronic pulmonary disease
	Pulmonary hypertension
	  Heartworm disease
	  Chronic mitral insufficiency

Right-ventricular inflow obstruction	Pericardial effusion
	  Idiopathic
	  Pericarditis
	    Idiopathic
	    Infectious
	  Neoplastic
	Pericardial constriction
	  Neoplastic
	Heart base tumor
	Intracardiac tumor
	  Right atrial myxoma
	  Sarcoma

from a dependent position. The vein should collapse at a level nearly parallel to the thoracic inlet (approximate level of the right atrium).

Distention of the jugular veins, the presence of a jugular pulse, and elevation of the jugular venous pressure are most often produced by right-sided congestive heart failure (Table 21-10). Right ventricular inflow obstruction may also produce elevation of the jugular venous pulse.

Cannon "a" waves are jugular pulses that occur when the right atrium contracts while the tricuspid valve is closed during right ventricular systole. They are associated with cardiac rhythm disturbances such as ventricular premature contractions, ventricular tachycardia, and complete heart block. Cannon "a" waves may occur in the presence or absence of right-sided congestive heart failure.

REFERENCES

1. Agostini E: Functional and histologic studies of the vagus nerve and its branches of the heart, lungs and abdominal viscera in the cat. J Physiol 135:182–185, 1957
2. Anderson MI, Castillo J: Cardiac innervation and synaptic transmission in the heart. In DeMellow WC (ed): Electrical Phenomena in the Heart. New York, Academic Press, 1972
3. Armour JA, Randall WC: Functional anatomy of canine cardiac nerves. Acta Anat 9:510–528, 1975

4. Baird JA, Robb JS: Study, reconstruction and dissection of the atrioventricular conducting system of the dog heart. Anat Sec 108:747–751, 1950
5. Berne RM, Levy MN: Cardiovascular Physiology. St Louis, CV Mosby, 1977
6. Kaye MP, Geesbrecht JM, Randall WC: Distribution of autonomic fibers to the canine heart. Am J Physiol 218:1025–1029, 1970
7. Liu SK, Tilly LP, Tushjian RJ: Lesions of the conduction system in the cat with cardiomyopathy. Recent Adv Stud Cardiac Struct Metab 10:681–693, 1975
8. Mizeres NJ: The anatomy of the autonomic nervous system in the dog. Am J Anat 96:290–926, 1966
9. Muir WW: Effects of atropine on cardiac rate and rhythm in dogs. J Am Vet Med Assoc 172:917–921, 1978
10. Myerberg RJ, Nillsson K, Celband H: Physiology of canine intraventricular conduction and endocardial excitation. Circ Res 30:217–243, 1972
11. Patterson DF, Detweiler DK, Hubben K, et al: Spontaneous abnormal cardiac arrhythmias and conduction disturbances in the dog. Am J Vet Res 22:355–369, 1961
12. Tilley LP: Essentials of Canine and Feline Electrocardiography, pp 164, 165, 371. Philadelphia, Lea & Febiger, 1985
13. Tilley LP: Transtelephonic analysis of cardiac arrhythymias in the dog. Vet Clin North Am 13:395–408, 1983
14. Truex RC, Smythe MQ: Comparative morphology of the cardiac conduction tissue in animals. Ann NY Acad Sci 127:19–33, 1965
15. Uhley HN, Rivkin L: Peripheral distribution of the canine A-V conduction system: Observations on gross morphology. Am J Cardiol 5:688–698, 1960

22

Heart Murmurs

CLAY A. CALVERT

PROBLEM DEFINITION AND RECOGNITION

Murmurs are audible successive sounds with distinct duration, as opposed to normal heart sounds, which are short transitory events. Cardiac murmurs result from turbulence created in laminar blood flow.[16] When the flow velocity of fluid within a pipe exceeds a certain value, turbulence develops and energy is dissipated, which generates audible vibrations. Turbulence may also arise when fluid passes through a small hole in a plate that partially occludes a pipe, when the pipe diameter changes abruptly, or when a jet of fluid strikes a surface. A critical level of turbulence must be achieved to produce a sound that is clinically evident. The characteristics of the murmur depend upon the velocity of blood flow and the surrounding structures that are caused to vibrate. Blood velocity and blood density variations can also produce turbulence within the heart and arteries.

CLASSIFICATION

Heart murmurs may be classified as (1) innocent, (2) functional, or (3) pathologic (Table 22-1). It is useful to categorize murmurs (Table 22-2) according to their timing in the cardiac cycle (Table 22-3). Accordingly, murmurs are identified as being systolic, diastolic, or continuous. A second aspect of the description of a heart murmur is its intensity (Table 22-4).[6] Unfortunately, murmur intensity does not necessarily indicate flow volume. Thus, although a very small jet does not usually generate a loud murmur, torrential flow through a large hole, as in a large ventricular septal defect, occasionally produces no murmur. The ear perceives higher-frequency noises as being louder than those of the same amplitude but of lower frequency. Third, the pitch or frequency of the murmur over each of the heart valves and at the thoracic inlet should be characterized. The fourth aspect of the characterization of a murmur is the modulation or shape of the

Table 22-1. Classification of Heart Murmurs and Examples

CLASSIFICATION	CHARACTERISTIC		
	Intensity	Frequency	Association
Innocent	I/VI–II/VI	Medium	Systolic ejection Puppies, kittens Thin-chested dogs
Functional	I/VI–III/VI	Medium to high	Systolic ejection Anemia Tachycardia Fever Hyperthyroidism High cardiac output
Pathologic	I/VI–VI/VI	Low to High	Congenital heart defects Acquired valvular disease Aortic outflow tract obstruction Systolic anterior mitral valve motion

Table 22-2. Description of Cardiac Murmurs Based on Auscultatory Criteria

CRITERIA	CHARACTERIZATION
Timing	Systole Diastole Continuous
Intensity	I/VI–VI/VI
Frequency (pitch)	Low Medium High Mixed
Modulation (shape)	Plateau Crescendo–decrescendo (diamond-shaped) Decrescendo
Location	Variable

Table 22-3. Cardiac Murmurs Based on Location Within the Cardiac Cycle (Timing) and Character (Modulation)

TIMING	MODULATION	ASSOCIATIONS
Systolic	Crescendo–decrescendo (diamond-shaped, ejection murmur)	Congenital pulmonic stenosis Congenital aortic stenosis Innocent murmurs
	Plateau holosystolic	Mitral regurgitation (insufficiency) Tricuspid regurgitation (insufficiency) Ventricular septal defect Functional
Diastolic	Decrescendo	Aortic regurgitation (insufficiency) Aortic valve bacterial endocarditis Secondary to chronic aortic stenosis Secondary to a high ventricular septal defect

Table 22-4. Classification of Cardiac Murmurs by Degree of Intensity

INTENSITY (GRADE)	DESCRIPTION
I/VI	Barely audible
II/VI	Audible after a few seconds of auscultation, low intensity
III/VI	Immediately audible, moderate intensity
IV/VI	Loud intensity without a precordial thrill
V/VI	Loud intensity with a precordial thrill
VI/VI	Loudest intensity, precordial thrill, audible with stethoscope slightly away from thoracic wall

murmur (Fig. 22-1). Although the holosystolic plateau murmur of mitral insufficiency (regurgitation) is relatively easy to recognize, not all plateau or ejection (crescendo–decrescendo or diamond-shaped) murmurs are easily discerned. A phonocardiogram is necessary to confirm the modulation of many murmurs. Last, the location of the murmur where the intensity is loudest and the area of radiation should be succinctly described. The classification of systolic murmurs[10] into systolic ejection murmurs and holosystolic (regurgitant systolic) murmurs is of clinical value.

PATHOPHYSIOLOGY

Systolic ejection murmurs imply turbulent blood flow at the time of right or left ventricular ejection into its corresponding great artery. They are typical of the murmurs produced by congenital aortic and pulmonic stenosis. The origin of such murmurs is likely to be along the ventricular outflow at the semilunar valve level or at the immediate artery (pulmonary or aorta). Since actual blood flow is an essential ingredient to the genesis of turbulence responsible for the murmurs, the murmur begins after semilunar valve opening and ends upon cessation of flow with the closure of the same semilunar valve. Such murmurs are crescendo–descrescendo or diamond-shaped (see Fig. 22-1, *B*).

Holosystolic or regurgitant systolic murmurs, that is, those associated with mitral or tricuspid valve regurgitation (insufficiency), begin as soon as the atrioventricular valve closes and continue beyond semilunar valve closure. Because

Fig. 22-1. (*A*) Phonocardiogram of a holosystolic, plateau murmur (*M*). The intensity of the murmur is constant between the first (*1*) and second (*2*) heart sounds. Holosystolic, plateau murmurs are associated with atrioventricular valvular insufficiencies and ventricular septal defects. (*B*) Phonocardiogram of a crescendo-decrescendo (diamond shaped) or ejection murmur (*M*). Such murmurs are associated with semilunar valve stenosis, usually congenital pulmonic or aortic valve stenosis. *1,* first heart sound; *2,* second heart sound. ▶

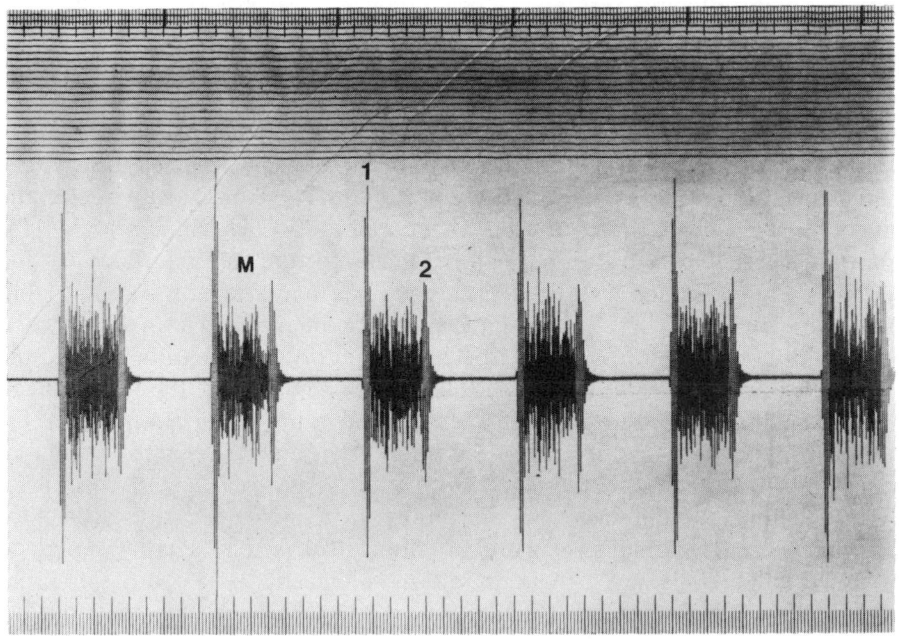

A

M 2

B

the pressure difference (gradient) between ventricle and recipient chamber (atrium) is considerable throughout systole, the murmur tends to have an even or plateau configuration (see Fig. 22-1, *A*). A holosystolic murmur is also typical of ventricular septal defect.

Innocent systolic ejection murmurs are produced by normal turbulent flow through the proximal great arteries at the time of ventricular ejection.[11] The intensity of the murmur, as influenced by stroke volume or velocity of ejection, and proximity of the great arteries to the chest wall determine whether the murmur is audible with the stethoscope. Such murmurs are typically heard in puppies, kittens, young lean dogs, and when a tachycardia exists. Puppies, kittens, and young lean dogs tend to have a brisk circulation and a smaller thoracic cage with a narrow transverse diameter. The murmur tends to be of medium frequency, peaks in early to mid-systole, usually ends before the second heart sound, and is best heard on the left side over the mitral or aortic valve or at the thoracic inlet. The murmur may be the result of turbulent flow into the pulmonary artery,[3] aorta,[17] or both.

Functional systolic murmurs are produced by increased velocity of blood within the cardiovascular system and by extracardiac factors.[6] Pleural or pericardial effusion, anemia, fever, hyperthyroidism, and tachycardia of any cause may produce functional murmurs. Such murmurs are often detected during anesthesia when a sinus tachycardia exists due to atropine administration.

Decreased blood viscosity and increased velocity of blood flow produce turbulence if the blood hemoglobin levels falls below 6 mg/dl (packed cell volume is usually less than 15% to 20%). The functional murmur of anemia is usually of low intensity and high frequency and occurs during early to mid systole. Anemic murmurs are best heard over the mitral valve or aortic valve area.[4,6]

Functional murmurs may be audible when high cardiac output states exist. Chronic anemia can lead to increased cardiac output, although the exact pathophysiology is not completely understood. The increased cardiac output is produced by both tachycardia and increased stroke volume. Reduction of blood viscosity is an important aspect of the increased cardiac output of anemia,[7] as is decreased peripheral resistance.[5] Thyrotoxicosis is characterized by an increased cardiac output. There is probably a direct effect of thyroid hormone upon the heart, producing a tachycardia. In addition, there is an increased sensitivity to circulating catecholamines and there may also be a decreased peripheral vascular resistance.[9,12,18]

Murmurs in diastole are unusual and occur in dogs and cats most often across the aortic valve. The murmur of aortic regurgitation (insufficiency) strongly implies the presence of aortic valvular bacterial endocarditis. The murmur begins immediately after aortic valve closure (second heart sound) and is usually of high frequency, with a decrescendo configuration (Fig. 22-2).

Continuous murmurs extend from systole into diastole. Such a murmur results from blood flow continuing from a high-pressure to a lower-pressure area despite semilunar valve closure. Patent ductus arteriosus is the prototype,

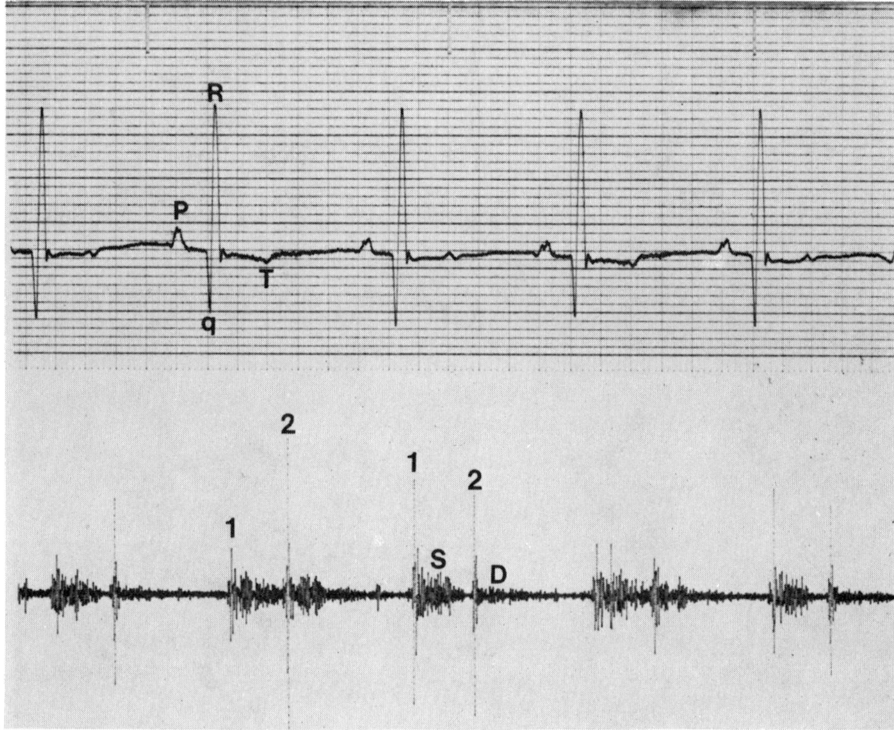

Fig. 22-2. Decrescendo murmur (*D*) resulting from aortic valvular regurgitation (insufficiency) in a 5-year-old male German shepherd with bacterial endocarditis. A systolic murmur (*S*) is also present and is the result of blood turbulence created by vegetations on the aortic valve. *1,* first heart sound; *2,* second heart sound.

and only common example in dogs and cats, of a continuous murmur that peaks in intensity at the second heart rate (Fig. 22-3).

CLINICAL ASSOCIATIONS

Mitral Insufficiency

The murmur of mitral insufficiency (regurgitation) is of mixed frequency and is usually harsh in character (Table 22-5). It is best ausculted from the mitral valve area to the left, caudal sternal border. Loud murmurs (IV/VI–VI/VI) are audible on the right thoracic wall and are difficult to distinguish in that location from concomitant tricuspid insufficiency. Occasionally these murmurs have a musical, high-frequency quality. The louder intensity mitral insufficiencies (IV/VI–VI/VI) do not necessarily correlate to the severity of valvular dysfunction. The first heart sound is often accentuated[8] and the second heart sound may be

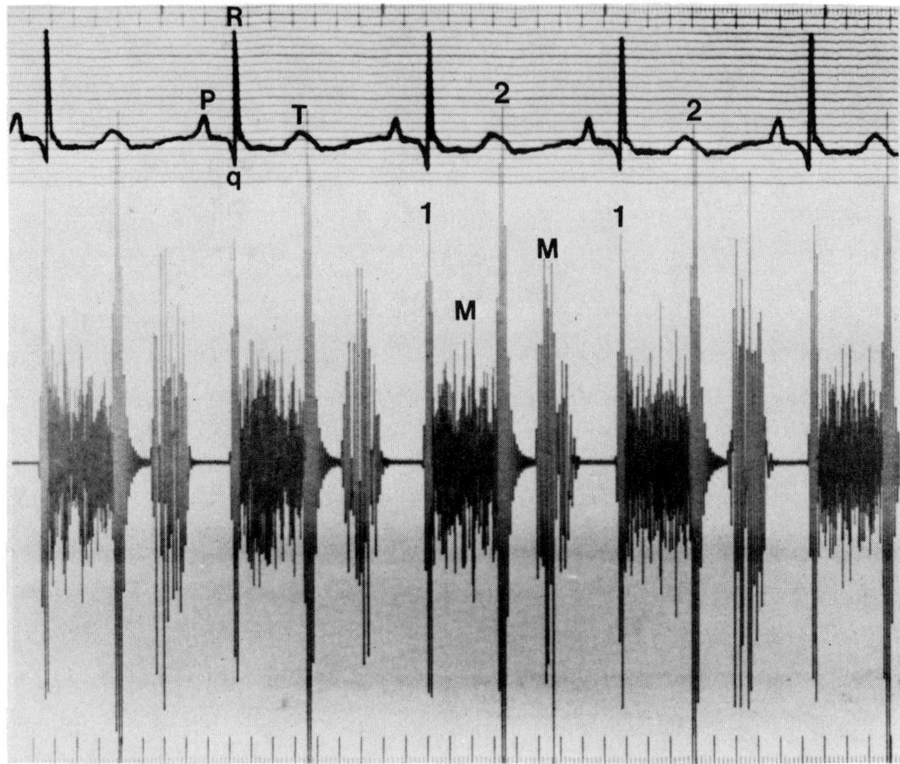

Fig. 22-3. Continuous murmur (*M*) associated with congenital patent ductus arteriosus. *1,* first heart sound; *2,* second heart sound.

difficult to detect (Fig. 22-4). Mitral insufficiency produces a sequential volume overload, dilatation and eccentric hypertrophy of the left ventricle, left atrial enlargement, pulmonary venous hypertension, and pulmonary edema (left-sided congestive heart failure). Eventually, pulmonary arterial hypertension with bilateral congestive heart failure may occur. By far, the most common clinical cause of mitral insufficiency is endocardiosis (fibrosis, polysaccharidosis) of the mitral valve of unknown etiology in middle-aged to older miniature, toy, small, and chondrodysplatic breeds, beagles, and spaniels.

Pulmonic Stenosis

The systolic ejection murmur of congenital pulmonic stenosis is best ausculted over the pulmonic valve area. The murmur is high frequency, and its intensity correlates with the degree of stenosis. The intensity of this crescendo–decrescendo murmur tends to peak early with mild stenosis and late with more severe stenosis. A palpable thrill is often detected over the left anterioventral precardium. The second heart sound is often split, but a phonocardiogram may be

Table 22-5. Characteristics of Cardiac Murmurs and Their Associations

MURMUR	TIMING	FREQUENCY	INTENSITY	MODULATION	ASSOCIATIONS*
Mitral insufficiency	Systolic	Mixed	Variable	Plateau (holosystolic)	Acquired in small breed dogs, spaniels, beagles, and chondrodysplastic breeds Congenital in large breed dogs, especially Great Danes Mitral valvular bacterial endocarditis Dilated congestive cardiomyopathy in cats and dogs Hypertrophic cardiomyopathy in cats Dysplasia (congenital) in cats
Pulmonic stenosis	Systolic	High	Variable	Crescendo–decrescendo	Congenital
Aortic stenosis	Systolic	High	Variable	Crescendo–decrescendo	Congenital
Patent ductus arteriosus	Continuous	Mixed	IV/VI–VI/VI	Crescendo–decrescendo	Congenital
Tricuspid insufficiency	Systolic	Mixed	Variable	Plateau (holosystolic)	Acquired in small breeds, especially dachsunds, and usually coexists with mitral insufficiency Acquired in Doberman pinschers Congenital in large breed dogs Congenital (dysplasia) in cats
Ventricular septal defect	Systolic	Mixed	Variable	Plateau (holosystolic)	Usually asymptomatic Common in dogs and cats Frequently associated with atrioventricular valvular defects in cats
Aortic insufficiency	Diastolic	High	I/VI–III/VI	Decrescendo	Aortic valve bacterial endocarditis Secondary to aortic stenosis and ventricular septal defects

* Most common associated conditions

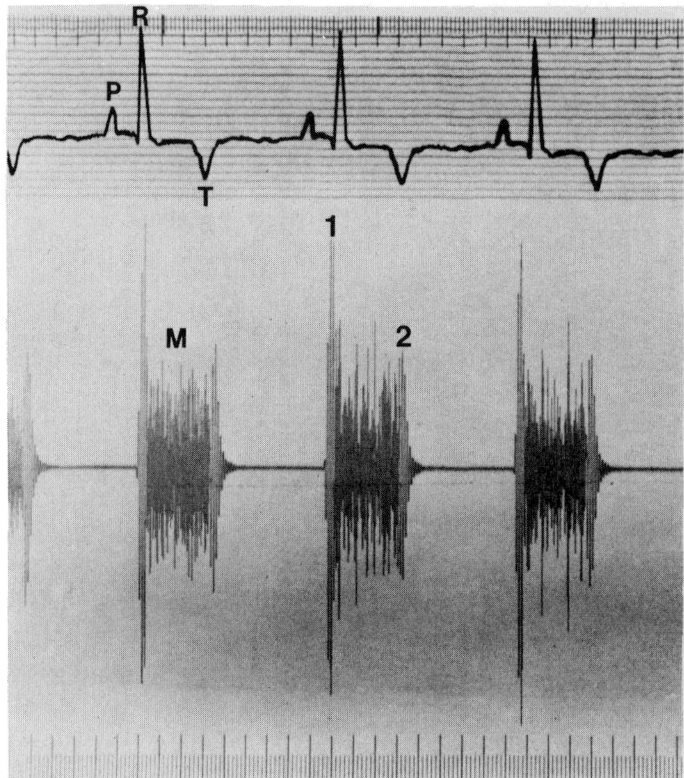

Fig. 22-4. Holosystolic (plateau) murmur (*M*) of mitral valvular insufficiency (regurgitation). Such murmurs are most often associated with valvular endocardiosis (fibrosis) in middle- and old-aged toy, miniature, and chondrodysplastic breeds, as well as beagles and spaniels. The valvular pathlogy is progressive, and left-sided congestive heart failure often occurs after several years. Tricuspid valvular insufficiency often occurs concomitantly.

required for detection since the murmur may obscure the second heart sound.[14] Congenital pulmonic stenosis occurs most often in English bulldogs, terriers, chihuahuas, miniature schnauzers, and brachycephalic breeds. Pulmonic stenosis is uncommon in cats. Clinically significant pulmonic stenosis is associated with electrocardiographic evidence of right ventricular hypertrophy. Radiographic evidence of a poststenotic dilation of the main pulmonary artery segment may be present. Decreased exercise tolerance, syncope, and right-sided congestive heart failure are the consequences of severe pulmonic stenosis. Heart failure, when it occurs, usually does so between the ages of 1 and 3 years.

Aortic Stenosis

The systolic ejection murmur of aortic stenosis is most audible over the aortic valve, although the murmur radiates along the aorta and is audible over the right cranioventral thoracic wall. A thrill is often palpable over the left cranial precordium. The murmur is usually detectable at the thoracic inlet and may be traced along the course of the carotid arteries to the angle of the mandible and, in some cases, to the top of the cranium. This congenital cardiac defect occurs most commonly in large breed dogs such as the Newfoundland, boxer, and German shepherd. It is also a relatively common defect in cats. Affected animals may remain asymptomatic, but many develop left-sided congestive heart failure between the ages of 3 and 6 years. Episodic weakness and sudden death are common in the Newfoundland dog and other breeds.[13,15] Atrial fibrillation may occur in middle-aged dogs due to secondary mitral insufficiency and left atrial enlargement. Radiographic and electrocardiographic evidence of chamber enlargement are uncommon until the patient reaches middle age. A poststenotic dilatation of the aorta may be seen radiographically.

A murmur of subaortic stenosis may be produced by left ventricular systolic outflow obstruction in some cats with hypertrophic cardiomyopathy.

Patent Ductus Arteriosus

The murmur of congenital patent ductus arteriosus (machinery-like murmur) is most audible over the aortic valve area, although this murmur is often audible over the entire thoracic wall. Often only a systolic murmur is detected over the left caudoventral thorax; the diastolic humming portion of the murmur may be only detected over the heart base on the left side. This murmur is usually audible at the thoracic inlet and frequently radiates up the carotid arteries. Breeds of dogs most often affected are the miniature and toy poodle, collie, Shetland sheepdog, Pomeranian, and German shepherd. This congenital defect is also relatively common in cats.

Patent ductus arteriosus produces a volume overload and subsequent enlargement of the left atrium and left ventricle. The electrocardiogram may be normal or reflect left atrial or ventricular enlargement. Lateral thoracic radiographs are characterized by enlargement of the cardiac silhouette, elevation of the trachea, and left atrial enlargement. The right ventricle is often enlarged and the cranial waist may be absent due to the widened aortic arch. Since the defect produces left-to-right shunting of blood, the right cranial lobar pulmonary artery is often larger than the corresponding vein. Severe pulmonary overcirculation is sometimes indicated by increased linear caudal lung lobe densities produced by enlarged arteries and veins. The dorsoventral radiograph typically reveals an elongated cardiac silhouette, partly due to the enlarged aortic arch. The right cranial border of the cardiac silhouette is characterized by enlargements of the descending aortic arch, main pulmonary artery segment, and left atrium.

Patent ductus arteriosus, if not surgically corrected, almost always produces left-sided congestive heart failure (coughing, exercise intolerance, dyspnea, pulmonary edema) before 3 years of age and often before 1 year of age.

Tricuspid Insufficiency

Tricuspid insufficiency (regurgitation) is usually detected in association with mitral insufficiency in middle-aged to old small breed and chondrodysplastic breeds. The dachshund often develops tricuspid insufficiency without an audible mitral valve murmur. Although right-sided congestive heart failure may develop, left-sided congestive heart failure is more commonly associated with this disorder because of concomitant mitral valve disease. Congenital tricuspid valve insufficiency, which is most common in large breed dogs such as Doberman pinschers, setters, and retrievers, often results in right-sided congestive heart failure.

Radiographic abnormalities associated with tricuspid valve insufficiency are right atrial and right ventricular enlargement. The electrocardiogram is often normal but may reveal high-voltage P waves (>0.4 mV in leads II and aVF) or, occasionally, evidence of right-ventricular enlargement. In large breed dogs with congenital tricuspid insufficiency, large Q waves are common and may produce a right axis deviation.

Aortic Insufficiency

The murmur of aortic insufficiency occurs during early diastole and is difficult to hear in most instances. This murmur is seldom loud and is most difficult to detect in the presence of a tachycardia. A phonocardiogram is often useful in confirming the presence of this murmur. Aortic insufficiency is most often detected in association with bacterial endocarditis affecting at least the aortic valve (Fig. 22-5). Congenital aortic stenosis is often associated with a mild aortic insufficiency, and the latter may be progressive as chronic blood flow turbulence produces abnormalities of the valve cusp margins. A high ventricular septal defect (most common type) may also result in a mild aortic insufficiency due to a loss of septal support of the septal leaflet of the aortic valve, resulting in a sagging effect.

Aortic insufficiency associated with bacterial endocarditis usually produces severe, intractable left-sided congestive heart failure. Aortic insufficiency secondary to aortic stenosis or ventricular septal defect usually does not result in clinical deterioration.

DIAGNOSTIC PLAN

The minimum data base for patients with cardiac murmurs is a complete physical examination and characterization of the murmur (timing, intensity, location, modulation). If the murmur is considered to be due to anemia or pathologic conditions, then the data base is extended (Table 22-6). The possibility of a

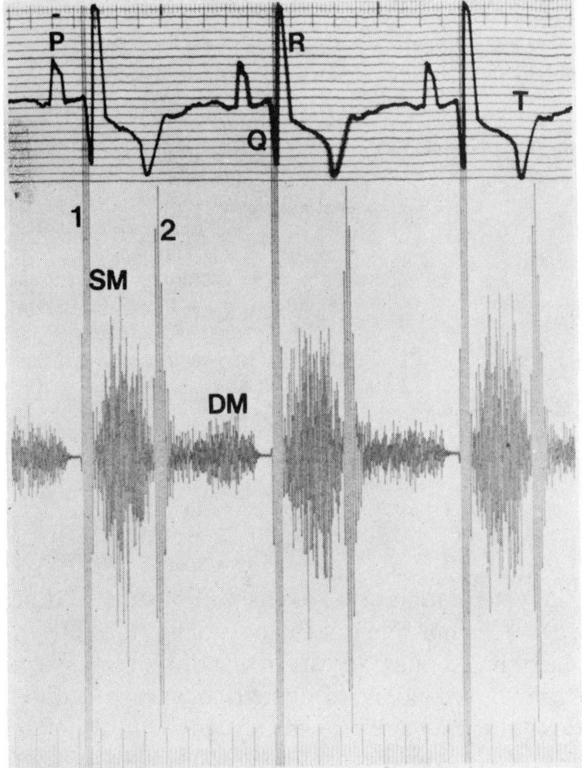

Fig. 22-5. Diastolic murmur (*DM*) associated with aortic valvular insufficiency (regurgitation). A systolic murmur (*SM*) is also present and may be due to blood flow turbulence caused by vegetations on the aortic and/or mitral valve leaflets. *1,* first heart sound; *2,* second heart sound.

cardiac murmur being due to a high cardiac output state (anemia, hyperthyroidism) depends on the history and physical examination findings.

If the cardiac murmur is felt to be pathologic, then the first steps that are indicated to generate a rank-ordered rule-out list are to consider the epizootiologic factors pertaining to the patient and to characterize the murmur. The age, breed (or type of dog), and historic evidence of a preexisting murmur should be assessed (Tables 22-7 and 22-8). Most puppies, kittens, and young dogs with loud murmurs (IV/VI–VI/VI) have a congenital heart defect. Most middle-aged to old small or miniature dog breeds, chondrodysplastic breeds, beagles, and spaniels with heart murmurs have acquired mitral valvular insufficiency, often with concomitant tricuspid valvular insufficiency. However, even middle-aged dogs of any breed or type may have a congenital defect, and the client may or may not be aware of its presence; therefore, such a history should be ascertained. Unfortunately, because of incomplete physical examinations or poor skill

Table 22-6. Minimum Data Base for Patients With Cardiac Murmurs

MURMUR INTENSITY	SUSPECTED ETIOLOGY	DATA BASE
I/VI–III/VI	Innocent	Sequential physical examination
	Functional	Sequential physical examination CBC, serum chemistry profile, UA if indicated by physical or historic findings
	Pathologic	CBC, serum chemistry profile, UA Thoracic radiographs Electrocardiogram Special tests*
IV/VI–VI/VI	Pathologic	As above

* Phonocardiogram, echocardiogram, nonselective angiogram, selective cardiac catheterization
CBC, complete blood count; UA, urine analysis

on the part of the veterinarian, the absence of a history of a heart murmur in animals of any age does not rule out the possibility of a congenital defect.

Giant and large breed dogs, 4 years of age or older, may develop murmurs of mitral insufficiency secondary to dilated congestive cardiomyopathy. Frequently, such dogs already manifest clinical signs of heart failure.

Dogs of any breed or type that are 7 to 9 years of age or older may develop a murmur of mitral insufficiency due to mitral valve endocardiosis (fibrosis).

Most commonly, heart murmurs associated with bacterial endocarditis are mitral in origin, but systolic aortic valve murmurs produced by vegetations and murmurs of aortic insufficiency are also common. The presence of a diastolic murmur should alert the clinician to the probability of bacterial endocarditis, especially when clinical and laboratory evidence is consistent with bacteremia.

Table 22-7. Common Rule Outs for Pathologic Heart Murmurs

AGE AND TYPE	MOST COMMON RULE OUTS
Puppies, kittens, young animals	Congenital
Adult	
Giant and large breed dogs	Cardiomyopathy (dilated congestive) Mitral insufficiency Tricuspid insufficiency Bacterial endocarditis
Small breed dog	Mitral insufficiency Tricuspid insufficiency Bacterial endocarditis
Cats	Cardiomyopathy Hyperthyroidism

Table 22-8. Differential Diagnosis of Common Disorders Associated With Pathologic Heart Murmurs

RULE OUT	MURMUR	TYPICAL BREED OR TYPE	AGE (USUAL)	POSSIBLE ASSOCIATED SIGNS	RADIOGRAPHIC[1] ABNORMALITIES	ECG[2] ABNORMALITIES
Acquired mitral valve endocardiosis	Holosystolic plateau	Toy, miniature, small, chondrodysplastic, spaniel, beagle	>7 yr	Asymptomatic Cough Exercise intolerance Dyspnea Crackles Syncope Ascites	↑ LA ↑ RCLPV Pulmonary edema Generalized cardiomegaly Chronic interstitial lung disease Collapsing trachea	None P > 0.04 sec ↑ LV SVPC VPC
Dilated congestive cardiomyopathy	Holosystolic plateau	Giant, Doberman pinscher, boxer, standard poodle, German shepherd, large dogs	>4 yr	Exercise intolerance Cough Dyspnea Crackles Syncope Pale mucous membranes Gallop heart rhythm Muffled heart, lung sounds Ascites Pulse deficits	Generalized cardiomegaly ↑ LA ↑ RCLPV Pulmonary edema Pleural effusion	P > 0.04 ↑ LV Atrial fibrillation VPC
Patent ductus arteriosus	Continuous (machinery)	Poodle, Shetland sheepdog, collie, German shepherd, many others	Puppy, kitten, young	None Exercise intolerance Cough Dyspnea Crackles	↑ LA ↑ RCLPA/V Pulmonary edema Elongated cardiac silhouette Aortic, pulmonic, LA bulges	None P > 0.04 sec ↑ LV

(Continued)

Table 22-8. Differential Diagnosis of Common Disorders Associated With Pathologic Heart Murmurs *(Continued)*

RULE OUT	MURMUR	TYPICAL BREED OR TYPE	AGE (USUAL)	POSSIBLE ASSOCIATED SIGNS	RADIOGRAPHIC[1] ABNORMALITIES	ECG[2] ABNORMALITIES
Pulmonic stenosis	Ejection (crescendo–decrescendo	Terrier, brachycephalic, miniature schnauzer, many others	Puppy, young	None Exercise intolerance Syncope Ascites	↑ RV ↑ Pulmonary artery segment	RVH
Bacterial endocarditis	Holosystolic or diastolic	Middle to large breeds	2–7 years	Fever ↑ WBC Monocytosis Lameness ↓ Albumin ↑ SAP Hypoglycemia	None Pulmonary edema Pneumonia	None VPC
Feline cardiomyopathy						
Hypertrophic	Systolic	Any	4–12 years	Dyspnea Gallop heart rhythm Crackles Rear limb monoparesis or paraparesis/paralysis	↑ LA–RA Pulmonary edema Pleural effusion (mild to moderate)	↑ Atria ↑ LV Atrial fibrillation SVPC
Dilated congestive	Systolic	Any, siamese	6–15 years	Dyspnea Muffled heart, lung sounds Rear limb monoparesis or paraparesis/paralysis	Generalized cardiomegaly Pleural effusion	↑ Atria ↑ LV VPC

ECG, electrocardiogram; LA, left atrium; RCLPV, right cranial lobar pulmonary vein; LV, left ventricle; SVPC, supraventricular premature contractions; VPC, ventricular premature contractions; RV, right ventricle; RVH, right ventricular hypertrophy; WBC, white blood cell count; SAP, serum alkaline phosphatase; RA, right atrium

Fever, leukocytosis, monocytosis, lameness, hypoalbuminemia, increased serum alkaline phosphatase activity, hypoglycemia, and bacteriuria are variably present in dogs with bacteremia.[1,2] The incidence of bacterial endocarditis in cats is unknown but is probably much lower than that in dogs.

Heart murmurs in middle-aged to older cats are most likely the result of cardiomyopathy. A careful history is necessary to rule out the possibility of the murmur having been present since birth (*i.e.*, congenital heart defect).

The most likely disorders associated with many cardiac murmurs can be quickly rank-ordered based on epizootiologic factors. The characteristics of the heart murmur are then determined during the physical examination. The character of the murmur associated with a patent ductus arteriosus in young animals is pathognomonic, and the diagnosis can usually be supported by thoracic radiograph findings. Young dogs, especially those of breed or type known to have an increased incidence of pulmonic stenosis, with cardiac murmurs that are clearly or suspected to be of pulmonic valve origin will usually have evidence of right-ventricular hypertrophy and a right-axis deviation on the electrocardiogram.

It is imperative that the patent ductus arteriosus and pulmonic stenosis be correctly diagnosed since surgical correction is feasible. For most practical purposes, the mere diagnosis of a congenital defect of other types is adequate. Special tests are usually required for a specific diagnosis, and surgical intervention is seldom feasible.

The character of the acquired mitral insufficiency in older, small breed dogs usually allows the clinical diagnosis to be made. Thoracic radiographs are indicated to assess the severity of cardiac enlargement and the therapeutic indications. The historic findings are also very important in assessing the indications for treatments.

The historic and physical findings in dogs with dilated congestive cardiomyopathy usually overshadow the significance of a cardiac murmur. The diagnosis is usually suspected during the physical examination and supported in most instances by radiographic and electrocardiographic abnormalities. Echocardiography is the safest and easiest method of confirming the diagnosis.

Feline cardiomyopathy and hyperthyroidism account for virtually all heart disease in the adult. The diagnosis is supported in almost all cases by abnormalities of thoracic radiographs, the electrocardiogram, or both. The diagnosis is confirmed by echocardiography and/or thyroid hormone assay.

Cyanosis in association with a heart murmur in a young animal is usually the result of a right-to-left shunt or severe left-sided congestive heart failure. In older dogs, cyanosis is associated with severe left-sided congestive heart failure.

REFERENCES

1. Calvert CA: Valvular bacterial endocarditis in dogs. J Am Vet Med Assoc 180:1080–1084, 1982
2. Calvert CA, Greene CE, Hardie E: Aerobic cardiovascular infections in dogs. J Am Vet Med Assoc 187:612–616, 1985
3. de Leon AC, Perloff JK, Twigg H, et al: The straight back syndrome. Circulation 32:193–203, 1965

4. Detweiler DK, Patterson DF: A phonograph record of heart sounds and murmur of the dog. Ann NY Acad Sci 127:322, 1965
5. Duke M, Abelmann WH: The hemodynamic response to chronic anemia. Circulation 39:503–515, 1969
6. Ettinger SJ, Suter PF: Heart sounds and phonocardiography. In Canine Cardiology. Philadelphia, WB Saunders, 1970, pp 29, 38
7. Fowler NO, Holmes JC: Blood viscosity and cardiac output in acute experimental anemia. J Appl Physiol 39:453–456, 1975
8. Gould L, Ettinger SO, Lyon AF: Intensity of the first heart sound and arterial pulse in mitral insufficiency. Dis Chest 53:545–549, 1964
9. Graettinger J, Muenster JJ, Silverstone LA, et al: A correlation of clinical and hemodynamic studies of patients with hyperthyroidism with and without congestive heart failure. J Clin Invest 38:1316–1321, 1959
10. Leatham A: A classification of systolic murmurs. Br Heart J 17:574–576, 1955
11. Lewis DH: Phonocardiology. In Handbook of Physiology. Bethesda, American Physiological Society, 1962
12. Lewis BS, Ehrenfeld EN, Lewis N: Echocardiographic LV function in thyrotoxicosis. Am Heart J 97:460–468, 1979
13. Patterson DF: Epidemiologic and genetic studies of congenital heart disease in the dog. Circ Res 23:171–202, 1968
14. Patterson DF, Detweiler DK: The diagnostic significance of splitting of the second heart sound in the dog. Zentralbl Veterinarmed 10:121–124, 1963
15. Patterson DF, Flickinger GL: Clinico-pathological conference. J Am Vet Med Assoc 180:1080–1084, 1982
16. Sabbah HN, Stein PD: Turbulent flow in humans: Its primary role in the production of ejection murmurs. Circ Res 38:513–525, 1976
17. Stein PD, Sabbah HN: Aortic origin of innocent murmurs. Am J Cardiol 39:665–671, 1977
18. Theilen EO, Wilson WR: Hemodynamic effects of peripheral vasoconstriction in normal and thyrotoxic subjects. J Appl Physiol 22:207–210, 1967

23

Pale Mucous Membranes

CLAY A. CALVERT

PROBLEM DEFINITION AND RECOGNITION

Pale mucous membranes (pallor) are a common clinical sign of a variety of disorders or diseases. Although pallor may be found when examining the skin, it is best evaluated by examination of the mucous membranes, primarily of the oral cavity. Physiologic vasoconstriction may result in visible pallor in normal cats and many nervous or apprehensive dogs. Other factors such as excitement and physical exertion can produce the appearance of a "healthier" color, particularly of the oral mucous membranes!

CLASSIFICATION

Pale mucous membranes are a manifestation of either decreased red blood cell mass (anemia) or decreased peripheral perfusion (see Classification of Disorders Producing Pale Mucous Membranes). Although moderate to severe anemia produces pale mucous membranes, many conditions result in pallor without a reduction of red blood cell mass.

Decreased peripheral perfusion may result from severe dehydration, loss of plasma protein resulting from severe thermal burn, or shock.

PATHOPHYSIOLOGY

The pathophysiology of anemia is discussed in a separate chapter. Anemia results from blood loss, blood destruction, or decreased erythrocyte production. The former two categories result in a bone marrow response (regenerative anemia), while the latter, by definition, results from atrophy of some component of the erythroid series of cells.

Classification of Disorders Producing Pale Mucous Membranes

- Anemia
- Decreased peripheral perfusion
  - Hypovolemic shock
    - Exogenous loss of fluid
      - Dehydration
      - Selective loss of plasma
      - Loss of whole blood
    - Endogenous loss of fluid
      - Exudative (peritonitis)
      - Modified transudative (heart failure)
      - Transudative (hypoalbuminemia)
    - Hypoadrenocortism
  - Cardiogenic shock
    - Myocardial failure
      - Dilated congestive cardiomyopathy
      - End-stage volume overload
        - Mitral insufficiency
        - Aortic insufficiency
        - Congenital defects (some)
    - Tachyarrhythmias
    - Cardiac tamponade
    - Pulmonary thromboembolism
  - Vasomotor shock
    - Septic
    - Neurogenic
    - Trauma
    - Pain
    - Anaphylaxis

Pale mucous membranes resulting from dehydration or selective loss of plasma protein are produced by peripheral vasoconstriction in an attempt to maintain sufficient blood pressure and blood perfusion of vital tissues and organs.

Shock is a complex group of acute cardiovascular syndromes that defy precise definition because of their varied origins. It is practical, however, to consider shock as a disturbance of circulation, resulting in ineffective or critical reduction of perfusion of vital tissues with associated hypoxia and a wide range of systemic effects. The clinical signs associated with shock are paleness of the mucous membranes, arterial hypotension, rapid and weak pulse, oliguria, and a tendency toward a progressive, refractory irreversible phase.

Pale mucous membranes in shock conditions result from hypovolemia, cardiac insufficiency (myocardial failure), and vasoconstriction. When a patient is in shock, several hemodynamic mechanisms are at work simultaneously, so continuous monitoring of multiple parameters of cardiovascular function is required. Hypovolemia and altered peripheral resistance may be significant factors in cardiogenic shock. Pump failure (myocardial failure) may be an important feature of severe hypovolemia.

Hypovolemic shock results from oligemia, hemorrhage, traumatic loss of fluids, or burns. There is a true diminution of blood volume due to loss of whole blood or constituents thereof from the intravascular compartment. Compensatory vasoconstriction temporarily reduces the intravascular fluid compartment, thereby maintaining adequate blood pressure. Peripheral vasoconstriction results in pallor.

Cardiogenic shock results from an inability of the left ventricle to perform effectively as a pump in maintaining adequate cardiac output. Pale mucous membranes result from poor peripheral perfusion and vasoconstriction.

Vasomotor shock may begin by expansion of the intravascular fluid compartment, resulting from vasodilation. This produces a relative inadequacy of blood volume. The increase capacitance results from widespread dilatation of the arteries and arterioles or from venous pooling. This so-called warm shock is not characterized by pale mucous membranes even though the arterial blood pressure is reduced and peripheral or splanchnic pooling of blood is occurring.

The most common form of vasomotor shock is septic shock. As septic shock proceeds, the typical clinical signs of shock (*e.g.*, tachycardia and pallor) develop as peripheral vasoconstriction occurs in an attempt to restore blood pressure and perfusion of vital tissues and organs.

Neurogenic factors elicited by trauma or pain may result in a type of vasomotor shock. Initially, epinephrine release results in tachycardia and vasoconstriction, which produce pallor. A reflex autonomic stimulation follows and produces splanchnic pooling of blood due to venous dilatation. A relative inadequacy of blood volume then exists. In the absence of hemorrhage or lung trauma, this type of vasomotor shock is self limiting.

Vascular shock may also result from anaphylaxis, histamine response, and arteriolar dilator drug therapy. All of these factors result in hypotension and pale mucous membranes.

DIAGNOSTIC PLAN

The diagnostic plan for pale mucous membranes varies with the severity of the patient's overall condition, history, and specific clinical findings (Table 23-1). The primary differential diagnosis is anemia versus shock. In most instances, the history and physical examination findings are consistent with one or the other of these problems. When anemia is not suspected to be the primary problem, then the differentiation of hypovolemic, septic, and cardiogenic shock is necessary.

SYMPTOMATIC THERAPY

The symptomatic therapy of pale mucous membranes is based on the history, physical examination, and initial diagnostic findings (Table 23-2). Severe anemia (packed cell volume $< 15\%$) usually requires blood transfusion. With the

Table 23-1. Diagnostic Plan for Pale Mucous Membranes

RULE OUT	DIAGNOSTIC PLAN
Anemia	Packed cell volume
	Reticulocyte count
Dehydration	Total solids
	BUN
	Urine specific gravity
Plasma loss	Total solids
	Total protein
	Albumin
Whole blood loss	Packed cell volume
	Total solids
Endogenous fluid loss	CBC
	Serum chemistry profile
	Urinalysis
	Cytology of effusion
	Radiographs
	Electrocardiogram
Cardiogenic shock	Thoracic radiographs
	Electrocardiogram
	Blood pressure
	Toe-web rectal temperature differential
Vasomotor shock	CBC
	Serum chemistry profile
	Urinalysis
	Blood pressure
	Toe-web rectal temperature differential
	Blood culture (if indicated)
	Urine culture (if indicated)

BUN, blood urea nitrogen; CBC, complete blood count

Table 23-2. Symptomatic Therapy for Pale Mucous Membranes

RULE OUT	THERAPY
Anemia	Blood transfusion if indicated
	Arrest blood loss
	Arrest blood destruction
Hypovolemic shock	Volume fluid replacement
	Whole blood
	Plasma
	Electrolyte solutions
Cardiogenic shock	
Myocardial failure	Preload reduction
	Furosemide
	Venodilator
	Inotrope therapy
	Digoxin
	Dopamine or dobutamine
Tachyarrhythmias	Antiarrhythmic therapy
Cardiac tamponade	Pericardiocentesis
Vasomotor shock	Volume fluid expansion

exclusion of cardiogenic shock, most other conditions outlined previously require selective fluid therapy. Cardiogenic shock is most often encountered with dilated congestive cardiomyopathy and is characterized by pleural effusion or pulmonary edema in addition to decreased cardiac output and hypotension. Both preload reduction and inotrope therapy are indicated. Although not well documented in dogs and cats, myocardial failure (pump failure) may also result from hypovolemic shock or septic shock. In such cases, inotrope therapy and fluid volume expansion are indicated.

24

Cyanosis

CLAY A. CALVERT

PROBLEM DEFINITION AND RECOGNITION

Cyanosis refers to a bluish color of the skin or mucous membranes, resulting from an increased amount of reduced hemoglobin, or hemoglobin derivatives, in the small blood vessels of those areas. The most superficial cutaneous capillaries contribute little to the color of the skin in most areas of the body.[8] The subpapillary venous plexus makes the largest vascular contribution to skin color.[8,10] Cyanosis is not synonymous with hypoxemia or hypoxia. The presence of cyanosis implies hypoxemia, but the absence of cyanosis does not preclude severe hypoxia. The degree of cyanosis is modified by the quality of cutaneous or mucosal pigments and the color of the blood plasma as well as by the state of the surface capillaries.

PATHOPHYSIOLOGY

Under normal conditions, during passage through the pulmonary capillaries, blood is exposed to an alveolar oxygen tension of approximately 100 mm Hg and leaves the capillaries in almost complete equilibrium with the alveolar gas. Normal blood leaves the lungs with an oxygen content of approximately 20 ml/dl. The arteriovenous blood oxygen difference under resting conditions is approximately 4 ml/dl.[5] Thus, the mixed venous blood in the pulmonary artery contains approximately 15 ml of oxygen per deciliter, which represents an oxyhemoglobin saturation of 75% and an oxygen tension of 40 mm Hg.

The increase in the amount of reduced hemoglobin in subpapillary venous plexuses, which produces cyanosis, may be brought about either by an increase in the quantity of venous blood in the cutaneous tissue as the result of dilatation of the vessels and venous ends of the capillaries or by a decrease in the oxygen saturation in the capillary blood. In general, cyanosis becomes apparent when the mean capillary concentration of reduced hemoglobin exceeds 5%.[6] The absolute rather than the relative amount of reduced hemoglobin is important in producing cyanosis. Thus, in severe anemia, the relative amount of reduced hemoglobin in the venous blood may be very large in relation to the total amount of hemoglobin. However, since the latter is severely lowered, the absolute amount of reduced hemoglobin may be small; therefore, patients with severe anemia and marked arterial desaturation do not display cyanosis. Conversely, patients with marked polycythemia, such as with polycythemia vera, tend to be cyanotic at higher levels of arterial oxygen saturation than patients with normal hematocrit values. Local passive congestion, which causes an increase in the total amount of reduced hemoglobin in the vessels of a given area, may cause cyanosis even though the average percentage arterial saturation is not altered. Cyanosis also is observed when nonfunctioning hemoglobin is present in the blood; as little as 1.5 g/dl of methemoglobin or 0.5 g/dl of sulfhemoglobin is sufficient to produce cyanosis.

CLASSIFICATION

True cyanosis may be divided into central and peripheral categories (Table 24-1). In the central type, there is arterial blood unsaturation or an abnormal hemoglobin derivative, and the warm mucous membranes and skin are both affected. Peripheral cyanosis is due to a slowing of blood flow to an area and abnormally great extraction of oxygen from normally saturated arterial blood. The most common type of peripheral cyanosis is the result of decreased blood flow through the peripheral capillary bed. This may result from cooling of the extremities, vasoconstriction of superficial vessels, polycythemia, thrombophlebitis and thrombosis, and low cardiac output. In low cardiac output states, the

Table 24-1. Causes of Cyanosis and Common Associations

CAUSE	ASSOCIATION(S)
Central	
Decreased arterial oxygen saturation	Impaired pulmonary function
	Alveolar hypoventilation
	Ventilation-perfusion mismatch
	Impaired oxygen diffusion from alveoli to capillaries
	Anatomic shunts
	Congenital heart defects
	Pulmonary arteriovenous shunting
Hemoglobin abnormalities	Methemoglobinemia
	Sulfhemoglobinemia
Peripheral	
Reduced cardiac output	Myocardial failure
Vasoconstriction	Cold exposure
Venous obstruction	Thrombophlebitis
Arterial obstruction	

arteriovenous oxygen differential is increased. During exercise, this differential increases because cardiac output does not increase appropriately. Consequently, cyanosis is more apparent during exertion. Peripheral cyanosis occurs usually on cool portions of the body such as digits, nose, and ears. In conditions such as cardiogenic shock with pulmonary edema, there may be a mixture of both types.

Hypoxemia, and therefore cyanosis, may occur when the normal state of gas exchange between alveolar air and pulmonary capillary blood is disturbed. Decreased arterial oxygen saturation results from a marked reduction in the oxygen tension of the arterial blood (PaO_2). Seriously impaired pulmonary function, through alveolar hypoventilation, ventilation perfusion mismatch (perfusion of poorly ventilated areas of the lung), or impaired oxygen diffusion can cause central cyanosis. Pneumonia, pulmonary edema, or chronic obstructive lung disorders, if severe, may produce cyanosis by these means. Alveolar hypoventilation may result from upper airway obstruction, laryngeal edema, or laryngeal paralysis. The latter is most commonly associated with recurrent laryngeal nerve palsy in old dogs, but has been seen as a hereditary disorder in young large breed dogs, especially the Bouvier des Flanders. Cyanosis occurs only when upper airway obstruction is nearly complete. Other causes of alveolar hypoventilation include inadequate ventilation during anesthesia and respiratory center depression from head trauma or cerebral edema. Ventilation–perfusion mismatch occurs in association with pulmonary edema, pulmonary thromboembolism, pneumonia, pulmonary contusion, and atelectasis. Decreased diffusion capacity of the alveolar-capillary membrane can result from alveolar destruction, severe pulmonary fibrosis, or infiltrative inflammatory or neoplastic diseases. Cyanosis is often absent in association with chronic lung disease with fibrosis and diminution of the capillary vascular bed because there is a decreased perfusion of underventilated areas. Blood flowing through the lungs without coming into contact with alveolar air can result from pulmonary arteriovenous shunts.

Cyanosis and Right-to-Left Shunts

Another cause of decreased arterial oxygen saturation is shunting of venous blood into the arterial circuit. Certain types of congenital heart defects, such as tetralogy of Fallot and Eisenmenger's complex, are associated with cyanosis. Since blood normally flows from a high-pressure to a low-pressure region, in order for a cardiac defect to result in a right-to-left shunt, it must ordinarily be combined with an obstructive lesion distal to the defect or with elevated pulmonary vascular resistance (Table 24-2). In patients with cardiac right-to-left shunts, the presence and severity of cyanosis depend on the size of the shunt relative to the systemic flow as well as on the oxyhemoglobin saturation of the venous blood. If the systemic blood flow is less than normal in a patient with cyanotic congenital heart disease, the arteriovenous oxygen difference is increased, and the mixed venous blood shunted into the arterial circuit is less saturated with oxygen. Under such circumstances, a small shunt may produce a significant degree of hypoxemia. The oxyhemoglobin saturation of mixed ve-

Table 24-2. Congenital Heart Defects With Associated Right-to-Left Shunting

OBSTRUCTION	DEFECT(S)
Pulmonic valve stenosis	Tetralogy of Fallot Pulmonic stenosis and ventricular septal defect
Pulmonary hypertension	Pulmonary hypertension associated with chronic left-to-right shunting occasionally results in reversal of shunting (right-to-left). Patent ductus arteriosus Ventricular septal defect

nous blood normally decreases during exercise; this decrease is exacerbated in congenital cyanotic heart disease, since the cardiac output cannot be increased appropriately. Some patients may not be cyanotic except during exercise. A useful means of differentiating cyanosis caused by a shunt in the heart or lungs from that caused by primary lung disease is to administer 100% oxygen. Cyanosis caused by a right-to-left shunt will be unaffected, whereas that due to parenchymal lung disease will decrease.

Cyanosis and Shock Lung

The syndrome known as shock lung (adult respiratory distress syndrome) can occur in association with a number of clinical problems. Classically, shock lung is associated with hypovolemic or septic shock, but an identical syndrome is also seen with head trauma, respiratory assisted ventilation, aspiration pneumonia, pancreatitis, electric cord bite, and seizures.

The onset of shock lung is characterized by an increase in tracheobronchial secretions, tachypnea, and cyanosis. The arterial partial pressure of oxygen (PaO_2) gradually decreases; the arterial partial pressure of carbon dioxide ($PaCO_2$) is initially low but may increase as the patient's condition deteriorates. Metabolic acidosis followed by combined metabolic and respiratory acidosis is common. The tidal volume becomes decreased as does the pulmonary compliance, requiring increased inspiratory pressure to maintain a given tidal volume.

No single cause of shock lung has been identified. The disorder probably is the result of several insults, including excessive fluid administration, oxygen toxicity, central nervous system injury, aspiration, disseminated intravascular coagulation, microembolization, and infection.

Cyanosis and Pulmonary Embolism

The incidence of pulmonary embolism in dogs is unknown, and this problem is often difficult to diagnose. Pulmonary embolism is most often identified in association with advanced heartworm disease and hyperadrenocorticism in dogs. Pulmonary embolism, when massive, is associated with a high mortality, but when diagnosed quickly by lung scanning or pulmonary angiography, appropriate therapy may reduce the mortality.

No clinical sign is pathognomonic for pulmonary embolism. Dyspnea, cough, and hemoptysis are commonly seen in association with severe heartworm disease. Tachypnea, crackles, and tachycardia are nonspecific signs that may be detected. With massive embolism, syncope, cyanosis, a gallop heart rhythm, or a splitting of the second heart sound may be detected.

Cyanosis and Abnormal Hemoglobins

Cyanosis is produced by small amounts of circulating methemoglobin[3] and by even smaller amounts of sulfhemoglobin, although such conditions are uncommon. Methemoglobinemia may be hereditary but is usually acquired via drug or chemical ingestion or contact. These agents preferentially oxidize hemoglobin and may overcome the normal reducing mechanism of the erythrocytes. Nitrates, after ingestion, may be converted to nitrites by intestinal bacteria. Certain sulfonamides such as sulfanilamide, sulfathiazole, and sulfapyridine may produce methemoglobinemia. Acetanilid and phenacetin readily cause methemoglobinemia and sulfhemoglobinemia in cats.[4] Local anesthetics containing benzocaine, when sprayed onto the larynx of cats prior to intubation, are capable of producing methemoglobinemia and sometimes cyanosis.[2] Cats treated with urinary antiseptics containing methylene blue often develop Heinz body (erythrocyte refractile body) anemia of variable severity with associated methemoglobinemia. Urinary tract compounds containing phenazopyridine (analgesic) can produce Heinz body anemia and methemoglobinemia when administered at high dosages.[1] In the dog, onion ingestion can produce methemoglobinemia via the major component of onion oil (alylpropyl disulfide).[7,9]

Peripheral Cyanosis

Peripheral cyanosis is uncommon in dogs and cats but may be caused by generalized vasoconstriction from cold exposure. Cutaneous vasoconstriction may occur in shock or congestive heart failure as a compensatory mechanism, so that blood is diverted to vital areas (kidneys, brain, heart). Even though the arterial blood may be normally saturated, the reduced peripheral blood flow through the surface vessels and the reduced oxygen tension at the venous end of the capillaries result in cyanosis. Peripheral cyanosis alone is not associated with cyanosis of warm mucous membranes such as the insides of the lips, cheeks, tongue, and conjunctiva.

Venous obstruction associated with thrombophlebitis produces stagnation of blood flow and increased oxygen extraction. Massage or warming of the cyanotic extremity will increase peripheral blood flow and abolish peripheral but not central cyanosis.

DIAGNOSTIC PLAN

The diagnostic plan indicated for the differential diagnosis of the cyanotic patient is dependent on the associated clinical signs (Tables 24-3 and 24-4). In most instances, the diagnosis of central cyanosis is assumed to be due to the presence of severe respiratory distress. Such dyspnea may result from severe pulmonary disease, congestive heart failure with associated severe pulmonary edema, or upper airway obstruction.

The auscultation of pulmonary crackles indicates parenchymal lung disease. Rule outs should include pulmonary interstitial fibrosis, especially in small terriers and miniature and toy breeds; pulmonary edema of cardiogenic or neurogenic origin; pulmonary contusion; pneumonia of various causes; heartworm disease with associated embolism; and shock lung. The presence of congestive heart failure is often suspected based on the age, breed, and history of the patient.

Central cyanosis in a young dog or cat without evidence of parenchymal lung disease raises the possibility of a right-to-left cardiac shunt. A cardiac murmur may or may not be present. Radiographic assessment may reveal evidence of pulmonary vascular overcirculation and hypertension. Hemoconcentration is often present, depending on the age of the patient and severity of the shunt. The degree of cyanosis is exacerbated with exercise. Arterial oxygen saturation (PaO_2) measurements will reveal hypoxemia.

Methemoglobinemia should be suspected in cyanotic patients with chocolate-brown blood. Anemia may be present and new methylene blue staining of a blood smear may reveal Heniz bodies. A drop of blood from a patient with cyanosis and methemoglobinemia will stain filter paper brown. Oxygen bubbled through a test tube containing blood from a cyanotic patient suspected of having methemoglobinemia will not produce oxyhemoglobin with its associated red color.

Table 24-3. Diagnostic Tests Often Indicated in the Cyanotic Patient

TEST	FINDING(S)	ASSOCIATION(S)
Arterial blood gas analysis	Reduced PaO_2	Central cyanosis
Thoracic radiographs	Enlarged arteries	Heartworm disease Right-to-left shunt
	Parenchymal disease	Pulmonary edema Pneumonia Contusion Shock lung Pulmonary embolism associated with severe heartworm disease
Electrocardiogram	Right ventricular hypertrophy	Severe heartworm disease Right-to-left shunt
Hematocrit	Elevated	Chronic hypoxemia Right-to-left shunt

Table 24-4. Diagnostic Plan and Differential Diagnosis of Cyanosis

DIAGNOSTIC TEST	FINDINGS	ASSESSMENT
Physical examination	Cyanosis of	
	Warm mucous membranes	Central cyanosis
	Cool extremities	Peripheral cyanosis
		Mixed cyanosis
	Crackles (severe)	Central or mixed
	Respiratory distress	Central or mixed
Thoracic radiographs	Severe disease	Central or mixed
	Pulmonary arterial	Heartworm disease
		Pulmonary embolism
	Parenchymal	Pulmonary edema
		Pneumonia
		Bacterial
		Fungal
		Aspiration
		Neoplasia
		Shock lung
		Heartworm disease
Blood analysis	Hemoconcentration	Central or mixed
		Right-to-left shunt
		Polycythemia vera
	Decreased PaO_2	Central
	Brown color	Central (methemoglobinemia)

Peripheral cyanosis alone is not associated with cyanosis of warm mucous membranes. The arterial oxygen saturation (PaO_2) is normal. Massaging or warming the affected tissues may abolish the cyanosis by increasing regional blood flow.

SYMPTOMATIC THERAPY

Symptomatic therapy of the cyanotic patient most often involves oxygen administration, relief of airway obstruction, bronchodilation, or diuretic therapy to relieve pulmonary edema (Table 24-5). Oxygen may be administered via an oxygen cage or through an intranasal catheter.

If methemoglobinemia is suspected, methylene blue can be administered at a rate of 1 to 2 mg/kg of a 1% solution administered as a single intravenous injection. In humans, the treatment is repeated if necessary. A published dosage of 8.8 mg/kg is a potentially toxic dose in the dog.[2] Acetylcysteine (1.4 mg/kg of a 10% solution) can be administered for the treatment of acetaminophen toxicity.[9]

Table 24-5. Symptomatic Therapy for Cyanosis

THERAPY	INDICATION(S)
Oxygen	Central cyanosis of all causes
Furosemide	Pulmonary edema
	Cardiogenic (left-sided congestive heart failure)
	Neurogenic
Bronchodilator	Bronchoconstriction
	Allergic bronchial spasms
	Irritant bronchial spasms
	Pulmonary edema
	Severe parenchymal lung disease
Methylene blue*	Methemoglobinemia

* This drug can produce toxicity, especially in cats. Consideration should be given to administering acetylcysteine for acetaminophen toxicity.

REFERENCES

1. Harvey JW, Kormick HP: Phenazopyridine toxicosis in the cat. J Am Vet Med Assoc 169:327–331, 1976
2. Harvey JW, Sameck JH, Bargard FJ: Benzocaine-induced methemoglobinemia in dogs. J Am Vet Med Assoc 175:1171–1175, 1979
3. Letchworth GJ, Bentinck-Smith J, Bolton GR, et al: Cyanosis and methemoglobinemia in two dogs due to NADH methemoglobin reductase deficiency. J Am Anim Hosp Assoc 13:75–79, 1977
4. Leyland A: Probable paracetamol toxicity in a cat. Vet Rec 94:104–105, 1974
5. Lukas DA: Cyanosis. In MacBryde CM, Backlow RS (eds): Signs and Symptoms. Philadelphia, JB Lippincott, 1970
6. Lundsgaard C, Van Slyke DD: Cyanosis. Medicine 1:1–5, 1923
7. Rebar AH, Lewis HB: Blood cells in disease. In Catcott EJ (ed): Canine Medicine. Santa Barbara, CA, American Veterinary Publications, 1979
8. Rothman S: Physiology and Biochemistry of the Skin. Chicago, University of Chicago Press, 1954
9. St. Omer UV, McKnight EB: Acetylcysteine for treatment of acetominophen toxicosis in the cat. J Am Vet Med Assoc 176:911–915, 1980
10. Winkelmann RK, Scheen SR, Pyka RA, et al: Cutaneous vascular patterns in studies with injections preparation and alkaline phosphatase reaction. In Montagna W, Ellis RA (eds): Advances in Biology of Skin. New York, Pergamon Press, 1961

Part Seven

RESPIRATORY PROBLEMS

25

Coughing

LARRY M. CORNELIUS

DEFINITION

Coughing is defined as a sudden noisy expulsion of air from the lungs.

PATHOPHYSIOLOGY

The function of coughing, a normal protective reflex, is to remove undesired material from the respiratory tract. Cough receptors in the respiratory system are most numerous in the large airways; none are present beyond the respiratory bronchioles. Afferent pathways for the cough reflex, located in the vagus, trigeminal, glossopharyngeal, and phrenic nerves, carry impulses to the coughing center in the medulla oblongata. Efferent conduction is carried out in the vagus, phrenic, and other spinal nerves which supply the larynx, tracheobronchial tree, diaphragm, and other respiratory muscles. A few cough receptors are also present in other locations such as the nose, paranasal sinuses, and pharynx. Cough receptors respond to both chemical and mechanical stimuli.

The beneficial effect of coughing is the clearing of the air passages, especially the trachea and large bronchi. Severe, persistent coughing, especially when dry and unproductive, may be harmful because it may (1) cause dissemination of infection, (2) further exacerbate inflammation and irritation of the respiratory mucosa, (3) cause overdistention of alveoli resulting in emphysema, (4) induce pneumothorax by causing rupture of bullae or airways, and (5) increase weakness and exhaustion in the patient.[2]

Causes of coughing can be grouped into three general classes by the location of the cause: (1) upper airway, (2) lower airway, and (3) cardiovascular (Table 25-1).

Table 25-1. Causes of Coughing in Dogs and Cats

UPPER AIRWAY	LOWER AIRWAY	CARDIOVASCULAR
Pharyngitis Tonsillitis Tracheitis Collapsed trachea (dogs) Neoplasia or trauma of pharynx, tonsils, or trachea	Acute or chronic bronchitis Bronchiectasis Pneumonia (including aspiration) Pulmonary fibrosis or abscess Hilar lymph node enlargement Allergic bronchitis; PIE Parasites (lungworms) Trauma or physical Bronchial foreign body Irritating gases or smoke Collapsing bronchi Neoplasia of mediastinum, bronchi, or lungs	Left-sided heart failure Left atrial enlargement Heartworm disease Pulmonary thrombosis Pulmonary edema

PIE, pulmonary infiltrates with eosinophils.

DIAGNOSTIC PLAN

History and Physical Examination

Other signs may be confused with coughing by owners. Gagging and expectoration of phlegm, regurgitation, and vomiting are often mistakenly reported as coughing. In many cases, an animal with a coughing problem can be induced to cough by vigorously manipulating the trachea. This should be done in the owner's presence to confirm that this is the sign they have observed.

It is important to ask about the pet's environment. If the animal has been in contact recently with groups of other dogs or cats, the likelihood of an infectious disease is increased. Environmental air pollutants, such as cigarette smoke and urban smog, may cause chronic coughing in dogs and cats. Indoor pets are less likely to have heartworm disease and other parasites, such as lungworms, than are outside animals.[1] Asking if the animal has shown other abnormal signs, such as depression, lethargy, anorexia, dyspnea, and exercise intolerance, often will help one decide which groups of rule outs should be pursued first (Table 25-2).

Certain characteristics of a cough may be of diagnostic value. A loud, harsh, dry cough is usually a sign of irritation or inflammation in the larynx, trachea, or mainstem bronchi and is a common observation in dogs with infectious tracheobronchitis (kennel cough) and cats with viral rhinotracheitis. A characteristic "goose-honk" cough is heard in many toy-breed dogs with collapsing trachea (Table 25-3).

Thoracic auscultation should be done carefully in the coughing animal. Both the heart and lungs should be carefully auscultated (see chapters 21 and 28). It is often helpful to induce coughing by tracheal manipulation and then reauscultate the thorax. Abnormal lung sounds are often heard for the first time or intensified after the animal has a series of coughs. Crackles, wheezes, and in-

Table 25-2. Differentiation of General Causes of Coughing

	CAUSE OF COUGHING		
	Upper Airway	Lower Airway	Cardiovascular
Depression/lethargy	Absent or mild	Mild to severe	Moderate to severe
Fever	Absent or mild	Mild to marked	None to marked
Dehydration	Absent	Mild to marked	Mild to marked
Inducible cough	Usually	Occasionally	Occasionally
Dyspnea	Usually absent	Mild to marked	Mild to marked
Exercise intolerance	Absent or mild	Mild to marked	Moderate to marked
Lung sounds	Normal	Abnormal	Abnormal
Heart sounds	Normal	Normal	Abnormal
White blood count	Normal	Increased or normal	Normal or increased
Thoracic radiographs	Normal	Abnormal	Abnormal

creased normal breath sounds are commonly heard in coughing patients. Cardiac murmurs and an abnormal heart rhythm may be auscultated in those animals with a cough caused by cardiac disease.

Laboratory Evaluation

A laboratory work-up should be done in most patients with signs of illness, such as fever, depression, anorexia, and dyspnea accompanying coughing, or if the coughing is chronic (>1 week in duration). A complete blood count and differential, serum biochemical profile, and urine analysis are usually indicated.

Radiography

Radiographic examination of the thorax is an extension of the physical examination in the coughing patient. Normal anatomy and disease conditions of the thorax are ideally suited for radiographic examination because of the natural contrast between the solid organs, such as the heart and large vessels, and the air-containing lung parenchyma. Proper radiographic technique, including two views, should be strictly followed.

Electrophysiologic Testing

If cardiac disease is suspected to be the cause of coughing, an electrocardiogram should be done. Other specialized tests, such as echocardiography, may need to be performed but are generally available only at referral centers.

Transtracheal Wash

An evaluation of the lining of the respiratory mucosa from the trachea to the alveoli can usually be obtained from a proper transtracheal wash. This can be

Table 25-3. Common Causes of Coughing in Dogs and Cats and Characteristic Findings

	HISTORY/PHYSICAL EXAMINATION	LABORATORY STUDIES	RADIOGRAPHS
DOGS			
Acute			
Pharyngitis/laryngitis	Hacking cough followed by gagging and swallowing of phlegm Hoarse voice Reddened pharynx and tonsils No systemic signs	Normal	Normal
Tracheitis	History of being in contact with a group of dogs Dry, hacking cough No systemic signs	Normal	Normal
Aspiration pneumonia	History of general anesthesia or megaesophagus Deep, moist cough Worsening dyspnea Fever	↑ WBC Neutrophilia and left shift or Stress leukogram	Consolidated alveolar pattern with cranioventral distribution
Chronic			
Infectious tracheobronchitis	History of exposure to a group of dogs Deep, dry, persistent cough No systemic signs	Normal	Normal
Tracheal collapse	Toy breed Obese "Goose-honk" cough Dyspnea May palpate collapsing trachea at thoracic inlet	Normal	Tracheal collapse, either intrathoracic or extrathoracic Best seen with fluoroscopy Bronchial collapse
Allergic bronchitis/PIE	Deep cough, dry or productive Mild to moderate dyspnea Crackles and wheezes on auscultation No systemic signs	Peripheral eosinophilia Eosinophilic inflammation on transtracheal wash	Prominent bronchial or interstitial pattern
Heartworm disease	Weight loss Persistent coughing Mild to severe dyspnea Exercise intolerance	Peripheral eosinophilia Hyperglobulinemia Microfilaria positive or Occult heartworm positive	Right-sided heart enlargement Pulmonary arterial enlargement, pruning, and tortuosity Focal consolidations in lungs, especially diaphragmatic lobes

Table 25-3. Common Causes of Coughing in Dogs and Cats and Characteristic Findings *(Continued)*

	HISTORY/PHYSICAL EXAMINATION	LABORATORY STUDIES	RADIOGRAPHS
Left-sided heart failure	Old, small breed dogs Cough most prominent at night Dyspnea and exercise intolerance	ECG variable, LVH pattern, PVCs	Left atrial enlargement Enlarged pulmonary veins Pulmonary edema around base of heart
CATS			
Acute			
Viral rhinotracheitis	Exposure to a group of cats Sneezing and red, watery eyes Oral ulcers	Normal or ↑ WBC with neutrophilia and left shift	Normal
Chronic			
Feline asthma	Deep, productive, paroxysmal cough with neck extended Severe dyspnea and cyanosis	Peripheral eosinophilia	Bronchial or interstitial lung pattern Hyperinflated lungs
Lungworms	Deep, productive, paroxysmal cough with neck extended Dyspnea Fever Positive FeLV test	Peripheral eosinophilia Ova or larvae in transtracheal wash or in the feces (Baermann technique)	Bronchial or interstitial lung pattern
Heartworms	Outside cat from endemic area Listless, decreased appetite Sporadic vomiting Occasional cough	Peripheral eosinophilia Hyperglobulinemia Microfilaria negative Occult heartworm positive	Enlarged caudal lobar pulmonary arteries Mildly enlarged right ventricle

↑ increased; WBC, white blood cell; PIE, pulmonary infiltrates with eosinophils; ECG, electrocardiogram; LVH, left-ventricular hypertrophy; PVCs, premature ventricular contractions; FeLV, feline leukemia virus

accomplished by using a tranquilizer (*e.g.*, acepromazine) and a local anesthetic and penetrating the cricothyroid membrane with a commercial flexible polyethylene intravenous catheter placement device. In small dogs and cats, many clinicians prefer to lightly anesthetize the patient with intravenous ketamine and diazepam and do the transtracheal wash through a sterile endotracheal tube. Sterile, isotonic fluid such as Ringer's lactate or 0.9% saline solution should be used to do the wash. The wash will usually be productive if the animal coughs vigorously during the procedure. Samples should be submitted for cytologic evaluation and culture/sensitivity.

Bronchoscopy

A bronchoscopic examination is sometimes indicated for the coughing patient but requires general anesthesia and relatively expensive equipment.

SYMPTOMATIC THERAPY

The beneficial and detrimental aspects of symptomatic therapy for coughing should be carefully considered. In general, potent cough suppressants should be used only in those patients having severe, persistent, dry, unproductive coughing. Other types of drugs may be safer and just as effective.

Bronchodilators

These compounds are beneficial in the treatment of cough associated with bronchospasm. The two most common categories of bronchodilators are the phosphodiesterase inhibitors and the sympathomimetics. The methylxanthine derivatives (theophylline, aminophylline) are phosphodiesterase inhibitors; they slow the breakdown of cyclic AMP and increase its concentration, which cause relaxation of bronchial smooth muscle. Aminophylline and theophylline also may increase the strength of diaphragmatic contractions in animals with respiratory distress and a weakened diaphragm and may improve mucociliary clearance. In humans, there is much variation in the dosages of aminophylline and theophylline needed to achieve therapeutic blood levels. The same is probably true for dogs and cats, and it is recommended that plasma theophylline levels be determined 1 to 2 hours after oral administration to be certain that appropriate concentrations are achieved and maintained. Since the drug must reach steady-state distribution in the plasma, the plasma theophylline level should not be measured until the second or third day after beginning treatment. The therapeutic range of plasma theophylline in humans is 10 μg to 20 μg/ml.

The sympathomimetic bronchodilators (terbutaline, metaproterenol, isoproterenol) are beta-adrenergic receptor agonists and act by increasing the intracellular conversion of adenosine triphosphate (ATP) to cyclic adenosine monophosphate (AMP). Cyclic AMP relaxes bronchial smooth muscle and increases mucocilary clearance in the respiratory tract. Sympathomimetic drugs should be used with caution or not all in animals with cardiac disease because of their stimulatory effects on the heart. Since the methylxanthines and beta-adrenergic receptor agonists cause bronchodilation by different mechanisms, it is often beneficial to use these drugs together for a synergistic effect. Aminophylline (10 mg/kg, three or four times per day, for dogs; 5 mg/kg, two or three times per day, for cats) and terbutaline (2.5 mg, three times per day for dogs; 1.25 mg, twice a day for cats) is a useful combination for bronchodilation in dogs and cats.[3]

Cough Suppressants

Antitussive drugs are grouped into the central and peripherally acting agents. Central cough suppression is achieved by depression of the medullary cough center, whereas peripheral cough suppressants act by increasing the threshold of cough receptors. Centrally acting antitussives include both narcotic and non-narcotic drugs and are much more effective than the peripherally acting drugs.

Hydrocodone bitartrate (Hycodan) is a narcotic cough suppressant that can be used at a dosage of 2.5 to 10 mg, two or three times per day, orally in dogs. It has the added benefit of causing sedation and allowing the animal to rest. Butorphanol tartrate (Torbutrol) is a centrally acting drug that is classified as a narcotic agonist-antagonist. It has potent analgesic and antitussive properties and can be administered both orally (0.5 mg/kg twice a day) and subcutaneously (0.05 mg/kg twice a day) to dogs.

Expectorants

Drugs that increase the volume of respiratory tract fluid, thus promoting the expulsion of secretions or exudates from the airways, are termed *expectorants.* The value of these agents in treating coughing is questionable. Maintenance of good patient hydration will probably be more effective in maintaining the proper volume and fluidity of respiratory tract secretions.

Antihistamines

Although used in many commercial cough preparations, antihistamines exert no substantial antitussive effects. They may be harmful because of their drying effects on mucous membranes, with resultant retained secretions and nonproductive coughing. Possible beneficial effects are the sedation and drowsiness that they produce, allowing the patient to rest.

Aerosol Therapy

The value of different forms of nebulization therapy for coughing and other respiratory problems is somewhat controversial. Inhaled water deposited in the bronchial tree helps to liquify thickened secretions. The particle size needed for deposition in the bronchioles and alveoli is in the range of 1 μm to 2 μm, which can be achieved only with certain types of nebulizers such as the ultrasonic varieties. In the hospital, aerosol therapy is usually done with a nebulizer and an enclosed cage or with a small hand-held nebulizer and face-mask unit. Either 0.45% or 0.9% saline solution, with or without aqueous antibiotics, such as gentamicin, are the most common solutions aerosolized. At home, aerosol or humidity therapy is usually done by exposing the animal to steam produced by a hot shower in the bathroom. Cool-mist or steam vaporizers can also be used, but caution must be exercised to prevent a burn or patient overheating from the latter device.

REFERENCES

1. Ettinger SJ: Differential diagnosis of coughing. In Ettinger SJ (ed): Textbook of Veterinary Internal Medicine, 2nd ed., pp 95–97. Philadelphia, WB Saunders, 1983
2. Head JR, Suter PF: Approach to the patient with respiratory disease. In Ettinger SJ (ed): Textbook of Veterinary Internal Medicine, pp 544–564. Philadelphia, WB Saunders, 1975
3. Papich MG: Bronchodilator therapy. In Kirk RW (ed): Current Veterinary Therapy IX—Small Animal Practice, 278–284. Philadelphia, WB Saunders, 1986

26

Dyspnea

LARRY M. CORNELIUS

DEFINITION

Dyspnea is a condition of a difficult or labored breathing.

PATHOPHYSIOLOGY

Dyspnea is a pathologic event, whereas tachypnea (increased rate of breathing) may be either physiologic (*e.g.*, due to exercise, heat, or anxiety) or pathologic. Labored breathing may occur for the following basic reasons: (1) need for additional oxygen, (2) compensation for metabolic acidosis, (3) excessive environmental heat (heatstroke), (4) damaged or diseased central nervous system (CNS) respiratory centers, (5) weakness of the respiratory muscles or dysfunction of the motor nerves of respiration, and (6) pain from structures involved in breathing (*e.g.*, pleura, spinal nerves, respiratory muscles, ribs).[1]

Lack of adequate oxygen can be caused by either diminished oxygen in the environment, disorders interrupting the transfer of oxygen from the environment to the blood (diseases of the upper or lower airway or restrictive diseases), or decreased oxygen-carrying capacity in the blood (anemia, methemoglobinemia). Compensation for metabolic acidosis involves the "blowing off" of CO_2 through the lungs and may cause an increase in both the rate and depth of respiration. Dogs and cats dissipate heat through the respiratory system by panting; therefore, an excessively hot environment may cause labored breathing. Any disorder causing damage to the CNS respiratory centers in the medulla (*e.g.*, head trauma, inflammation, mass) may disrupt control of breathing and cause dyspnea. Finally, decreased ventilation and labored breathing may result from disorders causing dysfunction of motor nerves and muscles involved in breathing, such as polyradiculoneuritis or diaphragmatic paralysis. Dyspnea may also be caused by painful processes of respiratory sensory nerves and muscles and other structures such as the pleura and ribs, which can be caused by trauma, pleuritis, or other factors. Causes of dyspnea in dogs and cats are shown in Table 26-1.

DIAGNOSTIC PLAN

History and Physical Examination

The history should include questions about whether the dyspnea was sudden in onset or slowly progressive. Asking if the animal is always confined or under the direct supervision of someone will help in the assessment of the possibility of trauma. Certain breeds are more prone to various disorders causing dyspnea. For example, brachycephalic dogs often have upper airway problems, and hunting dogs are more likely to have dyspnea caused by the deep mycoses. Age is also an important consideration. Neoplastic disorders are more likely in older animals.

Careful observation of the pattern of respiration may be of great help in localizing the cause of dyspnea. Upper airway disorders are associated with inspiratory dyspnea characterized by a prolonged, labored inspiratory effort and a quick, relatively easy expiratory phase. Lower airway diseases and restrictive

Table 26-1 Causes of Dyspnea in Dogs and Cats

UPPER AIRWAY	LOWER AIRWAY	RESTRICTIVE	MISCELLANEOUS

Stenotic nares
Rhinitis/sinusitis
Elongated soft palate
Laryngeal diseases
  Necrotic laryngitis
  Edema
  Paralysis of vocal folds
  Everted saccules
  Laryngeal collapse
Intraluminal tracheal or bronchial foreign body or mass
Extraluminal tracheal or bronchial obstruction
  Mediastinal mass
  Tracheal or bronchial collapse
  Hilar lymphadenopathy
	Bronchial diseases
	  Chronic obstructive pulmonary disease (COPD)
	  Allergic bronchitis (asthma, PIE)
	  Lungworms
	Pneumonia
	Pulmonary edema
	  Left heart failure
	  Hypoalbuminemia
	  Others
	Pulmonary thromboembolism
	  Heartworm disease
	  Hyperadrenocorticism
	  Others
	Pulmonary contusions (trauma)
	Pulmonary fibrosis
	Pulmonary granulomatosis
	Deep mycosis
		Pneumothorax
		Pleural effusion
		  Right heart failure
		  Neoplasia
		  Hypoalbuminemia
		  Hemothorax
		  Chylothorax
		  Pyothorax
		  Feline infectious peritonitis
		Pericardial effusion
		Diaphragmatic hernia
		Intrathoracic neoplastic mass
		Thoracic wall trauma
		  Flail chest
		Extreme obesity
		Severe hepatomegaly
		Marked ascites
		Large intra-abdominal mass
		Severe gastric distention (gastric volvulus)
			Anemia
			Methemoglobinemia
			Compensation for metabolic acidosis
			Heatstroke
			Damage to respiratory center
			  Head trauma
			  Encephalitis
			  Neoplasia
			Neuromuscular weakness
			  Polyradiculoneuritis (coonhound paralysis)
			  Diaphragmatic paralysis
			  Others
			Pain
			  Fractured ribs or vertebrae
			  Pleuritis
			  Others
			Paraquat poisoning

PIE, pulmonary infiltrates with eosinophils

disorders generally cause labored breathing characterized by both inspiratory and expiratory dyspnea with a rapid respiratory rate (Table 26-2).

A thorough examination of all systems is indicated to determine if other miscellaneous causes of dyspnea are present; however, care must be taken to not unduly stress a severely dyspneic animal, or death may occur. Allowing the animal to sit quietly in a high oxygen environment and other symptomatic treatment (see the section on symptomatic therapy) prior to diagnostic procedures may be necessary.

Laboratory Evaluation

A complete blood count, serum biochemical panel, and urine analysis are usually indicated but may be delayed until after thoracic radiographs are complete and essential symptomatic therapy has been given in some severely dyspneic animals. Other procedures such as testing for heartworms and feline leukemia virus and determination of feline infectious peritonitis titers should be done if appropriate (Table 26-3).

Radiography

Thoracic, and sometimes skull, radiographs should be taken (see chapter 25).

Cytology

If pleural effusion is observed on thoracic radiographs, a thoracocentesis should be done using aseptic technique and the fluid should be examined. The protein content can be measured by refractometry; a cell count and differential

(Text continues on p 222.)

Table 26-2. Differentiation of General Causes of Dyspnea

	CAUSE OF DYSPNEA			
	Upper Airway	Lower Airway	Restrictive	Miscellaneous*
Type of dyspnea	Inspiratory	Expiratory	Rapid, shallow	Rapid, shallow or deep
Fever	Absent	Variable	Variable	Variable
Dehydration	Absent	Present	Present	Present
Lung sounds	Referred from upper airway	Abnormal	Abnormal, often muffled	Increased normal breath sounds
Heart sounds	Normal	Variable	Variable	Usually normal
White blood count	Normal	Increased or normal	Increased or normal	Increased or normal
Thoracic radiographs	Normal	Abnormal	Abnormal	Usually normal

* See Table 26-1.

Table 26-3. Common Causes of Dyspnea in Dogs and Cats and Characteristic Findings

	HISTORY/PHYSICAL EXAMINATION	LABORATORY STUDIES	RADIOGRAPHS
Dogs			
Acute			
Aspiration pneumonia	Chronic vomiting or regurgitation Recent anesthesia	$\uparrow$ WBC Neutrophilia and left shift or Stress leukogram	Consolidated areas in lungs (alveolar and interstitial patterns), especially in ventral areas
Pulmonary thromboembolism	Recent heartworm treatment Rapid, shallow breathing Coughing Hemoptysis Fever Lethargy/depression	$\uparrow$ WBC Neutrophilia and left shift or Stress leukogram Biochemical panel variable	Evidence of heartworm disease (enlarged right ventricle and pulmonary arteries) Consolidated areas in lungs (alveolar and interstitial patterns), especially caudal lobes
Pulmonary contusions	Recent trauma Expiratory dyspnea or Rapid, shallow breathing Muffled lung sounds in certain lung fields Other signs of trauma	$\uparrow$ WBC Neutrophilia and stress leukogram Anemia $\downarrow$ Plasma protein	Patchy consolidation of lung lobes (alveolar and interstitial patterns) Pleural effusion
Pneumothorax	See pulmonary contusions.	$\uparrow$ WBC Neutrophilia and stress leukogram	Evidence of air in the pleural space with the heart apparently elevated off the sternum
Ethylene glycol poisoning	Consumption of antifreeze Ataxia Polydipsia/polyuria Severe depression or coma Deep, labored breathing Seizures	$\uparrow$ WBC Neutrophilia and stress leukogram $\downarrow$ TCO_2 $\uparrow$ Anion gap Hypocalcemia	Normal

Heatstroke	Exposure to hot environment Marked hyperthermia (temperature >107) Deep, rapid, labored breathing Signs of shock	↑WBC Neutrophilia and stress leukogram Evidence of DIC (prolonged clotting time and abnormal coagulogram)	Normal
Chronic			
Stenotic nares/elongated soft palate/laryngeal malformation or paralysis	Snoring/snorting type breathing Inspiratory dyspnea Brachycephalic breed	Normal	Normal
Mediastinal mass	Regurgitation Gagging Rapid, shallow breathing Decreased compressibility of thoracic inlet Muffled lung sounds	Hematology variable Cytology of fluid or tissue obtained by thoracentesis variable	Evidence of consolidation (mass) in anterior mediastinum Pleural fluid
Tracheal collapse	See Table 25-3.		
Allergic bronchitis/PIE	See Table 25-3.		
Heartworm disease	See Table 25-3.		
Left-sided heart failure	See Table 25-3.		
Deep mycosis	Hunting dog Labored breathing and tachypnea Fever Mucopurulent nasal discharge Lethargy and depression Crackles and wheezes	↑WBC Neutrophilia and left shift Mild to moderate nonregenerative anemia Biochemical panel variable	Nodular interstitial pattern diffusely throughout the lungs
Diaphragmatic hernia	Outside dog or history of trauma Rapid, shallow breathing Areas of reduced lung sounds on auscultation and areas of dullness on percussion	WBC usually normal Biochemical panel variable Increased SAP Hyperbilirubinemia	Indistinct diaphragmatic shadow Pleural effusion Intestinal loops, stomach, or liver in thoracic cavity

(Continued)

Table 26-3. Common Causes of Dyspnea in Dogs and Cats and Characteristic Findings *(Continued)*

	HISTORY/PHYSICAL EXAMINATION	LABORATORY STUDIES	RADIOGRAPHS
Cats			
Acute			
Pulmonary contusions	See pulmonary contusions in dogs.		
Pneumothorax	See pneumothorax in dogs.		
Ethylene glycol poisoning	See ethylene glycol poisoning in dogs.		
Cardiomyopathy	Expiratory dyspnea or rapid shallow breathing Muffled lung sounds or crackles Gallop rhythm Heart murmur Tachycardia Weak pulse Depression, weakness, lethargy	Hemogram variable Azotemia (prerenal) Arrhythmias and conduction disturbances on ECG Echocardiographic abnormalities	Pleural effusion or Pulmonary edema Enlarged heart, valentine shaped
Feline asthma	See Table 25-3.		
Acetaminophen intoxication	History of acetaminophen administration Tachypnea and labored breathing Cyanosis Pale mucous membranes Mild icterus Facial edema Severe depression	Anemia (nonregenerative if acute) Methemoglobinemia ↑ WBC Stress leukogram ↑ SAP and S-ALT	Normal

Chronic			
Rhinitis and sinusitis	Snoring noises Sneezing Naso-ocular discharge Nasal swelling Conjunctivitis	Hemogram and biochemical panel variable Cytology of nasal exudate variable FeLV test often positive	Increased fluid density in nasal passages and sinuses Variable bony lysis and proliferation of nasal and frontal bones
Mediastinal mass	See mediastinal mass in dogs.		
Feline asthma	See Table 25-3.		
Lungworms	See Table 25-3.		
Diaphragmatic hernia	See diaphragmatic hernia in dogs.		
Pyothorax	Depression and lethargy Fever or hypothermia Tachypnea and labored breathing Muffled lung sounds Dull sounds on percussion of thorax	WBC variable Neutrophila and left shift or Neutropenia and degenerative shift with toxic neutrophils Nonregenerative anemia FeLV test often positive Biochemical panel variable Cytology of pleural fluid—septic, purulent exudate	Pleural effusion
Feline infectious peritonitis	Depression and anorexia Rapid, shallow breathing Fever Weight loss Abdominal effusion Uveitis CNS signs (*e.g.,* ataxia, paresis)	WBC variable Moderate nonregenerative anemia Hyperglobulinemia FIP titer variable Pleural and abdominal fluid Protein >3.5 g/dl Cell count <5000/cm^3	Pleural effusion Abdominal effusion

↑, increased; WBC, white blood cells; ↓, decreased; TCO_2, total carbon dioxide; DIC, disseminated intravascular coagulation; PIE, pulmonary infiltrates with eosinophils; SAP, serum alkaline phosphatase; S-ALT, serum alanine transaminase; FeLV, feline leukemia virus; CNS, central nervous system

should be recorded. A portion of the fluid should be submitted for bacterial and (sometimes) fungal culture.

If a mass is observed radiographically, a percutaneous, fine-needle aspirate should be obtained if the mass is not located near the heart or large vessels. Sedation and local anesthesia may be used if necessary to prevent excessive patient movement. After appropriate aseptic preparation, a 22-gauge, 1- or 1.5-inch needle and a 6-ml syringe are used to aspirate the mass. Several slides should be prepared for staining with Wright-Giemsa and other special stains as needed.

Electrophysiologic Testing

If cardiac disease is suspected, electrocardiography, and sometimes echocardiography are indicated.

SYMPTOMATIC THERAPY

Appropriate symptomatic treatment of dyspnea will depend upon the cause. As discussed previously, severely dyspneic animals should not be unduly stressed. Administering oxygen with an oxygen cage, face mask, or indwelling nasal tube may be necessary.

It is very important to determine whether there is restrictive disease (pleural effusion, pneumothorax, or an intrathoracic mass) or pulmonary edema present early in the diagnostic work-up so that appropriate corrective measures can be taken without undue delay. Pleural fluid can be removed by thoracocentesis using a 22-gauge, 1-inch needle, three-way connecting valve, and a 20-ml syringe. Alternatively, polyethylene intravenous catheters, either rigid or flexible, can be used. Sometimes it is better to place one or two indwelling chest tubes and periodically aspirate the pleural fluid. Air in the pleural space can be removed by similar methods.

Hypoalbuminemia often results from excessive removal of pleural fluid and will cause more rapid formation of pleural effusion. When repeatedly removing large quantities of pleural fluid, the serum albumin concentration should be measured at least twice weekly. If the serum albumin level decreases to <2.0 g/dl, the amount of pleural fluid removed should be decreased. Intermittent use of furosemide may help control the amount of pleural fluid formation. Use of plasma or whole blood transfusions may be required for severe hypoalbuminemia (serum albumin <1.0 g/dl).

Bronchodilators are often helpful for symptomatic treatment of dyspnea caused by lower airway, restrictive, and cardiac disorders. The most common types of bronchodilators are discussed in chapter 25. In addition to their bronchodilating effects, the theophylline derivatives increase strength of diaphragmatic contractions, improve mucociliary function in the respiratory mucosa, and cause mild diuresis, all of which may be helpful in dyspneic patients.

For symptomatic treatment of pulmonary edema, furosemide should be used either intravenously (for severely dyspneic animals) or orally. Side-effects of furosemide are dehydration, azotemia, and hypokalemia; therefore, the drug should be used at the lowest effective dosages and for the shortest period of time possible. Intermittent (every 2 to 3 days) usage is sometimes adequate and reduces the incidence of side-effects. Morphine sulfate may be administered parenterally to dyspneic dogs (not cats) at a dosage of 4 to 6 mg repeated as required to cause sedation and lessen the severity of the labored breathing. Tranquilizers such as acetylpromazine can be used parenterally in both dogs and cats (0.1 mg/kg) for the same purposes. Due to the peripheral vasodilating effects of tranquilizers, hypotension may develop and fluid therapy may be required.

REFERENCE

1. Ettinger SJ: Dyspnea and tachypnea. In Ettinger SJ (ed): Textbook of Veterinary Internal Medicine, 2nd ed, pp 97–99. Philadelphia, WB Saunders, 1983

27

Hemoptysis

LARRY M. CORNELIUS

DEFINITION

The coughing up of blood is termed *hemoptysis.*

PATHOPHYSIOLOGY

Hemoptysis is the result of one or more of the following basic abnormalities: (1) damage to blood vessels, (2) severe pulmonary hypertension, or (3) a clotting or bleeding problem. Vascular damage can be the result of inflammation (infectious or noninfectious), necrosis, neoplasia, or trauma. Pulmonary hypertension is usually the result of pulmonary thromboembolism (arteriolar hypertension) or left ventricular failure (venous hypertension). Clotting or bleeding disorders are caused by abnormalities of clotting factors or platelets (see chapter 19 and Causes of Hemoptysis in Dogs and Cats).

Hemoptysis usually results in minimal blood loss; however, if it is chronic, blood loss anemia can develop. Occasionally, massive hemoptysis occurs and may cause death due to asphyxiation or hypovolemia.

DIAGNOSTIC PLAN

History and Physical Examination

Before proceeding with an extensive diagnostic work-up of hemoptysis, it is important to localize the source of bleeding. Expectoration of blood may be the result of bleeding from the nasopharynx or from the respiratory or gastrointestinal tract. Aspiration of blood from the nasopharynx, or of regurgitated or vomited blood from the gastrointestinal tract, may lead to hemoptysis.

Careful questioning of the client may help localize the site of bleeding. Severe persistent sneezing with a bloody nasal discharge prior to the onset of hemoptysis usually indicates that the source of bleeding is the nasal cavity. A history of severe coughing or dyspnea preceding hemoptysis suggests that the blood is coming from the respiratory tract. Animals with a history of serious gastrointestinal disease (*e.g.*, vomiting, diarrhea, weight loss) may vomit blood and aspirate the vomitus, leading to hemoptysis.

A thorough physical examination should be done to evaluate all systems. The lips, oral cavity, and nasopharynx should be carefully observed for signs of recent bleeding (due to inflammation, masses, foreign bodies, or other factors) as well as for the presence of petechiae. Thoracic auscultation is important to help determine the possible involvement of the cardiopulmonary system.

Laboratory Evaluation

If hemoptysis is not massive and life-threatening, thoracic radiographs should be obtained after the history and physical examination are completed. Depending on the results, further tests to consider are a complete blood count, platelet count, serum biochemical panel, urinalysis, heartworm testing, clotting

Causes of Hemoptysis in Dogs and Cats

- Cardiovascular
  - Pulmonary thromboembolism
    - Heartworm disease
    - Hyperadrenocorticism
    - Others
  - Left heart failure
- Inflammatory
  - Chronic bronchitis (chronic obstructive pulmonary disease)
  - Pneumonia
  - Deep mycosis
    - Blastomycosis
    - Histoplasmosis
  - Lung abscess
- Neoplastic
  - Bronchogenic carcinoma
  - Others
- Miscellaneous
  - Trauma
  - Clotting or bleeding disorder
  - Foreign body
  - Transtracheal wash or bronchoscopy
  - Needle biopsy

panel, blood gas analysis, electrocardiogram, transtracheal wash, bronchoscopy, and fine needle aspirate sampling.

For massive, life-threatening hemoptysis, diagnostic procedures should be delayed until the patient's condition is stabilized. After stabilization thoracic radiographs should be taken and other tests considered as previously outlined.

SYMPTOMATIC THERAPY

For mild, non-life-threatening hemoptysis, symptomatic treatment may not be needed. If severe, persistent coughing is the cause of hemoptysis, the use of cough suppressants and bronchodilators may be helpful (see chapter 25). The patient should be kept quiet, and the use of phenothiazine tranquilizers to cause sedation and mild hypotension should be considered. Indiscriminate use of prophylactic antibiotics for hemoptysis is not warranted.

When massive hemoptysis occurs, emergency measures may be necessary to save the patient's life. Primary consideration should be given to maintaining a patent airway, restoring blood volume, and preparing the patient for surgery to find the source of bleeding if necessary. Anesthesia and tracheal intubation should be done so that blood in the airway can be continually suctioned out and oxygen can be administered. Lactated Ringer's solution can be used intravenously to help restore vascular volume, but if the packed cell volume decreases to <15 or if a clotting or bleeding defect is present, whole blood should be administered. Caution must be used in the volume of fluid or blood administered to avoid excessively raising blood pressure and causing continued hemorrhage. In some patients, bronchoscopy or exploratory thoracotomy is necessary to localize the site of hemorrhage and correct the problem.

REFERENCE

1. Howard WJ: Hemoptysis—causes and a practical management approach. Postgrad Med 77:53–57, 1985

28

Abnormal Lung Sounds

LARRY M. CORNELIUS

DEFINITION

Abnormal lung sounds are heard upon auscultation of the thorax in many patients with diseases of the airway.

PATHOPHYSIOLOGY

The exact origin of normal breath sounds is not well understood. Lung sounds are believed to be produced by oscillations of solid respiratory tissue and by rapid fluctuations of gas pressure.[1] Sounds produced are filtered and dampened as they travel within the lung outward toward the thoracic wall. Thus, normal lung sounds heard by thoracic auscultation are a composite of individual noises generated from multiple sites within the lungs. Normal lung sounds originate primarily from the trachea and lobar and segmental bronchi. It is a common misconception that normal lung sounds are generated in the alveoli. Flow at the acinar and alveolar levels is laminar with low velocity; therefore, neither turbulence nor sound is produced.

Normal lung sounds differ according to the age of the animal, respiratory pattern, thickness of the thoracic wall, site of auscultation, and pattern of respiration. Sound intensity in young or thin animals is louder, apparently because of less attenuation of sound by fewer intervening alveoli and thinner thoracic walls. In older or obese animals, normal breath sounds may be barely detectable. Variation in normal breath sounds may be caused by changes in the respiratory pattern such as panting (increased intensity) and neuromuscular weakness (decreased intensity). Abnormal sounds produced by pathologic processes within the tracheobronchial tree and lungs are termed *adventitious sounds.* The point of maximal intensity is usually near the diseased area. Adventitious sounds may be either discontinuous (crackles) or continuous (wheezes).

Crackles are intermittent explosive sounds that have no recognizable musical tone. Crackles are often characterized as "coarse" and "fine." Coarse crackles are bubbling or gurgling sounds, whereas fine crackles have been described as Velcro or cellophane-type sounds. One of the mechanisms responsible for coarse crackles is bursting bubbles of secretions within airways; fine crackling is generally caused by various lung diseases in which some airways remain closed for a portion of inspiration and then suddenly open. Course crackles associated with bursting of fluid bubbles may occur with severe pulmonary edema, bronchitis, and bronchopneumonia, in which copious secretions are present within the airways (Table 28-1). Fine crackling heard during the sudden opening of airways during inspiration is due to the rapid equalization of gas pressure upstream and downstream from the closed airway section. Persistent fine crackling is often a sign of fibrosis, inflammation, and interstitial pulmonary edema (see Table 28-1).

Wheezes are continuous musical or whistling sounds generated by air passing through a narrowed airway and causing a regular vibration or oscillation of the airway wall. Wheezing noises occur when an airway lumen is narrowed. If conditions are right, the airway wall flutters between open and nearly closed to produce a continuous sound. The amplitude, pitch, and duration of the wheeze depend on the velocity of airflow and mechanical properties of the airway involved. A common misconception is that the pitch of the wheeze depends on the

Table 28-1. Causes of Abnormal Lung Sounds in Dogs and Cats

CRACKLES	WHEEZES	SILENT LUNG
Coarse	Inspiratory	Pneumothorax
Severe pulmonary edema	Laryngeal obstruction	Pleural effusion
Left heart failure	Necrotic laryngitis	Right heart failure
Hypoalbuminemia	Laryngeal paralysis	Neoplasia
Others	Laryngeal edema	Hypoalbuminemia
Bronchopneumonia	Laryngeal collapse	Hemothorax
Pulmonary contusions (trauma)	Tracheal stenosis	Chylothorax
	Tracheal foreign body	Pyothorax
Fine	Extrathoracic tracheal collapse	Feline infectious peritonitis
Interstitial pulmonary edema	Extraluminal tracheal compression	Diaphragmatic hernia
Chronic interstitial pneumonia	Neoplastic mass	Intrathoracic neoplastic mass
Chronic interstitial fibrosis	Lymphadenopathy	Consolidated lung lobe
	Expiratory	Abscess
	Bronchitis	Granuloma
	Allergic (asthma, PIE)	Neoplasm
	Infectious	Lung lobe torsion
	Bronchopneumonia	Extreme obesity
	Chronic obstructive pulmonary disease (COPD)	Neuromuscular weakness
	Pulmonary contusions	Polyradiculoneuritis (coonhound paralysis)
	Lungworms	Diaphragmatic paralysis
	Pulmonary granulomatosis	Others
	Deep mycosis	
	Heartworm disease	

PIE, pulmonary infiltrates with eosinophils; COPD, chronic obstructive pulmonary disease

size of the diseased airway. The pitch is actually determined by the mass and elasticity of the solid structures set into oscillation, as well as the linear velocity of the airflow through the stenosed airway.

Wheezing is much more common during expiration than during inspiration. Causes of expiratory wheezes include bronchospasm, mucosal edema, mucous plugging, foreign bodies, tumors, and hilar lymphadenopathy (see Table 28-1). Lower pitched wheezes are often caused by secretions in the airways, such as occur with bronchopneumonia, and change markedly after a deep cough. Inspiratory wheezing, sometimes termed *stridor,* is associated with a rigid stenosis of the upper airway, trachea, or mainstem bronchi, such as laryngeal edema or inflammation, tracheal foreign body, or segmental tracheal stenosis (see Table 28-1).

Other abnormal sounds that may be heard upon thoracic auscultation include pleural friction rub and silent lung. A pleural friction rub is characterized by a loud, coarse sound resembling creaking or rubbing of new leather and is not commonly heard in dogs and cats. Muffled lung sounds or silent lung are often the result of fluid or air in the pleural space. Obesity, diaphragmatic hernia, space-occupying thoracic lesions, emphysema, diffuse terminal airway disease, and weak, shallow breathing from neuromuscular diseases are other causes of muffled lung sounds (see Table 28-1).

DIAGNOSTIC PLAN

History and Physical Examination

The signs most often reported by owners of animals with abnormal lung sounds are coughing, difficult breathing, and wheezing (see chapters 25 and 26). The wheezing described by clients is often due to abnormal sounds originating from the nasal passages and upper airway. Careful questioning should be done to avoid confusion.

A thorough physical examination should be performed in a quiet area so that meaningful thoracic auscultation can be accomplished. Heart and lung sounds should be evaluated while the patient is standing. If the animal is panting, an assistant should intermittently close the animal's mouth while auscultation is done. Purring in a cat can usually be stopped for a short period of time by either exerting moderate pressure on the animal's larynx or distracting the cat by turning on water flow in a sink. Skin and hair noises can be minimized by first wetting the hair over the area to be ausculted and holding the head of the stethoscope firmly against the thoracic wall. Both sides of the thorax should be ausculted in several areas to evaluate each lung field. Referred sounds from the nasal passages and pharyngeal/laryngeal areas can be differentiated by alternating the site of auscultation from the thorax to the laryngeal area back and forth and comparing the quality and intensity of sounds. If referred sounds from these areas are being heard during thoracic auscultation, the sounds will be similar except less intense over the thorax. After listening to each lung field, it is often helpful to induce coughing with digital pressure on the trachea and then reevaluate lung sounds.

Laboratory Evaluation

Diagnostic procedures for evaluation of a patient with abnormal lung sounds are similar to those used for animals with coughing and dyspnea (see chapters 25 and 26).

SYMPTOMATIC THERAPY

Symptomatic treatment of abnormal lung sounds is not necessary. See chapters 25 and 26 for a discussion of symptomatic therapy of the related problems of coughing and dyspnea.

REFERENCE

1. Roudebush P: Lung sounds. J Am Vet Med Assoc 181:122–126, 1982

29

Sneezing and Nasal Discharge

MICHAEL R. LAPPIN

PROBLEM DEFINITION

Sneezing is a superficial reflex that originates in the mucous membranes lining the nasal cavity and is easily induced by chemical or mechanical stimuli. The sneeze results in forceful expulsion of air that passes through the airways with great velocity.[3] This airstream helps clear the respiratory passages, which is the primary function of the sneeze.

Nasal discharge is any material that escapes the respiratory passageways via the external nares. Discharges are classified by their physical characteristics as serous, mucoid, purulent, hemorrhagic, or a combination of these types. Food or fluid that had been previously ingested may occasionally be passed secondary to conditions affecting the oronasal cavities. The nasal discharge may be unilateral or bilateral, continuous or intermittent, or present only associated with sneezing.

PATHOPHYSIOLOGY

The afferent impulses generated by stimulation of the nasal mucous membranes are carried via the trigeminal nerve to the medulla of the brain, where a complex automatic sequence of events is initiated. After rapid inspiration, the vocal folds and epiglottis close, followed by forceful contraction of the abdominal, external intercostal, and other respiratory muscles, which greatly elevates the air pressure within the respiratory passageways. The epiglottis and vocal folds then open rapidly, allowing the passage of air, which results in the sneeze.

Sneezing and nasal discharge occur primarily with conditions directly affecting the nasal cavity and secondarily to pharyngeal or more distal respiratory passageway disease. The nasal cavity function includes olfaction and the filtration, warming, humidification, and conduction of air. The nasal cavity is composed of cartilagenous turbinates covered by a ciliated pseudocolumnar epithelium. This epithelium is primarily respiratory peripherally and olfactory caudomedially and caudodorsally. The lamina propria of the respiratory portion contains serous, mucous, and mixed tubuloalveolar glands. Goblet cells are also present throughout the nasal cavity. The lateral nasal gland is a serous gland in the lateral mucosa that functions primarily in heat exchange. Paranasal sinuses, including the maxillary recess, the frontal sinus, and the sphenoidal sinuses, are connected with the respiratory passageways and occasionally are primarily or secondarily involved with diseases resulting in nasal discharge and sneeze.[4]

The nasal cavity can only respond to insult in a limited number of ways. Most conditions leading to inflammation of the nasal mucosa result in glandular secretions that generally progress from a serous discharge early in the course of disease to a mucoid or mucopurulent discharge as chronicity and secondary bacterial infection develop. Hemorrhage can occur with trauma, coagulopathies, any acute deep insult to the richly vascularized nasal mucosa, chronic erosive or invasive disease, or acute multiple sneezing induced by any etiology. Food or water draining from the external nares may be present due to a communication of the oral and nasal cavities or by passage of ingesta from the nasopharynx into the nasal cavity.

RULE OUTS AND DIAGNOSTIC PLAN

The causes of sneeze and nasal discharge in the dog and cat are listed in Table 29-1. The signalment, history, physical examination, and physical characteristics of the nasal discharge, if present, will help direct the veterinary clinician to appropriate diagnostic procedures and subsequent therapy.

Signalment

Animal signalment occasionally will suggest likely etiologies. Young, very old, and immunosuppressed animals tend to be more susceptible to infectious agents. Clinical signs associated with congenital diseases often appear in the very young. Brachycephalic breeds often have nasal discharge directly related to stenotic nares or may have nasal discharge secondary to poor handling of ingesta or respiratory secretions in the pharyngeal region caused by an elongated soft palate. Nasal neoplasia and dental disease are more common in older dogs and cats. Medium to large breed dogs with a long nose may have an increased frequency of nasal neoplasia. Nasal foreign bodies and fungal disease are more likely to occur in free-roaming animals.

History

Acute sneezing or nasal discharge accompanied by ocular discharge is suggestive of viral disease. Congenital abnormalities or pharyngeal disorders cause clinical signs soon after the animal eats or drinks. Recurrent sneeze and nasal discharge that respond to antibiotic therapy are suggestive of bacterial rhinitis secondary to any etiology, including trauma, allergic disease, nasal foreign body, fungal infection, and neoplasia. Seasonal bilateral serous to mucoid nasal discharge accompanied by sneezing and ocular discharge is consistent with allergic rhinitis. Nasal foreign bodies often lead to acute violent sneezing accompanied by pawing or rubbing of the face. Neoplasia and fungal infection often present with a history of nasal discharge that slowly changed in character from serous to mucopurulent to hemorrhagic. Animals with a history of chronic otitis externa/media will occasionally present with nasal discharge and sneeze due to communication of the middle ear with the nasopharynx via the eustachian tube. Gagging is commonly reported by the owners of animals with pharyngeal disease. Foreign bodies, nasopharyngeal polyps in cats, neoplasia (including tonsilar), cricopharyngeal dysphagia, and inflammation of any etiology may present with a history of gagging and nasal discharge. Sneezing is much more common with acute disease than in chronic disorders.

Physical Examination

A thorough examination of the entire animal, with emphasis on the respiratory system, eyes, and oropharyngeal cavity, is indicated in any animal with sneezing and nasal discharge. Stenotic nares, cleft palate, traumatic oronasal fistula, otitis externa or media, dental disease, and elongated soft palate may be detected on examination of the head and mouth. Redness of the oropharynx or red and enlarged tonsils can occur with many diseases leading to sneezing and nasal discharge. Facial or palate deformity is most consistent with severe fungal disease or neoplasia. Fractures of the bones overlying the nasal cavity often can be palpated. *Pneumonyssus caninum* is occasionally seen crawling from the external nares.

Many upper respiratory disorders (*e.g.*, infectious disease, allergy, and facial deformities) also cause ocular discharge. Feline viral rhinotracheitis may cause dendritic corneal ulceration, anorexia, and ptyalism secondary to oral ulceration. Both canine distemper and cryptococcocosis can cause chorioretinitis; cryptococcosis may cause anterior uveitis.[6]

Unilateral nasal discharge is most consistent with neoplasia, fungal disease, foreign bodies, tooth root abscess, and oronasal fistulas. Aggressive neoplasia or severe chronic fungal infection may invade both sides of the nasal cavity, leading to bilateral discharge. Bilateral nasal discharge occurs with infectious diseases, congenital deformities, pharyngeal diseases, and allergic rhinitis. Dullness on percussion of the nasal cavity and paranasal sinuses is often present with many diseases but is most consistent with fungal granulomas and neoplasia. Diminished airflow through one or both external nares occurs with most nasal diseases.

Pulmonary parenchymal sounds may be abnormal in disseminated fungal disease or neoplasia, in primary pulmonary disease resulting in secondary nasal discharge, or in diseases affecting both upper and lower respiratory systems (canine distemper virus). Coagulopathies may have symptoms of bleeding in

(Text continues on p 238.)

Table 29-1. Common Causes of Sneeze and Nasal Discharge in the Dog and Cat

CAUSE	SIGNALMENT	HISTORY	PE*	DISCHARGE	Dxp†	COMMENTS
Congenital						
Stenotic nares	Brachycephalic dogs	Snoring	Stenotic nares	Serous to mucoid	Physical examination	Often without respiratory signs
Cleft palate	Young, all breeds	Poor suckling Milk from nares Chronic discharge postweaning	Cleft palate Abnormal lung sounds with aspiration pneumonia	Food or fluid Mucopurulent with secondary infection Usually bilateral	Physical examination	Less common in cats
Elongated soft palate	Brachycephalic dogs	Gagging, snorting ± association with eating	Elongated soft palate Reddened pharynx Inflamed tonsils	Food or fluid Serous to mucopurulent Usually bilateral	Physical examination	Diagnosis may require sedation; often without respiratory signs
Dysphagia	All breeds Congenital—young Acquired—older	Coughing, gagging Multiple swallowing attempts	Reddened pharynx Inflamed tonsils Abnormal lung sounds with aspiration pneumonia	Food or fluid Serous to mucopurulent Usually bilateral	Physical examination Fluoroscopy Metabolic workup Electromyogram	Many acquired etiologies, often without respiratory signs
Infectious‡						
Viral						
Feline viral rhinotracheitis (FVR)	All breeds All ages; more common in young	Animal contact Poor vaccination history Anorexia common Pytalism	± oral ulcers ± conjunctivitis ± dendritic ulcer ± abnormal lung sounds Fever common	Mucopurulent	Direct fluorescent antibody staining of conjunctival scraping	Often severe clinical disease; abortion and bronchopneumonia common
Feline calcivirus	All breeds All ages (more common than FVR)	Animal contact Poor vaccination history Anorexia common Pytalism	Oral/nasal ulcers ± conjunctivitis ± abnormal lung sounds Fever common	Mucopurulent	Diagnosis by clinical signs and exclusion	Ulcers and bronchopneumonia more common than FVR Oculonasal discharge less common than FVR

Reovirus	Cats—all breeds and ages	Mild symptoms	Fever rare Often ocular signs alone	Rare	Diagnosis by exclusion	Generally mild respiratory signs
Canine distemper virus	All breeds, all ages	Poor vaccination history Animal contact Multiple system involvement (CNS, gastrointestinal)	Fever ± vomiting/diarrhea ± abnormal lung sounds ± CNS disease ± ophthalmologic changes ± foot pad hyperkeratosis	Mucopurulent	Clinical signs Complete blood cell count (lymphopenia) Direct fluorescent antibody staining of conjunctival scraping Serology Characteristic cerebrospinal fluid	Immunosuppressive disease with multiple system involvement
Bacterial						
Many species	All breeds—dogs Common in cats All ages	Chronic sneeze Snuffling respiration Often 2° to a primary inflammation	Decreased air flow Dull percussion Signs of primary etiology ± anorexia and dehydration	Mucopurulent Usually bilateral	Clinical signs History of primary etiology Culture occasionally valuable	Generally a secondary disease Often secondary to virus, trauma, fungus, congenital, and neoplasia
Chlamydia	Cats All breeds, all ages More frequently in young	Animal contact Usually no polysystemic illness	Mild conjunctivitis	Serous to mucopurulent Usually bilateral	Cytology Exclusion History	Frequently recurrent Mildest feline infectious upper respiratory disease
Mycoplasma	All breeds, all ages	Usually no polysystemic illness	Mild conjunctivitis	Rare Serous, if it occurs	Cytology Culture	Primarily conjunctivitis
Fungal						
Aspergillus and *Penicillium*	Brachycephalic less common All ages	Progressive Secondary to trauma (15%)	Fever—rare Facial or palate deformity rare Decreased air flow Dull percussion ± lymphadenopathy or anorexia	Mucoid, mucopurulent, or hemorrhagic ⅓ unilateral ⅔ bilateral	Cytology Culture Serology Radiographic changes	Difficult to distinguish from neoplasia Not recognized in cats

(Continued)

Table 29-1. Common Causes of Sneeze and Nasal Discharge in the Dog and Cat *(Continued)*

CAUSE	SIGNALMENT	HISTORY	PE*	DISCHARGE	Dxp†	COMMENTS
Cryptococcus neoformans	Dog and cat All ages	Upper respiratory signs Polysystemic progression	± fever ± CNS signs ± abnormal lung sounds due to dissemination ± ophthalmologic changes	Mucoid to mucopurulent	Cytology Serology Culture	Most common mycotic infection in cats
Trichosporon sp.			Nasal polyp or granuloma			Rare
Rhinosporidium seeberi			Nasal polyp or granuloma			Rare
Parasitic						
Linguatula serrata	Dogs—all ages	Mild sneezing	None	Serous to none	Cytology (isolation)	Often subclinical
Pneumonyssus caninum	Dogs—all ages	Mild sneezing	None	Serous to none	Cytology (isolation)	Often subclinical
Neoplastic	Dog—common Cats—rare Older animals	Progressive	Decreased air flow Dull percussion ± exophthalmos ± facial or palate deformity	Progressive from mucopurulent to hemorrhagic	Cytology Radiographic changes Biopsy	Facial deformity, exophthalmos, unilateral more common than fungal
Allergic	Dog and cat Usually young	Acute, mild signs Seasonal	± conjunctivitis ± dermatologic change	Serous	History	May predispose to secondary bacterial infection
Inflammatory polyps	Cats—young	Gagging Dysphagia ± respiratory signs	± reddened pharynx ± reddened tonsils	Serous to mucopurulent	Caudal pharyngeal examination	Likely congenital and arise from the middle ear

Dental disease	All animals More common in old	Halitosis Paroxysms of sneezing Pawing face	Fistula Gingival recession Dental calculi Facial abscess Halitosis	Unilateral Mucopurulent Occasionally blood tinged	Physical examination Skull radiographs	
Otitis media	All animals	Mild signs Otitis externa	Keratoconjunctivitis sicca Otic lesions	Dry, crusty	Otoscopic examination Aspirate and culture	Damage to chorda tympani or facial nerves leads to decreased nasal mucosal gland secretion.
Trauma	All animals	Acute History of trauma	Fractures often palpable	Hemorrhagic Unilateral or bilateral	History Radiographs	Secondary bacterial osteomyelitis common
Foreign body	All animals Cats less likely	Acute paroxysms of sneezing Head-banging Free-roaming	Nonspecific	Serous to mucopurulent, depending on chronicity Occasionally hemorrhagic	Sedation and nasal and caudopharyngeal examination	Secondary bacterial infection common Commonly secondary to plant materials
Coagulation abnormalities	All animals Dogs more frequently	Hemorrhage without trauma Hemorrhage in other areas	Pale mucous membranes ± hemothorax ± hemoperitoneum ± petechiae/ecchymoses Dependent on etiology	Hemorrhagic	Platelet count Activated coagulation time Bleeding time Factor VIII–related antigen	Multiple etiologies—can occur with thrombocytopenia, platelet dysfunction, or factor deficiency

* Physical examination
† Diagnostic plan
‡ Feline leukemia virus immunosuppression may be involved with recurrent upper respiratory infections.

other areas, including petechiation or ecchymoses of the skin and mucous membranes, abdominal distension due to hemoperitoneum, dull heart and lung sounds due to hemothorax, or joint swelling due to hemarthrosis.

Physical Characteristics of the Nasal Discharge

Serous nasal discharge is present in the initial stage of most diseases affecting the nasal cavity. Continuous or long-term serous discharges are most consistent with mild irritative disease such as allergy or nasal parasitism. Viral infection or any long-term inflammatory disease process with secondary bacterial overgrowth produces a mucopurulent discharge. Hemorrhage is present most often with neoplasia, trauma, coagulopathies, and fungal infection.

Diagnostic Plan

Diagnostic procedures with the greatest potential yield include cytology, serology, culture and sensitivity, oral or nasal examination under sedation, thoracic and nasal radiographs, direct fluorescent antibody techniques, coagulation profiles, caudal nasal cavity examination with a dental mirror, endoscopy, and nasal biopsy.

Cytology characterizes the type of nasal discharge present and occasionally will detect fungal elements, neoplastic cells, or parasites. Direct swabs can be evaluated; if deep disease is suspected, nasal flushing with sterile saline may be indicated. Airflow through the nasal cavities can be semiquantitated by holding a cool microscope slide in front of the external nares and observing for vapor formation. Cats with chronic nasal discharge or recurrent sneezing should be assessed for feline leukemia virus infection.

Direct fluorescent antibody staining of cells obtained by conjunctival scrapings can be used to detect viral elements of canine distemper virus and feline viral rhinotracheitis. *Chlamydia* and *Mycoplasma* inclusion bodies may be detected on cytologic evaluation of conjunctival scrapings.

Bacterial and fungal cultures are usually of low yield in that the nasal cavity has a wide population of normal bacterial flora and *Aspergillus* and *Penicillium* may be isolated from normal animals. Occasionally, chronic bacterial sinusitis and rhinitis in cats will yield a pure bacterial culture that may be useful in determining appropriate antibiotic therapy.

Serologic assays to detect circulating antibodies to *Aspergillus, Penicillium,* and *Cryptococcus* are now available.[2,5] Unfortunately, a positive titer may reflect previous exposure and may not be indicative of ongoing or active disease.

Radiographs of the head and thoracic cavity are often indicated in animals with chronic nasal discharge or signs of polysystemic involvement. Thoracic radiographs are best performed in an awake animal, but anesthesia is desirable when evaluating the nasal cavities and paranasal sinuses because fine detail is imperative. Destruction of the nasal turbinates or nasal bones can be detected radiographically; its presence is most consistent with neoplasia and fungal disease. Destruction of the lamina dura is indicative of dental disease.

If destructive disease is present radiographically, biopsy is indicated. Biopsy of nasal masses has been described utilizing endoscopy, open surgical exploration, and techniques utilizing various biopsy punches.[7] Often, surgery is required to make a definitive diagnosis.

If a hemorrhagic discharge is present with or without signs of polysystemic disease, coagulation should be evaluated. This is best done in a practice situation by performing a platelet count, an activated coagulation time, and a bleeding time. In certain breeds, primarily the Doberman pinscher, a Factor VIII–related antigen assay should be performed in animals with spontaneous idiopathic hemorrhagic nasal discharge to help rule out von Willebrand's disease.[1]

SYMPTOMATIC THERAPY

Primary control of sneezing and nasal discharge is attained by removal of the initiating cause. This stresses the importance of an accurate diagnosis. Specific treatment modalities for each etiologic diagnosis have been extensively described elsewhere. Symptomatic control can be used while completing diagnostic procedures. Medications are most commonly delivered to the respiratory tract by systemic or topical methods or nebulization.

Decongestants can be utilized either topically or systemically in the treatment of nasal discharge. Commonly used drugs include oxymethazoline HCl (Afrin) topically and pseudoephedrine (Sudafed [up to 30 mg every 8 to 12 hours orally]) systemically. These drugs induce vasoconstriction of the nasal vasculature by virtue of their sympathomimetic effect. Heart disease is a potential contraindication for the use of these compounds. The major side-effect with topical decongestants is rebound congestion, which can be avoided by alternating nostrils every 2 to 3 days.

Antibiotics may be administered topically, systemically, or via nebulization and may be beneficial in most causes of mucopurulent nasal discharges. Care must be taken not to let partial antibiotic response mislead the normal diagnostic process. The author has had success utilizing ophthalmic antibiotic preparations intranasally in cats with chronic rhinitis. Systemic antibiotics also may decrease nasal discharge with primary or secondary bacterial involvement. A major problem with antibiotic therapy is poor penetration into thick nasal secretions.

Corticosteroids are helpful when used in allergic rhinitis. Topical application of corticosteroids have no proven beneficial effect. Corticosteroids are contraindicated in infectious diseases and should not be used in animals with mucopurulent nasal discharge.

Nasal hemorrhage can often be controlled by quieting the animal (occasionally requiring tranquilization), applying cold nasal compresses, or instilling four or five drops of 1 : 50,000 epinephrine intranasally. If epinephrine is used, the animal should be carefully monitored for adverse cardiovascular effects. Some cases will require sedation and packing of the internal and external nares.

Humidification of the airways can be helpful in all causes of mucoid or mucopurulent nasal discharge. Systemic hydration should be maintained with parenteral fluid therapy if dehydration is present. Nebulization of saline, the use of a mist tent with a humidifier, or placing the animal in a bathroom filled with steam from the shower three to four times daily may help loosen and mobilize respiratory secretions.

REFERENCES

1. Dodds WJ: Von Willebrand's disease in dogs. Mod Vet Pract 65:681–686, 1984
2. Harvey CE, O'Brien JA: Nasal Aspergillosis-Penicillosis. In Kirk RW (ed): Current Veterinary Therapy VIII, pp 237–241. Philadelphia, WB Saunders, 1983
3. Jenson D: The Principles of Physiology, pp 227, 739. New York, Appleton-Century-Crofts, 1976
4. Miller ME: Anatomy of the Dog, pp 716–719. Philadelphia, WB Saunders, 1964
5. Prevost E, et al: Successful medical management of severe feline cryptococcosis. J Am Anim Hosp Assoc 18:111–114, 1982
6. Slatter DH: Fundamentals of Veterinary Opthalmology, pp 701–703, 228. Philadelphia, WB Saunders, 1981
7. Withrow SJ et al: Aspiration and punch biopsy techniques for nasal tumors. J Am Anim Hosp Assoc 21:551–554, 1985

Part Eight

DIGESTIVE PROBLEMS

30

Ptyalism

LARRY M. CORNELIUS

DEFINITION

Ptyalism is excessive secretion of saliva. This condition is also called hypersialosis. Drooling may be the result of either excessive production of saliva or reduced or abnormal swallowing (See chapter 31). It may be difficult to distinguish between true ptyalism and inadequate swallowing of normal quantities of saliva. In this discussion, ptyalism will be used to describe any condition characterized by excessive loss of saliva from the mouth.

PATHOPHYSIOLOGY

Saliva is normally produced by four major paired salivary glands: the parotids, mandibulars, sublinguals, and zygomatics. Both sympathetic (inhibitory) and parasympathetic (stimulatory) nerves supply the salivary glands, with the latter being through cranial nerves V, VII, and IX. Salivation is stimulated by both taste and tactile stimuli from the tongue and other areas of the mouth. Salivation also occurs in response to reflexes originating in the gastrintestinal tract when certain gastrointestinal diseases are present. Salivation can be stimulated by impulses originating in higher centers of the brain as a result of conditioned reflexes (pavlovian response).

The saliva of dogs and cats has no significant enzyme content. Saliva's function is to soften and lubricate food in preparation for its passage through the pharynx and esophagus into the stomach. Evaporation of saliva from the oral mucosa is also important for heat loss in dogs.

Ptyalism may be caused by several disorders that can be categorized as (1) conformational disorders of the lips and mouth; (2) morphologic disorders of the gastrointestinal system; (3) metabolic disorders; (4) neurologic disorders; and (5) drugs or toxins.

Conformational disorders of the lips and mouth causing drooling are often seen in giant breed dogs. Morphologic disorders of the gastrointestinal system may cause ptyalism by causing pain and nausea. Drooling is most often caused by reluctance to swallow due to painful lesions such as stomatitis, pharyngitis, and esophagitis. Less commonly, ptyalism is caused by neuromuscular disorders affecting the oral, pharyngeal, or esophageal stages of swallowing and is associated with dysphagia (see chapter 31). Inflammatory, infiltrative, and obstructive lesions of the gastrointestinal tract stimulate receptors, which may cause nausea and drooling. Diseases of the salivary glands are usually characterized by swelling of the glands rather than ptyalism.

Metabolic disorders such as hepatic encephalopathy and uremia often cause excessive salivation, but the mechanism is not defined. Increases in the blood of ammonia, urea, and other nitrogenous wastes may cause nausea, which in turn causes ptyalism.

As previously mentioned, salivation aids in heat loss in dogs. Overheating due to a hot, humid environment or nervousness and excitement cause ptyalism.

Neurologic disorders causing ptyalism include neuromuscular swallowing disorders (see chapter 31), nausea caused by excessive stimulation of the vestibular apparatus (motion sickness), and conditioned reflexes (pavlovian response). The neurologic effects of the rabies virus cause drooling due to interruption of swallowing.

Several drugs and toxins may cause ptyalism by different mechanisms. Oral drugs or toxins may have a bitter or noxious taste or be caustic. Other agents such as apomorphine cause nausea by stimulating the chemoreceptor trigger zone or the vomiting center in the midbrain. Organophosphates result in parasympathetic stimulation of salivary secretion.

Prolonged, severe ptyalism, especially when accompanied by decreased appetite and water intake, may cause dehydration. Electrolyte and acid–base balance is minimally affected.

DIAGNOSTIC PLAN

History and Physical Examination

Morphologic lesions of the lips, mouth, or pharynx account for most cases of ptyalism. The diagnosis can often be established by history and physical examination (Table 30-1). Access to drugs, toxins, or caustic agents should be established. Associated signs such as nausea, retching, and vomiting are indications for a work-up for either a gastrointestinal or metabolic cause of vomiting (see chapter 32). A history of "staring into space," depression, head-pressing, and intermittent blindness is typical of hepatoencephalopathy. Weight loss, coughing, and difficulty in eating often are reported in animals with swallowing disorders (see chapter 31). Rabies vaccination history and possible exposure to unvaccinated animals should always be established prior to physical examination.

(Text continues on p 248.)

Table 30-1. Characteristic Findings of Common Disorders Causing Ptyalism

DISORDER	CLINICAL SIGNS OTHER THAN PTYALISM	HEMATOLOGY	BIOCHEMISTRY	SPECIAL TESTS
CONFORMATIONAL DISORDERS OF THE LIPS (GIANT BREEDS)	Secondary cheilitis	Normal	Normal	None
LESIONS OR DISORDERS OF THE MOUTH AND PHARYNX				
Gingivitis/Stomatitis				
Pemphigus vulgaris	Anorexia Fever ± Mucocutaneous ulcerative lesions Painful mouth	Normal or Leukocytosis with neutrophilia and left shift	Normal or ↑ globulin	Biopsy of mucocutaneous lesions for histopathology and immunofluroresence testing
Secondary infection due to FeLV in cats	Anorexia Depression Pale membranes Sneezing and naso-ocular discharge ± Oral inflammation Painful mouth	Nonregenerative anemia Leukopenia with inappropriate left shift ±	Variable	FeLV test on blood
Viral upper respiratory infection	Anorexia Depression Fever Sneezing Naso-ocular discharge Oral ulcers Painful mouth	Normal or Mild nonregenerative anemia Mild leukocytosis with mature neutrophilia	Normal	None
Uremia	Anorexia Depression Vomiting Oral ulcers Polydipsia/polyuria ±	Variable	Variable BUN ↑ TCO_2 ↓	Variable Urine culture Abdominal radiographs IVP Renal biopsy

(Continued)

Table 30-1. Characteristic Findings of Common Disorders Causing Ptyalism *(Continued)*

DISORDER	CLINICAL SIGNS OTHER THAN PTYALISM	HEMATOLOGY	BIOCHEMISTRY	SPECIAL TESTS
Ingestion of caustic agent	Anorexia Vomiting Diarrhea Oral ulcers Painful mouth	Normal or Stress leukogram	Normal	None
Foreign Body	Anorexia Pawing at mouth Painful mouth	Normal	Normal	Radiograph mouth and neck
Neoplasm	Anorexia Oropharyngeal mass	Variable	Normal or ↑ globulin	Radiograph mouth and thorax
Functional Disorder of the Pharynx or Cricopharynx	Dysphagia (see chapter 31.)			
ESOPHAGEAL DISORDERS	Dysphagia (see chapter 31.)			
OTHER GASTROINTESTINAL DISORDERS				
Gastroenteritis	Nausea Vomiting Diarrhea Depression	See chapters 32 and 33.		
METABOLIC DISORDERS				
Hyperthermia	Hot, humid environment Marked panting Polydipsia	Normal or PCV and plasma protein ↑ Stress leukogram	Normal or ↑ albumin and globulin	None

Hepatoencephalopathy Congenital portosystemic shunt Acquired portosystemic shunt (liver disease) Hepatic failure	Head pressing Apparent blindness Stupor/coma	See chapter 51		Plasma ammonia or an ammonia tolerance test BSP retention Portal venography
Uremia	See above.			
DRUGS OR TOXINS				
Bitter or Disagreeable Taste	Anorexia Excessive licking and swallowing Shaking head	Normal	Normal	None
Organophosphates	Vomiting Diarrhea Muscle trembling Miosis Seizures Other CNS signs	Normal or Stress leukogram	Normal	Serum cholinesterase level (decreased)
NEUROLOGIC DISORDERS				
Rabies	Depression Paresis/paralysis Aggressiveness Others	Normal	Normal	None before death Fluorescent antibody evaluation of brain after death
Disorders Causing Dysphagia	See chapter 31.			
Conditioned Reflex (Pavlovian Response)	None	Normal	Normal	Normal

±, present or absent; FeLV, feline leukemia virus; BUN, blood urea nitrogen; TCO_2, total carbon dioxide; IVP, intravenous pyelogram; PCV, packed cell volume; BSP, bromosulfophthalein; CNS, central nervous system; ↑, increased

Protective gloves should be worn and caution used whenever rabies is a possible cause of drooling.

Sedation or general anesthesia may be required to adequately examine the oral and pharyngeal cavities, but this should be delayed until laboratory results are obtained if a systemic or metabolic cause is likely. Thorough palpation should include the salivary glands and the abdomen. Neurologic examination is indicated if a neurologic disorder is suspected.

Laboratory Evaluation

Laboratory tests needed depend upon the suspected cause of ptyalism (Table 30-1). For some oropharyngeal lesions, such as a foreign body or stomatitis caused by a caustic substance, further evaluation may not be needed. Biopsy of oral ulcers for histopathology and immunofluorescence testing is sometimes indicated. Other causes, such as suspected hepatoencephalopathy, require a complete blood count, urine analysis, biochemical profile, and special tests such as blood ammonia, an ammonia tolerance test, and bromosulfophthalein (BSP) retention. Radiographic studies of the oral and pharyngeal cavities or other parts of the gastrointestinal tract may be needed (see chapters 31 and 32).

SYMPTOMATIC THERAPY

Symptomatic treatment of ptyalism is only necessary whenever excessive salivation is severe and prolonged. Methods to reduce flow of saliva should not mask other signs of the underlying disorder and delay a diagnosis.

The objectives of symptomatic treatment for ptyalism are to reduce excessive salivation; keep the mouth, lips, and face as clean as possible; and protect the lips from excoriation and inflammation or infection due to constant wetness. Atropine (0.05 mg/kg three times daily) may be given orally or subcutaneously to decrease flow of saliva. Twice-daily washing with dilute hexachlorophene-containing soaps will help reduce odor and prevent secondary dermatitis of the face and lips.

Application of clear petrolatum jelly to the portions of the lips and face exposed to constant wetness is indicated to reduce the chances of moist dermatitis. If moist dermatitis develops, soaking the affected areas with an astringent solution for 10 minutes two or three times a day will help dry the lesions. If dehydration is present, parenteral lactated Ringer's solution should be administered.

REFERENCE

1. Harvey CE et al: Oral, dental, pharyngeal, and salivary gland disorders. In Ettinger SJ (ed): Textbook of Veterinary Internal Medicine, 2nd ed, pp 1126–1191. Philadelphia, WB Saunders, 1983

31

Dysphagia

LARRY M. CORNELIUS

DEFINITION

Dysphagia is difficulty in swallowing.

PATHOPHYSIOLOGY

Swallowing is a complex reflex action coordinating many muscular functions, including those of the tongue, hard and soft palate, pharynx, esophagus, and gastroesophageal junction. It is coordinated by cranial nerves V, VII, IX, X, and XI and their nuclei in the brain stem, which in turn are controlled by the swallowing center in the reticular formation of the brain.[1]

The normal swallowing sequence has been divided into three phases for detailed study: (1) oropharyngeal, (2) esophageal, and (3) gastroesophageal. The oropharyngeal phase is subdivided into oral, pharyngeal, and cricopharyngeal phases.[1] During the oral stage, the bolus is accumulated at the base of the tongue. Rostral to caudal pharyngeal contractions then propel the bolus from the base of the tongue to the cricopharyngeal passage (pharyngeal stage). The cricopharyngeal stage consists of the relaxation of the cricopharyngeal sphincter, passage of the bolus into the cranial esophagus, closure of the upper esophageal sphincter, and relaxation of the pharyngeal muscles.

As the esophagus receives the bolus, the esophageal phase starts. Both primary and secondary peristaltic waves have been observed in the esophagus.[3] The final phase of swallowing is the gastroesophageal phase, during which the lower esophageal sphincter relaxes and the bolus passes into the stomach. This phase overlaps prior phases.

Swallowing disorders can result from morphologic lesions or functional disorders of any of the structures involved at any time during the passage of a bolus from the mouth to the stomach (Table 31-1). Structural changes that

(Text continues on p 254.)

Table 31-1. Characteristic Findings of Selected Disorders Causing Dysphagia

DISORDER	CLINICAL SIGNS OTHER THAN DYSPHAGIA	HEMATOLOGY	SPECIAL TESTS
Oral			
Morphologic			
Gingivitis, stomatitis	Decreased appetite Weight loss Drooling Halitosis	Normal	Consider biopsy for histopathology and immune fluorescent studies.
Foreign body	Evidence of oral pain (*e.g.*, pawing at mouth) Drooling Gagging	Normal	Radiographs of head may show foreign body.
Neoplasia	Decreased appetite Weight loss Halitosis Gagging Enlarged submandibular lymph nodes	Variable	Radiographs of thorax may show metastasis. Biopsy of mass by needle aspiration or wedge
Functional			
Myopathies			
Eosinophilic myositis	Anorexia Depression Difficulty in opening mouth Late atrophy of masticatory muscles	Usually normal	Biopsy of masticatory muscles may show eosinophilic inflammatory response.
Neuromuscular junction—myasthenia gravis	Weakness worsened with exercise Coughing Dyspnea Weight loss Voice change or loss of voice Regurgitation	Normal or Leukocytosis with neutrophilia and left shift	Transient regaining of strength after 0.1–0.5 mg Tensilon* IV. EMG and repetitive nerve stimulation show decremental response, which disappears after Tensilon.

Neuropathies (cranial nerves V, IX, XII)			
Hydrocephalus	Brachycephalic and toy breeds Open fontanelle Mild depression to severe seizures Visual deficits and motor dysfunction	Normal	Skull radiography including pneumoventriculography EEG
Trauma	Variable		
Idiopathic bilateral trigeminal palsy	Dropped jaw, unable to close mouth Signs usually transient for 1–2 weeks	Normal	EMG of masseter and temporalis muscles
Pharyngeal			
Morphologic			
Pharyngitis/tonsillitis	Depression Anorexia Fever ± Weight loss	Variable—leukocytosis with neutrophilia and left shift	None
Retropharyngeal abscess	See pharyngitis/tonsillitis. Swelling in pharynx	Leukocytosis with neutrophilia and left shift	Fine needle aspirate of pharyngeal swelling shows septic, purulent exudate.
Foreign body	See oral foreign body.		
Neoplasia	See oral neoplasia.		
Functional			
Myopathies—polymyositis	Variable ↓ Exercise tolerance Lameness Stiff gait Painful muscles Weakness Loss of muscle mass Regurgitation with signs of aspiration pneumonia (cough, dyspnea)	Normal or Leukocytosis with neutrophilia and left shift (due to aspiration pneumonia)	Contrast radiographs of pharynx following barium swallow show retention of barium in pharynx and cranial esophagus ↑ CPK ± EMG may show positive waves, fibrillation potentials, and bizarre high-frequency discharges.

(Continued)

Table 31-1. Characteristic Findings of Selected Disorders Causing Dysphagia *(Continued)*

DISORDER	CLINICAL SIGNS OTHER THAN DYSPHAGIA	HEMATOLOGY	SPECIAL TESTS
			Muscle biopsy may show muscle necrosis and lymphocytic inflammation. Immunofluorescence may show staining along muscle sarcolemma.
Neuromuscular junction—myasthenia gravis	See oral.		
Cricopharyngeal			
Functional			
Cricopharyngeal achalasia	Often in puppies Repeated attempts to swallow food Nasal reflux of liquids Coughing Dyspnea Gagging Poor growth rate	Variable Neutrophilic leukocytosis with left shift (due to aspiration pneumonia)	Contrast radiographs of pharynx following barium swallow show retention of barium in pharynx. Fluoroscopy of cricopharyngeal area shows nonopening of the upper esophageal sphincter during a forceful contraction of the pharynx (barium swallow). Laryngotracheal aspiration is observed.
Cricopharyngeal incoordination	See cricopharyngeal achalasia.		Fluoroscopy of pharynx following barium swallow shows opening and closing of the upper esophageal sphincter at inappropriate times, causing retention of barium in pharynx. Laryngotracheal aspiration is observed.

Cricopharyngeal chalasia			
Myasthenia gravis	See oral.		Barium contrast studies show a continuous column of barium from the pharynx into the cranial esophagus. Megaesophagus is often present. Fluoroscopy shows esophagopharyngeal reflux of barium.
Following general anesthesia			
Following cricopharyngeal myotomy			
Esophageal	See chapter 32.		
Morphologic			
Esophagitis			
Stenosis			
Perforation			
Diverticulum			
Neoplasia			
Parasitic (*Spirocerca lupi*)			
Foreign body			
Vascular ring anomaly			
Functional—megaesophagus, congenital and acquired			
Gastroesophageal	See chapter 32.		
Morphologic			
Esophagitis			
Sliding hiatal hernia			
Intussusception			
Neoplasia			
Pharyngostomy tube			
Functional—neuromuscular disorders			
Megaesophagus			
Myasthenia gravis			

* Trade name for edrophonium chloride

IV, intravenously; EMG, electromyogram; EEG, electroencephalogram; ±, present or absent; CPK, creatine phosphokinase

interfere with swallowing include foreign bodies, traumatic lesions, strictures, or mass lesions, either inflammatory or neoplastic. Functional or motility disorders affecting swallowing include failure, spasticity, or incoordination of muscular contractions and are due to neurologic, neuromuscular junction, or muscular diseases. They may be either congenital or acquired.[2]

Disorders affecting the oropharyngeal phase of swallowing usually cause more clinically pronounced dysphagia, whereas abnormalities of the esophageal and gastroesophageal stages are typified by regurgitation (see chapter 32). Discussion in this chapter will be limited to oropharyngeal dysphagia.

DIAGNOSTIC PLAN

Because treatment and prognosis are different, careful differentiation between oral, pharyngeal, and cricopharyngeal dysphagias has been stressed.[1] Swallowing disorders are complex and therefore should be approached systematically.

History and Physical Examination

The chief complaints and presenting clinical signs of swallowing disorders in dogs and cats often are more directly related to the secondary effects of dysphagia than to the swallowing problem itself. Gagging, drooling, "vomiting," coughing, dyspnea, excessive mandibular or head motion while eating, dropping food from the mouth while eating, reluctance to eat, and weight loss or failure to grow may be the main signs reported by the owner. It is very important to consider a swallowing disorder in an animal with any of these signs, so that appropriate diagnostic procedures can be done to document the exact cause.

A thorough physical examination should include a neurologic examination. The gag reflex should be evaluated by placing a finger in the pharynx. Sedation or general anesthesia is often required to thoroughly examine the oropharyngeal regions for morphologic lesions such as foreign bodies and masses.

Laboratory Evaluation

A complete minimum data base (complete blood count, biochemical profile, urine analysis, and fecal parasite examination) should be done to rule out associated problems. An increased serum creatine phosphokinase may be present in some animals with polymyositis. An antinuclear antibody titer and lupus erythematosus cell test should be performed if an immune-mediated disorder is suspected. Neuropathy due to primary hypothyroidism can be ruled out by doing a thyroid-stimulating hormone stimulation test with pre- and post-serum T_4 levels.

Special Studies

Survey radiographs of the mouth and upper cervical area are usually helpful for recognizing gross morphologic abnormalities causing oropharyngeal dysphagia.

For functional (motility) disorders of the pharynx, cricopharyngeal sphincter, and esophagus, special studies (cinefluorography or videofluorography) are needed. The barium swallow must be done using both liquids and solids. Manometry, electromyography, and biopsy are required in some cases to establish a diagnosis.

SYMPTOMATIC THERAPY

Appropriate symptomatic care of dysphagia depends upon the anatomic area involved. Handfeeding or feeding from an elevated platform facilitates intake of food. Use of a pharyngostomy or gastrostomy tube may be needed for a period of time in some cases to maintain nutrition. Aspiration pneumonia is uncommon with oral dysphagia; therefore, either gruels or solids can be fed. Surgical removal of morphologic lesions may be helpful.

Pharyngeal dysphagia is caused by weakened pharyngeal contraction and results in pharyngeal retention of ingested food. Aspiration pneumonia is common. Symptomatic treatment should consist of handfeeding or feeding from an elevated platform. Gruels are more likely to be aspirated and, if fed, should be given slowly in small quantities. Semimoist foods in small chunks are preferred. Aspiration pneumonia should be treated with appropriate antibiotics, preferably selected based upon culture and sensitivity of a transtracheal wash. Bronchodilators may also be helpful. Myotomy of the upper esophageal sphincter is contraindicated.

Cricopharyngeal dysphasia is usually caused by either failure of cricopharyngeal muscles to relax during pharyngeal contraction while swallowing (pharyngeal-cricopharyngeal incoordination) or nonopening of the cricopharyngeal passage (cricopharyngeal achalasia). Signs of cricopharyngeal dysphagia may be reduced or abolished by cricopharyngeal myotomy. However, concurrent weakness of pharyngeal or upper esophageal contraction is a contraindication for surgery. Symptomatic care consists of managing aspiration pneumonia. Feeding from an elevated platform is usually not effective.

If the cause of oropharyngeal dysphagia can be determined, other treatment may be indicated. For example, polymyositis may respond to immunosuppressive dosages of glucocorticoids; however, extreme care must be used to avoid exacerbation of aspiration pneumonia.

REFERENCES

1. Suter PF, Watrous BJ: Oropharyngeal dysphagia in the dog: A cinefluorographic analysis of experimentally induced and spontaneously occurring swallowing disorders. I. Oral stage and pharyngeal stage dysphagias. Vet Radiol 21:24–39, 1980
2. Watrous BJ: Esophageal disease. In Ettinger SJ (ed): Textbook of Veterinary Internal Medicine, 2nd ed, pp 1191–1233 Philadelphia, WB Saunders, 1983
3. Watrous BJ, Suter PF: Oropharyngeal dysphagias in the dog: A cinefluorographic analysis of experimentally induced and spontaneously occurring swallowing disorders. II. Cricopharyngeal stage and mixed oropharyngeal dysphagias. Vet Radiol 24:11–24, 1983

32

Vomiting and Regurgitation

LARRY M. CORNELIUS

DEFINITION

Vomiting is the forceful ejection of food or fluid through the mouth from the stomach and, sometimes, the proximal duodenum. Regurgitation is more passive and results in expulsion of food or fluid from the oral or pharyngeal cavity or the esophagus.

PATHOPHYSIOLOGY

The Vomiting Reflex

Vomiting is a reflex act that requires a coordinated effort of the gastrointestinal, musculoskeletal, and nervous systems. Stimulation of the vomiting center in the medulla causes vomiting. The neurons of the vomiting center can be activated directly by certain blood-borne drugs or toxins or indirectly through afferent nerves or the chemoreceptor trigger zone (CTZ) located on the floor of the fourth ventricle. Stimulation of receptors in abdominal viscera as well as many other sites throughout the body may result in vomiting. Impulses travel along afferent nerve fibers located in the vagus and sympathetic nerves and synapse in the vomiting center. Receptor activation can occur as a result of inflammation, irritation, distention, or hypertonicity, among other factors. The CTZ can be thought of as a receptor because the vomiting center must be functional for the animal to vomit when the CTZ is stimulated. The CTZ is stimulated by blood-borne drugs or toxins such as apormorphine and uremic toxins and by impulses from the inner ear during motion sickness.

Electrolyte and Acid–Base Changes

Vomiting may result in dehydration because of water loss in secretions of the gastrointestinal tract and lack of dietary intake. Potassium depletion, which is a frequent complication of profuse vomiting (see following discussion), may impair renal tubular concentrating ability and worsen dehydration. Prerenal azotemia may develop if dehydration is severe. In patients with preexisting borderline renal insufficiency, dehydration caused by vomiting may cause decompensation and renal failure.

Electrolyte and acid-base changes caused by vomiting are variable and difficult to predict in both magnitude and direction. Deficits of body sodium, potassium, and chloride are likely, but the plasma concentrations depend upon the amount of ion lost relative to the quantity of plasma water lost.

Hyponatremia is commonly associated with persistent vomiting despite the lower concentration of sodium in gastric juice than in plasma. Hyponatremia probably occurs as a result of dilution of extracellular fluid caused by the patient's consumption of water. Clinical signs attributable to hyponatremia generally are not obvious. Dehydration associated with hyponatremia is termed *hypotonic dehydration*. Extracellular fluid is hypotonic, and water is transferred from the extracellular space into the cellular compartment by osmotic attraction. This type of dehydration markedly reduces the volume of extracellular fluid because this compartment has lost volume to the external environment and to the cells. Therefore, such patients are more prone to vascular collapse (shock) and warrant prompt and aggressive fluid therapy.

Deficit of body potassium and hypokalemia are frequent during profuse vomiting. Clinical signs due to potassium deficit include weakness, ileus, and impaired renal concentrating ability. Potassium losses during vomiting are primarily the result of excretion of potassium in urine caused by alkalemia and loss of potassium in vomitus. Lack of dietary intake may contribute to this depletion. Alkalemia also causes transfer of potassium from extracellular to intracellular fluid in exchange for hydrogen ions, thus worsening hypokalemia.

Serum chloride levels and acid–base status of blood during profuse vomiting depend upon the source of the majority of fluid lost and are difficult to predict without laboratory data. Loss of mostly gastric secretions, as occurs with functional or structural causes of pyloric outlet or high duodenal obstruction, results in loss of mostly hydrochloric acid. Pancreatic and biliary secretions contain large quantities of bicarbonate. Obstruction of pancreatic and biliary flow, as may occur during pancreatitis and cholestatic disorders, can significantly reduce the amount of bicarbonate entering the duodenum. Vomitus produced as a result of obstructive disorders of the pancreas and biliary system is more acidic. Acute pancreatitis may also impede pyloric outflow (due to pressure caused by swelling), resulting in loss of mostly hydrochloric acid in vomitus. The usual outcome is hypochloridemia, high serum bicarbonate concentration (metabolic alkalosis), and sometimes metabolic alkalemia (see Causes of Vomiting Usually Associated With Increased Plasma Bicarbonate [TCO_2]). Paradoxical aciduria (urine $pH < 7.0$) may be observed as the kidneys preferentially reabsorb bicarbonate ions to defend against anion (chloride) deficit. Thus, body defense against metabolic alkalemia caused by vomiting is inadequate.

Plasma bicarbonate concentration may be increased, normal, or decreased, and blood pH may be increased, normal, or low during vomiting. As mentioned

Causes of Vomiting Usually Associated With Increased Plasma Bicarbonate (TCO_2)

- Gastric atony with sequestration of fluid in stomach
- Pyloric outlet obstruction
  - Pyloric stenosis
  - Pylorospasm
  - Gastric foreign body
  - Neoplasm (intramural or extramural)
- High duodenal obstruction
  - Foreign body
  - Neoplasm
  - Others
- Acute pancreatitis
- Biliary obstructive disorders

above, the location of the lesion causing vomiting and the acidity of vomitus affect the plasma bicarbonate concentration. Other concurrent abnormalities may affect acid–base balance (see Causes of Vomiting Usually Associated With Normal or Decreased Plasma Bicarbonate [TCO_2]). For example, dehydration may cause poor renal perfusion and retention of metabolic acids. Lactic acidosis can also result from poor tissue perfusion caused by dehydration or any condition causing hypoxia (such as aspiration pneumonia secondary to vomiting). Net plasma bicarbonate will be determined by the process that is quantitatively more severe.

Regurgitation usually does not cause severe changes in electrolyte or acid-base status. Dehydration and weight loss may result primarily from lack of dietary intake.

DIAGNOSTIC PLAN

History and Physical Examination

Signs of vomiting are often confused with those of regurgitation, dysphagia, gagging, and coughing (Fig. 32-1). In none of these disorders, except for vomiting, are hypersalivation, retching, and forceful contractions of the abdominal

Causes of Vomiting Usually Associated With Normal or Decreased Plasma Bicarbonate (TCO_2)

- Gastroenteritis
- Uremia
- Toxins or drugs
- Hypoadrenocorticism
- Others

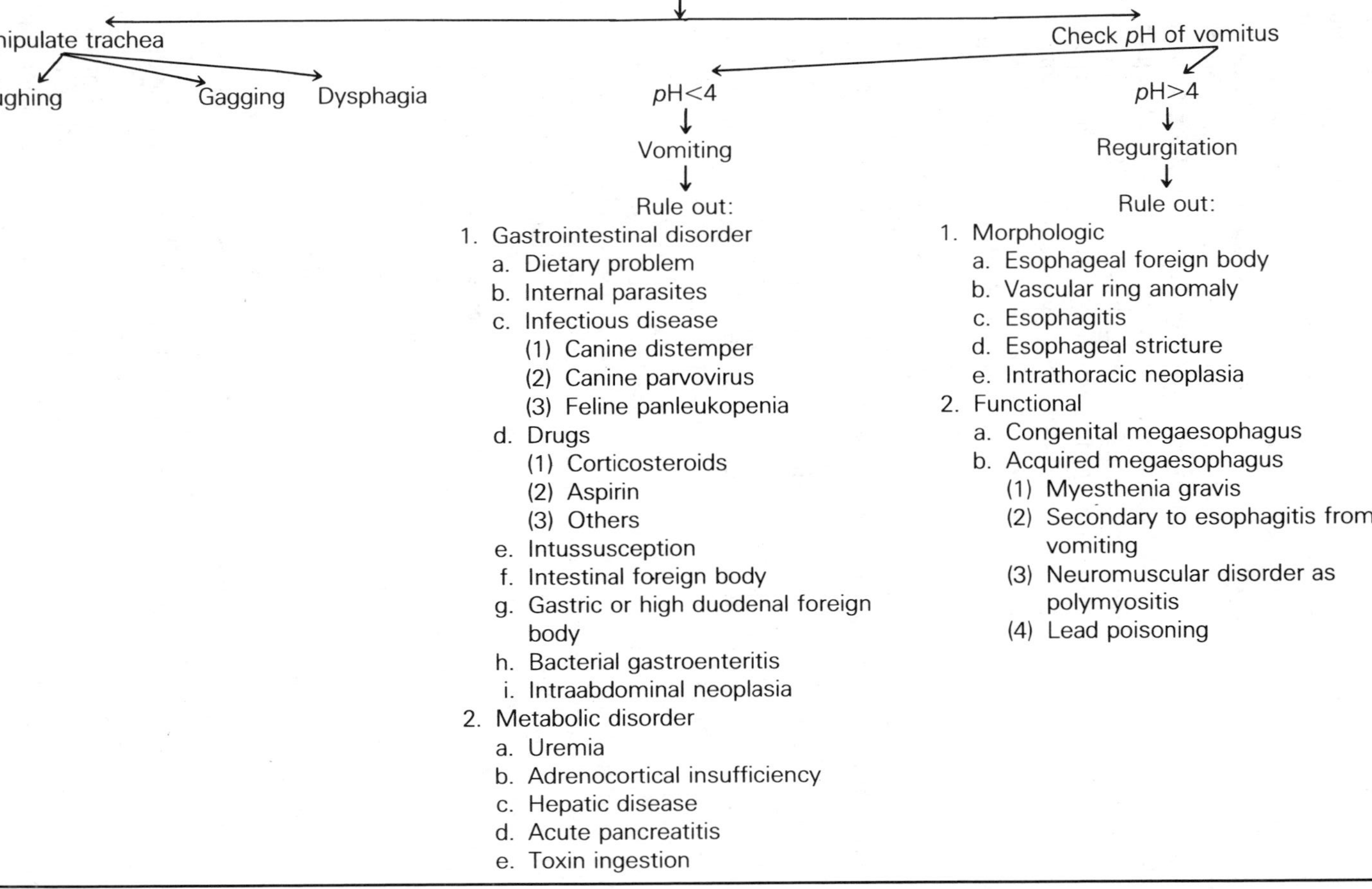

Fig. 32-1. Initial plan for evaluating vomiting.

muscles and diaphragm present. Regurgitation is the effortless expulsion of fluid or food from the pharyngeal cavity or esophagus. By measuring the *p*H of the material regurgitated, it may be possible to determine if the material has been in the stomach. Usually vomitus contains hydrochloric acid and has a *p*H of 3 or less, whereas fluid regurgitated from the esophagus has a *p*H of 4 or more. Gagging may be followed by either regurgitation or vomiting. Dysphagia means difficulty in swallowing and is most commonly observed during eating or drinking. Drooling of saliva often accompanies dysphagia (see chapter 31). Coughing is often misinterpreted as vomiting, especially when it is characterized by expectoration of excessive phlegm. Paroxysmal coughing may also be followed by regurgitation or vomiting, making the situation even more confusing for the client and sometimes the veterinarian. Coughing can often be elicited by firm palpation of the trachea. This should be done while the client is present so that the animal's problem can be confirmed or denied.

A carefully taken history is well worth the time required. If doubt still exists about which sign is present, it is very important to hospitalize the animal to observe the abnormal signs. If possible, to save time and money, this should be done prior to initiating a laboratory work-up.

Since it is not feasible to hospitalize and work-up every vomiting animal, initial efforts should be directed at distinguishing those patients requiring only symptomatic care from those with more serious disorders. For this purpose, it is helpful to consider the duration (acute versus chronic) and frequency of vomiting and the presence or absence of associated signs. Whenever vomiting has been of short duration (less than 3 or 4 days) and infrequent (once or twice daily) and there are no associated signs, the work-up may consist of a minimum data base, including only history and physical examination (emphasis on thorough abdominal palpation) followed by symptomatic therapy. Chronic vomiting (more than 3 or 4 days), increased frequency of vomiting (more than one or two times daily), and vomiting of blood, as well as associated signs such as depression, fever, dehydration, abdominal pain, and signs of shock, often indicate a potentially serious or life-threatening disorder and require an immediate, in-depth laboratory work-up.

Laboratory Evaluation

The initial diagnostic consideration for those patients hospitalized because of vomiting is to distinguish primary gastrointestinal causes from metabolic or nongastrointestinal causes (Fig. 32-1, Table 32-1). History may or may not be helpful. Careful abdominal palpation and abdominal radiography are the diagnostic methods of choice to rule out gastrointestinal causes of vomiting. Metabolic causes are best ruled out by an initial data base consisting of a complete blood count, serum biochemical profile, and urine analysis. Ideally, complete arterial blood gas/*p*H analysis is needed for thorough evaluation of a vomiting animal. Because of difficulties in obtaining these data, measurement of plasma bicarbonate is an acceptable alternative. Plasma total CO_2 (TCO_2) consists mostly of bicarbonate and, for clinical purposes, can be substituted for plasma bicarbonate. Automated methods for measuring TCO_2 are routinely available, and TCO_2 should always be included whenever a plasma biochemical profile is requested on a vomiting patient. Special laboratory tests such as determination of serum lipase activity and ammonia level may be needed in some cases. Common causes of regurgitation and associated clinical signs are shown in Table 32-2.

SYMPTOMATIC THERAPY

Treatment of Vomiting

Vomiting is a sign of many different disorders involving several organ systems, and treatment will vary depending upon the specific cause. The use of antiemetics is usually discouraged unless vomiting is so persistent and profuse that associated dehydration and electrolyte and acid–base imbalance cannot be controlled. Antiemetics may mask signs of a potentially fatal disorder and delay diagnosis and treatment. When antiemetics are used, it should be remembered that those acting on both the CTZ and the vomiting center are the most effective.

Symptomatic management of acute vomiting is done by confining the animal and not permitting any oral intake for at least 12 to 24 hours. Allowing the animal to lick ice cubes may help relieve thirst without inducing further vomiting. If dehydration is present, parenteral fluid therapy with a multielectrolyte solution is indicated. Ideally, the choice of the particular solution to be used is based upon knowledge of the patient's acid-base and electrolyte values. Ringer's solution or 0.9% saline solution are high in chloride, contain neither lactate nor bicarbonate, and are preferred for treatment of dehydration associated with metabolic alkalosis. With either normal acid-base values or metabolic acidosis, lactated Ringer's solution is the fluid of choice. Lactated Ringer's solution is similar in electrolyte composition to extracellular fluid. Lactate is converted by the liver to bicarbonate, thereby helping to correct metabolic acidosis. If laboratory data are unavailable, Ringer's solution is preferred. If urine output is normal, potassium should be added to the fluid being used whenever vomiting has been persistent and profuse or whenever hypokalemia is suspected or confirmed. The minimum dosage of potassium is estimated at 1 to 3 mEq/kg/day; serum potassium is measured every 24 to 48 hours to evaluate the need for further potassium supplementation. With severe potassium depletion (serum potassium < 2.5 mEq/liter), it may be necessary to administer up to three times the above amount of potassium. It is safer to administer the potassium-enriched fluid (35 mEq potassium/liter) subcutaneously. If this solution is given intravenously, the rate of administration should not exceed 0.5 mEq of potassium per kilogram per hour without electrocardiographic monitoring. Excessively rapid intravenous administration of potassium can cause fatal cardiotoxicity. After 24 hours, small quantities of water followed by bland food (broth, baby food, prescription diet I-D [Hill's Pet Products, Topeka, KS 66601]) can be offered every 3 or 4 hours. If no vomiting occurs, the amount of food should be gradu-

(*Text continues on p 267.*)

Table 32-1. Characteristic Findings of Common Disorders Causing Vomiting

DISEASE	CLINICAL SIGNS OTHER THAN VOMITING	HEMATOLOGY	URINE ANALYSIS	BIOCHEMISTRY	SPECIAL TESTS
Gastrointestinal disorders					
Dietary problem	Few systemic signs Diarrhea and flatulence are sometimes present.	Normal	Normal	Normal	None
Internal parasites	Weight loss and poor hair coat Diarrhea	May have regenerative anemia Eosinophilia	Normal	Normal	Fecal flotation or sedimentation X 3
Drugs					
Corticosteroids	Polyuria Polydipsia Melena Dermatologic changes (alopecia, thin skin)	Regenerative anemia ± (blood loss) Stress leukogram	Specific gravity 1.010–1.030	↓ Albumin and globulin ± (blood loss) ↑ SAP and ALT	None
Aspirin	Melena	Regenerative anemia	Normal	↓ Albumin and globulin ± (blood loss)	None
Others					
Infectious disease Canine distemper Canine parvovirus Feline panleukopenia	See Table 33-1.				

Intussusception	Anorexia Depression Dehydration Abdominal pain Palpable abdominal mass	↑ PCV and plasma protein Stress or inflammatory leukogram Toxic granulation of neutrophils ±		Normal albumin and globulin Electrolytes and acid–base variable ↑ BUN (prerenal)	Abdominal radiographs show gas distended intestinal loops, indicative of intestinal obstruction.
Intestinal foreign body		Same as intussusception			Abdominal radiographs show gas-distended bowel loops, indicative of intestinal obstruction.
Gastric or high duodenal foreign body	Chronic intermittent vomiting with few other signs or acute, profuse vomiting Dehydration Anorexia Depression	Normal or ↑ PCV and plasma protein Stress leukogram	Variable specific gravity Paradoxical aciduria	Normal or ↑ albumin and globulin ↑ BUN (prerenal) ↓ Na^+ ↓ K^+ ↓ Cl^- ↑ TCO_2	Abdominal radiographs may show fluid- and gas-distended stomach and gastric or high duodenal foreign body. Upper gastrointestinal study may show delayed gastric emptying.

(Continued)

Table 32-1. Characteristic Findings of Common Disorders Causing Vomiting (*Continued*)

DISEASE	CLINICAL SIGNS OTHER THAN VOMITING	HEMATOLOGY	URINE ANALYSIS	BIOCHEMISTRY	SPECIAL TESTS
Bacterial gastroenteritis	Anorexia Depression Dehydration Fever ± Diarrhea	↑ PCV and plasma protein Variable WBC Stress or inflammatory leukogram and toxic granulation of neutrophils ±	Normal	↑ Albumin and globulin ↑ BUN (prerenal) Electrolytes, acid–base variable	Fecal cultures positive for *Salmonella* or *Campylobacter* in some cases.
Intra-abdominal neoplasia	Decreased appetite Lethargy Weight loss Palpable abdominal mass ± Vomiting ± Diarrhea ±	Mild nonregenerative anemia ± Variable WBC	Normal	Variable	Abdominal radiographs may show evidence of a mass. Thoracic radiographs may show metastatic disease.
Metabolic disorders					
Uremia	Anorexia Depression Dehydration Weight loss Polyuria/polydipsia Oliguria/anuria ±	PCV variable ↑ Plasma protein WBC variable—stress leukogram ±	Variable depending on cause	↑ Albumin and globulin ↑ BUN Electrolytes variable ↓ TCO_2	Depends on cause

Adrenocortical insufficiency	Lethargy Weakness Intermittent diarrhea Bradycardia Collapse and shock ±	↑ PCV and plasma protein Eosinophilia and lymphocytosis ±	Normal	↑ Albumin and globulin ↑ BUN ↓ Na^+ ↑ K^+ Na^+/K^+ ratio < 23 to 1	↓ Baseline plasma cortisol and no response to ACTH stimulation
Hepatic disease	Depression, anorexia Head pressing, stupor, coma ± Polyuria, polydipsia ± Icterus Ascites Diarrhea, melena ±	Variable Stomatocytosis ±	Variable ↓ Specific gravity ± Bilirubinuria Ammonium biurate crystals ±	Variable ↓ Albumin and ↑ globulin ± ↓ BUN ± ↑ Bilirubin ± ↑ ALT and SAP ± ↓ Glucose ±	↑ BSP retention ↑ Plasma NH_3 ↓ NH_3 tolerance
Acute pancreatitis	Depression, anorexia, dehydration Obesity Vomiting Abdominal pain upon palpation ± Diarrhea, melena ± Icterus ± Dyspnea ±	↑ PCV and plasma protein ↑ WBC with either inflammatory or stress leukogram Toxic granulation of neutrophils ±	Usually normal Bilirubinuria ± Proteinuria ± Casts ±	↑ Albumin and globulin ↑ BUN ± ↑ SAP ± ↑ ALT ↓ K^+ ± ↓ Cl^- ± ↓ Ca^+ ± ↑ TCO_2	↑ Serum lipase Abdominal radiographs may show lack of contrast in pancreatic area and displacement of cranial duodenum.
Toxin ingestion	Variable depending upon the toxin ingested.				

±, present or absent; ↓, decreased; ↑, increased; SAP, serum alkaline phosphatase; ALT, alanine transaminase; PCV, packed cell volume; BUN, blood urea nitrogen; WBC, white blood cells; TCO_2, total CO_2; ACTH, adrenocorticotropic hormone; BSP, bromosulfophthalein

Table 32-2. Characteristic Findings of Common Disorders Causing Regurgitation

DISEASE	CLINICAL SIGNS OTHER THAN REGURGITATION	HEMATOLOGY	URINE ANALYSIS	BIOCHEMISTRY	SPECIAL TESTS
Morphologic					
Esophageal foreign body	See megaesophagus.				
Vascular ring anomaly	Young animal Failure to gain weight See megaesophagus.	See megaesophagus.			
Esophagitis	History of persistent vomiting Coughing Dyspnea Dehydration Weight loss	Variable ↑ PCV and plasma protein ↑ WBC with inflammatory leukogram	Normal	↑ Albumin and globulin ± Electrolytes and acid–base variable	Esophagoscopy for visualization of esophageal mucosa
Esophageal stricture	See megaesophagus.				
Intrathoracic neoplasia	Coughing Dyspnea Weight loss Anorexia Depression Dehydration	Mild to moderate nonregenerative anemia ± WBC and leukogram variable	Normal	↑ Albumin and globulin ±	Thoracic radiographs may show mass. Barium swallow for esophageal study
Functional					
Megaesophagus, congenital and acquired	Coughing Dyspnea Drooling ± Weight loss	WBC and leukogram variable	Normal	Normal	Esophagoscopy Barium swallow for esophageal study

↑, increased; PCV, packed cell volume; ±, present or absent; WBC, white blood cell

ally increased. Over a 2- or 3-day period, the animal's regular food should be gradually mixed in with the bland food in increasing proportions until the regular food is being fed exclusively.

Client education should emphasize that if vomiting persists during the 24 hours of restricted oral intake or returns whenever food and water intake is reinstated, the client should inform the veterinarian without delay. In this situation, it is likely than an in-depth work-up is indicated to rule out a more serious cause of vomiting.

Treatment of Regurgitation

Since regurgitation usually does not cause serious electrolyte and acid-base changes, parenteral fluid therapy may not be necessary. Lactated Ringer's solution is the preferred fluid to correct dehydration in the regurgitating patient.

Regurgitation is often chronic, necessitating caloric replacement. With megaesophagus, attempts should be made to supply calories by feeding the animal from an elevated position. Semimoist or chunk food are less likely to be aspirated than are gruels. Depending upon the cause of chronic regurgitation, it may be necessary to place either a pharyngostomy or a gastrostomy tube. A thin gruel can be prepared by mixing canned dog or cat food with water in a blender. This mixture can be administered through the pharyngostomy or gastrostomy tube to meet calculated water and caloric requirements.

33

Diarrhea

LARRY M. CORNELIUS AND MICHAEL D. LORENZ

DEFINITION

Diarrhea is a change in one or more of the characteristics of the bowel movement: increased frequency, increased fluidity, or increased volume. Disease involving the small or large intestine or both may result in diarrhea. Many diseases produce similar pathophysiologic changes that culminate in diarrhea. The management of diarrhea often is based on these altered physiologic mechanisms.

PATHOPHYSIOLOGY

A common abnormality found in diarrhea is increased fecal water. Most of the diseases that produce diarrhea cause an increased concentration of fecal water. Several pathophysiologic mechanisms, including hypersecretion, altered permeability, altered motility, and malabsorption, result in increased fecal water.[5] Diarrhea of small bowel origin usually results from fluid being delivered to the colon at a rate or volume that overwhelms normal colonic absorptive capacity (colon overload). Diarrhea of large bowel origin usually occurs because fluid normally delivered to the colon is not absorbed due to decreased colonic absorptive capacity.

Hypersecretion

Hypersecretion occurs in several enteric bacterial diseases of domestic animals. In the normal small intestine, fluid and electrolytes are secreted by immature cells in the base of the intestinal villi. This fluid and electrolytes are promptly absorbed by the mature epithelial cells lining the tips of the villi. This process is called ''bidirectional flux,'' and in the normal animal, absorptive flux always exceeds the secretory flux so that a net absorption of fluid and electrolyte occurs. In certain diseases, secretion of fluids is stimulated to such a degree that the absorptive capacity of the small and large intestine is overwhelmed, allowing a marked increase in fecal water. Enterotoxigenic bacteria such as *Escherichia coli* produce substances that stimulate hypersecretion and watery diarrhea even though the gut appears intact structurally. In small animals, hypersecretion is of less importance than in large animals; however, in certain diseases, hypersecretion is partially responsible for increased fecal water.

Altered Permeability

Many enteric diseases dramatically alter gut permeability. Small changes in permeability result in the secretion of electrolyte-rich, protein-poor fluid. Greater permeability changes produce the exudation of fluid containing considerable quantities of plasma proteins. An example of this process is lymphangiectasia, a protein-losing enteropathy. Characteristically, both albumin and globulin are lost in equal amounts, resulting in both hypoalbuminemia and hypoglobulinemia. Structural damage to mucosal integrity produces tremendous permeability changes. A 10,000-fold increase in gut permeability produces hemorrhagic exudates and suggests that the gut defense barriers have been greatly compromised.

Altered Motility

Unfortunately, many veterinarians were taught that diarrhea resulted from hypermotility of the gut. Certainly, in diarrhea, luminal contents are transported aborally at an accelerated rate. However, hypermotility is not the primary cause; rather, hypomotility is the usual intestinal response when disease is present. Two major intestinal movements are normally present: rhythmic contractions or segmentations and peristalsis. Rhythmic segmentations retard the passage of ingesta through the intestine, thereby aiding digestion and absorption. In diarrheal states, the strength of these contractions is greatly reduced, resulting in decreased resistance to the flow of ingesta. Anticholinergic drugs tend to further decrease the strength and rate of segmental contractions, further complicating the hypomotile condition of the diseased gut. Peristaltic waves move ingesta in the aboral direction. There is little evidence to support the widely held concept that peristaltic activity is exaggerated in diarrheal states. In fact, when resistance to flow is decreased by lack of rhythmic contractions, very little peristaltic activity is required to move luminal contents a great distance. In summary, one should view the diseased gut as a hypomotile tube with decreased resistance to the aboral movement of luminal contents. Therapy regarding alteration of motility should be predicated on this assumption.

Malabsorption

Both structural and biochemical mechanisms may produce malabsorption. Diseases that destroy the villous integrity result in malabsorption of fluid, electrolytes, and basic nutrients. The enteric corona and parvoviruses are examples of this mechanism. Altered permeability, hypomotility, and even hypersecretion (which occurs in the recovery phase of these diseases) are also encountered. Gluten enteropathy is another example of a disease that decreases the absorptive surface of the intestine via villous atrophy. Infiltrative disease of the gut wall (inflammatory or neoplastic) may also cause malabsorption. Forms of malabsorption have been recognized in dogs that have little structural abnormality in their gut. In these cases, biochemical malabsorption has been suspected (deficiency of brush border enzyme systems, lymphatic obstruction or malfunction, failure of active transport systems). On a clinical basis, biochemical malabsorption is extremely difficult to prove.

There are several sequelae to intestinal malabsorption. Volume overload of the colon is a common mechanism; however, several other mechanisms come together to increase the volume of fecal water. Malabsorbed basic nutrients (*e.g.*, carbohydrates, fatty acids) create significant osmotic effects in the gut lumen. These osmotically active substances tend to hold water in the gut lumen and may even stimulate the secretion of fluid into the lumen. Bacterial action on carbohydrate and fats in the gut lumen may produce substances (*e.g.*, lactic acid, hydroxy fatty acids) that are osmotically active but also irritative to the intestinal mucosa. These substances aggravate the diarrheal state by enhancing gut secretion of fluid and electrolytes. Malabsorption of bile salts may contribute to hypersecretion and decreased fat digestion, because the bile acid pool may become depleted.

Intestinal Resistance to Pathogens

Immunologic Mechanisms

Both antibody-mediated and cell-mediated immune mechanisms are important. IgA is a secretory antibody produced by plasma cells in the gut wall. It contains a unique protein called "secretory component" that promotes transport through epithelial cells to the mucosal barrier and protects the antibody from enzymatic digestion. Although IgA has little opsonic, complement-fixing, or bacteriocidal activity, it functions by preventing adherence of organisms to the intestinal mucosa. Other immunoglobulins (IgM, IgG, IgE) are present in low concentrations in the gut lumen unless inflammation of the bowel wall allows their exudation.

The role of cell-mediated immunity in intestinal defense against pathogens is not well defined. It is known that animals with T-cell dysfunction are susceptible to gastrointestinal disease. Deficient cell-mediated immunity may play a role in the villous atrophy of chronic nonspecific enteritis.

Nonimmunologic Mechanisms

Gastric acidity may render inactive a number of organisms and their toxins before they reach the lower portions of the intestine. Mucins in the mucous coat of the gastrointestinal mucosa act as receptors for organisms or their toxins, thus protecting the epithelium by competitive binding. Lysozymes and bile salts have been shown to inhibit bacterial growth *in vitro.* Peristalsis helps prevent bacterial overgrowth in the gut. The role of altered intestinal motility in the pathophysiology of diarrhea has been discussed previously.

The intestinal microflora is a very important host defense mechanism against bacterial pathogens. It is normally quite stable; after disruption, it rapidly returns to its previous state. Many diarrheal conditions are treated symptomatically with antimicrobial drugs even though a primary bacterial pathogen is not suspected. The normal gut flora serves as a primary defense barrier for the host. Bacterial pathogens must attach to the target cell before they can produce disease either by invasion or secretion of enterotoxins. Normal gut bacteria inhibit this attachment by occupying spaces available to pathogenic bacteria. Reduction of the normal gut flora with antimicrobial agents decreases this beneficial competition, allowing pathogenic bacteria to attach to target cells, proliferate, and potentially invade the gut mucosa. Proliferation of enteric pathogens such as *Salmonella* is enhanced when antibiotics are given. In certain situations, such as intestinal ileus, overgrowth of bacteria may contribute to diarrheal states. The use of antimicrobial drugs should be limited to conditions in which gut permeability has been greatly increased. Parenteral antibiotics should then be used as opposed to poorly absorbed luminal antibiotics.

DIAGNOSTIC PLAN

The initial step in the diagnosis of diarrhea is to localize the problem to either the small or large intestine. This is accomplished by history, physical examination, and gross fecal examination (Table 33-1). Small bowel diarrhea is characterized by increased fecal volume (either watery or bulky). The frequency of defecation is increased; however, tenesumus is absent. Mucus and fresh blood are not prominent, except in young puppies or kittens. In adults, blood is usually di-

Table 33-1. Localization of Diarrhea From History and Physical Examination

	SMALL BOWEL	LARGE BOWEL
Fecal volume	Increased	Decreased or normal
Frequency of defecation	Increased	Markedly increased
Tenesmus	Absent	Present
Blood in feces	Melena	Hematochezia
Mucus in feces	Absent or small amount	Large amount
Steatorrhea	Present in some	Absent
Associated signs	Vomiting marked weight loss, dehydration	Less severe weight loss and dehydration

gested, resulting in melena. Associated clinical signs include vomiting, rapid weight loss, and dehydration. Gross steatorrhea is pathognomonic of small bowel disease or pancreatic exocrine insufficiency.

Large bowel diseases produce stools that are soft, semiformed, occasionally watery, or even excessively firm. The hallmark of large bowel disease is tenesmus, with fresh blood and mucus in the feces.

The follow-up diagnostic plan will depend upon whether diarrhea is acute or chronic and the particular diseases being considered (Figs. 33-1 and 33-2, Table 33-2).

SYMPTOMATIC THERAPY

Whenever possible, a precise diagnosis should be made and the inciting cause of diarrhea treated specifically.[2]

Small Bowel Diarrhea

Concepts regarding symptomatic treatment of small bowel diarrhea have changed dramatically in the past few years because of better knowledge of the pathophysiologic mechanisms involved.

Fluid Therapy

When the animal will drink and when vomiting and severe dehydration are not present, oral fluid and electrolyte therapy is cheaper, more convenient, and usually effective in restoring hydration and electrolyte balance. Shown in Table 33-3 is the recipe for "WHO juice," a glucose-electrolyte solution recommended by the World Health Organization for the oral treatment of secretory diarrhea. Active absorption of glucose facilitates absorption of sodium and water, thus effectively restoring extracellular fluid volume. In contrast to commercial products such as Gatorade, WHO juice tastes almost like water and is likely to be consumed by dogs and cats. Parenteral fluid therapy is necessary if dehydration is severe or if the patient refuses to drink. Lactated Ringer's solution is generally preferred to rehydrate the animal and correct the metabolic acidosis sometimes present. If hypokalemia is present and urine output is adequate, potassium chloride should be added to the lactated Ringer's solution (1–3 mEq potassium/kg/day). The rate of intravenous potassium administration should not exceed 0.5 mEq of potassium per kilogram per hour.

Antibiotics

The normal intestinal microflora is an important host defense mechanism against enteric pathogens. Improper use of antibiotics can cause an imbalance in the microflora and favor the replication of pathogens. In general, the use of antibiotics in diarrhea should be restricted to those conditions associated with

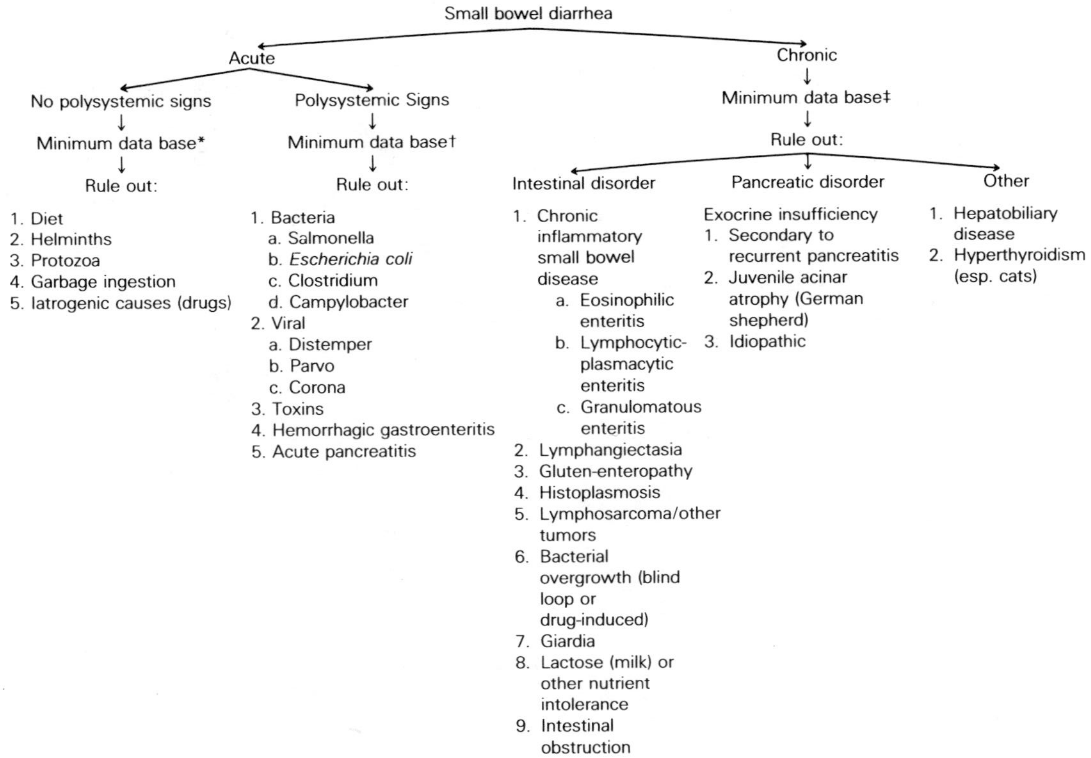

Small bowel diarrhea

Acute

No polysystemic signs
↓
Minimum data base*
↓
Rule out:

1. Diet
2. Helminths
3. Protozoa
4. Garbage ingestion
5. Iatrogenic causes (drugs)

Polysystemic Signs
↓
Minimum data base†
↓
Rule out:

1. Bacteria
   a. Salmonella
   b. *Escherichia coli*
   c. Clostridium
   d. Campylobacter
2. Viral
   a. Distemper
   b. Parvo
   c. Corona
3. Toxins
4. Hemorrhagic gastroenteritis
5. Acute pancreatitis

Chronic
↓
Minimum data base‡
↓
Rule out:

Intestinal disorder

1. Chronic inflammatory small bowel disease
   a. Eosinophilic enteritis
   b. Lymphocytic-plasmacytic enteritis
   c. Granulomatous enteritis
2. Lymphangiectasia
3. Gluten-enteropathy
4. Histoplasmosis
5. Lymphosarcoma/other tumors
6. Bacterial overgrowth (blind loop or drug-induced)
7. Giardia
8. Lactose (milk) or other nutrient intolerance
9. Intestinal obstruction

Pancreatic disorder

Exocrine insufficiency
1. Secondary to recurrent pancreatitis
2. Juvenile acinar atrophy (German shepherd)
3. Idiopathic

Other

1. Hepatobiliary disease
2. Hyperthyroidism (esp. cats)

* History, physical examination (thorough abdominal palpation), fecal flotation x3, protozoal exam x3.
† As above plus CBC, urine analysis, biochemical profile, electrolytes, lipase, fecal culture.
‡ As for acute small bowel diarrhea with polysystemic signs plus microscopic examination of feces for fat and starch, fecal trypsin, fat absorption (plasma turbidity) test, D-xylose absorption test, BT-PABA test, serum trypsin-like immunoreactivity, intestinal biopsy.

Fig. 33-1. Initial diagnostic plan for small bowel diarrhea.

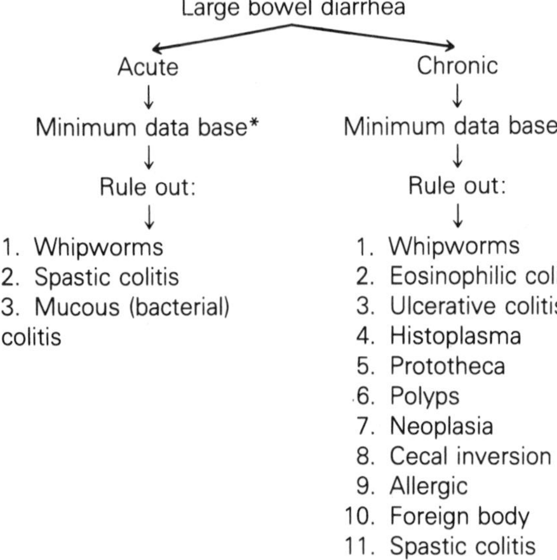

Fig. 33-2. Initial diagnostic plan for large bowel diarrhea.

severe disruption of the intestinal mucosa (bloody diarrhea) or polysystemic signs such as fever, dehydration, depression, and inflammatory leukograms. Parenteral antibiotics (cepahlosporins, ampicillin, penicillin, chloramphenicol, gentamicin) or well-absorbed oral antibiotics (trimethroprim-sulfa, ampicillin, cephalosporins, chloramphenicol) are preferred because they are more effective and less likely to damage the intestinal microflora than are the poorly absorbed oral antibiotics such as neomycin and kanamycin. In dogs, tylosin is helpful in chronic diarrhea due to inflammatory bowel disease.[6] Metronidazole and clindamycin are effective against enteric anaerobic bacteria.

Antimotility Drugs

Since most diarrheal conditions are accompanied by a hypomotile gut (see pathophysiology), the use of anticholinergic drugs (*e.g.*, atropine, hyoscyamine, and methscopolamine) should be condemned. Their use, especially if for more than a few days, may cause severe ileus and intestinal stasis, which favor replication of pathogens and absorption of endotoxins.

Narcotic analgesic drugs, such as diphenoxylate (Lomotil) and paregoric, increase rhythmic segmentation activity of the small bowel, thereby retarding flow of luminal contents. Short-term use of these drugs may be helpful in alleviating diarrhea, but their use in severe bacterial enteritis due to toxin-producing

(*Text continues on p 282.*)

Table 33-2. Characteristic Findings of Common Disorders Causing Diarrhea

DISEASE	CLINICAL SIGNS OTHER THAN DIARRHEA	HEMATOLOGY	BIOCHEMISTRY	SPECIAL TESTS
ACUTE SMALL BOWEL DIARRHEA				
Diet change or lactose intolerance	Few polysystemic signs Flatulence often present	Normal	Normal	None
Intestinal parasites	Melena Hematochezia Weight loss Dry hair coat "Unthrifty" appearance	May have regenerative anemia (hookworms, coccidia) Eosinophilia	May have ↓ plasma protein	Fecal flotation or sedimentation × 3
Garbage ingestion	Vomiting ± Few polysystemic signs	Normal	Normal	None
Bacterial enteritis				
Salmonella	Anorexia Depression progressing to signs of shock Fever progressing to subnormal temperature Dehydration Vomiting Melena Hematochezia Abdominal pain	↑ PCV and plasma protein Leukopenia with inappropriate left shift Toxic neutrophils Thrombocytopenia	↓ Albumin ± ↑ Globulin ↑ SAP ± ↓ Glucose ±	Fecal and blood cultures for *Salmonella*
Escherichia coli, Clostridium	Anorexia Depression Fever Dehydration Vomiting Abdominal pain	Neutrophilic leukocytosis with left shift ↑ PCV and plasma protein	See *Salmonella.*	None

(*Continued*)

Table 33-2. Characteristic Findings of Common Disorders Causing Diarrhea (*Continued*)

DISEASE	CLINICAL SIGNS OTHER THAN DIARRHEA	HEMATOLOGY	BIOCHEMISTRY	SPECIAL TESTS
Campylobacter	Those of *E. coli* and *Clostridium* + hematochezia and mucus in feces	See *E coli.*	↑ Albumin and globulin	Fecal culture for *Campylobacter*
Viral enteritis				
Parvo in dogs	Anorexia Depression Vomiting Dehydration Abdominal pain Fever	Leukopenia (neutropenia with left shift)	Electrolytes variable	ELISA test on feces
Panleukopenia in cats	See parvo.	Leukopenia (neutropenia)	See parvo.	None
Distemper	See parvo. Naso–ocular discharge Chorea Seizures Paresis Chorioretinitis	Neutrophilic leukocytosis with left shift ↑ PCV and plasma protein	↑ Albumin and globulin	Fluorescent antibody test on conjunctival smear
Toxin (*e.g.*, arsenic, thallium)	Anorexia Depression Vomiting Dehydration Abdominal pain Others depending on toxin	Leukocytosis (stress leukogram)	↑ Albumin and globulin ↑ BUN ↓ TCO_2	Analysis of vomitus, feces, urine for toxin

Hemorrhagic gastroenteritis	Melena Anorexia Depression progressing to signs of shock	Markedly ↑ PCV (60–80%) and plasma protein Leukocytosis (stress leukogram)	↑ BUN ↑ Albumin and globulin ↓ TCO_2	None
CHRONIC SMALL BOWEL DIARRHEA				
Lymphocytic–plasmacytic enteritis	Weight loss Variable appetite	Mild nonregenerative anemia ↓ Plasma protein	↓ Albumin and globulin ↓ Ca^{++}	D-Xylose absorption decreased Small intestinal biopsy
Lymphangiectasia	See lymphocytic–plasmacytic enteritis.	As for lymphocytic–plasmacytic enteritis ↓ Lymphocytes	↓ Albumin and globulin ↓ Ca^{++}	Small intestinal biopsy
Small intestinal neoplasia (*e.g.,* lymphosarcoma)	Severe weight loss Variable appetite Sporadic vomiting	As for lymphocytic–plasmacytic enteritis	↓ Albumin and globulin Ca^{++} variable	Abdominal radiographs show thickened bowel loops. Small bowel biopsy
Eosinophilic enteritis	Mild weight loss Sporadic vomiting Melena Hematochezia	Eosinophilia	Normal	Fecals negative for parasites Small bowel biopsy—infiltration with eosinophils Rapid response to glucocorticoids
Intestinal parasites (giardiasis)	Light colored "cow-flop" stools Mild weight loss "Unthrifty" appearance	Normal	Normal	Direct smears of fresh diarrheal feces for motile trophozoites Fecal sedimentation × 3 for cysts Duodenal aspirates Therapeutic trial with metronidazole for 5 days

(Continued)

Table 33-2. Characteristic Findings of Common Disorders Causing Diarrhea (*Continued*)

DISEASE	CLINICAL SIGNS OTHER THAN DIARRHEA	HEMATOLOGY	BIOCHEMISTRY	SPECIAL TESTS
Histoplasma enteritis	Severe weight loss Variable appetite Fever	Neutrophilic leukocytosis Eosinophilia ± Basophilia ± ↓ Plasma protein Histoplasma organisms in monocytes of peripheral blood or bone marrow ±	↓ Albumin Globulin variable	Complement fixation titer Small bowel and mesenteric lymph node biopsies
Pancreatic exocrine insufficiency	Severe weight loss Ravenous appetite "Unthrifty" appearance Bulky, light, greasy feces	Mild nonregenerative anemia	Normal	Plasma turbidity test Negative 1–4 hr after fatty meal Positive 1–4 hr after fatty meal + pancreatic enzyme supplement Fecal exam × 3 X-ray film test—negative for trypsin Lugol's iodine stain—positive for starch Sudan IV stain—positive for undigested fat

				BT-PABA test—decreased chyomtrypsin activity Decreased serum trypsin-like immunoreactivity Therapeutic trial on pancreatic enzyme supplement for 1 month
Iatrogenic (antibiotic and antimotility drug abuse)	Mild weight loss Variable appetite	Normal		Stop all drug administration and feed bland diet for 1 week.
ACUTE LARGE BOWEL DIARRHEA				
Spastic (nervous) colitis	Tenesmus Hematochezia Mucus in feces Nervous animal	Normal	Normal	Fecal negative for parasites
CHRONIC LARGE BOWEL DIARRHEA				
Whipworms	Hematochezia Mucus in feces Intermittent depression and abdominal pain	Eosinophilia ±	Normal	Fecal flotation × 3 (commonly negative) Response to anthelmintic therapy

(*Continued*)

Table 33-2. Characteristic Findings of Common Disorders Causing Diarrhea (*Continued*)

DISEASE	CLINICAL SIGNS OTHER THAN DIARRHEA	HEMATOLOGY	BIOCHEMISTRY	SPECIAL TESTS
Eosinophilic ulcerative colitis	Mild weight loss Sporadic vomiting Tenesmus Hematochezia Mucus in feces	Eosinophilia	Normal	Fecals negative for parasites Proctoscopy and colonic biopsy—infiltration with eosinophils Rapid response to glucocorticoids
Histocytic ulcerative colitis (granulomatous colitis)	Mostly in Boxer dogs Weight loss may be severe. See eosinophilic ulcerative colitis.	Normal	Normal	Proctoscopy and colonic biopsy
Idiopathic ulcerative colitis	See eosinophilic ulcerative colitis.	Normal	Normal	Proctoscopy and colonic biopsy
Histoplasma colitis	Fever Depression Weight loss may be severe. See eosinophilic ulcerative colitis	See chronic small bowel diarrhea, histoplasma enteritis.		Colonic biopsy

Prototheca colitis	Fever Depression Severe weight loss Uveitis Tenesmus Hematochezia Mucus in feces	Neutrophilic leukocytosis with left shift	Normal	Examine rectal scrapings stained with Wright-Giemsa. Proctoscopy with colonic biopsy
Rectal polyps	Tenesmus Hematochezia Mucus in feces Digitally palpable masses in rectum	Normal	Normal	Proctoscopy and rectal biopsy
Neoplasia	Variable weight loss Tenesmus Hematochezia Mucus in feces Palpable mass in colon or rectum	Normal		Proctoscopy and biopsy
Cecal inversion	See neoplasia. Palpable mass in caudal abdomen ±	Normal	Normal	Survey abdominal radiographs followed by barium enema study

↓, decreased; ±, present or absent; PCV, packed cell volume; SAP, serum alkaline phosphatase; ELISA, enzyme-linked immunosorbent assay; ↑ increased; BUN, blood urea nitrogen; TCO_2, total CO_2; BT-PABA, N-benzoyl-L-tyrosyl-p-aminobenzoic acid

Table 33-3. Recipe for "WHO Juice" (World Health Organization) (1 Gallon)

INGREDIENT	ELECTROLYTE CONTENT
Sodium chloride—14 g	Na^+—90 mEq/liter
Sodium bicarbonate—10 g	K^+—32 mEq/liter
Potassium chloride—6 g	Cl^-—92 mEq/liter
Dextrose—80 g	HCO_3^-—30 mEq/liter
Deionized water—1 gallon	Dextrose—111 mosm/liter

Procedure: Weigh NaCl, KCl, and $NaHCO_3$ into gallon container. Add 3 liters of deionized water. Place on stir plate and stir well with magnetic stirrer. Slowly add dextrose to stirring water and allow to dissolve (if dextrose is added too quickly or before water, it will clump). Fill to 1 gallon.
Store in refrigerator until used. Expiration of final product is 3 months from date of manufacture.

Caution! WHO Juice tends to become contaminated easily. Check solution before dispensing.

For oral use only.

bacteria is not warranted because retarding luminal flow may allow increased production and absorption of bacterial toxins.

Antisecretory Drugs

For bacterial diarrhea characterized by intestinal hypersecretion, drugs that inhibit secretory activity are effective. Little information is available regarding use of these agents in canine and feline diarrhea, but it is likely that they will be helpful, as in humans and other species. Bismuth subsalicylate (Pepto Bismol) and the alpha-adrenergic blockers chlorpromazine and phenoxybenzamine have been shown to reduce diarrhea caused by hypersecretion.[1,3,4]

Protectants

Kaolin and pectin are often used as coating and protecting agents for diarrhea. It is doubtful whether they are effective for this purpose. Kaolin may activate clotting and may be useful in diarrhea characterized by intraluminal hemorrhage. Barium sulfate used for radiographic contrast studies of the gastrointestinal tract sometimes alleviates diarrhea, which may be the result of a protectant effect.

Cimetidine is indicated for diarrhea characterized by melena because it inhibits gastric HCl secretion, thereby decreasing HCl-induced irritation in the upper small bowel.

Diet

Feeding a patient with diarrhea depends upon the cause and severity of the disease. Food should not be given for at least 1 to 2 days in animals with a severely compromised intestinal mucosa (hemorrhagic diarrhea) and in vomiting patients. Otherwise, most animals with diarrhea can tolerate bland foods (*e.g.*, boiled hamburger, rice, cottage cheese, and prescription diet I-D*) fed in small quantities at frequent intervals. Foods containing lactose (milk) and large quantities of fat should be restricted, because malabsorption of these nutrients is often present in diarrhea. Scientific studies have failed to confirm any benefit of feeding lactobacillus-containing preparations for reestablishing intestinal microflora. In cats with chronic small bowel diarrhea, changing the diet from dry food to canned food such as prescription diet C-D* will sometimes alleviate the diarrhea. The semimoist food Tender Vittles† seems to control diarrhea in some cats. It is not known why such dietary changes are beneficial.

Large Bowel Diarrhea

Dehydration and electrolyte imbalance are not as likely with large bowel diarrhea. See the previous section for suggested therapy. For hemorrhagic colitis, antibiotics can be used, as previously discussed. Salicylazosulfapyridine (Azulfidine) may be helpful in idiopathic ulcerative colitis. Antimotility drugs, antisecretory drugs, and protectants are not recommended.

It is now generally accepted that the diet for most patients with large bowel diarrhea should be high in fiber, not low as previously recommended. High fiber in the colon apparently helps maintain normal colonic motility, thereby improving function. Commercial foods high in poorly digestible fiber, bran, and commercial fiber products for people have been used successfully in dogs and cats with large bowel diarrhea. However, low-fiber, low-bulk diets are better in severe acute colitis because they are less likely to further irritate the colonic mucosa.

REFERENCES

1. Dupont HL, et al: Symptomatic treatment of diarrhea with bismuth subsalicylate among students attending a Mexican university. Gastroenterol 73:715–718, 1977
2. Dupont HL: Intervention in diarrheas of infants and young children. J Am Vet Med Assoc 173:649–652, 1978
3. Hood DM, Stephens KA, Bowen MJ: Phenoxybenzamine for the treatment of severe nonresponsive diarrhea in horses. J Am Vet Med Assoc 180:758–762, 1982
4. Lonroth I, et al: Chlorpromazine reverses diarrhea in piglets caused by enterotoxigenic *Escherichia coli.* Infec Immun 24:900–905, 1979
5. Moon HJ: Mechanisms in the pathogenesis of diarrhea: A review. J Am Vet Med Assoc 172:443–448, 1978
6. Van Kruiningen HJ: Clinical efficacy of tylosin in canine inflammatory bowel disease. J Am Anim Hosp Assoc 12:498–501, 1976

* Hill's Pet Products, Topeka, KS
† Ralston Purina Co., St. Louis, MO

34

Constipation

MICHAEL D. LORENZ

PROBLEM DEFINITION AND RECOGNITION

Constipation is the infrequent or difficult passage of feces. Feces may be excessively hard, firm, or dry. Obstipation is intractable constipation and results in severe fecal impaction throughout the rectum and colon. Obstipated animals cannot eliminate the impacted fecal mass. Megacolon is a clinical disorder characterized by marked dilatation and hypomotility of the rectum and colon. Megacolon may cause obstipation and fecal impaction. In dogs and cats, the disorder is usually acquired; congenital defects may cause megacolon in humans.

The clinical signs of constipation include tenesmus with little or no passage of feces. Defecation may be painful. The fecal mass can be palpated through the abdomen or by digital examination of the rectum.

PATHOPHYSIOLOGY

In dogs and cats, the colon absorbs water and electrolytes from ingesta passing from the small intestine. The colon stores fecal matter until it can be eliminated through the process of defecation. It is believed that the proximal half of the colon serves primarily an absorptive function, whereas the distal colon is more involved with storage. Rhythmic segmental contractions mix ingesta within the colon and increase the absorption of water and electrolytes. Segmental contractions thus tend to decrease the rate of movement of luminal contents through the colon. Occasionally, these contractions may weakly propel the fecal mass towards the rectum. The primary propulsive wave within the colon is a "mass movement." These movements occur only a few times each day and propel feces into the rectum, stimulating the desire for defecation.

When feces enter the rectum, a weak defecation reflex is stimulated. Distention of the rectal wall stimulates afferent signals that spread through the myenteric plexus to initiate mass movements in the descending colon and rectum. Neurologically coordinated relaxation of the anal sphincter allows the fecal column to pass through the anus. This intrinsic defecation reflex is enforced by a second reflex mediated via parasympathic nerves from the sacral spinal cord segments. This sacral reflex greatly enforces the strength of the colonic movements and may allow complete evacuation of the colon. In house-trained pets, relaxation of the anal sphincter is voluntarily controlled by the cerebral cortex. Therefore, house-trained pets can inhibit the defecation reflex until they find an appropriate place.

Any condition or disease that promotes fecal stasis and increased water absorption may cause constipation (see Causes of Constipation).[1] As feces are retained in the colon, they harden and dry due to water absorption. As the colon impacts with feces, the colonic wall is stretched and may develop irreversible degenerative changes. Megacolon may result from any disease that causes chronic constipation.

Idiopathic megacolon is disease of unknown etiology that affects primarily adult dogs and cats. It is most likely a disease of altered myoneural function affecting the smooth muscle of the colon. Decreased motility causes chronic constipation, which causes further degeneration of the colonic wall. In this syndrome, there is no anatomic or inflammatory basis for the constipation. The perineal reflex is normal and anal sphincter tone is usually good.

The sequelae of obstipation include weight loss, dehydration, anorexia, weakness, and depression. These signs have been ascribed to the absorption of toxins produced by colonic bacteria.[1] Paradoxic diarrhea may occur in some cases, perhaps due to hypersecretion by the colonic mucosa. The diarrheal feces can bypass the fecal impaction.

DIAGNOSTIC PLAN

The diagnostic plan for constipation is based on the cause. The diet, defecation habits, exercise patterns, drug therapy, and history of pelvic, lumbar, or coccygeal trauma should be recorded. The physical examination should emphasize palpation of the caudal abdomen, pelvis, tail, perianal tissue, prostate, and rectum. Neurologic examination with emphasis on the L4–S3 spinal cord segments should be performed. Survey radiographs of the abdomen and pelvis help establish the severity of fecal impaction and the presence of mechanical obstruction due to a fractured pelvis.

A complete blood count, urine analysis, and biochemical profile should be performed. These tests help evaluate the metabolic and endocrine status of the animal and also help evaluate the side-effects of chronic constipation.

Colonoscopy and barium enemia studies for the presence of intraluminal obstruction must be delayed until the constipation or fecal impaction is removed.

Causes of Constipation

- Dietary
  - Foreign material
    - Hair
    - Bones
    - Rocks, sand
  - Low fiber
- Environment
  - Lack of exercise
  - Failure to provide adequate time and place for defecation
  - Dirty cat litter
- Colonic obstruction
  - Intraluminal
    - Foreign body
    - Neoplasia
    - Perineal hernia
  - Extraluminal
    - Healed fractured pelvis
    - Prostatic enlargement
    - Pelvic and perianal neoplasia
- Neurologic disease
  - Spinal cord disease L4–S3
  - Bilateral pelvic nerve injury
  - Idiopathic megacolon
- Perirectal pain
  - Anal sacculitis
  - Anal abscess
  - Perianal fistula
  - Anal stricture
  - Rectal foreign body
  - Pseudocoprostasis
- Metabolic and endocrine diseases
  - Hypothyroidism
  - Hyperparathyroidism
  - Pyrexia
  - Generalized debility
- Drug-induced
  - Anticholinergics
  - Antihistamines
  - Anticonvulsants
  - Barium sulfate
  - Opiates

SYMPTOMATIC THERAPY

The fecal impaction should be gently softened with mild, soapy water enemas. Phosphate enemas should be avoided in cats and the soap must not contain hexachlorophene. Mineral oil enemas may help lubricate the fecal mass and facilitate its passage. In some animals, the fecal impaction is so severe that forceps extraction and colonic irrigation are required. These animals must be carefully evaluated, and any dehydration or electrolyte imbalances must be corrected. Forceps extraction is painful; therefore, deep sedation or anesthesia is warranted. The "clamshell" forceps must be used gently to avoid severe colonic damage. By alternating colonic irrigation with forceps manipulation, the fecal mass can usually be removed.

The long-term management of constipation should reestablish normal colonic motility and defecation habits. Bran added to the diet is helpful. Commercial bulking agents such as methylcellulose and dioctyl sodium are no more effective but are more expensive than bran. Animals should be exercised frequently and litter boxes should be kept clean.

Megacolon is very difficult to manage since recurrent constipation almost always occurs. Owners must carefully watch their pets during defecation and estimate the volume of feces passed. Owners should be taught to palpate the colon in the caudal abdomen for constipation before severe fecal impaction occurs. Bethanechol hydrochloride may stimulate colonic motility in cats with megacolon. This drug should not be given until the colonic impaction has been relieved.

Surgical correction of obstructive lesions is indicated; however, megacolon, if present, may be permanent in chronic cases.

REFERENCE

1. Burrows CF: Diarrhea and constipation. In Ettinger SJ (ed): Textbook of Veterinary Internal Medicine, 2nd ed. Philadelphia, WB Saunders, 1983

35

Flatulence

MICHAEL D. LORENZ

PROBLEM DEFINITION AND RECOGNITION

Flatulence is distention of the stomach or the intestines with air or gases. Flatus is the gas expelled from a body opening. Ordinarily, the terms *flatus* and *flatulence* pertain to the expulsion of intestinal gas through the anus. The problem is easily recognized in house pets from the quantity or quality of gas expelled or by the constant rumbling noises created by gas movement in the intestines.

PHYSIOLOGY OF GAS PRODUCTION

Gas production or accumulation in the gastrointestinal tract is a normal physiologic event. Excessive production may not be indicative of any pathophysiologic event. However, in certain gastrointestinal diseases, the normal production of gas may be increased and excessive flatulence may result. Diagnostic plans and management are based on our current knowledge of intestinal gas production and composition.

Gas contained in the stomach is very similar to atmospheric air, whereas the composition of flatus is quite variable. Gastrointestinal gas comes from four primary sources: aerophagia (swallowed air), bacterial fermentation of substrates, diffusion of gas from the blood into the intestinal tract, and the reaction of acids with basic compounds in the upper intestinal tract. Generally, flatus contains mostly nitrogen (N_2) with far lesser quantities of hydrogen (H_2), carbon dioxide (CO_2), oxygen (O_2), and methane (CH_4). Nitrogen and, to a lesser extent, oxygen come from swallowed air that moves into the intestinal tract. Since the concentrations of CO_2, CH_4, and H_2 in flatus are often greater than in atmospheric air, these gases are partially derived from other sources. Methane production by dogs and cats is thought to be very rare; 30% of the human population may be methane producers.

In dogs, most of the H_2 and CO_2 in intestinal gas is produced by bacterial fermentation of nonabsorbable oligosaccharides such as stachyose and raffinose. Soybeans contain large quantities of the nonabsorbable oligosaccharides. Production of H_2 and CO_2 is greatly increased in the intestinal tract of dogs fed a commercial diet high in soybean content. The rapid growth of bacteria supporting this fermentation process is enhanced by diets high in soybean content.

Diffusion of gas from the bloodstream into the intestinal tract or production of gas from acid–base reactions add only small amounts of gas to the total volume contained in the gastrointestinal tract. These reactions are not clinically important in small animals.

Diets that contain carbohydrates, such as the oligosaccharides in soybean meal, increase gas production. Diets high in fiber may cause poor carbohydrate digestion in the small intestine; thus, more of this fermentable substrate reaches the colon, where it is subject to bacterial fermentation. Diets that are low in fiber and easily digested produce less flatus than diets high in fiber, poorly digested carbohydrates, or fat. Diseases of the small bowel that cause maldigestion or malabsorption may cause flatulence since increased amounts of carbohydrate are available for bacterial fermentation. Diseases that cause intestinal ileus, obstruction, or luminal stasis of ingesta may favor the rapid growth of fermenting bacteria such as clostridial species. The combined effects of luminal stasis and increased fermentation largely explain the gaseous distention of intestinal loops observed in these disorders.

The odor of flatus is attributed to minute quantities of ammonia, hydrogen sulfide, indole, skatole, volatile amines, and short-chain fatty acids. The major components of flatus are nonodorous.

DIAGNOSTIC PLAN

The diagnosis of flatus is usually evident from the history. A thorough examination for other signs suggestive of digestive tract disease should be made (*e.g.*, vomiting, diarrhea, weight loss). The owner should be questioned carefully concerning the patient's diet, eating habits, and bowel eliminations. Greedy eaters are subject to aerophagia and can produce flatulence. Fecal retention or constipation may cause chronic flatulence. The diet should be closely inspected for the substrates that are potentially gas producers (*e.g.*, soybean meal, high fiber content).

If specific signs of digestive system disease are present, intestinal parasitism and malassimilation syndromes should be considered. The feces must be inspected for mucus, blood, fat, volume, and consistency. Microscopic examinations for parasites, fat droplets, muscle fibers, starch, and blood cells sould be made. If indicated, tests for maldigestion (fecal trypsin test, BT-PABA test) and malabsorption (blood D-xylose absorption test, oral fat absorption test) should be made. Rarely, dietary allergy may cause diarrhea and flatulence. A trial of hypoallergic food is given for 2 to 3 weeks when dietary allergy is suspected. Diets containing large amounts of lactose may cause flatulence, especially in cats and puppies. In cats, hyperthyroidism may cause maldigestion, steatorrhea, and flatulence. Signs of restlessness, hyperactivity, weight loss, and polyphagia are usually apparent.

SYMPTOMATIC THERAPY

The most important factor in therapy is to rule out small intestinal disease, malabsorption, or maldigestion syndromes. When present, these diseases should be definitively treated.

Aerophagia is difficult to control; however, feeding smaller meals two to three times a day may be helpful. Easily digested low fiber diets may be helpful but may not totally relieve the problem. Enteric antibiotics (*e.g.*, neomycin and phthalylsulfathiazole [Sulfathalidine]) are effective in decreasing gas production in all regions of the intestinal tract since they inhibit putrefactive bacterial growth. Long-term use of enteric antibiotics may cause fungal or yeast overgrowth in the gut lumen; neomycin can create villous atrophy and malabsorption in humans. Enteric antibiotics are only indicated in the actue management of flatulence. Pancreatic enzymes, bile salts, and carminatives are usually ineffective.

Simethicone may be useful since it reduces the surface tension of intestinal mucus, thereby liberating mucus-entrapped gas, which facilitates absorption or elimination. It does not prevent gas production; rather, it helps prevent gas accumulation. Twenty to 40 mg orally every 8 hours is recommended.

Vigorous exercise helps expel colonic gas and encourages colonic evacuation. In summary, symptomatic therapy should focus on the diet and proper exercise. Simethicone is reserved for those cases not adequately responding to these changes.

REFERENCE

1. Richards EA et al: Relationship of bean substrates and certain intestinal bacteria to gas production in the dog. Gastroenterology 55:502–509, 1968

36

Abdominal Pain

LAINE A. COWAN

Abdominal pain may be the chief presenting complaint of the pet owner or, more frequently, may require a thorough history and physical examination by the veterinarian for detection. A painful abdomen may be the only indication of inflammation or organ dysfunction; hence, it is an important (though nonspecific) finding.

An astute veterinarian must not forget that extraabdominal lesions can mimic abdominal pain (Table 36-1). This may be due to similarity of signs of pain in other locations.

Abdominal pain can be subdivided into true visceral pain, deep somatic pain, and referred pain. In visceral pain, the abdominal organs, excluding the peritoneum, are the source of the noxious stimuli. Deep somatic pain, on the other hand, eminates from the parietal peritoneum or the mesentery and may be aggravated by movement (which causes torsion or tension on the peritoneum). Referred pain occurs when the stimuli is perceived as if it were coming from a site distant from the actual stimuli; it may accompany deep somatic or visceral pain.

PATHOPHYSIOLOGY

Abdominal pain is usually due to one of four basic mechanisms: (1) distention of a hollow viscus, (2) traction on the peritoneum or mesentery, (3) ischemia, or (4) inflammation. Much less frequently, pain can be secondary to direct invasion of afferent neurons by tumor[1] or another mass lesion. The abdominal pain can then be modified by previous alterations in blood supply or inflammation; these reduce the pain threshold[5] (see chapter 46).

There are no specific pain receptors in the viscera; neuronal excitation begins in bare nerve endings.[4] The viscera is sparsely innervated, and localized stimuli rarely cause pain. Diffuse involvement is necessary for visceral pain. This

Table 36-1. Conditions That Mimic Abdominal Pain

MIMICKING CONDITION	BASIS FOR DIFFERENTIATION FROM ABDOMINAL PAIN
Pleuritis	Auscultation of thorax, thoracic radiographs, shallow respirations
Severe pneumonia	Auscultation of thorax, thoracic radiographs
Spinal or paraspinal pain	Neurologic exam, careful digital palpation along the vertebrae, spinal radiographs
Polyarthritis	Palpation, arthrocentesis, radiographs
Apprehensive patient	History, reevaluate without owner present
Myositis	Generalized (potentially) involvement; evaluate muscle enzymes and a muscle biopsy
Vasculitis	Generalized edema

low density of pain fibers may also contribute to the poor localization of abdominal visceral pain.[1,4]

As detailed in chapter 46, the sensory neurons from the viscera reach the spinal cord via splanchnic nerves, the pelvic nerve, and the mesenteric plexii and then travel in the lateral spinothalamic tract to the cerebral cortex.[5] In humans, this type of pain tends to be a dull aching pain and is probably similar in animals, although this is impossible to ascertain. Pain in solid viscera is due to the organ capsules, which, when rapidly stretched, create a noxious stimulus.

Noxious stimuli to the parietal peritoneum or mesentery cause deep somatic pain. The parietal peritoneum is innervated by spinal nerves; the afferents travel in the cerebrospinal pathways. In humans, disease of the parietal peritoneum results in a very sharp, intense pain.[1,4]

Frequently, visceral pain is felt at the skin surface. One explanation for this phenomenon is that visceral pain fibers, once in the spinal cord, utilize some of the same interneurons as skin pain fibers. This results in an animal feeling pain as if it were originating in the skin.[4]

Rigidity of the abdominal muscles is frequently associated with deep abdominal pain. This is due to a reflex muscle contraction that is sustained. When the abdominal wall is involved in the origin of pain, the resulting muscle tension is very prominent. Pain from hollow viscera, however, may not elicit this reflex[7]; thus, abdominal pain may result from a combination of decreased blood supply to the muscles (secondary to prolonged contraction) in addition to the underlying abdominal disease.

Specific Organs (Table 36-2)

Stomach

Gastritis, ulcers, dilatation–volvulus, and perforation are common causes of gastric pain. Besides the noxious stimuli of chemical irritation (ulcer) and distention seen in these syndromes, most gastric pain is due to muscular spasm, which results in decreased organ perfusion.[1] Gastric pain tends to localize in the cranial abdomen.

Intestine

Small intestinal pain is better localized than that in the large bowel.[5] The most common stimulus for pain in this organ is bowel distention. Enteroviruses may cause pain also, but usually it is of less severity. It may or may not be possible to localize pain to a specific region, depending on the diffuseness of the lesion.

Pancreas

Pancreatic pain is multifactorial but includes distention of the pancreatic duct and vascular spasms with ischemia or inflammation. Cranial abdominal pain is one of the hallmarks of acute pancreatitis.

Hepatic and Biliary System

Hepatic pain is due to rapid distention of the liver, resulting in stretching of the liver capsule. Bile duct and gall bladder distention are other noxious stimuli. In humans, this pain is referred to the right scapular margin.[4] No such precise referral regions are commonly reported in veterinary medicine.

Urinary Tract

Distention is the main cause of pain in the urinary tract. Acute renal parenchymal distention can occur in acute renal failure or acute obstruction. The resulting capsular stretching is the noxious stimulus. Pain in this region may be referred to the paraspinal muscles. "Flank pain" is not recognized routinely in veterinary species with renal pain. Ureteral pain can be produced by a rapid increase in lumenal pressure with subsequent reflex peristalis and muscular spasms.[3] Pain in the urinary bladder is stimulated by overdistention or irritation of the bladder mucosa.[6] Muscular spasms of the bladder after mucosal irritation may also contribute to the pain.

Both prostatic parenchyma and the surrounding capsule are innervated.[2] Whether pain originates in the parenchyma or is secondary to stretch within the capsule is unknown.

DIAGNOSIS

Signalment

Younger animals tend to acquire more infectious diseases, more dietary indiscretion, and fewer malignancies in general than a similar older pet. Likewise, breed and sex predispositions occur for many abdominal disease syndromes.

(*Text continues on p 296.*)

Table 36-2. Diagnosis of Abdominal Pain Caused by Disorder of Specific Organ

ORGAN	LOCATION OF PAIN	ADDITIONAL CLUES TO SUGGEST THIS ORGAN	ANCILLARY DIAGNOSTIC TESTS	COMMONLY ASSOCIATED DISEASE PROCESSES
Pancreas	Cranial abdomen	Obese, high fat diet, vomiting/diarrhea, diabetes mellitus	Amylase, lipase	Acute pancreatitis Tumor
Stomach	Dorsal or ventral cranial abdomen	Abdominal distention, vomiting, hematemesis, melena	Upper GI contrast studies, endoscopy, fecal occult blood	Dilatation/volvulus Gastric ulcer Rupture Foreign body Toxin Tumor Nonspecific inflammation
Small intestine	Midabdomen—variable Diffuse	Vomiting, diarrhea, melena, history of garbage ingestion	Upper GI contrast studies, rectal scraping, multiple biopsies (exploratory)	Foreign body Tumor Intussusception Parasites Perforation Toxin Torsion Fungal, bacterial, viral
Large intestine	Mid to caudal abdomen	Tenesmus, diarrhea, mucus, hematochezia, constipation, obstipation	Rectal scraping, barium enema, proctoscopy, biopsy	Infection Tumor Inflammatory Foreign body Perforation Obstruction

Liver	Cranial abdomen	Icterus, coagulopathy	Bilirubin (serum), BSP percent retention, ammonia tolerance, coagulogram	Congestion Tumor Infectious Inflammatory
Spleen	Cranial to mid abdomen	Circulating nucleated red blood cells	Ultrasound, abdominocentesis	Torsion Tumor Abscess
Kidneys/ureters	Cranial dorsal (canine) to midabdomen (feline)	Uremia, oliguria/anuria	Excretory urogram, ultrasound, renal biopsy, angiogram	Acute renal failure due to Toxin Obstruction Vascular Trauma
Bladder	Caudal abdomen	Anuria, stranguria, pollakiuria	Cystogram, ultrasound	Infection Tumor Calculi
Ovaries/uterus	Cranial dorsal to caudal abdomen	Estrous cycle, vaginal discharge, polyuria, polydipsia	Vaginal exam, ultrasound	Pyometra Tumor Abscess Granuloma Endometritis
Testicles	Variable if not descended—cranial dorsal to caudal abdomen	Cryptorchid	Ultrasound abdomen	Torsion Abscess Granuloma Tumor Inflammation
Prostate	Caudal abdomen	Tenesmus, urethral discharge, recurrent urinary tract infections	Ejaculate, prostatic massage, urethrogram/cystogram, biopsy, ultrasound	Infection Tumor Cyst Abscess

GI, gastrointestinal; BSP, bromosulfophthalein

History

The owner may notice trembling, reluctance to move, inappetence, crying, or abnormal posture, which may suggest that the animal is experiencing pain. Some animals assume specific postures in attempts to relieve some of the discomfort. This is known as the "position of relief." An animal with peritonitis may refuse to move and have shallow respirations in attempt to minimize peritoneal movement. The praying posture (extended outstretched forelimbs, normal standing position of hindlimbs, with head and neck resting on the forelimbs) has been described in dogs with abdominal pain.[8]

The owner should be questioned about the presence of emesis, diarrhea, melena, and hematochezia and about the animal's environment. Possible exposures to infectious diseases, toxins, or dietary indiscretions must be ascertained.

Duration, intensity, and the time sequence of the pain may be helpful. Unfortunately, even the most astute veterinarian may have difficulty in thorough characterization of the pain, due to its subjective nature and the lack of communicative ability of pets.

Physical Examination

The goal of a physical examination in a pet with apparent abdominal pain is to exclude the extraabdominal disorders that mimic abdominal pain (Table 36-1). Once the problem is localized to the abdomen, the pain should be regionalized as specifically as possible.

Findings that suggest abdominal pain include the animal crying out when lifted on to the examination table and splinting of the abdominal musculature during gentle palpation in a calm animal. Nonspecific findings such as body condition may suggest the nature of the disease process (*e.g.*, obesity may attend pancreatitis in the animal with the appropriate signalment; an animal with a chronic systemic disease process such as neoplasia may be emaciated). Gas- or fluid-filled bowel loops, foreign bodies, intussusception, organomegaly, abdominal masses, organ displacement, lymphadenopathy, and ascites need to be specifically assessed during the physical examination. The abdominal examination must be complete (including a rectal exam), and extra-abdominal evaluation is essential.

Once abdominal pain is identified, attempts should be made to specifically localize the pain. Dividing the abdomen into cranial, middle, and caudal regions may be helpful in determining the origin of the pain (Table 36-3). Not all pain, however, can be localized into just one region. Diffuse pain is seen with generalized peritonitis due to any cause. Sedation or analgesics may aid in palpation of the patient in pain.

Tests

The appropriate laboratory tests are dependent on the acuteness, severity, and localization of the pain (Table 36-2). Other physical or historical findings will also influence the choice of tests. Acute, mild discomfort may only warrant

Table 36-3. Detection of Origin of Pain by Location in the Abdomen

DORSOCRANIAL	VENTROCRANIAL	MIDABDOMEN	CAUDAL
Adrenals	Stomach	Intestines	Urinary bladder
Kidneys	Liver	Uterus	Prostate
Ovaries	Gallbladder	Spleen	Colon
Lymph nodes	Pancreas	Left (and right) kidney	Uterus
Spleen	Spleen	Ovaries (cat)	Retained testicle
Stomach		Lymph nodes	Lymph nodes
Caudate/right liver lobes			
Retained testicle			

observation of the pet initially. On the other hand, any severe or chronic pain of undetermined or unlocalized cause necessitates a complete blood count, chemistry profile (including BUN, alanine aminotransferase, alkaline phosphatase, albumin, total protein, calcium, sodium, and potassium), and urine analysis. These will help rule out generalized inflammatory, infectious, and systemic disease processes. Abdominal radiographs may be of low yield if the abdominal palpation was unremarkable. However, even in those cases, radiographs can help confirm extravisceral diseases such as a small peritoneal effusion or diskospondylitis. Radiographs are also indicated when a thorough palpation is impossible due to the pain or when an abnormality was detected during palpation.

Ancillary tests may include four-quadrant abdominocentesis, diagnostic peritoneal lavage, abdominal ultrasound, and more specific laboratory evaluation (Table 36-2).

TREATMENT

Treatment is aimed at relieving or treating the underlying disease process. If analgesia is needed, it should be administered, but the clinician should keep in mind that it may mask some of the progression or deterioration of the underlying problem. The severity of the pain is proportional to the diffuseness or acuteness of the process; therefore, the cases that are extremely painful and warrant analgesic intervention are usually the ones in which prompt diagnosis is essential. Refer to chapter 46 for a discussion of the recommended analgesics.

REFERENCES

1. Aach D: Abdominal pain. In Blacklow RS (ed): MacBryde's Signs and Symptoms, 6th ed, pp 165–179. Philadelphia, JB Lippincott, 1983
2. Blacklock WJ: Surgical anatomy. In Chisholm GD, Williams DI (eds): Scientific Foundations of Urology, 2nd ed, pp 473–485. Chicago, Year Book Medical Publishers
3. Carlton CE: Initial evaluation including history, physical exam, and urinalysis. In Harrison JH, Gettes RF, Perlmutter A et al (eds): Campbell's Urology, 4th ed, pp 203–221. Philadelphia, WB Saunders, 1978

4. Guyton AC: Somatic sensations: Pain, visceral pain, headache, and thermal sensations. In Guyton AC (ed): Textbook of Medical Physiology, 6th ed, pp 611–625. Philadelphia, WB Saunders, 1981
5. Menaker GJ: The physiology and mechanism of acute abdominal pain. Surg Clin North Am 42:241–248, 1962
6. Perlmutter AD, Blacklow R: Urinary tract pain. In Blacklow RS (ed): MacBryde's Signs and Symptoms, 6th ed, pp 181–194. Philadelphia, JB Lippincott, 1983
7. Ruch: Pathophysiology of pain. In Ruch TC, Patton HD, Woodbury JW, Towe AL (eds): Neurophysiology, 2nd ed, pp 345–363. Philadelphia, WB Saunders, 1965
8. Thrall DE, Bovee KC, Biery DN: Demonstration of a "position of relief" in dogs with lesions of the stomach or small bowel. J Am Anim Hosp Assoc 14:343–347, 1978

37

Icterus

LARRY M. CORNELIUS

DEFINITION

Icterus is a syndrome characterized by hyperbilirubinemia and deposition of bile pigment in tissues, including the skin and mucous membranes.

PATHOPHYSIOLOGY

Approximately 70% of bilirubin is derived from the death of senescent erythrocytes in reticuloendothelial cells mainly in the spleen and liver; another 10% is derived from ineffective erythropoiesis in the bone marrow.[2] Most of the remaining bilirubin is derived from hepatic cytochromes, catalase, peroxidase, and myoglobin.

Bilirubin is the only major breakdown product that requires excretion. The protein and iron components of the heme molecule enter the body pool and are reused.

Newly formed unconjugated bilirubin is insoluble in water and bound to circulating albumin. In addition to allowing transport of bilirubin via the blood to the liver, binding prevents diffusion of the large bilirubin–albumin complex across cell membranes and thus tends to retain bilirubin in the vascular space. In humans, the plasma-binding capacity of albumin is about 20 to 25 mg bilirubin per deciliter.[1,8] Beyond this capacity, or if binding capacity is reduced, unbound bilirubin may cross cell membranes and enter tissues. Central nervous system toxicity termed *kernicterus* occurs in neonates whenever unconjugated bilirubin crosses the blood–brain barrier, but toxic effects in older patients are unknown. Bilirubin-binding capacity of albumin may be reduced by (1) decreased plasma albumin, (2) decreased binding sites on the albumin molecule, caused by competition for sites by drugs (*e.g.*, sulfonamides or salicylates), and (3) decreased affinity of albumin for bilirubin, caused by acidosis.[1]

Bilirubin dissociates from albumin before entry into the liver cell.[2] A carrier mechanism has been postulated but is unproven. The flow of bilirubin between plasma and liver is bidirectional, with approximately one third of the unconjugated bilirubin that enters the liver cell ultimately returning to the plasma unaltered. Hepatic uptake of unconjugated bilirubin is apparently unaffected by severe impairment of hepatic conjugation or excretion of bilirubin.[2] Hepatic bilirubin uptake is subject to competitive inhibition by bromosulfophthalein (BSP) but not by bile acids. Once inside the hepatocyte, specific proteins termed *Y* (or ligandin) and *Z* bind bilirubin. These proteins also bind other anions such as drugs and steroids.[3]

Hepatic conjugation of bilirubin with glucuronic acid to form bilirubin monoglucuronide and diglucuronide is catalyzed by the enzyme glucuronyl transferase. The importance of conjugation is that bilirubin is transformed from a lipid-soluble to a water-soluble compound. Water solubility is mandatory for excretion of bilirubin in the urine. Lipid insolubility limits back-diffusion of bilirubin into hepatocytes and reabsorption from the intestine, causing it to be excreted through bile into the feces.

Conjugated bilirubin is excreted from the liver cell into the bile canaliculus by a system that appears to have the properties of active, carrier-mediated transport. BSP also competes with bilirubin for hepatocellular excretion into the bile canaliculus. The transport mechanism involved is different than that for hepatocellular secretion of bile salts. Hepatic excretion of conjugated bilirubin is the rate-limiting step in the overall capacity of the liver to move bilirubin from blood to bile. In contrast to uptake and conjugation, which are well preserved in the presence of hepatocellular injury, the excretory transport system is very sensitive to various types of liver damage. Hence, an increase in plasma-conjugated bilirubin occurs early in the course of hepatocellular injury. However, total plasma bilirubin concentration may not increase until later in dogs with hepatocellular injury, because dogs have a low renal threshold for conjugated bilirubin, and significant bilirubinuria occurs soon after hepatocellular injury. Trace to 1+ amounts of conjugated bilirubin may also appear in the urine of normal dogs, especially in concentrated urine samples. In cats, the renal threshold for bilirubin is significantly higher. Bilirubinuria in cats is nearly always pathologic, indicating either cholestasis or hepatocellular damage.

The bacteria of the lower intestinal tract reduce most of the conjugated bilirubin to a group of chromagens termed *urobilinogen.* Much of the urobilinogen is excreted in the feces, but some is reabsorbed from the colon and carried via portal blood back to the liver. Most urobilinogen is subsequently reexcreted into bile, but a small amount may gain entrance to systemic circulation and be excreted in the urine.

Hyperbilirubinemia and Cholestasis

Bilirubin uptake, conjugation, and excretion are controlled by hepatocellular mechanisms that are separate from the conjugation and excretion of bile acids.[2] Disturbances in bilirubin transport are recognized by hyperbilirubinemia and icterus. Cholestatic syndromes (reduced bile flow) are characterized by marked bile acidemia, usually with normal to slightly elevated bilirubin levels. Severe cholestasis can, however, cause icterus. Measurement of serum bile acids is a reliable procedure for the detection of cholestasis and is a sensitive test of hepatic function. Increased serum alkaline phosphatase and gamma glutamyl transpeptidase (GGT) activities also result from cholestasis.

Hyperbilirubinemia may be caused by increases in unconjugated or conjugated bilirubin in plasma. The van den Bergh test is used to fractionate plasma bilirubin into indirect (unconjugated) and direct (conjugated) reacting bilirubin. This test is of value only when total serum bilirubin is increased (greater than 1.0 mg/dl). One can generally observe a yellow color of plasma in a microhematocrit tube when total plasma bilirubin is increased.

Unconjugated Hyperbilirubinemia

Increased plasma unconjugated bilirubin can result from increased pigment production (hemolysis or ineffective erythropoiesis) or impaired hepatic uptake or conjugation of bilirubin. Increased pigment production (hemolysis) probably accounts for most instances of unconjugated hyperbilirubinemia in icteric dogs and cats. The liver normally has a large reserve capacity for uptake, conjugation, and excretion of bilirubin (30–60 times basal rate[3]). It has been shown in humans that a plasma unconjugated bilirubin concentration in excess of 4 mg/dl suggests reduced hepatic bilirubin clearance (due to liver disease) irrespective of the presence or absence of hemolysis.[2] In hemolytic icterus, hyperbilirubinemia is initially characterized by a preponderance of unconjugated bilirubin. Three to 4 days after the hemolytic crisis, however, the plasma-conjugated bilirubin concentration may equal or exceed unconjugated bilirubin (total serum bilirubin still increased, although less than during the hemolytic crisis). Therefore, at certain stages of hemolytic icterus, relative concentrations of conjugated and unconjugated bilirubin may overlap those observed in hepatocellular disease and biliary obstruction. Although incompletely understood, it has been suggested that increases in conjugated bilirubin later in hemolytic icterus may be due to compromise of the excretory system of a previously normal liver injured by anemic anoxia.[6] In this situation, it is assumed that hepatocellular uptake and conjugation of bilirubin remain relatively normal. With lack of excretion, regurgitation from the hepatocyte into blood would occur. Another possible explanation is that excessive hepatocellular production of conjugated bilirubin causes bile inspissation. This results in intrahepatic biliary obstruction and regurgitation of conjugated bilirubin into blood.[6] It is doubtful that serum alkaline phosphatase activity would help differentiate these two possible mechanisms, since it takes 7 to 8 days of total biliary obstruction to produce maximum serum alkaline phosphatase increases.[11] Patients with hemolytic icterus would be expected to have anemia characterized by signs of regeneration (reticulocytosis, anisocytosis, or poikilocytosis), provided that the bone marrow is functional and 3 to 5 days have elapsed since the hemolytic crisis. If hemolysis occurs intravascularly (as opposed to extravascularly in reticuloendothelial cells) and is sufficiently rapid, the plasma may be red due to the presence of increased amounts of free hemoglobin. Normally, a plasma protein termed *haptoglobin* binds the free circulating hemoglobin and prevents it from entering urine. With rapid, massive hemolysis, all haptoglobin may be saturated with hemoglobin, and the unbound hemoglobin is filtered by the glomerulus and appears in the urine, where it causes the urine to be red (port-wine colored). Few or no intact erythrocytes are present in the urine to account for the red color and strongly positive occult blood test results. One would not expect significant increases in serum levels of leaked enzymes (alanine aminotransferase [ALT]) or overproduced enzymes (alkaline phosphatases, GGT) in hemolytic disease. It is conceivable, however, that anemic anoxia might cause hepatocellular membrane damage and increases in serum ALT. It is possible that biliary obstruction due to bile inspissation, as previously mentioned, could eventually cause increases in serum alkaline phosphatase.

Conjugated Hyperbilirubinemia

Hepatocellular disease and biliary obstruction (intrahepatic or extrahepatic) may result in an increase in plasma conjugated and unconjugated bilirubin, with the former predominating. It is not usually possible to distinguish hepatocellular disease from biliary obstruction on the basis of laboratory data. Ongoing hepatocellular disease is often associated with marked increases in serum ALT. Other laboratory abnormalities that may be present with severe hepatic dysfunction include decreased serum concentrations of urea nitrogen, albumin, and glucose and increased plasma ammonia. Conjugated bilirubin appears in the urine in increased amounts.

Biliary obstruction is better characterized by marked increases in serum alkaline phosphatase as a result of induction of synthesis of large amounts of alkaline phosphatase by hepatocytes and biliary epithelial cells.

Conjugated Bilirubin Increases in Urine

Hepatocellular disease and partial biliary obstruction (usually intrahepatic) frequently coexist in diseased patients. Clinical signs are usually more severe with hepatocellular disease than with biliary obstruction. Bacterial sepsis and endotoxemia may cause impaired hepatic secretion of conjugated bilirubin and decreased bile flow. Increased serum alkaline phosphatase activity and conjugated hyperbilirubinemia may result.[10]

Cholestasis

Cholestasis refers to decreased bile flow and is characterized by increased serum bile acid levels and alkaline phosphatase activity and, in more severe cases, by hyperbilirubinemia.[2] Causes of cholestasis include partial or complete biliary obstruction and drug administration. Drugs thought to cause cholestasis in dogs include corticosteroids and anticonvulsants (diphenylhydantoin [Dilantin], phenobarbital, and primidone). Their mechanisms have not been completely worked out, although it is known that corticosteroids induce a characteristic hepatopathy in some dogs with associated hepatomegaly.

DIAGNOSTIC PLAN

History and Physical Examination

Initially efforts should be made to categorize icterus into hemolytic, hepatocellular, or obstructive causes, keeping in mind that combinations of these basic causes frequently occur in clinical disease states. History and physical examination may sometimes suggest one of these categories, but laboratory evaluation is usually necessary (Table 37-1).

Table 37-1. Initial Plan for Diagnosis of Icterus in Dogs and Cats

DATA BASE	RULE OUT*	MOST COMMON FINDINGS	
History (Hx), physical examination (PE), CBC, reticulocyte count, microfilariae check (dogs only), urine analysis, BUN, ALT, SAP, total protein, albumin, globulin, glucose, total, conjugated and unconjugated serum bilirubin, fecal examination	Hemolytic	Hx and PE	Sudden onset of weakness and exercise intolerance, very pale mucous membranes with slight yellow tinge, holosystolic mitral murmur common (anemic)
		Lab	PCV < 15, ↑ reticulocytes and NRBCs if 3–4 days since onset, WBC variable, slightly ↑ urine bilirubin, increased total bilirubin with >50% unconjugated (3–4 days after onset may have >50% conjugated), ALT normal or slightly ↑ (2–5× normal), rest of data base normal
	Hepatocellular	Hx and PE	Lethargy, anorexia, vomiting, diarrhea, dehydration, mild to marked icterus
		Lab	PCV normal or ↑, WBC variable, moderately to markedly ↑ urine bilirubin, increased total bilirubin with >50% conjugated, ALT moderately to markedly ↑ (5–50× normal), SAP mildly to moderately ↑ (2–10× normal, dog; 2–5× normal, cat), total protein variable, albumin normal or ↓, globulin normal or ↑, BUN normal or ↓
	Obstructive	Hx and PE	Mild to moderate lethargy, variable appetite, occasional vomiting and weight loss, mild to marked icterus
		Lab	PCV normal, WBC variable, moderately to markedly ↑ urine bilirubin, ↑ total bilirubin with >50% conjugated, ALT mildly to moderately ↑ (2–10× normal), SAP moderately to markedly ↑ (5–100× normal, dog; 5–15× normal, cat), rest of data base variable

* Combinations of these three basic types of icterus are frequently present in clinical cases.

CBC, complete blood count; BUN, blood urea nitrogen; ALT, alanine aminotransferase; SAP, serum alkaline phosphatase; PCV, packed cell volume; ↑, increased; WBC, white blood cells; ↓, decreased

(Cornelius LM: Icterus. In Proceedings of the 49th Annual Meeting of the American Animal Hospital Association, 1982)

Laboratory Evaluation

Follow-up diagnostic plans for an icteric dog or cat will depend upon which category or categories are suspected after results of initial tests are returned (Tables 37-2, 37-3, and 37-4). With hemolytic icterus, further history for toxin or drug ingestion is indicated. Careful examination for blood parasites should be done, as well as a Coomb's test, lupus erythematosus (LE) prep, and antinuclear antibody titer if autoimmune disease is suspected.

Other Diagnostic Procedures

For hepatocellular disease, abdominal radiographs are usually indicated. Plasma ammonia or the ammonia tolerance test can be used to evaluate liver function. Hyperbilirubinemia interferes with BSP uptake and excretion by the liver and falsely increases BSP retention values. It is often helpful to repeat initial serum biochemical analysis to monitor the progress of hepatic disease.[5] Half-life of serum ALT is 2.5 hours. If either no improvement or actual deterioration in clinical appearance or laboratory data is observed, liver biopsy is indicated. If the liver is noticeably enlarged, percutaneous needle biopsy is easy and relatively safe. If the liver is normal in size or small, biopsy via laparoscopy or celiotomy is preferred. Ultrasonography allows evaluation of liver size and consistency and permits accurate placement of the percutaneous biopsy needle. All liver biopsy procedures should be preceded by laboratory evaluation of clotting and a platelet count.

Follow-up plans for icterus due to biliary obstruction are similar to those discussed for hepatocellular disease. It is safer to biopsy via laparoscopy or celiotomy rather than risk bile peritonitis from puncture of a distended gallbladder or bile duct during blind percutaneous liver biopsy with a needle. Ultrasonic guidance of a percutaneous biopsy need is also reasonably safe.

(*Text continues on p 317.*)

Table 37-2. Follow-up Plan for Icterus in Dogs and Cats

RULE OUT	DATA BASE*
Hemolytic	Further history, blood parasite check, Coomb's test, antinuclear antibody, blood cultures
Hepatocellular	Abdominal radiographs, repeat biochemistry profile, plasma ammonia, feline leukemia virus test (cats only), consider blood cultures, biopsy liver (coagulogram first) by laparoscopy, ultrasonically guided needle, or celiotomy
Obstructive	Abdominal radiographs, repeat biochemistry profile, consider serum amylase/lipase, biopsy liver by laparoscopy, ultrasonically guided needle, or celiotomy.

* May repeat all or part of initial data base (Table 37-1)

(Cornelius LM: Icterus. In Proceedings of the 49th Annual Meeting of the American Animal Hospital Association, 1982)

Table 37-3. Selected Causes of Icterus in Dogs and Associated Findings

CAUSE	HISTORY	PHYSICAL EXAMINATION	LABORATORY DATA
Hemolytic*			
Autoimmune hemolytic anemia	Sudden onset of severe weakness and possibly collapse in an adult dog	Very pale mucous membranes. Icterus, when present, is mild. Weakness, tachycardia, holosystolic murmur (anemic), splenomegaly	Severe anemia (PCV < 15) that is regenerative provided 3–4 days have elapsed since onset of hemolysis. Leukocytosis with neutrophilia and left shift; spherocytes common; autoagglutination of erythrocytes may be present, most are Coomb's positive
Heartworm disease—postcaval syndrome	Sudden onset of weakness and collapse	Signs of shock. Icterus is mild to moderate. Evidence of impaired coagulation due to DIC may be present (*e.g.*, petechiae, ecchymoses, melena).	May be positive or negative for microfilariae. Often positive on ELISA or fluorescent antibody test. Leukocytosis, usually with stress leukogram, is present. Hemoglobinemia (red plasma) and hemoglobinuria (port-wine colored urine) may be marked. BUN and ALT may be markedly ↑. If DIC is present, see ↑ ACT, PT, PTT, TT, and fibrin degradation products and ↓ platelet numbers and fibrinogen. Thoracic radiographs show enlarged right ventricle and pulmonary arteries.

(Continued)

Table 37-3. Selected Causes of Icterus in Dogs and Associated Findings (*Continued*)

CAUSE	HISTORY	PHYSICAL EXAMINATION	LABORATORY DATA
Hemolytic bacteremia/septicemia	Depression, anorexia, weakness. May have history suggesting a likely source of bacteria such as bite wounds (other common sources are dental disease, bacterial endocarditis, prostatitis, diskospondylitis, and indwelling venous catheters).	Fever, depression, dehydration, and possibly signs of shock. Icterus is usually mild. May see signs of DIC	Nonregenerative anemia, neutropenia, and thrombocytopenia may be present. Icteric plasma or hemoglobinemia may be found. Mild to markedly ↑ SAP (2–15× normal) is sometimes present. Blood cultures may be positive. Evidence of DIC may be found.
Incompatible blood transfusion	Depression, anorexia, occasional vomiting, history of multiple blood transfusions	Depression, mild to severe icterus	Mild to moderate anemia, usually nonregenerative, ↑ WBC with either a stress or inflammatory leukogram; SAP and ALT usually normal.
Hepatocellular*			
Cholangitis/Cholangiohepatitis	Usually a chronic course of lethargy, decreased appetite, sporadic vomiting, and diarrhea	Depression, mild fever (103–103.5°F), mild to moderate dehydration, and weight loss; mild to severe icterus. Later may see signs of hepatic failure (stupor, headpressing, apparent blindness, ascites, melena)	PCV and plasma total solids are normal to slightly increased, moderately ↑ WBC (20,000–30,000/cm^3 with inflammatory leukogram, BUN may be ↓, albumin sometimes ↓ and globulin ↑, ALT mildly to moderately (2–10× normal), SAP moderately ↑ (5–15× normal), blood glucose may be ↓, plasma ammonia tolerance ↓. Ascitic fluid, when present, is a low protein (<2.5 g/dl) transudate.

Chronic active hepatitis	Similar to hepatic copper accumulation		
Hepatic copper accumulation (hereditary in Bedlington terriers). Also reported in Doberman pinschers	Most are asymptomatic. Early have sporadic anorexia and vomiting with weight loss. Later have severe depression, vomiting, and diarrhea	Most show no signs or only slight weight loss. Later severe depression, mild to severe dehydration, weight loss, icterus, ascites, melena, and signs of hepatic encephalopathy are seen.	PCV and WBC usually normal. ↑ ALT is the earliest abnormality (2–100× normal). Later have ↑ SAP (100–150× normal), ↓ albumin, ↓ BUN, ↑ ammonia, or ↓ ammonia tolerance and evidence of impaired coagulation (↑ ACT, PT, PTT, TT). Hepatic copper ↑ (5–50× normal)
Drugs or toxins			
Thiacetarsamide (Caparsolate)	Within a few hours of drug administration, depression, anorexia, vomiting	Depression, dehydration, mild to severe icterus in some cases	PCV and plasma total protein normal to ↑ (dehydration), WBC mildly ↑ with a stress leukogram, ALT markedly ↑ (15–50× normal), SAP normal to slightly ↑ (2–5× normal)
Aflatoxins (molds from grain-type foods)	Chronic lethargy, anorexia, weight loss, sometimes polydipsia and polyuria	Depression, weight loss, dehydration, severe icterus, bloody vomiting, melena	PCV and WBC variable, slightly ↑ ALT and SAP (2–5× normal), ↓ BUN, albumin, glucose, and cholesterol, evidence of DIC (↑ ACT, PT, PTT, TT, FDPs), and ↓ platelet numbers), high levels of aflatoxins in food
Mebendazole (Telmintic) (possibly others such as oxibendazole)	Within a few days of drug administration, anorexia, depression, dehydration, and vomiting	Depression, dehydration, moderate to severe icterus; in some, signs of hepatic failure (hepatic encephalopathy, bloody vomitus, melena)	PCV and plasma total protein normal to ↑ (dehydration), ↑ WBC with stress or inflammatory leukogram, ALT and SAP markedly ↑ (10–50× normal), plasma ammonia sometimes ↑, bilirubinuria

(Continued)

Table 37-3. Selected Causes of Icterus in Dogs and Associated Findings (*Continued*)

CAUSE	HISTORY	PHYSICAL EXAMINATION	LABORATORY DATA
Anticonvulsants—especially primidone	Takes 2–3 years of continuous therapy	Anorexia, weakness, ascites, no icterus or mild	Albumin ↓, ALT and SAP moderately to markedly ↑ (5–30×) BSP ↑, ascitic fluid is a low protein (<2.5 g/dl) transudate
Hepatic fibrosis ("cirrhosis")	Chronic course of depression, decreased appetite, weight loss, sporadic vomiting and diarrhea, and in some cases polydipsia, polyuria, head pressing, stupor, apparent blindness, and seizures	Depression, weight loss, icterus usually mild, ascites, melena, and, in some, signs of hepatoencephalopathy	Usually a mild nonregenerative anemia (PCV 20–30), WBC normal, BUN ↓, albumin severely ↓ (<1.5 g/dl), globulin normal to ↑, glucose ↓, ALT normal, SAP normal to moderately ↑ (5–10× normal), ↑ plasma ammonia or ↓ ammonia tolerance, clotting may be abnormal, ascitic fluid is a low protein (<2.5 g/dl) transudate, liver is small radiographically
Bacteremia/septicemia (usually gram-negative)	See hemolytic bacteremia/septicemia.	See hemolytic bacteremia/septicemia.	See hemolytic bacteremia/septicemia. Some bacterial endotoxins (especially *Escherichia coli*) apparently interfere with hepatocyte secretion of conjugated bilirubin into the bile canaliculus.
Infectious canine hepatitis	Severe depression, vomiting, weakness, sometimes seizures or collapse	Depression, weakness, fever (103–105°F), scleral injection, abdominal pain, hepatomegaly, "blue-eye" occasionally, evidence of DIC in some (*e.g.*, petechiae, melena, hematuria). Icterus is uncommon.	PCV variable, WBC ↓ (neutropenia), moderately to markedly ↑ ALT (10–50× normal), mildly to moderately ↑ SAP (2–10× normal), in some cases, ↓ blood glucose and ↑ plasma ammonia, proteinuria in the absence of cells, bilirubinuria, evidence of DIC

Leptospirosis	Severe depression, weakness, anorexia, vomiting, sometimes polydipsia, polyuria, and stiff gait	Depression, weakness, dehydration, scleral injection, fever (103–105°F), mild to severe icterus, sometimes muscle pain and oral ulcers	PCV and plasma total solids ↑, WBC ↑, inflammatory leukogram, platelet numbers may be ↓, BUN ↑ (frequently > 100), ALT and SAP moderately ↑ (5–10× normal), urine may have isosthenuric specific gravity (1.008–1.012) despite dehydration, may have coarse and fine granular casts, proteinuria and bilirubinuria, may be *Leptospira* (spirochetes) in urine by darkfield microscopy, may see rising *Leptospira* titer (two paired titers 7–10 days apart)
Hepatic neoplasia, primary or metastatic	Chronic course of lethargy, decreased appetite, moderate to severe weight loss, sporadic vomiting and diarrhea, and, in some cases, head pressing, stupor, apparent blindness, and seizures	Depression, mild to moderate dehydration, mild to severe icterus, abdominal enlargement due to hepatomegaly, palpable intraabdominal mass, or ascites in some cases	Mild to moderate nonregenerative anemia (PCV 18–25), ↑ WBC with either inflammatory or stress leukogram, BUN variable, albumin variable, globulin may be ↑, ALT normal to mildly ↑ (2–5× normal), SAP normal to markedly ↑ (20× normal), ↑ plasma ammonia or ↓ ammonia tolerance. Abdominal radiographs show hepatomegaly, abnormal masses, or ascites. Ascitic fluid is a high protein (>2.5 g/dl), modified transudate containing nondegenerate neutrophils, erythrocytes, macrophages, and mesothelial cells, but rarely neoplastic cells.

(*Continued*)

Table 37-3. Selected Causes of Icterus in Dogs and Associated Findings (*Continued*)

CAUSE	HISTORY	PHYSICAL EXAMINATION	LABORATORY DATA
Obstructive*			
Intrahepatic			
Cholangitis/cholangiohepatitis	See cholangitis/cholangiohepatitis (hepatocellular).		
Hepatic fibrosis (cirrhosis)	See hepatic fibrosis (hepatocellular).		
Neoplasia	See neoplasia (hepatocellular).		
Extrahepatic			
Acute pancreatitis—bile duct compression	Depression, anorexia, vomiting, restlessness, sometimes after a fatty meal	Often obese, depression, mild to moderate dehydration, mild fever (103–104°F), abdominal pain upon palpation in some cases, mild to moderate icterus in some	PCV and plasma total solids often increased (dehydration), fasting hyperlipemia in many cases, ↑ WBC with inflammatory leukogram, mild to moderate ↑ BUN, mild to moderate ↑ ALT (2–5× normal) and SAP (2–15× normal) in some cases, mild hypocalcemia, focal peritonitis, ileus, displaced bowel loops seen radiographically in some cases, ↑ serum amylase or lipase
Neoplasm compressing bile duct	Chronic course of lethargy, decreased appetite, weight loss, sporadic vomiting and diarrhea	Depression, weight loss, mild to moderate dehydration, severe icterus, may palpate abdominal mass	PVC variable, WBC normal to ↑, may be an inflammatory leukogram, mild to moderate ↑ ALT (2–5× normal), markedly ↑ SAP (10–50× normal), may see abdominal mass radiographically

Traumatic rupture of gall bladder or bile duct	History of trauma followed in 12–24 h by depression, anorexia, and vomiting	Depression, fever (103–105°F), icterus, abdominal pain	PCV and plasma total solids slightly ↑ (dehydration), ↑ WBC with inflammatory leukogram, moderately to markedly ↑ ALT (5–20× normal) due to hepatic trauma, SAP usually normal, decreased contrast of serosal surfaces radiographically (peritonitis), mild fluid accumulation in abdomen in some cases, (high protein [>2.5 g/dl] nonseptic exudate with mostly neutrophils [nondegenerate]), bilirubin in abdominal fluid higher than in plasma
Cholelithiasis	Intermittent episodes of depression, anorexia, and vomiting	Most are asymptomatic. Some show depression, dehydration and moderate to severe icterus.	PCV and plasma total solids sometimes ↑ (dehydration), WBC normal to ↑ with inflammatory leukogram, ALT normal to mildly ↑ (2–5× normal), SAP mildly to moderately ↑ (2–15× normal), may see cholelith radiographically

* See Table 37-1 for general characteristics.

PCV, packed cell volume; DIC, disseminated intravascular coagulation; BUN, blood urea nitrogen; ALT, alanine aminotransferase; ↑, increased; ACT, activated clotting time; PT, prothrombin time; PTT, partial thromboplastin time; TT, thrombin time; ↓, decreased; SAP, serum alkaline phosphatase; WBC, white blood cells; FDP, fibrin(ogen) degradation products

Table 37-4. Selected Causes of Icterus in Cats and Associated Findings

CAUSE	HISTORY	MAJOR CHARACTERISTICS AND ASSOCIATED FINDINGS	
		Physical Examination	Laboratory Data
Hemolytic*			
Hemobartonellosis	Lethargy, weakness, anorexia, often associated with stress such as fighting and abscesses	Fever (103–105°F), depression, dehydration, pale mucous membranes; icterus, when present, is mild	Regenerative anemia (unless associated with feline leukemia virus), variable WBC, organisms seen in erythrocytes intermittently, mildly ↑ ALT (2–5× normal)
Drugs 1. Acetaminophen 2. Methylene blue	Depression, weakness, dyspnea, vomiting, drug administration	Severe depression; pale or cyanotic mucous membranes; icterus, when present, is mild; subnormal body temperature; dyspnea	Hemoglobinemia, stress leukogram, anemia (too acute for regenerative response), markedly ↑ ALT (5–20× normal), Heinz bodies in erythrocytes with methylene blue
Bacteremia/septicemia	Depression, anorexia, weakness	Subnormal temperature or fever; depression; dehydration; icterus, when present, is mild. Sources of infection may be observed (*e.g.*, abscess, purulent vaginal discharge)	Nonregenerative anemia, neutropenia with inappropriate left shift, thrombocytopenia, mildly ↑ ALT (2–5× normal), mild to moderately ↑ SAP (2–5× normal), positive blood cultures in some cases

Hepatocellular*			
Feline leukemia virus-associated diseases (lymphosarcoma, myeloproliferative disorders, immune suppression with bacterial infection)	Lethargy, anorexia, vomiting, weight loss	Fever, depression, dehydration, icteric mucous membranes, sometimes hepatomegaly	Nonregenerative anemia, neutropenia with inappropriate left shift, neoplastic cells sometimes present in blood, thrombocytopenia, normal to slightly ↑ ALT (2–3× normal), moderately to markedly ↑ SAP (3–10× normal), feline leukemia virus positive, neoplastic mass or effusion observed on radiographs. Malignant lymphocytes may be observed in the effusion with Wright-Giemsa stain.
Cholangitis/cholangiohepatitis	Intermittent episodes of decreased appetite, lethargy, weight loss, occasional vomiting	Depression, unkept appearance, icteric mucous membranes, thin, hepatomegaly±. (Some are asymptomatic except for mild, intermittent lethargy and anorexia.) Fever ±, ascites ±	Mild nonregenerative anemia (PCV 20–25), WBC normal or ↑ (neutrophilia with left shift), moderately ↑ ALT (5–10× normal), mild to moderately ↑ SAP (2–5× normal), in some cases ↓ albumin, ↑ globulin, ↓ BUN, ↑ plasma ammonia or ↓ ammonia tolerance, ↑ BSP retention, and positive bacterial culture of bile (usually *Escherichia coli*). Ascitic fluid is a transudate.

(*Continued*)

Table 37-4. Selected Causes of Icterus in Cats and Associated Findings (*Continued*)

CAUSE	HISTORY	MAJOR CHARACTERISTICS AND ASSOCIATED FINDINGS	
		Physical Examination	Laboratory Data
Hepatic lipidosis			
Idiopathic	Chronic, total anorexia, history of obesity, lethargy, weight loss, stress	Depression, unkempt appearance, icteric mucous membranes, dehydrated. May still be obese.	Mild nonregenerative anemia (PCV 20–25), WBC normal, mild to moderately ↑ ALT (2–5× normal), moderately to markedly ↑ SAP (5–15× normal), ↓ albumin, ↓ BUN, ↑ plasma ammonia or ↓ ammonia tolerance, ↑ BSP retention time, in some cases ↑ activated clotting time, ↑ prothrombin time, ↑ partial thromboplastin time, and ↑ thrombin time
Secondary to diabetes mellitus	Polydipsia, polyuria, polyphagia See idiopathic (above)	See idiopathic (above).	Hyperglycemia, glucosuria. See idiopathic (above).
Feline infectious peritonitis	Chronic lethargy, decreased appetite, weight loss	Depression, dehydration, fever (103–105°F), icteric mucous membranes in a few cases, abdominal enlargement (ascites) and dyspnea (pleural effusion) in effusive form, anterior and posterior uveitis in some cases	Mild to moderate nonregenerative anemia (PCV 18–25), WBC variable, ALT and SAP normal, ↑ globulin in some cases, ascitic and pleural fluids are modified transudates with high protein (>3.0 g/dl), FIP titer variable, feline leukemia virus test positive in half

Bacteremia/endotoxemia	See bacteremia/septicemia under hemolytic (above).		Hepatocyte secretion of conjugated bilirubin is impaired, resulting in functional cholestasis. Mildly to moderately ↑ SAP (2–5× normal), normal or mildly ↑ ALT (1½–2× normal)
Drugs or toxins			
Acetaminophen	See acetaminophen under hemolytic (above).		
Neoplasia			
Feline leukemia virus–related (lymphosarcoma, reticuloendotheliosis)	See feline leukemia virus–associated diseases under hepatocellular (above).		
Others (primary or metastatic)	Depression, decreased appetite, weight loss, sporadic vomiting and diarrhea	Depression, weight loss, icteric mucosa, palpably enlarged liver, abdominal mass. Ascites in a few	Mild to moderate nonregenerative anemia (PCV 18–25), normal to ↑ WBC with either inflammatory or stress leukogram, ALT usually normal to slightly ↑ (1½–2× normal), SAP normal to markedly ↑ (5–15× normal), neoplastic mass, ascites, or hepatomegaly observed radiographically in some. The ascites is a modified transudate with moderate protein content (3.0–4.5 g/dl) and a preponderance of nondegenerate neutrophils.
Obstructive*			
Intrahepatic			
Cholangitis/cholangiohepatitis	See cholangitis/cholangiohepatitis under hepatocellular (above).		
Neoplasia (primary or metastatic)	See neoplasia under hepatocellular (above).		

(*Continued*)

Table 37-4. Selected Causes of Icterus in Cats and Associated Findings (*Continued*)

		MAJOR CHARACTERISTICS AND ASSOCIATED FINDINGS	
CAUSE	HISTORY	Physical Examination	Laboratory Data
Extrahepatic			
Neoplasm compressing bile duct	See neoplasia under hepatocellular (above).		
Trauma-ruptured gall bladder or bile duct	History of trauma or opportunity for trauma, depression, anorexia, vomiting	Fever 103–104°, depression, dehydration, icteric mucosa, abdominal pain upon palpation	↑ PCV and total solids (dehydration), ↑ WBC with neutrophilia and left shift, moderately to markedly ↑ ALT (5–20× normal), normal to slightly ↑ SAP (2× normal), abdominal fluid observed radiographically Fluid is a moderate protein (3.0–4.5 g/dl), nonseptic exudate with a preponderance of nondegenerative neutrophils. Bilirubin concentration of fluid is higher than in plasma in acute stage.
Cholelithiasis	Usually secondary to chronic cholestasis and bile inspissation associated with cholangitis/cholangiohepatitis (see above).		

* See Table 37-1 for general characteristics and associated findings.
WBC, white blood cells; ↑, increased; ALT, alanine aminotransferase; SAP, serum alkaline phosphatase; PCV, packed cell volume; ±, present or absent; ↓, decreased; BUN, blood urea nitrogen; BSP, bromosulfophthalein
(Cornelius LM, Rogers KS: Finding the cause of jaundice in cats. Mod Vet Pract 66:166–170, 1985)

SYMPTOMATIC THERAPY

With hemolytic icterus, it is important to allow the animal to rest and to avoid stress. Blood transfusion should be avoided unless it is absolutely necessary. Immune-mediated hemolysis of transfused blood may occur, resulting in release of hemoglobin and erythrocyte membrane fragments, both of which are potentially deleterious to the patient. Maintenance of hydration by fluid therapy will help maintain urine flow. The latter is especially desirable if hemoglobinuria is present, because hemoglobin nephrosis can occur.

Symptomatic therapy of hepatocellular disease may include fluid therapy with Ringer's solution. Glucose (5%–10%) and potassium (1–3 mEq/kg/day) may be added to the Ringer's solution. Multiple vitamins, especially fat-soluble vitamins A, D, E, and K, should be given. If antibiotics are used, those concentrated in bile and effective against enteric organism (gram-negative and anaerobes) are best. Ampicillin and cephalosporins are good for anaerobes and are concentrated in bile. Gentamicin is best for gram-negative organisms, but because of its nephrotoxicity, this drug should be used only with evidence of severe illness or when culture and sensitivity results indicate resistance to other drugs. If hepatic encephalopathy is present, protein in the diet should be restricted to less than 1 g of protein per 20 calories per day. Cottage cheese and rice should be the mainstays of the diet.[9] If no signs of hepatic encephalopathy are present, protein content of the diet should be high and of good biologic value to aid in hepatic regeneration.

For icterus due to biliary obstruction, antibiotics may be used as described for hepatocellular disease. If biliary obstruction is partial instead of complete, use of a choleretic may be helpful. Certain bile acids stimulate flow of watery bile, thereby thinning bile that may have become inspissated secondary to cholestasis. Dehydrocholic acid (Decholin) is a hydrocholeretic. Dosage is extrapolated from the dose for people. The usual dosage is 10 to 15 mg/kg every 8 hours for 7 to 10 days. The drug may be continued until bilirubinuria is no longer present.

REFERENCES

1. Badley BWD: A physiologic approach to jaundice. Clin Biochem 9(3):144–148, 1976
2. Berk PD: Hyperbilirubinemia and cholestasis. Am J Med 64:311–326, 1978
3. Bissel DM: Formation and elimination of bilirubin. Gastroenterology 69:519–538, 1975
4. Cornelius LM: Icterus. In Proceedings of the 49th Annual Meeting of the American Animal Hospital Association, 1982
5. Dusol M, Jr, Schiff ER: Clinical approach to jaundice. Postgrad Med 57:118–123, 1975
6. Maldonado JE, Kyle RA, Schoenfield LJ: Increased serum conjugated bilirubin in hemolytic anemia. Postgrad Med 55:183–190, 1974
7. Rogers KS, Cornelius LM: Feline icterus. Compend Cont Ed Pract Vet 7(5):391–399, 1986
8. Schmid R: Bilirubin metabolism in man. N Engl J Med 287:703–709, 1972
9. Strombeck DR: Chronic hepatitis, chronic active hepatitis, chronic copper toxicity, hemochromatosis. In Strombeck DR (ed): Small Animal Gastroenterology, pp 425–449. Davis, CA, Stonegate Co, 1979

10. Utili R, Abernathy CO, Zimmerman HJ: Cholestatic effects of Escherichia coli endotoxin on the isolated perfused rat liver. Gastroenterology 70:248–253, 1976
11. Van Vleet JF, Alberts JO: Evaluation of liver function tests and liver biopsy in experimental carbon tetrachloride intoxication and extrahepatic bile duct obstruction in the dog. Am J Vet Res 29:2119–2131, 1968

Part Nine

UROLOGIC PROBLEMS

38

Abnormal Micturition: Dysuria, Pollakiuria, and Stranguria

MICHAEL D. LORENZ

PROBLEM DEFINITION AND RECOGNITION

Dysuria is painful or difficult urination. Pollakiuria is frequent urination, and stranguria is slow and painful discharge of urine due to spasm of the bladder and urethra. These clinical signs are frequently encountered in small animals and are caused by disease of the lower urinary tract or genital tract. They must be differentiated from polyuria (increased urine volume). When in doubt, direct observation of the patient and quantitation of urine output should be performed early in the diagnostic process. Disease of the lower urinary and genital tract usually results in a combination of these three clinical signs. Throughout this chapter, dysuria will be used for all three clinical problems.

PATHOGENESIS

The urinary bladder is innervated by the pelvic and hypogastric nerves. The pelvic nerve originates from sacral cord segments S1, S2, and S3 and is comprised of efferent and afferent parasympathetic fibers. The efferent fibers innervate the detruser muscle and provide motor function for coordinated voiding. The afferent fibers mediate the sensation to void, proprioception, and pain. The hypogastric nerve provides sympathetic innervation to the bladder; however, it has little influence on normal micturition. Sympathetic afferents provide some awareness of bladder distention and pain. Sensory receptors are located in the bladder mucosa and are most abundant in the ureterovesical junction and bladder neck. Initiation of inflammation of the mucosa or contraction of the bladder wall may cause pain, an urgency to urinate even though the bladder may be empty or partially filled, bladder wall spasm, or a burning sensation.

The urethra receives its nerve supply from the pudenal nerve, which arises from sacral cord segments. The pudenal nerve is a mixed somatic nerve that contains motor fibers to the external urethral sphincter. Stimulation of these motor fibers contracts the urethral sphincter and maintains continence as the bladder fills with urine. During normal micturition, nerve impulses to the external urethral sphincter are inhibited, allowing the sphincter to dilate for the passage of urine. Sensory receptors within the urethra respond to flow, urethral distention, and thermal sensation. The awareness of voiding is from these urethral sensations and traction on the bladder neck and trigone. Irritation or inflammation of the urethra causes pain, burning sensations, and spasms of the urethral sphincter. In male dogs, disease of the prostate usually involves the urethra and bladder and produces dysuria by the mechanisms previously described.

CAUSES

Any disease of the lower urinary tract (bladder and urethra) or lower genital tract (prostate, vagina) that results in mucosal irritation or inflammation will produce dysuria. In addition, diseases that cause urethral or bladder neck obstruction also cause dysuria. The causes of dysuria are usually associated with hematuria, pyuria, or both because of mucosal inflammation or infection. Hematuria is described in chapter 39 (Discolored Urine). General causes of dysuria (calculi, neoplasia, and feline urologic syndrome) frequently cause urethral obstruction, a life-threatening emergency. Certain forms of urinary incontinence may also produce signs similar to dysuria (see chapter 40).

DIAGNOSTIC PLAN

The initial data base includes a complete history regarding micturition characteristics and urine color, physical examination that emphasizes bladder and prostatic palpation, and midstream voided and cystocentesis samples for urine analysis (Fig. 38-1). If the bladder is distended with urine, urethral obstruction should be strongly suspected. A catheter is passed to relieve the obstruction and obtain urine for analysis and culture. If the animal is depressed, anorexic, or vomiting, uremia may be present and should be confirmed with biochemical tests (blood urea nitrogen [BUN], creatinine, potassium, and total CO_2). In male dogs, rectal palpation for an enlarged or painful prostate gland identifies urethral obstruction due to prostatic disease.

If bladder distention is absent, the bladder is carefully palpated for calculi, neoplasia, or thickening of the wall. The prostate should be carefully palpated, since many dogs with prostatic disease are not obstructed. A voided midstream urine sample is collected for initial analysis. A second urine sample collected by cystocentesis is also analyzed. The results of these urine analyses are compared. The presence of blood, white blood cells (WBC), and bacteria in the cystocentesis sample suggests disease in the bladder or prostate. The absence of blood, WBC, and bacteria in the cystocentesis sample in animals with abnormalities in the voided sample suggests disease in the urethra or lower genital tract.

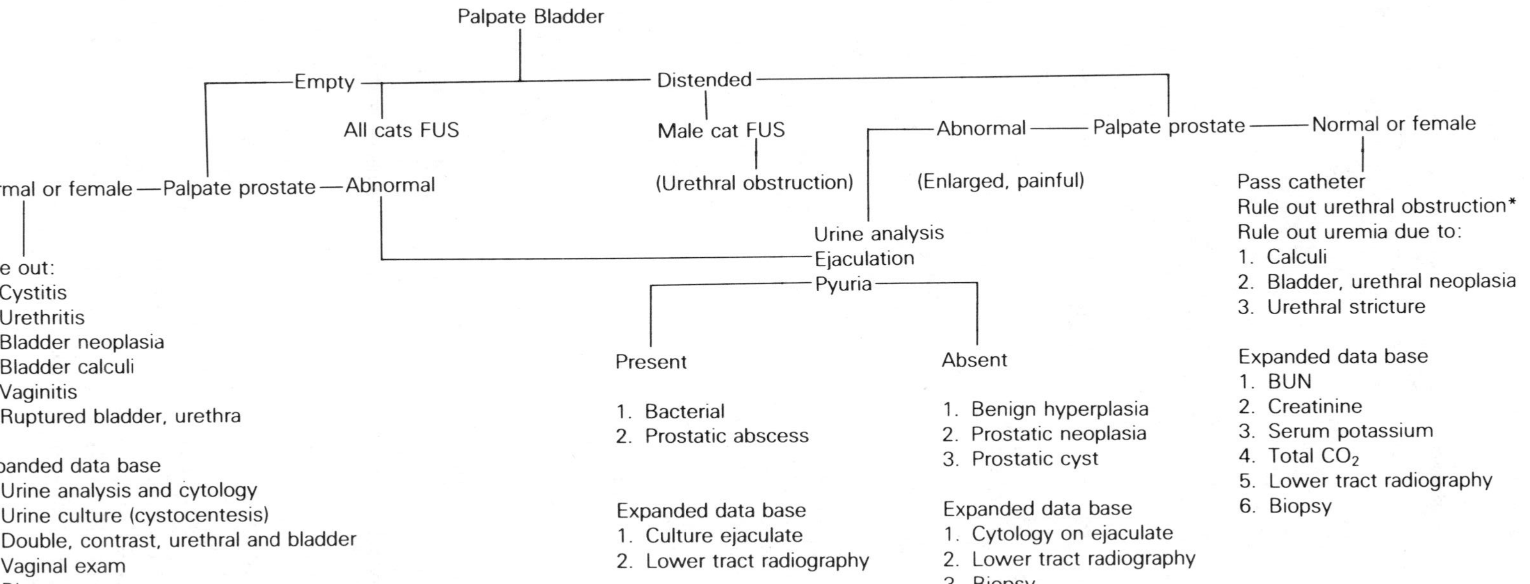

* If no obstruction exists, pursue bladder detrusor or neurologic dysfunction. See chapter 40.

Fig. 38-1. Algorithm for the differential diagnosis of dysuria.

Causes of Dysuria

- Infection
  - Bacterial cystitis
  - Urethritis
  - Bacterial prostatitis
  - Prostatic abscess
  - Vaginitis
- Calculi
  - Cystic
  - Urethral
- Neoplasia
  - Bladder
    - Transitional cell carcinoma
    - Rhabdomyoma or sarcoma
  - Prostate
    - Carcinoma
    - Adenocarcinoma
    - Squamous cell carcinoma
  - Urethra
    - Transitional cell carcinoma
    - Transmissible veneral tumor
  - Vagina, penis
    - Transmissible veneral tumor
    - Fibromas
    - Sarcomas
- Trauma
  - Ruptured bladder, urethra
  - Urethral stricture
- Inflammation
  - Benign prostatic hyperplasia
  - Feline urologic syndrome
- Neurologic
  - Certain forms of incontinence (*e.g.*, vesicular-urethral asynchronization: reflex dysergia)

The genital organs, vagina, uterus, penis, and testicles are thoroughly examined for pain, masses, or abnormal discharge. If traumatic rupture of the urinary tract is a possibility, the abdomen is carefully palpated for pain and the patient is assessed for uremia.

In male dogs with palpably abnormal prostate glands, the initial data base should be expanded to include cytology and microbiologic examination of an ejaculate. Lower tract radiography is also useful for estimating the extent and potential causes of the enlarged or painful prostate. Noninfectious inflammatory or neoplastic conditions may require prostatic biopsy to establish the definitive diagnosis.

In male dogs with normal prostate glands or in all nonobstructed small animals, the initial data base is expanded to further define the etiology of dysuria. A urine culture from a cystocentesis sample, urine cytology, double contrast urethral and bladder radiography, and vaginal endoscopy are indicated. If neoplasia or calculi are present, cystotomy and biopsy are indicated for therapeutic and diagnostic purposes.

If traumatic rupture of the bladder or urethra is likely, the initial data base is expanded to assess the patient for uremia (BUN, creatinine, serum potassium, total CO_2). Abdominal fluid collected by abdominocentesis is analyzed for creatinine concentration. With intra-abdominal rupture of the urinary tract, creatinine levels in abdominal fluid are usually higher than serum concentrations, since creatinine from urine leaking into the abdomen equilibrates rather slowly with intravascular fluid. Lower urinary tract radiography (positive contrast urethrocystogram) is also useful for identification of rents in the lower tract. The presence of normal urine from catheterization does not rule out urinary tract rupture.

Assessment of Urinary Tract Infection

Urinary tract infection (UTI) is a very common cause of dysuria and is often associated with urinary tract calculi or prostatitis. It is also a common complication with urinary incontinence and repeated bladder catheterization. For causes of UTI except urethritis, urine samples should be collected for analysis by cystocentesis. This is especially important for microbiologic studies. Urine should be placed in culture media within 30 minutes after collection to prevent the rapid growth of nonpathogenic, contaminating organisms. If possible, quantitative urine cultures should be performed. In properly obtained cystocentesis samples, organism numbers in excess of 1000 indicate probable UTI; this diagnosis should be pursued by repeating the procedure or through appropriate therapy. Organisms in excess of 100,000 in quantitated culture of a cystocentesis sample indicate definitive UTI. These animals are treated accordingly.

The contraindications for cystocentesis include extreme bladder distention or possible necrosis of the bladder wall. Prolonged obstruction, detrusor muscle paralysis, or severe infection may result in abnormal urine leakage following cystocentesis.

Dysuria Versus Incontinence

In certain cases, dysuria as previously described may be difficult to distinguish from urinary incontinence due to detrusor muscle or neurologic dysfunction. When the previously described diagnostic plan for dysuria does not establish an etiologic diagnosis, the clinician should pursue incontinence as the probable problem. Incontinence is described in chapter 40.

SPECIFIC DISEASES

The clinical and diagnostic characteristics of the specific diseases that cause dysuria are listed in Table 38-1.

(Text continues on p 330.)

Table 38-1. Summary of the Diseases That Produce Dysuria

DISEASE	PREDOMINANT CLINICAL SIGNS OTHER THAN DYSURIA	HEMATOLOGY	URINE ANALYSIS	BIOCHEMISTRY	SPECIAL DIAGNOSTIC TESTS
Bacterial cystitis (UTI)	Palpably thickened bladder wall in some cases	Usually normal unless associated with pyelonephritis	Hematuria Pyuria Bacteruria ↑ Protein Alkaline *p*H	Normal	Cystocentesis for quantitative urine culture >1000 organisms/ml of urine on cystocentesis sample Thickened bladder wall on cystography
Feline urologic syndrome	In male cats, may result in urethral obstruction Inflammation of bladder and urethra	Normal	Hematuria ↑ Protein Crystalluria	Normal	Urine cultures negative unless sample is contaminated or cat has been previously catherized to relieve obstruction
Obstructive uropathy of any cause	Failure to void urine Severe stranguria Distended bladder Dribbling urine If prolonged, uremic signs	Early: normal Late: ↑ PCV ↑ WBC	Hematuria Pyuria ± Bacteruria ↑ Protein Crystalluria	Early: normal Prolonged: ↑ BUN, creatinine ↑ Potassium ↑ TCO_2 (acidosis)	Failure to easily pass catheter Positive double-contrast urethrocystography Urine culture positive in cases complicated by UTI
Cystic neoplasia	See cystitis and obstructive uropathy. Chronic hematuria despite appropriate therapy for UTI	See cystitis.	See cystitis.	Normal unless obstruction occurs	Cytology of urine sediment Positive double-contrast cystography Urine cultures usually negative

					Abnormal excretory urogram (especially with transitional cell carcinoma of bladder neck)
Prostatitis, bacterial	Acute signs Fever Tenesmus Enlarged *painful* prostate	↑ WBC	See cystitis (rarely, the urine analysis is normal).	Normal	Ejaculate or prostatic massage Cytology—septic exudate Culture—positive Positive-contrast urethrocystography is usually normal. *Brucella* titer
Prostatic abscess	Chronic signs Asymmetric prostatic enlargement Prostatic pain ± Tenesmus	↑ WBC	See cystitis.	Normal	Ejaculate or prostatic massage Cytology—septic exudate Culture—positive Brucella titer Positive contrast urethrocystography Prostatic enlargement Dye reflux into prostate
Benign prostatic hypertrophy	Acute signs Symmetric prostatic enlargement Usually *nonpainful* Tenesmus	Normal	Hematuria or normal	Normal	Ejaculate or prostatic massage Cytology—hemorrhagic exudate Culture—negative
Prostatic cyst	Chronic signs Asymmetric prostatic enlargement. *Fluctuant prostatic mass* Dribbling blood from penis Tenesmus	Normal	Hematuria, mild pyuria	Normal	Ejaculate or prostatic massage Cytology—hemorrhagic exudate Culture—negative Positive contrast urethrocystography: reflux of dye into cyst. Prostatic biopsy: squamous metaplasia

(*Continued*)

Table 38-1. Summary of the Diseases That Produce Dysuria (*Continued*)

DISEASE	PREDOMINANT CLINICAL SIGNS OTHER THAN DYSURIA	HEMATOLOGY	URINE ANALYSIS	BIOCHEMISTRY	SPECIAL DIAGNOSTIC TESTS
Prostatic neoplasia	See prostatic cyst. *Palpable mass is firm.*	Normal	Hematuria	Normal	Ejaculate or prostatic massage Cytology—hemorragic exudate Tumor cells may be found Pelvic radiograph ↑ Prostate ↑ Sublumbar lymph nodes Exostosis or lysis of pelvic brim Biopsy
Traumatic rupture of bladder or urethra	History of trauma or prolonged obstruction Abdominal pain Uremic signs	↑ PCV ↑ WBC	Normal or hematuria	Early: normal Late: ↑ BUN, creatinine ↑ Potassium ↓ TCO_2 (acidosis)	Abdominocentesis Cytology—nonseptic purulant or hemorrhagic exudate Creatinine on fluid greater than plasma Positive contrast urethrocystogram—dye spillage into abdomen Abdominal radiography—evidence of peritonitis

Urethritis (bacterial)	No consistent findings May see swelling or inflammation of urethral meatus Unknown incidence in dogs and cats	Normal	See cystitis.	Normal	Difficult to confirm with special diagnostic tests currently available
Vaginitis	Vaginal discharge History of recent estrus Common in prepuberital bitches Rare in cats	Normal	Hematuria and pyuria on voided sample Normal on cyststocentesis	Normal	Vaginoscopy—swelling, inflammation, or exudate Cytology—purulent exudate Culture—positive
Transmissible venereal tumor	Cauliflower-like growth on penis, in vagina, may involve urethra Persistent hemorrhagic penile or vaginal discharge	Normal	Hematuria	Normal	Vaginoscopy Exfoliative cystology Biopsy
Neurogenic-induced dysuria	Inability to void urine Distended bladder Various degrees of incontinence	Normal	Hematuria and pyuria if secondarily infected	Normal	Cystometrograms Urethral pressure profiles Lower tract radiography Neurologic examination (see chapter 40)

UTI, urinary tract infection; ↑, increased; PCV, packed cell volume; WBC, white blood cells; ±, variable; BUN, blood urea nitrogen; ↓, decreased; TCO_2, total CO_2

SYMPTOMATIC THERAPY

Several drugs may be used to relieve dysuria caused by muscle spasm of the bladder or urethra. The majority of the compounds currently available contain hyoscyamine, a belladonna alkaloid with parasympatholytic activity (antimuscurinic) similar to atropine. These drugs reduce smooth muscle spasm in the urinary tract by antagonizing parasympathetic control. Unlike other smooth muscle–containing organs, the bladder exhibits less dramatic response. In recent years, the synthetic parasympatholytic agent propantheline has been used to effectively inhibit or reduce detrusor muscle hyperactivity in the dog. Dosages of 5 to 15 mg three times a day are recommended. In obstructive uropathies, these drugs can increase urinary retention. They are contraindicated in animals with diminished detrusor muscle function. Flavoxate hydrochloride, exybutymin, and diaplomine are synthetic antispasmodics that exert their effects directly on smooth muscle. Their use is contraindicated in obstructive uropathies of the lower urinary tract. Phenazopyridine hydrochloride is a urinary tract analgesic. It is excreted in the urine, where it exerts a topical analgesic effect on the urinary tract mucosa. This action may help to relieve burning, pain, and urgency associated with mucosal inflammation. Its use is contraindicated in renal insufficiency and may cause methemoglobinemia and hemolytic anemia. Its safety in cats has not been established. Phenazopyridine hydrochloride is also available in combination with hyoscyamine hydrobromide.

39

Discolored Urine

MICHAEL D. LORENZ

Urine is yellow to amber in color. The depth of color is related to urine volume. Dark urine does not necessarily mean concentrated urine. Urine pigments, being rather large molecular structures, add little to urine osmolality. Therefore, urine pigments are assessed by strip reagents and specific gravity with a refractometer or hydrometer. The differential diagnosis and causes of discolored urine are listed in Figure 39-1. Simple diagnostic procedures (urine occult blood test, urine sediment examination, and urine bilirubin test) are required to complete this algorithm. In succeeding sections, the diagnosis of red and brown colored urine is discussed.

RED URINE

Many animals are presented for diagnostic evaluation of red urine. There are several basic causes for red urine and diverse etiologies for each of these basic causes. Figure 39-1 is a diagnostic plan for finding the basic cause of red urine. The initial step requires the collection of a voided urine sample and analysis for occult blood. The occult blood test will be positive for blood, hemoglobin, and myoglobin and negative for red pigments such as porphyrins, pyridium, or red dyes in some dog foods. The urine sample is centrifuged and the supernatant and sediment are tested for occult blood. The sediment is also examined microscopically for red blood cells (RBCs). A negative occult reaction in the sediment coupled with the absence of RBCs suggests that hemoglobin or myoglobin is present. A positive occult test on the sediment with the presence of RBCs in the sediment confirms the presence of hematuria. Plasma in a capillary tube should be examined for the presence of a red color. The presence of hemoglobinemia further differentiates causes of red urine. Myoglobinemia does not impart any color change to plasma.

The color of urine containing different pigments of red hue is dependent on the amount of pigment and urine *p*H. Hemoglobin in an acidic urine is often

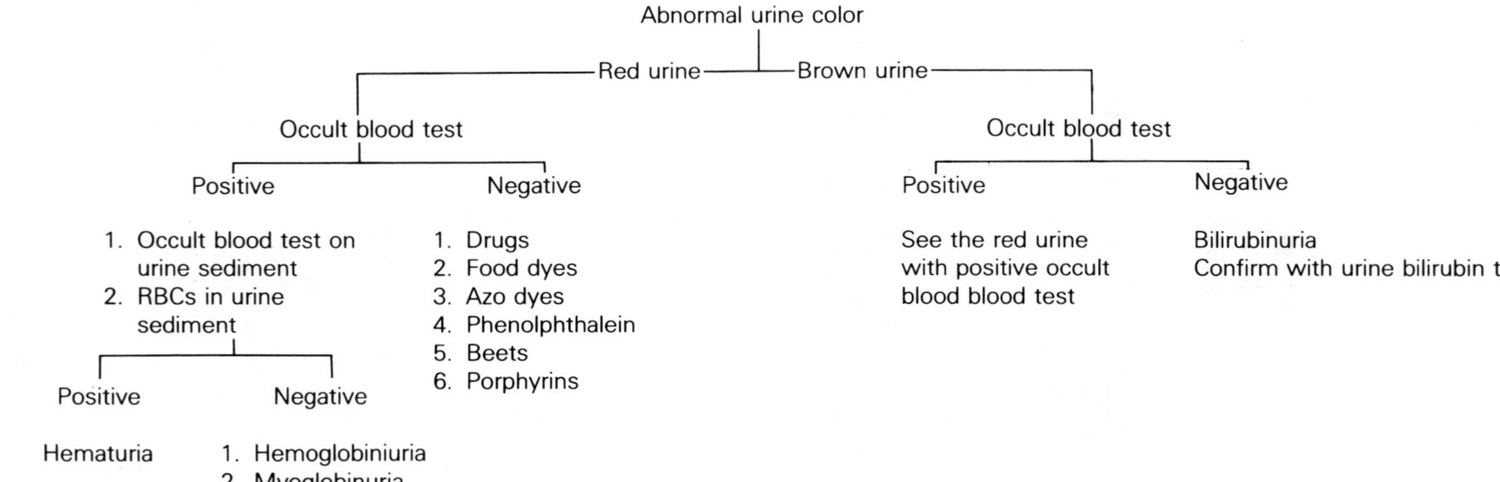

Fig. 39-1. Algorithm for the diagnosis of discolored urine.

brown or smokey; in an alkaline urine, the color is red. The causes of red urine are discussed in subsequent sections.

Hematuria

Hematuria is the presence of blood in the urine. It occurs as a clinical sign in variety of diseases affecting the urogenital tract (Table 39-1). The various types of hematuria are listed in Classification of Hematuria. In healthy animals, RBC excretion in urine is about 3000 per minute, which amounts to less than two to

Table 39-1. Causes of Hematuria in Dogs and Cats Classified by Anatomical Site of Origin

SITE	DISEASES
Kidney	Pyelonephritis
	Glomerulopathy
	Neoplasia
	Calculi
	Renal cysts
	Infarction
	Trauma
	Benign renal bleeding
	Hematuria of Welsh corgis
	Dioctophyma renale
	Microfilaria of *D. immitis*
	Chronic passive congestion
Bladder, ureter, urethra	Infection
	Calculi
	Inflammation—feline urologic syndrome
	Neoplasia
	Trauma
	Capillaria plica
	Cyclophosphamide
Any site	Coagulation disorders
	Heatstroke, DIC
Extraurinary causes (genital tract or spurious hematuria)	Prostate
	Neoplasia
	Infection
	Hypertrophy
	Uterus
	Estrus
	Subinvolution
	Infection
	Neoplasia
	Vagina
	TVT
	Trauma
	Penis
	TVT
	Trauma

DIC, disseminated intravascular coagulation; TVT, transmissible venereal tumor

Classification of Hematuria

- *Essential:* hematuria for which no cause can be identified after complete diagnostic evaluation
- *False:* redness of urine due to pigments other than blood
- *Macroscopic:* hematuria detectable by gross observation of the urine. Macroscopic hematuria occurs when more than 1 million RBCs are excreted per minute.
- *Microscopic:* hematuria detectable only by microscopic examination of urine. The finding of more than two to four RBCs per high-power field is abnormal.
- *Morphologic:* hematuria originating from a particular site

Kidney	Urethra
Ureter	Prostate
Bladder	Genital tract

four RBCs per high power field in the urine sediment. Because of the numerous potential causes for hematuria listed in Table 39-1, a systemic diagnostic plan must be followed if an accurate diagnosis is to be made.

Diagnostic Plan

There are three steps in the diagnostic plan for the problem of hematuria: (1) collection of the initial data base, (2) localization of hematuria to an anatomic site, and (3) identification of the cause. Figure 39-2 shows algorithms for the diagnosis of hematuria in the presence and absence of dysuria.

The Initial Data Base

The initial data base includes a medical history, complete physical examination, observation of micturition, and analysis of the urine. The initial data base will detect hematuria, help localize the site of bleeding, and help dictate further diagnostic procedures.

Historical information should include duration and severity of hematuria; when blood appears during urination; the presence of other urinary tract signs such as dysuria, stranguria, or pollakuiria; and any medication the patient may be taking. The owner's observations should be verified by the clinician. A complete physical examination is given; particular attention is given to palpation of the kidneys, bladder, prostrate and uterus. The animal is carefully searched for evidence of a generalized coagulation problem. The penis or vagina is carefully examined for evidence of bleeding, trauma, or tumors.

A urine analysis is performed early in the evaluation process since subsequent diagnostic procedures are predicated in many cases by these findings.

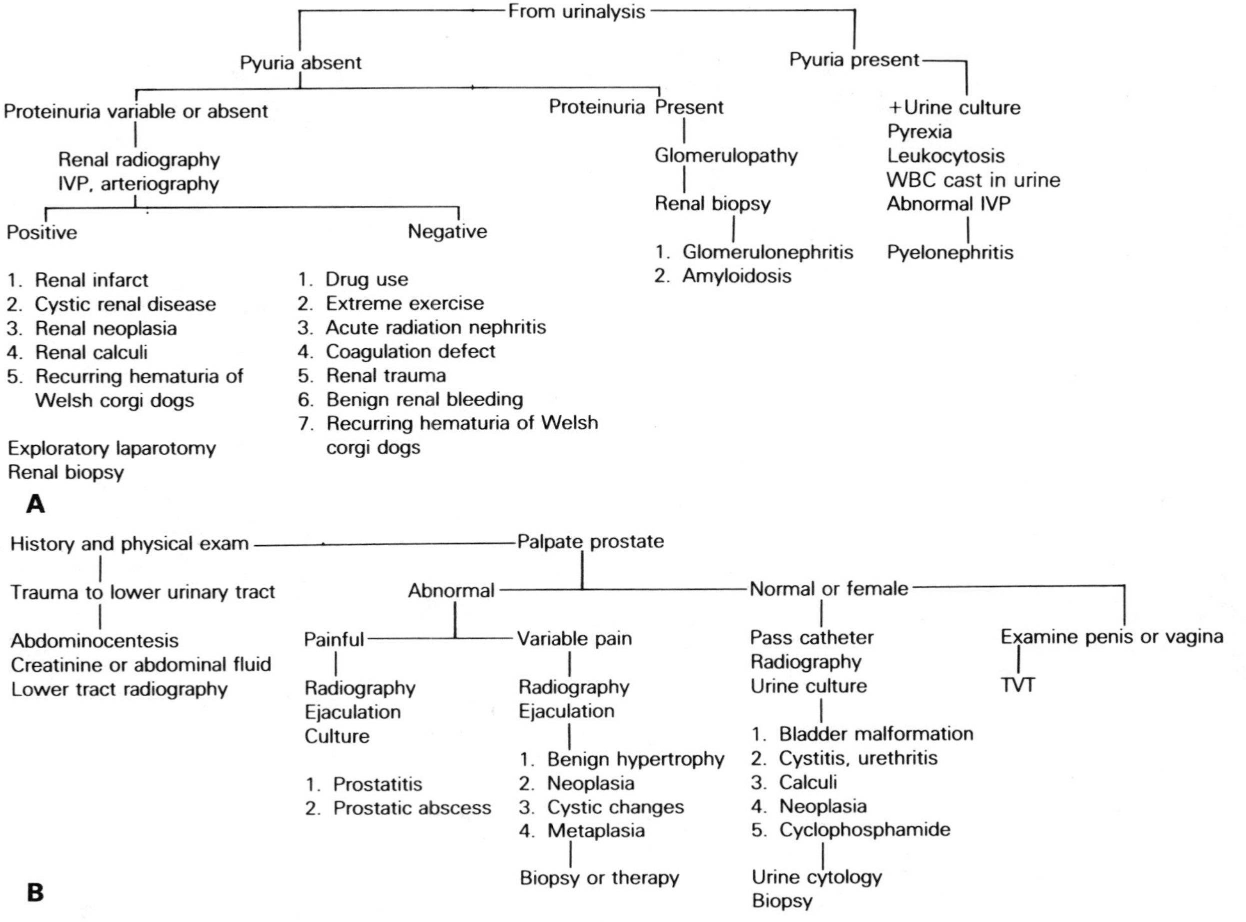

Fig. 39-2. Algorithms for the differential diagnosis of hematuria when the animal does not have (*A*) and does have (*B*) dysuria.

Urine collection techniques may affect the presence and amount of blood in the urine. The initial urine analysis should be a midstream voided sample since no trauma is involved in collection and the urine has traversed the entire urogenital tract. However, blood, bacteria, and white blood cells may be contributed to urine by disease in the genital tract, and these findings may be confused with disease in the urinary tract. Collection of urine by catheterization or manual expression is not encouraged, since catheterization invites infection and some trauma, whereas manual expression usually produces some hematuria and is technically difficult in male dogs and cats. Cystocentesis is safe and does not produce significant iatrogenic hematuria if 22-gauge needles are used. The results of the voided urinalysis are compared with the cystocentesis specimen. This procedure helps localize the site of hematuria.

Urine specimens are examined within 30 minutes after collection since RBCs begin to disappear within minutes after their addition to urine. Refrigeration of urine helps delay RBC degradation if examination must be delayed. RBCs, free hemoglobin, and myoglobin give positive occult blood tests. Dip sticks for occult blood fail to detect intact RBCs. Both the urine sediment and the supernatant are examined with the dip stick for occult blood and the sediment is examined microscopically for intact or lysed RBCs. Red urine that does not give a positive occult blood test is suggestive of pigmentation by porphyrins or red dyes used in some commercial dog foods. A positive occult blood test to the supernatant but negative to the sediment indicates hemoglobinuria or myoglobinuria. When examining the urine sediment, two to four RBCs per high power field are considered normal. The presence of RBC casts in the sediment localizes the hematuria to the kidneys.

Localization of Hematuria to an Anatomic Site

Animals with gross hematuria can be divided into two groups, depending upon the presence or absence of dysuria, stranguria, and pollakuiria. The presence of these signs indicates disease of the bladder, urethra, prostate, or vagina. When dysuria is absent, disease of the kidneys or uterus is suspected. Blood that is present throughout urination indicates disease of the kidneys, ureters, or bladder or prostatic reflex into the bladder. Hematuria at the beginning of micturition suggests disease in the prostate, urethra, penis, uterus, or vagina. Hematuria at the end of micturition is characteristic of bladder or prostatic disease. Hematuria detected in voided samples but absent in cystocentesis samples suggests disease of the urethra or genital tract. Although considerable overlap occurs among the various sites, the astute clinician is able to localize the source of hematuria to a general region of the urogenital tract.

Identification of the Cause of Hematuria

Following the procedures outlined in Figure 39-2, a clinical diagnosis is made following completion of radiographic, cytologic, microbiologic, and endoscopy procedures. These procedures comprise the expanded data base for the problem of hematuria. Table 39-2 lists the various causes of hematuria and characterizes them relative to clinical findings. There is no effective symptomatic therapy for hematuria.

(Text continues on p 340.)

Table 39-2. Causes and Differential Diagnosis of Hematuria

DISEASE	CLINICAL SIGN(S)	URINE ANALYSIS	HEMATOLOGY	BIOCHEMISTRY	SPECIAL TEST(S)
Glomerulopathy Glomerulonephritis SLE Amyloidosis	Early—no consistent signs Late—signs of chronic renal failure P&P Vomiting Ascites Edema	Primary protenuria Hyaline casts Microscopic hematuria Late—↓ specific gravity	Variable PCV, N or ↑ WBC, N or ↑	Early—normal Late ↓ Albumin ↑ BUN	24-hr urine protein quanitation Urine electrophoresis Renal biopsy
Acute pyelonephritis	Pyrexia Perirenal pain Vomiting P&P	Pyuria White cell casts or clumps Bacteruria ↓ Specific gravity Hematuria in acute cases	WBC ↑ (polymorphonuclear leukocytosis)	Early—normal Late—↑ BUN	Urine culture IVP Renal function tests
Renal calculi	Perirenal pain Late—may progress to chronic renal failure	Hematuria—gross or microscopic Variable pyuria Variable bacteruria	Normal	Variable BUN, N or ↑	IVP Exploratory laparotomy Nephrotomy
Renal neoplasia	No consistent signs Perirenal pain Asymmetric renal enlargement	Hematuria—gross or microscopic	Normal	No consistent clues	IVP Renal arteriogram Renal biopsy
Renal cysts	No consistent signs May palpate enlarged kidneys	Hematuria—gross or microscopic	Normal	No consistent clues	IVP Renal arteriogram
Renal infarction	Small infarcts—no consistent signs Large infarcts—may produce primary renal failure	Small infarcts—microscopic hematuria Large infarcts—gross hematuria	Variable—depends upon cause of infarction	No consistent clues	IVP Renal arteriogram

(*Continued*)

Table 39-2. Causes and Differential Diagnosis of Hematuria (*Continued*)

DISEASE	CLINICAL SIGN(S)	URINE ANALYSIS	HEMATOLOGY	BIOCHEMISTRY	SPECIAL TEST(S)
Recurring macroscopic hematuria of Welsh corgi dogs	No apparent signs of illness	Hematuria—gross	Normal	No consistent clues	IVP Arteriogram Renal biopsy
Benign renal bleeding	No consistent signs Cause is unknown	Hematuria—gross	PCV, N	No consistent clues	IVP, Arteriogram, Biopsy } negative
Dioctophyma renale infection	No consistent signs History of eating raw fish	Hematuria—gross Parasite ova in sediments	Normal	No consistent clues	None
Lower urinary tract disorders					
Cystitis	Dysuria Urethral obstruction	Gross hematuria Triple phosphate crystals	PCV, N or ↑	BUN, N or ↑ K, N or ↑	Urine culture
Bladder calculi	Dysuria Bladder mass on palpation Incontinence	Gross hematuria Pyuria	Normal	Normal	Double contrast cystography Pneumocystography
Bladder neoplasia	See cystitis.	See cystitis.	Normal	Normal	See cystitis. Urine cytology for neoplastic cells
Urethral diseases					
Urethritis	Edema or inflammation of urethral orifice Blood dripping from urethra	Hematuria—gross	Normal	Normal	Voiding urethrocystogram Urine culture Cytology of urethral fluid
Urethral rupture	Depression Abdominal pain Vomiting	Gross hematuria	PCV	↑ BUN ↑ Creatinine	Urethrogram Abdominocentesis Creatinine analysis on fluid

	Subcutaneous fluid and inflammation of ventral abdominal skin				
Urethral calculi Urethral neoplasia	Stranguria Urethral obstruction Urinary incontinence	Hematuria—gross	Normal	Normal unless obstructed. Then: ↑ BUN ↑ K	Catheterization Retrograde urethrogram
Genital diseases					
Prostatic infection Bacterial Abscess	Palpably painful enlarged prostate Pyrexia	Gross hematuria Pyuria	WBC ↑ (neutrophilic leukocytosis)	No consistent clues	Ejaculation Culture fluid Cytology Biopsy
Prostatic neoplasia	Prostate enlarged—surface may be irregular Prostate adhered to pelvic structures	Gross hematuria at tip of penis	Normal	No consistent clues	See prostatic infection. Add retrograde urethrogram
Benign hypertrophy	Prostate enlarged, nonpainful Bleeding from tip of penis	Gross hematuria	Normal	No consistent clues	See prostatic infection.
Prostatic cyst	Prostate asymmetrically enlarged Palpatable fluctuating areas Usually nonpainful	Gross hematuria	Normal	No consistent clues	See prostatic infection.
Transmissible venereal tumor	Bloody vaginal or penile discharge Vaginal or penile masses	May be normal or show hematuria	Normal	No consistent clues	Vaginal exam Penis exam Exfolative cytology

SLE, systemic lupus erythematosus; P&P, polydipsia and polyuria; ↓, decreased; PCV, packed cell volume; N, normal; ↑, increased; WBC, white blood cells; BUN, blood urea nitrogen; IVP, intravenous pyelogram

Hemoglobinuria

Hemoglobinuria is the presence of free hemoglobin in urine, arising from two basic sources: (1) hemoglobin filtered by the glomerulii and (2) hemoglobin released by the lysis of RBCs in dilute urine or aged urine. These two causes of hemoglobinuria are differentiated by examining the urine sediment for RBCs (hematuria causing hemoglobinuria). In this section, true hemoglobinuria is discussed.

Causes

Hemoglobin is a metalloprotein of molecular weight 64,500 and is barely small enough to pass the glomerular filter. True hemoglobinuria is caused by the intravascular destruction of RBCs with released hemoglobin into the plasma. When intravascular hemolysis is moderate to severe, free hemoglobin passes the glomerular filter and appears in the urine. Most of the free hemoglobin in plasma is probably excreted in urine as a dimer with a molecular weight of approximately 32,000. Since true hemoglobinuria results from intravascular hemolysis, the condition is usually accompanied by other clinical problems such as pale mucous membranes, rapid respiratory rate, rapid heart rate, and, in some cases, cyanosis. The presence of true hemoglobinuria necessitates an immediate search for the presence and cause of intravascular hemolysis. The causes of hemolytic anemia (see list) are discussed in chapter 23. Hemoglobinuria results from hemolytic anemia only when red cells are destroyed within the vascular system at a rate that exceeds the capacity for conversion of hemoglobin to bilirubin. Therefore, many patients with hemolytic anemia will not have hemoglobinuria but predictively have bilirubinuria and icterus (chapter 37).

Symptomatic Therapy

Large amounts of hemoglobin in urine may be toxic to renal tubules. Therefore, patients with moderate to severe hemoglobinuria must have renal functions supported with intense fluid therapy.

Myoglobinuria

Myoglobinuria is characterized by brownish red urine, a positive occult blood test, and no erythrocytes in the urinary sediment. Myoglobin does bind significantly to plasma proteins and is excreted in the urine before reaching levels that discolor the plasma. Myoglobin is released from muscle following severe muscle necrosis or trauma. Myoglobinuria is observed in generalized muscle diseases such as exertional rhabdomyolysis (greyhound cramps) and extensive crushing injuries to heavy muscle. It is rarely observed in acute polymyositis or generalized degenerative myopathies. The presence of myoglobinuria indicates the immediate search for clinical or laboratory evidence of muscle disease. Generalized muscle pain, muscle weakness, muscle swelling, and elevated muscle enzymes (creatine phosphokinase, serum glutamic–oxaloacetic transaminase, and lactic

Causes of Hemolytic Anemia

- Intravascular hemolysis (more likely to cause hemoglobinuria)
  - Bacteria
    - *Leptospira* spp
    - Clostridial spp
  - RBC parasites
    - *Babesia* spp
  - Chemicals
    - Phenothiazine
    - Methylene blue
    - Acetaminophen
    - Copper
    - Ricin
  - Immune-mediated
    - Neonatal isoerythrolysis
    - Incompatible transfusion
  - Hypo-osmolality
    - Cold-induced hemoglobinuria
- Extravascular hemolysis (less likely to cause hemoglobinuria)
  - RBC parasites
    - *Hemobartonella* spp
  - Immune-mediated
    - Autoimmune hemolytic anemia
    - Systemic lupus erythematsus
    - Cold agglutinin disease
  - Intracorpuscular defects
    - Pyruvate kinase deficiency
      - Besenji
      - Beagle
    - Congenital porphyria—cats
    - Hereditary stomatocytosis—Malamute
  - Fragmentation (microangiopathic disorders)
    - Disseminated intravascular coagulation
    - Cirrhosis of the liver

dehydrogenase) are findings indicative of muscle disease. A muscle biopsy is often necessary for identification of the etiology.

Myoglobin may be extremely toxic to renal tubules. Animals with myoglobinuria must have renal function supported with intense fluid therapy.

BROWN URINE

Brown or reddish brown urine suggests the presence of bilirubin, myoglobin, or heme products in acid urine. With the exception of bilirubin, these products give a positive occult blood test and have been previously discussed.

Bilirubinuria

Conjugated bilirubin is water soluble and freely filtered by the glomeruli. Nonconjugated bilirubin does not pass the renal filter in significant quantities to be detected in urine. Reagent strips and the tablet method both employ the diazotization method for detection of bilirubin. Urine colors may interfere with reading the reagent strips; however, no interference occurs with the tablet method. Both tests are very reactive with conjugated bilirubin but insensitive to free bilirubin. Since bilirubin is oxidized on exposure to light, excessive delay in analysis may produce a negative test. Trace to +1 reactions are found in concentrated urine from normal dogs. Levels above this concentration or +1 reactions in dilute urine are abnormal. In cat urine, +1 reactions are always considered abnormal.

Causes

Bilirubinuria indicates the regurgitation of conjugated bilirubin into the blood. This may occur in hemolytic anemia, primary hepatocellular disease, or cholestatic disorders. Bilirubinuria may precede hyperbilirubinemia and clinical icterus. See chapter 37 for a complete discussion of icterus.

40

Urinary Incontinence

JEANNE A. BARSANTI

DEFINITION

Urinary incontinence is defined as the lack of voluntary control of micturition. Incontinence must be distinguished from inappropriate urination since they appear similar to the client. With inappropriate urination, urination occurs at the wrong place or time (as defined by the owner) but is under the voluntary control of the pet. Problems associated with inappropriate urination include nocturia, dysuria, polyuria, urine spraying, submissive urination, and other behavioral problems. A thorough history or direct observation of the problem is necessary to determine whether the problem is incontinence or inappropriate urination. This chapter deals only with incontinence. Please see chapters referring to the other problems listed.

PHYSIOLOGY

Normal micturition requires storage and emptying phases. During the storage phase, the bladder slowly fills via the ureters as urine is produced by the kidneys. The detrusor muscle of the bladder adjusts to filling by stretching, with no increase in intravesicular pressure. The sympathetic system facilitates detrusor relaxation via beta receptors. The external urethral sphincter (urethral musculature) maintains resting tone, which can increase with sudden increases in intra-abdominal pressure (*e.g.*, coughing). The urethral musculature comprises both striated and smooth muscle. The pudendal nerve innervates the striated muscle, while the sympathetic system via alpha receptors innervates the smooth muscle. Continence is also maintained by an internal sphincter that consists of spiralling detrusor muscle fibers at the bladder neck. These fibers are automatically pulled closed as the bladder distends.

The emptying phase begins when stretch receptors in the bladder wall detect bladder fullness. Impulses are relayed via the pelvic nerves to the sacral segments of the spinal cord and up the spinal cord to the brain stem (Fig. 40-1). A reflex occurs at this level back down the spinal cord to the sacral parasympathetic nucleus. Impulses are sent via the pelvic nerve to the detrusor muscle. In the detrusor muscle, excitation spreads via tight junctions between muscle fibers. Contraction pulls the bladder neck open. Simultaneously, the pudendal motor neurons are inhibited, resulting in relaxation of the external urethral sphincter. Urine is evacuated. When the bladder is empty, the afferent discharge from the pelvic nerve stops, the pelvic motor neurons cease their discharge, pudendal motor activity is no longer blocked, and external sphincter tone resumes.

Voluntary control of this reflex pathway is via the cerebral cortex to the brain stem. The cerebellum has an inhibitory effect on the brain stem micturition center.

DIAGNOSTIC PLAN

The diagnostic approach to incontinence should start with a thorough history. The age of onset of the problem, reproductive status of the pet, relationship between the onset of incontinence and neutering, chronologic course of the

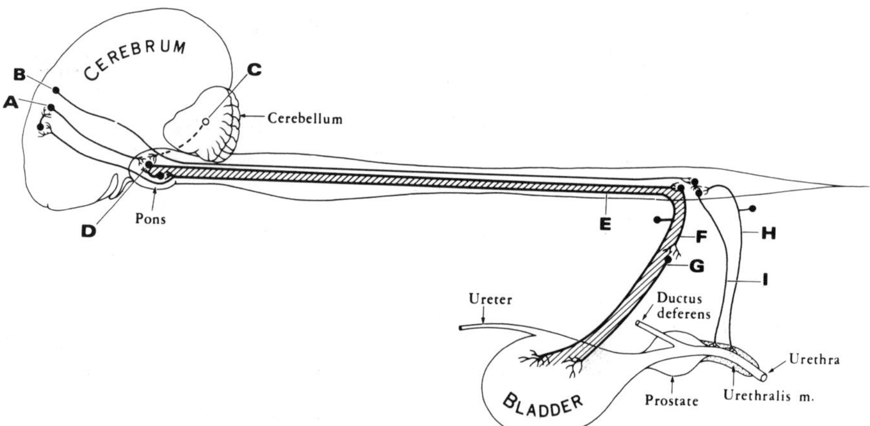

Fig. 40-1. Neurophysiology of micturition. The cerebrum controls voluntary micturition by inhibitory and facilitory influences on the brain stem micturition reflex area. The cerebellum also has an inhibitory influence on the micturition reflex. The pelvic nerve carries both afferent and efferent fibers between the bladder and the sacral spinal cord. The reflex between these fibers is in the brain stem. Efferent fibers are also carried by the hypogastric nerve (sympathetic system, not shown) and pudendal nerve. The hypogastric nerve supplies beta-adrenergic fibers to the bladder and alpha-adrenergic fibers to the bladder neck and urethra. The pudendal nerve innervates the striated muscle of the urethra. (Oliver JE, Osborne CA: Neurogenic urinary incontinence. In Kirk RW [ed]: Current Veterinary Therapy, 7th ed, p 1123. Philadelphia, WB Saunders, 1980)

incontinence, associated urinary tract problems, history of other neurologic abnormalities, whether normal micturition occurs at all, and when incontinence occurs in relation to micturition are all especially important as well as any drug usage or dietary changes. Any drug or dietary change that stimulates polyuria (*e.g.*, glucocorticoids, high salt diet) could precipitate a latent predisposition to incontinence.

A complete physical examination should follow. Special attention should be paid to the bladder. Is it large and distended, small and contracted, or normal? In a male dog, the prostate should be palpated. Anal tone and the integrity of the perineal reflex should be evaluated. Any abnormal neurologic signs should be pursued by a complete neurologic examination. Micturition should be observed and residual volume determined if there is any question about the ability of the bladder to empty. Normal residual volume is less than 10 ml, although some male dogs may want to repeatedly mark territory before the bladder is completely emptied. If complete micturition occurs, the empty bladder should be palpated for calculi, soft tissue masses, and wall thickness. Any yellow fluid found dripping from the urethra should be compared with urine, since in male dogs fluid from a prostatic cyst communicating with the urethra may have the same color as urine.

After the history and physical examination, the incontinence should be classified as neurogenic (associated with other neurologic problems) or nonneurogenic (see Causes of Incontinence).

Neurogenic Incontinence

If neurologic abnormalities are detected, a complete neurologic examination is essential to localize the lesion site so that appropriate diagnostic tests can be chosen.

With cerebral lesions, micturition will be normal except for loss of voluntary control. The pet cannot be housetrained or loses its former training. Associated neurologic signs might include change in mental attitude, possible loss of other cerebral functions such as vision (with normal pupillary light responses) or hearing, and decreased postural reactions in spite of a normal-appearing gait. Segmental reflexes may be normal or hyperactive.

With cerebellar diseases, there is some loss of inhibition of micturition; thus, urination may occur at the wrong place or time, even though voluntary control is maintained. Signs of diffuse cerebellar disease such as ataxia and intention tremors should be present.

With brain stem and spinal cord lesions cranial to the first sacral spinal cord segment (fifth lumbar vertebra in the dog and seventh in the cat), the micturition reflex is lost, but sphincter tone remains. The bladder fills, but sensation of this cannot be relayed to the reflex center. As a result, the bladder overdistends with urine and bladder pressure markedly increases. When bladder pressure exceeds urethral pressure, some urine will dribble from the urethra. There may be attempts by the detrusor muscle intrinsically to contract. These contractions occur against resting external urethral tone. Such contractions are usually ineffectual in emptying the bladder. The bladder is distended on physical examination, and attempts to express it will be difficult because the external sphincter does not relax. Passage of a urinary catheter is easy, since no anatomic urethral obstruction exists. With brain stem lesions, other neurologic abnormalities may include changes in mental attitude, posture, and gait; cranial nerve abnormalities; and postural reaction deficits in the limbs, with normal or hyperactive segmental reflexes. With spinal cord lesions, mental attitude and cranial nerve function are normal, but postural reaction deficits are present in the limbs at or caudal to the lesion. See the chapter on paresis and paralysis for further help in localizing spinal cord lesions.

With sacral spinal cord lesions, sacral root lesions, and peripheral nerve lesions, the micturition reflex is lost and the external sphincter is atonic. The bladder overdistends, and urine dribbles out when bladder pressure exceeds urethral pressure. The detrusor muscle will intrinsically contract when stretched. Such contractions may be more successful in voiding urine, since resting urethral tone is decreased. However, complete voiding is rare, and loss of the tight junctions between detrusor muscle fibers by overdistention may prevent effective bladder contraction. On physical examination, the bladder will be overdistended but easy to express. Research in small animals suggests that spinal root and peripheral nerve lesions must be *bilateral* to disrupt bladder function. Associated neurologic abnormalities with lesions at these sites include fecal incontinence, loss of the perineal reflex, paralysis of the tail, and possible evidence of sciatic nerve dysfunction such as knuckling the paw, decreased stifle flexion, decreased flexor reflex, and loss of sensation in the limb, especially on the dorsal surface of the paw, which is solely innervated by branches of the sciatic nerve.

Once the lesion is localized by neurologic examination and characterization of the abnormality in micturition, further diagnostic tests could include skull or spinal radiographs, myelography, cerebrospinal fluid analysis, electroencephalogram, and other tests based on lesion localization (refer to the chapter on paresis/paralysis).

Non-neurogenic Incontinence

Non-neurogenic incontinence is incontinence unassociated with other neurologic abnormalities on neurologic examination. Some etiologies that have a local neurologic cause (such as detrusor dysfunction) are included in this category. Non-neurogenic incontinence is best approached diagnostically by subdividing it into two categories on the basis of the physical examination: a distended bladder with inability to void or a normal bladder with ability to void (see Causes of Incontinence).

Bladder Distended

A partial or complete urethral obstruction should be the first consideration in any animal with a distended bladder and inability to void, especially if the animal tries to urinate. In dogs, the urethra should be carefully palpated. This

Causes of Incontinence

- Neurogenic
  - Cerebral lesions
  - Brain stem lesions
  - Spinal cord lesions (cervical, thoracic, lumbar)
  - Lesions of the sacral spinal cord, sacral spinal roots, pelvic or pudendal nerves
- Non-neurogenic
  - Bladder distended
    - Urethral obstruction
    - Mass in the bladder neck area
    - Detrusor–urethral dyssynergia
  - Bladder not distended
    - Ectopic ureter(s)
    - Patent urachus
    - Reproductive hormone responsive incontinence
    - Urethral incompetence
    - Mass in the bladder neck area
    - Reduced bladder capacity

will involve percutaneous palpation in males and rectal palpation in both males and females. After palpation, a urinary catheter should be passed as aseptically as possible. If an obstruction is encountered, it is characterized as to location and consistency. Survey and contrast radiographs are often necessary to further characterize the obstruction. Laboratory work, including serum urea nitrogen (BUN), serum creatinine, serum electrolytes, and urine analysis should be obtained to determine the degree of post-renal azotemia and to evaluate for the presence of urinary tract infection. If a urolith is the cause of the obstruction, survey radiographs of the abdomen are necessary to determine if other uroliths are present in the kidneys, ureters, or bladder.

Ability to pass a urinary catheter to the bladder does not preclude the presence of an anatomic obstruction. An obstruction may prevent urine passage retrograde via bladder contraction but not markedly inhibit passage of a catheter antegrade. Examples include prostatic diseases, masses in the area of the bladder neck, and small uroliths. Retrograde urethrography and contrast cystography are necessary to document such obstructions. Once the obstruction has been localized and characterized, a biopsy may be required to identify the cause precisely.

Once an anatomic obstruction has been *excluded,* two general etiologies are considered: (1) detrusor dysfunction and (2) failure of the urethral musculature to relax during detrusor contraction.

Detrusor dysfunction occurs most commonly due to loss of tight junctions from prolonged bladder overdistention. Bladder overdistention may result from urethral obstruction, neurologic dysfunction (*e.g.*, intervertebral disk disease), with unwillingness to void with forced recumbancy (*e.g.*, after pelvic trauma), and, we suspect, with development of polyuria in well housetrained dogs with limited access to the outdoors. One cause of detrusor atony in cats described in Great Britain is feline dysautonomia, an autonomic polygangionopathy (Key-Gaskell syndrome). The bladder dysfunction in this syndrome consists of apparent inability to contract the bladder in spite of efforts to do so, but the bladder is easily expressed manually. Other signs such as persistent pupillary dilation, decreased tear production, chronic regurgitation due to megaesophagus, and constipation are more common than bladder atony. In some animals, the cause of detrusor dysfunction cannot be determined. Detrusor dysfunction is suspected on the basis of the history, physical examination, and the exclusion of an anatomic obstruction to urine outflow. Cystometry is necessary to confirm detrusor dysfunction (Fig. 40-2).

Lack of relaxation of the urethral musculature, preventing micturition despite detrusor contraction, is very difficult to confirm in veterinary medicine. There are two possible causes: urethral spasm due to inflammation of any cause and urethral dyssynergia, in which the urethra contracts rather than relaxes as

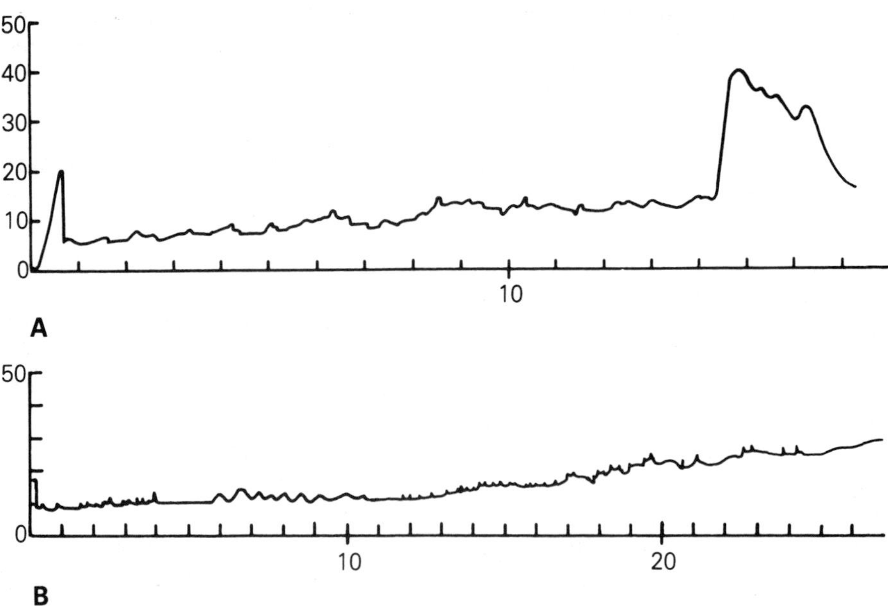

Fig. 40-2. Comparison of a normal cystometrogram (*A*) with a cystometrogram (*B*) indicating detrusor dysfunction. Intravesicular pressure (cm H_2O) is on the vertical axis, and time to contraction during CO_2 infusion (ml/min) is on the horizontal axis. The normal cystometrogram (*A*) shows little increase in pressure as the bladder fills. As the bladder contracts, intravesicular pressure rises dramatically and then falls as the CO_2 is expelled. The cystometrogram from a dog with detrusor dysfunction (*B*) shows a gradual rise in intravesicular pressure with no sharp increase in pressure because the detrusor muscle could not contract even though the bladder filled.

micturition is initiated. The typical history with detrusor-urethral dyssynergia is that the dog initiates urination, but urination ceases immediately thereafter in spite of continued efforts to urinate. The condition has only been noted in male dogs. In humans, dyssynergia is documented by urethral pressure profilometry at rest and during micturition in correlation with measurement of the volume and strength of the urine stream. The cause in humans is usually a spinal lesion that may or may not be associated with other neurologic signs. A urethral pressure profile can also be performed in dogs. However, since it is performed under sedation or resting and not during micturition, it may be normal, even though a problem exists during micturition. There is currently no adequate method to confirm a diagnosis of urethral spasm or dyssynergia in veterinary medicine. One can only rely on physical examination, observation of micturition, and cystometry to exclude detrusor dysfunction. If dyssynergia is suspected, spinal radiographs and a myelogram or epidurogram of the sacral area may be warranted.

Bladder Not Distended

If an animal is presented for incontinence and if the bladder is normal or empty on physical examination, there are two major categories to consider: (1) the urethral sphincter is not competent or is being bypassed or (2) the bladder is contracting involuntarily at low volumes.

The urethral sphincter may be bypassed with a patent urachus or an ectopic ureter, both usually congenital defects in young animals. A patent urachus should be recognizable on physical examination. An ectopic ureter is suspected when urine dribbling occurs in spite of apparent normal micturition in a puppy or kitten. Female dogs are most commonly affected, but cases in male dogs and in cats of both sexes have been reported. The lesion may be unilateral or bilateral. The ureter may terminate in the urethra or in the vagina in females. Most cases are diagnosed by excretory urography to visualize the course of the ureters. Interpretation is difficult in some cases, since the ureters may enter the serosa at the normal site and then tunnel subserosally to enter the urethra. Positive contrast vaginourethrography identifies this defect. Cases in which the ureter exits into the vagina may be visualized by vaginoscopy. An advantage of excretory urography is that the kidneys and ureters can be examined for other associated problems such as hydroureter, pyelonephritis, and abnormal kidney size or shape. A complete blood count, BUN, or serum creatinine, urine analysis, and urine culture should be performed prior to surgical correction of an ectopic ureter.

A urethral sphincter of decreased competence is the most likely cause of incontinence associated with neutering in dogs. Commonly called "spay incontinence," this also occurs in neutered males; a more descriptive term is "reproductive hormone responsive incontinence." Affected dogs have been found to have decreased resting urethral pressures on urethral pressure profilometry (Fig. 40-3). Diagnosis is usually made on the basis of history, physical examination, and urine analysis. Suggestive historical findings include a neutered female or

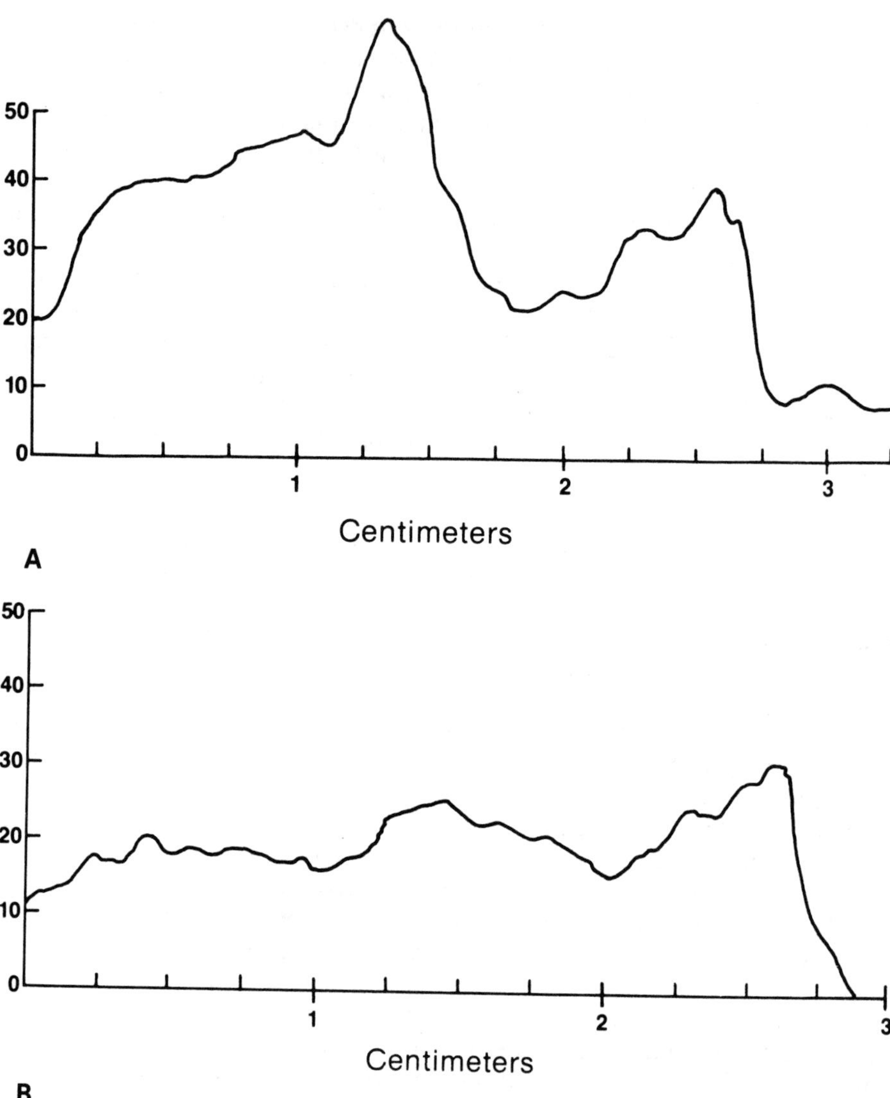

Fig. 40-3. Comparison of a normal urethral pressure profile in a female dog (*A*) and a urethral pressure profile from a female dog with urethral incompetence (*B*). Profiles were recorded with xylazine restraint. Urethral pressure (cm H_2O) is on the vertical axis, and urethral length is on the horizontal axis. The abnormal urethral pressure profile (*B*) had markedly lower pressures than the normal profile (*A*).

male dog that leaks urine while sleeping or lying down but otherwise urinates normally. The condition has also been described in two neutered female cats. Male dogs often have been neutered for treatment of a prostatic disease. The physical examination is normal, except for urine scalding in some cases. The urine analysis is normal. A similar condition may occur in juvenile bitches of any breed and in intact bitches, particularly of the Doberman breed. The proposed cause is decreased urethral competence, which has been associated with an anatomically short urethra (*i.e.*, intrapelvic bladder position on cystography). However, this association is still unproven, since intrapelvic bladder location can be present in normally continent dogs. Urethral incompetence has also been mentioned as a rare sequel to perineal urethrostomy in cats.

A similar type of incontinence occurs in cats of both sexes, neutered or not. The cat typically dribbles urine while relaxed but otherwise urinates normally. Physical examination may be normal, or the cat may have anisocoria. These cats are usually feline leukemia virus positive, although the relationship of the viremia to the incontinence is unknown. Whether the incontinence is due to urethral incompetence or unrestrainable detrusor contractions at low bladder volumes has not been determined.

A mass in the area of the bladder neck may cause incompetence of the internal urethral sphincter. Diagnosis may be suspected by an associated history of dysuria or hematuria, a palpable abnormality (not always detectable), or abnormalities in the urine sediment (possibly hematuria, pyuria, or abnormal cells). Cystography or retrograde urethrography are necessary to confirm the mass. A biopsy is usually required to determine its nature.

Unrestrainable detrusor contractions at low bladder volumes (urge incontinence) result in incontinence that appears very similar to urethral incompetence. Causes include severe chronic cystitis and prior cystectomy with markedly reduced bladder volume. Further study is needed to determine whether the incontinence in cats associated with feline leukemia is due to uninhibited detrusor contractions or to urethral incompetence. Diagnosis is based on palpating an abnormal bladder, abnormalities on urine analysis, or an abnormal cystogram and a small bladder threshold volume on cystometry.

SYMPTOMATIC THERAPY

Bladder Distended

Regardless of cause, a distended bladder must be emptied and kept empty to avoid postrenal uremia, renal injury from increased intraurinary tract pressures, detrusor muscle damage, and possible sepsis if the urine is infected. Aseptic, atraumatic, urinary catheterization is the usual mechanism of relieving bladder distention. Once the bladder is emptied, the catheter is removed when the cause of the distention has been rectified (*e.g.*, obstructing material has been removed). For recurrent bladder distention, the catheter may be left in place (indwelling urinary catheter) or passed intermittently (usually three or four times a day). The advantage of an indwelling catheter, in addition to saving time, is less urethral trauma; however, a major disadvantage is the likelihood of urinary tract infection. Infection can occur from movement of bacteria alongside the catheter as well as through it. Use of a closed system (catheter connected via sterile tubing to a sterile bottle) will delay development of infection. Antibiotic use may also delay development of infection but may result in infections with antibiotic-resistant bacteria. For this reason, antibiotic therapy is not recommended during catheterization unless other systemic signs of infection are present. Urine analysis, urine culture, or both are performed when the catheter is removed. Any infection is appropriately treated then.

Parasympathetic stimulants such as bethanechol are used to try to stimulate detrusor function in animals with atonic bladders as long as no urethral obstruction is present (see Pharmacology of the Lower Urinary Tract and Drugs Used in the Management of Micturition Disorders). The drug seems most efficacious in people with partial lower motor neuron injuries. Changes in efficacy with lesion

Pharmacology of the Lower Urinary Tract

- Drugs that increase bladder contractility
  - Parasympathomimetics
    - Bethanechol
- Drugs that decrease bladder contractility
  - Parasympatholytics
    - Propantheline
  - Antispasmodics
    - Flavoxate
    - Oxybutynin
    - Dicyclomine
  - Beta-adrenergic agonists
    - Terbutaline
  - Alpha-adrenergic antagonists
  - Prostaglandin inhibitors
  - Calcium antagonists
  - Imipramine
- Drugs that increase urethral pressure
  - Alpha-adrenergic agonists
    - Phenylpropanolamine
    - Ephedrine
  - Beta-adrenergic antagonists
    - Propranolol
  - Estrogens
  - Imipramine
- Drugs that decrease urethral pressure
  - Alpha-adrenergic antagonists
    - Phenoxybenzamine
  - Diphenylhydantoin
  - Dantrolene
  - Diazepam
  - Baclofen

Drugs Used in the Management of Micturition Disorders

- Detrusor atony
  - Bethanechol
  - Bethanechol plus phenoxybenzamine or diazepam
- Detrusor–urethral sphincter dyssynergia
  - Phenoxybenzamine
- Urethral incompetence
  - Reproductive hormones
    - Estrogen in females
    - Testosterone in males
  - Alpha-adrenergic agonists
    - Ephedrine
    - Phenylpropanolamine
    - Phenylephrine
  - Imipramine
- Urge incontinence
  - Propantheline

localization have not been evaluated in clinical cases in dogs, but experimental work in dogs and cats suggests they would respond similarly. The efficacy of oral bethanechol therapy has never been proven. This may partially explain the wide dosage range. Initial doses of 2.5 mg for a cat or small dog to 10 mg for a large dog are suggested. The drug is administered orally every 8 hours. A response should occur in 30 to 60 minutes. An appropriate area for urination should be provided and urination, if it occurs, should be documented. The bladder should not be allowed to overdistend if the bethanechol is ineffective. The dosage should be gradually increased to 7.5 mg for a small dog or cat or 25 mg for a large dog unless side effects such as salivation, vomiting, diarrhea, abdominal straining, or bradycardia appear.

Drugs to relax the urethra (see lists) can be used in conjunction with parasympathetic stimulants. These regimens have not been evaluated for efficacy or toxicity in small animals. Drugs that relax urethral skeletal muscle include diazepam. Those that relax smooth muscle include the alpha blockers such as acepromazine and phenoxybenzamine. The drug combination of bethanechol and phenoxybenzamine has reversed bladder atony in some humans. Side effects of phenoxybenzamine include hypotension, tachycardia, and gastrointestinal irritation. One recommended dosage for phenoxybenzamine is 0.5 mg/kg orally per day divided into two doses.

Phenoxybenzamine (0.5 mg/kg orally per day divided into two doses) is currently the drug of choice for detrusor-urethral dyssynergia. A trial period of at least a week is recommended before the dosage is increased. Dosage requirements may decrease with time.

Bladder Not Distended

Surgical therapy is required for patent urachus or ectopic ureters.

Reproductive hormone responsive incontinence is treated by estrogen administration in females and testosterone in males (see lists of drugs). Diethylstilbestrol (DES) is given orally at 0.5 to 1 mg per day for 3 to 5 days and then as needed. If signs of estrus are induced, the dosage must be reduced. One severe potential side effect of prolonged DES administration is aplastic anemia. In medium-sized research dogs, 1 mg per day for 270 days was required to induce this effect. Nevertheless, DES should always be used with caution and at the lowest effective dose for the shortest time. In most dogs, a few days of therapy will result in resolution of signs for months, so that constant therapy is not required. Approximately 50% of juvenile bitches with sphincteric incompetence have been reported to become continent with onset of estrus.

With neutered males, 2.2 mg/kg of injectable testosterone proprionate is usually effective. If the duration of action is too short, testosterone cypionate (depotestosterone) can be used at the same dose. Because of rapid hepatic degradation, oral testosterone is often ineffective unless dosages as high as 22 mg/kg are used. If the dog was neutered because of a testosterone-related problem such as a prostatic disease, the disease may recur with testosterone administration.

Alpha-adrenergic drugs may also be used to stimulate urethral tone in dogs with hormone responsive incontinence or urethral incompetence (see lists of drugs). These drugs have the disadvantage of requiring at least twice a day administration, but they may have the advantage of fewer side effects. Examples are phenylpropanolamine (1.5 mg/kg every 8 to 12 hours) or ephedrine (25 to 50 mg every 12 hours). These drugs are combined with antihistamines or caffeine in some over-the-counter cold and diet remedies. Potential side effects include hypertension, urine retention, and cardiac arrhythmias. In women, the effects of estrogen and alpha-adrenergic agents can be additive.

Drugs to treat bladder hyperactivity or urge incontinence include propantheline, oxybutynin, dicyclomine, and flavoxate (see lists of drugs). The dosage of propantheline is 7.5 to 15 mg as needed. In cats, a single dose of propantheline apparently has a duration of action of 2 to 3 days. In dogs, the dosage should be repeated two to three times a day. Potential side effects include light sensitivity (from dilated pupils), constipation, and urine retention. In humans, the combined use of propantheline and phenoxybenzamine gave better results in one study than propantheline alone.

SUGGESTED READINGS

Barsanti JA, Downey R: Urinary incontinence in cats. J Am Anim Hosp Assoc 20:979–982, 1984

Downie JW: Bethanechol chloride in urology: discussion of issues. Neurourology and Urodynamics 3:211–222, 1984

Holt PE: Urinary incontinence in the bitch due to sphincter mechanism incompetence: Prevalence in referred dogs and retrospective analysis of sixty cases. J Small Anim Pract 26:181–190, 1985

Holt PE, Gibbs C, Latham J: An evaluation of positive contrast vagino-urethrography as a diagnostic aid in the bitch. J Small Anim Pract 25:531–550, 1984

Khanna OP: Disorders of micturition: Neuropharmacologic basis and results of drug therapy. Urology 8:316–328, 1976

Lees GE, Moreau PM: Management of hypotonic and atonic urinary bladders in cats. Vet Clin North Am 14:641–647, 1984

Rosin AE, Barsanti JA: Diagnosis of urinary incontinence in dogs: Role of the urethral pressure profile. J Am Vet Med Assoc 178:814–822, 1981

Sharp NJH, Nash AS, Griffiths IR: Feline dysautonomia (the Key-Gaskell Syndrome): A clinical and pathological study of 40 cases. J Small Anim Pract 25:599–615, 1984

Part Ten

REPRODUCTIVE PROBLEMS

41

Vaginal and Preputial Discharges

JEANNE A. BARSANTI

DEFINITION AND RECOGNITION

Vaginal and preputial discharges can be normal or abnormal. They can originate from the external genitalia, the reproductive system, or the distal urethra. To determine the cause of a discharge, a thorough history, physical examination, and cytology of the discharge are required. In the history, the age of onset of the discharge, the breeding record, and, in the female, relationship of the discharge to estrus or pregnancy are especially important. The entire reproductive tract should be examined as carefully as possible. In the bitch, tranquilization may be required to perform an adequate vaginal examination using a sterile vaginal speculum. The discharge should be applied to a slide, dried, stained, and examined microscopically. In this chapter, the causes of vaginal and preputial discharges (see corresponding lists of rule outs) will be reviewed based on their cytologic characteristics. Discharges will be classified as to whether they are primarily mucus, blood, or pus.

CLASSIFICATION AND DIAGNOSIS

Vaginal Discharges

Mucoid

An occasional, mild mucoid discharge is normal in bitches and queens, whether pregnant or not. Normal vaginal cytology contains epithelial cells, a few neutrophils, and bacteria. Usual numbers of bacteria are low, but higher numbers may be seen during estrus. A heavier mucoid discharge is normal in metestrus, and the mucus may contain large numbers of nondegenerate neutrophils. A heavier mucoid discharge may also be associated with an irritative lesion in the vagina such as a tumor. The diagnostic plan for a heavy mucoid discharge in a nonmetestral bitch should include a thorough vaginal examination.

Rule Outs for Vaginal Discharge

- Mucoid
  - Normal
  - Metestrus
  - Intravaginal irritative lesion
- Hemorrhagic
  - Proestrus
  - Postpartum
  - Impending abortion
  - Subinvolution of pacental sites
  - Neoplasia
  - Cystic endometrial hyperplasia
  - Coagulopathy
  - Trauma
- Purulent
  - Metestrus
  - Vaginitis
  - Acute metritis
  - Pyometra

Hemorrhagic

A hemorrhagic discharge is normal during proestrus in the bitch and for up to 6 weeks postpartum. The normal postpartum discharge is nonodorous and greenish to greenish-red for the first 2 to 3 weeks. It gradually becomes more serosanguineous and decreases in amount.

If a hemorrhagic discharge develops during pregnancy, abortion may be imminent. The animal should be closely confined to enforce rest and to permit observation for abortion.

If a hemorrhagic discharge persists longer than 6 weeks postpartum in a dog, the most likely cause is subinvolution of placental sites. The affected bitch is usually young (<3 years) and is otherwise normal. The uterus may have palpable areas of nodular enlargement. Occasionally the hemorrhage may be severe enough to cause blood-loss anemia or iron-deficiency anemia. Rarely, the uterine placental sites will rupture. Diagnosis is by history, physical examination, and vaginal cytology. There is no specific treatment, but the perivulvar area should be kept as clean as possible. Iron supplementation may be warranted. If severe anemia develops, transfusion may be required. If the dog is not a valuable breeding animal, ovariohysterectomy should be performed.

Another cause for a hemorrhagic or serosanguineous discharge is neoplasia of the vagina, uterus, or distal urethra. The most common tumor is transmissible venereal tumor. Transitional cell carcinoma of the urethra can cause a urethral discharge, which will be evident to the owner as a vaginal discharge. A leiomy-

Rule Outs for Preputial Discharge

- Hemorrhage
  - Preputial lesion
    - Trauma
    - Neoplasia
    - Foreign body
  - From urethral orifice
    - Distal urethra
      - Urethral prolapse
      - Neoplasia
      - Trauma
      - Urolith
    - Prostate
      - Cystic hyperplasia
      - Bacterial prostatitis
      - Neoplasia
- Purulent discharge
  - Preputial
    - Balanoposthitis
    - Foreign body
    - Neoplasm
  - Urethral
    - Prostatic disease
      - Acute prostatitis
      - Chronic prostatitis
      - Abscess formation
      - Neoplasia
- Serous
  - Urethral
    - Prostatic cyst

oma of the uterus or vagina is not uncommon in older, intact bitches and may or may not be accompanied by a vaginal discharge. Diagnosis of neoplasia is based on identifying a mass by vaginal examination or uterine palpation and determining the type of cytology, impression smear, or biopsy. A transmissible venereal tumor is usually diagnosed by cytology, due to its characteristic large, round cells which easily exfoliate. Treatment is based on tumor type.

In intact but not frequently bred dogs, cystic endometrial hyperplasia has been reported to cause a mild serosanguineous discharge with no other signs. This condition can only be suspected by history and by eliminating other causes of the discharge. Confirmation requires uterine biopsy.

A coagulopathy should also be considered a possible cause for vaginal bleeding of unknown origin. Refer to the chapter on hemostasis for a diagnostic plan.

Purulent

A mucoid discharge with a large number of nondegenerate neutrophils is normal in metestrus in the bitch. Bacteria may be seen in vaginal cytology from normal bitches at any time, and relatively high numbers may be present during estrus. Vaginal cultures are almost always positive (>98%) in normal bitches, and the organisms found are varied and include all the common pathogens of the reproductive and urinary tracts, with the exception of *Brucella canis.* Contrary to some breeders' understanding, organisms such as beta-hemolytic streptococci and hemophilus can be cultured from normally fertile bitches and are only transiently transmitted to the stud dog.

With a purulent discharge in an intact female, it is important to determine whether the origin of the discharge is the vagina or the uterus. This differentiation is based on the history, physical examination, vaginal examination, and complete blood count (CBC). Ultrasound of the abdomen and abdominal radiography may also be helpful. Uterine infections are usually associated with signs of systemic illness; vaginal infections are not.

The principal signs of vaginitis are a purulent vaginal discharge, vulvar licking, and, occasionally, attraction of males. Vaginitis does not result in any signs of systemic illness such as fever, depression, or leukocytosis. Large numbers of degenerate and nondegenerate neutrophils and bacteria are found on vaginal cytology. Vaginitis is common in puppies and usually resolves with the first estrus due to estrogen stimulation of keratinization of mucosal cells. No further diagnostic work is usually needed in puppies. In older bitches, a complete vaginal examination should be done to identify lesions and rule out a foreign body or space-occupying mass such as a neoplasm. A vaginal culture may also be indicated, although results will be difficult to interpret because of the normal vaginal flora. A culture should be taken by cleaning the vulva, inserting a sterile vaginal speculum, and passing a culturette through the speculum into the proximal vagina. The culture can be relied upon to have identified the pathogen only if large numbers of a single organism are found. Vaginitis may be due to organisms other than the commonly cultured aerobic bacteria. If a bacterial infection is confirmed or strongly suspected, a culture of urine collected by cystocentesis is indicated, since ascent of bacteria to the bladder is common. Symptomatic therapy for vaginitis is based upon local therapy with vaginal douches such as 10% povidone-iodine. Most systemic antibiotics do not reach significant concentrations in the vagina, with the exception of trimethoprim.

Acute metritis and pyometra are uterine causes of a purulent vaginal discharge. Acute metritis is a bacterial infection of the uterus, which usually occurs early postpartum but can also occur postabortion or postbreeding. The usual causative organisms are gram-negative aerobic bacilli such as *Escherichia coli,* but anaerobes such as bacteroides may also be causative agents. Predisposing factors to infection include prolonged labor, retained placental or fetal tissues, vaginitis, and improper manipulation or use of instruments. The discharge is usually copious and foul smelling. The animal is usually systemically ill with fever, depression, and anorexia and may neglect her young. Sepsis may develop. The uterus is usually mildly enlarged and doughy. The white blood cell count indicates an inflammatory disease with either a regenerative or degenerative left shift. The diagnostic plan should include abdominal radiographs to determine the presence of retained fetal tissues and a brucella titer if the problem follows abortion in a bitch. Treatment requires antibiotics and supportive fluid therapy as needed. Initial choice of an antibiotic is often ampicillin/amoxicillin or chloramphenicol. Because of the risk of nephrotoxicity, aminoglycosides should be reserved for animals that are septic and nonresponsive to the initial drugs. Prostaglandin $F_{2\alpha}$ (0.1 mg/kg Luteolyse subcutaneously daily for two to five injections) may help evacuate the uterus, although in the majority of cases it has not been necessary. Side-effects of prostaglandins include vomiting, salivation, anxiety, bradycardia, dyspnea, and diarrhea.

Pyometra usually occurs several weeks postestrus or after estrogen or progesterone therapy. Pyometra is usually the final stage of the cystic endometrial hyperplasia/endometritis complex, which is very common in intact, but not bred, bitches. Infection with *E. coli* is common but is secondary to the underlying changes in the uterine wall. Pyometra is referred to as "open" or "closed" in relation to the cervix. An open pyometra is accompanied by a profuse, purulent vaginal discharge; no vaginal discharge is evident with a closed cervix. Dogs with a closed cervix are usually very ill. Clinical signs include depression, vomiting, dehydration, and anorexia. The enlarged uterus should be palpable. A neutrophilic leukocytosis is common. Abdominal radiographs or ultrasound may be necessary to distinguish pyometra from pregnancy or another illness. Standard treatment of pyometra is supportive fluid therapy, antibiotics, and ovariohysterectomy. If the owner wants to save the bitch for breeding purposes, prostaglandins can be tried if the bitch's condition is stable. If the bitch's condition is critical, delaying surgery may be fatal.

Preputial Discharge

Hemorrhagic

The major causes of a hemorrhagic discharge are penile/preputial trauma, neoplasia within the sheath, distal urethral injury, neoplasia or urolith, and prostatic disease. The diagnostic plan should include a complete history and physical examination, including rectal palpation of the prostate in dogs and complete examination of the sheath. In dogs, this involves complete protrusion of the penis and may require tranquilization.

The most common bleeding preputial lesions in dogs are trauma and neoplasia. The most common neoplasms of the prepuce and penis are transmissible venereal tumor, papillomas, and carcinomas. Transmissible venereal tumors can usually be diagnosed by finding the typical large round cells on impression smear. Biopsy is usually required to diagnose the other types of tumors. Treatment depends on tumor type.

If the bleeding is from the urethral orifice, urethral diseases such as a urethral prolapse, neoplasm, urolith, trauma, or other cause of inflammation are possible causes. Urethral prolapse should be evident on physical examination. The other urethral diseases should be accompanied by other signs such as dysuria. A retrograde urethrogram may be necessary to further investigate these possibilities.

The most common cause of a hemorrhagic urethral discharge without other clinical problems, except perhaps hematuria, is cystic hyperplasia of the prostate. Other prostatic diseases such as acute or chronic bacterial prostatitis and neoplasia can also cause a hemorrhagic urethral discharge. History, physical examination, CBC, urine analysis, abdominal radiography, ultrasonography, and prostatic fluid and tissue evaluation may be needed to differentiate these possibilities. Prostatic cystic hyperplasia is predominantly characterized by blood in urine and prostatic fluid. The prostate is enlarged but nonpainful, and the enlargement is often mild to moderate and symmetric. The predominant finding with bacterial prostatitis is infection of urine and prostatic fluid. Systemic signs of illness may accompany acute prostatitis and prostatic abscess. With prostatic neoplasia, the prostate is usually markedly enlarged and irregular or contains firm nodules. Prostatic fluid often contains red and white blood cells but is usually not infected. The dog may be in pain, depressed, and anorectic. Because these signs may overlap, a tissue biopsy is often necessary for a definitive diagnosis. Treatment depends on the disease process.

Purulent

A purulent discharge from the prepuce should be determined to be preputial or urethral in origin by a careful physical examination. The entire sheath should be examined.

If the discharge is preputial, the most common cause is balanoposthitis. Balanoposthitis is characterized by a thick, creamy discharge with lymphoid follicular hyperplasia in the sheath. This condition is so common in dogs that a mild discharge is considered normal. New owners of male dogs need to be educated in this regard. If the discharge is copious, symptomatic therapy with 10% povidone-iodine douches or intramammary infusion preparations can be used. A careful physical examination is indicated to rule out foreign body or space-occupying masses, such as a neoplasm, which may be acting as a source of irritation.

If the discharge is urethral, an inflammatory prostatic disease such as acute or chronic prostatitis, abscess formation or neoplasia should be considered. The diagnostic plan should include thorough prostatic palpation, CBC, urine analysis, urine culture, cytology and culture of prostatic fluid, and abdominal radiography or ultrasonography. Therapy would depend on cause.

Urethritis as a cause of a purulent urethral discharge independent of other urinary tract disease is rarely recognized in dogs and cats.

Serous Fluid

Serous fluid may drip from the urethral orifice when prostatic cysts communicate with the urethra. This discharge is difficult to differentiate from urinary incontinence by visual examination alone. The diagnostic plan should include a "urine analysis" of the discharge and analysis of urine from the bladder to determine if the two are identical.

SUGGESTED READINGS

Allen WE, Dagnall GJR: Some observations on the aerobic bacterial flora of the genital tract of the dog and bitch. J Small Anim Prac 23:325–336, 1982

Baba E, Hata MSH, Fukata T, et al: Vaginal and uterine microlora of adult dogs. Sm J Vet Res 44:606–609, 1983

Barsanti JA: Genitourinary tract infections. In Greene CE (ed): Clinical Microbiology and Infectious Diseases of the Dog and Cat, pp 269–283. Philadelphia, WB Saunders, 1984

Barton CL: Canine vaginitis. Vet Clin North Am 7:711–714, 1977

Johnston SD: Management of the post-partum bitch and queen. In Kirk RW (ed): Current Veterinary Therapy VIII, pp 959–961. Philadelphia, WB Saunders, 1983

Ling GV, Ruby AL: Aerobic bacterial flora of the prepuce, urethral, and vagina of normal adult dogs. Am J Vet Res 39:695–698, 1978

Nelson RW, Feldman EC, Stabenfeldt GH: Treatment of canine pyometra and endometritis with prostaglandin F_2. J Am Vet Med Assoc 181:899–903, 1982

Osbaldiston GW: Bacteriological studies of reproductive disorders of bitches. J Am Anim Hosp Assoc 14:363–367, 1978

Schall WD, Duncan JR, Finco DR, et al: Spontaneous recovery after subinvolution of placental sites in a bitch. J Am Vet Med Assoc 159:1780–1782, 1971

42

Abnormalities of the External Genitalia

JEANNE A. BARSANTI

This chapter describes external genitalia abnormalities that are detectable by physical examination. Abnormalities of the vulva, mammary glands, scrotal sac, and prepuce are presented in the lists of abnormalities on subsequent pages.

VULVAR ABNORMALITIES

Small Size

A relatively small vulva can be due to immaturity, neutering at a young age, or hypoplasia.

Swelling

A generalized swelling of the vulva can be characterized as turgid, soft, or pitting. The vulva is swollen and turgid in proestrus, occasionally with vaginitis or in association with perivulvar dermatitis. The vulvar swelling becomes softer with onset of estrus and as a pregnant bitch nears parturition. Pitting edema of the vulva may be due to hypoalbuminemia. Diagnosis of the cause of generalized vulvar swelling can usually be made by history of estrus cycle stage, physical examination, and vaginal cytology. If pitting edema of the perineal area is present, a complete blood count, blood chemistry profile, and urine analysis are indicated.

Vaginal Mass

A mass protruding from the vulva may be vaginal hyperplasia, a vaginal neoplasm, or a prolapsed uterus.

Vaginal hyperplasia occurs during estrus, principally in large breed dogs. The vaginal mucosa becomes markedly swollen during estrus in affected dogs

Abnormalities of the Female External Genitalia

- Vulva
  - Small
    - Immaturity
    - Neutering at a young age
    - Hypoplasia
  - Generalized swelling
    - Proestrus
    - Vaginitis
    - Perivulvar dermatitis
    - Estrus
    - Nearing parturition
    - Edema
  - Mass
    - Vaginal hyperplasia
    - Vaginal tumors
    - Prolapsed uterus
  - Congenital
    - Anovulvar cleft
    - Clitoral hypertrophy
  - Vaginal Trauma
- Mammary glands
  - Galactosis
  - Mammary hypertrophy/hyperplasia
  - Mastitis
  - Neoplasia

and protrudes through the vulvar lips as a red fleshy mass. The condition tends to recur with each estrus. The most effective therapy is ovariohysterectomy. Local therapy to prevent trauma and desiccation of the protruding vaginal mucosa may also be required.

Vaginal tumors such as leiomyoma or transmissible venereal tumor may also protrude through the vulvar lips. Differentiation from vaginal hyperplasia can usually be made from history of estrus cycle stage, physical appearance of the mass, and impression smears; biopsy is occasionally required. Leiomyomas are usually pedunculated. Diagnosis is based on cytologic examination of impression smears, biopsy, or both. Transmissible venereal tumors can usually be diagnosed on impression smear by the characteristic uniform population of large round cells.

A prolapsed uterus is uncommon in the dog and cat. It can occur at or within 48 hours of parturition, when the cervix is open. Diagnosis is made from the history of recent parturition and physical examination. The entire uterus or only one horn may prolapse. Manual reduction after cleansing should be attempted. If unsuccessful, therapy is surgical removal, with careful attention paid

Abnormalities of Male External Genitalia

- Scrotum
    - Dermatitis
    - Edema
    - Tumor
- Testicles
    - Cryptorchidism
    - Small testicles
        - Degeneration
        - Chronic inflammation
        - Atrophy
    - Enlarged Testicles
        - Acute orchitis
        - Testicular torsion
        - Neoplasia
- Epididymis
    - Epididymitis
- Prepuce/Penis
    - Balanoposthitis
    - Trauma
    - Tumors
    - Phimosis
    - Paraphimosis
    - Congenital defects
    - Urethral prolapse

to the location and preservation of the urethral orifice. In contrast to vaginal hyperplasia, uterine prolapse rarely recurs after the uterus is replaced.

Others

Other vulvar abnormalities that may be detected by physical examination include congenital defects, clitoral hypertrophy, and trauma. An anovulvar cleft results from incomplete closure of the skin from the dorsal vulvar commissure to the anus. Clitoral hypertrophy occurs in hermaphrodites, pseudohermaphrodites, normal females receiving androgenic drugs, and, rarely, animals with hyperadrenocorticism.

MAMMARY GLAND ABNORMALITIES

Mammary gland enlargement can be due to milk accumulation, hypertrophy, inflammation, or neoplasia.

Galactosis

Galactosis describes mammary accumulation of milk. Such accumulation is normal in advanced pregnancy and lactation. During weaning and in pseudopregnancy, such accumulation may increase to the point that the mammae become painful and warm. There are no signs of systemic illness, and the white blood cell count is normal. Diagnosis is made from the history, physical examination, and cytology of mammary fluid. Fluid expressed from the teats will appear as milk. Microscopically it may contain some neutrophils and macrophages with engulfed milk fat. Symptomatic treatment includes cool soaks, compresses, and decreased caloric intake. The milk should *not* be expressed, because this stimulates continued lactation. In severe cases, mild doses of diuretics or glucocorticosteroids may be indicated. The condition can be prevented in lactating bitches by more gradual weaning.

Mammary Hypertrophy/Hyperplasia

Mammary hypertrophy/hyperplasia is a hormone-dependent, dysplastic change in the mammary glands of cats. Young pregnant queens are most commonly affected, but the condition also occurs in nonpregnant intact queens and in neutered males or females receiving progesterone therapy such as megestrol acetate. In queens, the mammary enlargement starts in the first 2 weeks of pregnancy rather than in late pregnancy, as is normal.

Signs of mammary hypertrophy are painless, marked enlargement of one or more mammae. The overlying skin may ulcerate in severely swollen glands. There are no systemic signs of illness, except those related to the marked swelling, unless the ulcerated glands become secondarily infected. Diagnosis is based on the history and physical examination. The condition resolves with removal of the influence of progesterone such as delivery of kittens, ovariohysterectomy, or discontinuation of progesterone therapy. Local symptomatic therapy can include soaks, antibiotics, and drainage as needed. In breeding queens, the problem may recur in subsequent pregnancies but may not be as severe.

Mastitis

Mastitis occurs 24 hours to 6 weeks postpartum. One or more mammae become hot, swollen, and painful. Associated systemic signs include anorexia, depression, and fever. The neonates may become systemically ill and die from bacteremia or toxemia. Diagnosis is based on the history of recent parturition, physical examination, and cytology of exudate expressed from the affected glands. The milk usually appears purulent or hemorrhagic with degenerative neutrophils and bacteria on cytologic examination. Affected bitches usually have an inflammatory hematologic response. The diagnostic plan should include culture and antibiotic sensitivity testing of the affected milk.

Treatment involves hot soaks, lancing abscessed areas (avoiding the nipple), not allowing the young to nurse affected glands, and systemic antibiotics. Initial recommended antibiotics include chloramphenicol, ampicillin, or amoxicillin. Tetracycline should be avoided if the young continue to nurse the bitch, since this antibiotic may stain developing teeth.

Neoplasia

Mammary gland neoplasia is common in dogs and is as often benign as malignant. Mammary gland neoplasia is less common in cats but is usually malignant. Clinical signs include firm, nodular masses in one or more mammae. The affected female is otherwise normal unless severe metastatic disease (such as lung metastasis) has already occurred. The differential diagnosis should include areas of glandular fibrosis or chronic inflammation. Diagnosis usually requires excisional biopsy and histopathology. The diagnostic plan should include thoracic radiographs to check for lung metastasis. Primary treatment is surgical removal.

ABNORMALITIES OF THE SCROTUM

The most common lesions of the scrotum include dermatitis, edema, and neoplasia.

Dermatitis

Scrotal dermatitis can be associated with a generalized dermatitis, can be due to local irritation, or can be secondary to orchitis. The sensitive scrotal skin may become inflamed by contact with soaps, dips, and disinfectants. An underlying orchitis may result in scrotal licking and secondary dermatitis. For this reason and because of its public health significance and contagious nature, infection with *Brucella canis* should always be considered in dogs with scrotal dermatitis.

Edema

Scrotal edema may result from local irritation or as part of a systemic tendency toward edema due to hypoalbuminemia or vasculitis. Edema may be more evident in the scrotum than in other body parts of animals with these systemic causes. Examples are vasculitis due to Rocky Mountain spotted fever and hypoalbuminemia due to chronic hepatic failure or proteinuric renal diseases.

Neoplasia

Certain tumors are prone to affect the scrotal skin. These include mast cell tumors and melanomas. Impression smears of ulcerated scrotal skin should be performed to establish the diagnosis. Biopsy specimens should be taken from areas that are slow to heal and that give nondiagnostic impression smears.

TESTICULAR ABNORMALITIES

Cryptorchidism

The testicles in dogs and cats generally descend into the scrotum within the first 2 weeks after birth. Until puberty, the testicles normally can move or be moved between the external inguinal ring and the scrotum. After puberty, the testicles remain in the scrotum. If both testicles have not descended to the scrotum by puberty (6 months of age), the animal is cryptorchid. The retained testicle(s) may be either abdominal or at or within the inguinal canal. The condition is considered hereditary and affected males should not be bred. Bilateral cryptorchid males are sterile because of thermal deterioration of spermatogenesis but will develop masculine appearance and behavior since testosterone production is normal. Diagnosis is based on physical examination. Recommended treatment is castration, since affected animals should not be bred and since retained testicles have a higher incidence of neoplasia. One study showed that the incidence of tumor development in intra-abdominal testicles was especially high in the Pekinese breed.

Small Testicles

A decrease in testicular size can be due to degeneration with aging, chronic inflammation and fibrosis, atrophy secondary to abnormal hormone production by a neoplastic testicle, or atrophy secondary to endocrinopathies such as hyperadrenocorticism and hypothyroidism. Sertoli cell tumors are commonly associated with atrophy of the other testicle. The diagnostic plan for small testicles should include thorough palpation for testicular tumors and semen evaluation for evidence of inflammation and abnormal sperm production. No therapy is needed for aging change. Castration is recommended for neoplasia. Therapy for inflammation depends on its severity.

Testicular Enlargement

An increase in testicular size can be associated with acute orchitis, testicular torsion, or testicular neoplasia.

Acute Orchitis

Acute orchitis can result from infection or trauma. Clinical signs include testicular swelling, pain, and heat. Signs of systemic illness may or may not be present. Diagnosis is based on history and physical examination. Infection with *B. canis* should always be considered and appropriate laboratory tests performed. The diagnostic plan should include urine analysis and urine culture since infection can spread via the spermatic cord to and from the urinary tract. Treatment includes cool soaks and systemic antibiotics. Sequelae can include abscesses, fibrosis, and decreased fertility. If only one testicle is involved and the animal is valuable for breeding, the affected testicle should be surgically removed to protect the remaining testicle from spread of infection and thermal degeneration. If the animal is not used for breeding, castration plus systemic antibiotics will usually be curative.

Testicular Torsion

Testicular torsion is uncommon in intrascrotal testicles in dogs and cats. Clinical signs include pain, vomiting, lethargy, anorexia, diarrhea or constipation, tenesmus, and mild fever. The torsed testicle becomes markedly swollen, and the scrotum may have mild edema. Diagnosis is based on the physical signs, but differentiation from acute unilateral orchitis may be difficult. Signs of systemic illness and pain are usually greater with testicular torsion. Aspiration of the affected testicle may help rule out infection but is often not performed because of the degree of testicular pain. Treatment is surgical removal of the affected testicle.

Testicular Tumors

Testicular tumors are common in older male dogs. The usual types are interstitial cell tumors, seminomas, and Sertoli cell tumors. Testicular tumors are rare in cats, but Sertoli cell tumors have been noted. The rate of metastasis is low for all types, but Sertoli cell tumors and seminomas have the potential for malignancy. Growth is usually slow. Physical examination indicates an intratesticular nodule that is neither painful nor hot and that is very similar to fibrotic or chronic inflammatory nodules.

Approximately 15% to 40% of dogs with Sertoli cell tumors develop signs of feminization, including loss of libido, pendulous prepuce, gynecomastia, contralateral testicular atrophy, and attraction of male dogs. Other signs that may develop include alopecia and hyperpigmentation, prostatic squamous metaplasia, and, rarely, bone marrow aplasia. Alopecia and hyperpigmentation have also been reported with seminomas. Serum testosterone concentrations are low. Diagnosis may be suspected by physical examination and confirmed by castration and histopathology. Treatment is also castration.

ABNORMALITIES OF THE EPIDIDYMIS

The most common problem with the epididymis is enlargement due to epididymitis. This is most often associated with orchitis. Diagnosis is by history, physical examination, semen cytology and culture, and possibly aspiration or tissue evaluation. *B. canis* infection should always be evaluated by serologic testing.

PREPUTIAL/PENILE ABNORMALITIES

The most common preputial/penile abnormalities are balanoposthitis, trauma, tumors, phimosis, paraphimosis, congenital defects, and urethral prolapse. The first three problems are discussed in chapter 41.

Phimosis

Phimosis is the inability to protrude the penis due to a stricture at the preputial orifice. A stricture may be congenital or acquired due to trauma. Treatment is surgical correction of the stricture.

Paraphimosis

Paraphimosis is the inability to withdraw the penis into the prepuce. This occurs normally in male dogs with erection, usually after coitus or masturbation, and may be especially pronounced in young dogs. A small preputial orifice or constricting preputial hairs may be predisposing factors. Prolonged erection may lead to severe penile injury, desiccation, necrosis, and urethral obstruction. The dog should be removed from the source of sexual stimulation and allowed a period of rest in isolation. Cool water soaks may be used to reduce penile swelling. In severe cases, general anesthesia and penile lubrication may be needed to relieve the paraphimosis. If this is not effective, surgery should be performed to enlarge the preputial orifice. In cases of severe necrosis, penile amputation with careful preservation of the urethra may be required.

Congenital Defects

Hypospadias is the most common developmental abnormality of the male external genitalia. It occurs when the urogenital folds fail to fuse, causing incomplete closure and formation of the penile urethra. On physical examination, the external urethral orifice is displaced to the ventral midline of the penis. The penis is underdeveloped and the prepuce is incomplete ventrally. Urine scalding of the ventral abdomen may occur. Treatment is surgical correction.

Other congenital defects include curvature of the penis and a persistent penile frenulum. The penile frenulum is a fine band of connective tissue that attaches the penis to the prepuce ventrally. It usually ruptures prior to puberty; however, when rupture does not occur, the dog may have pain on erection and may lick at the prepuce.

Strangulation of the penis can occur from foreign bodies (*e.g.*, rubber bands) or a constricting ring of preputial hairs. The penis becomes swollen, necrotic, and painful. The dog will lick the area and become dysuric.

Urethral prolapse appears as a small, red, pea-shaped mass at the end of the penis. It is not uncommon in bulldogs and Boston terriers. It may also occur with urinary tract diseases associated with marked dysuria.

SUGGESTED READINGS

Barsanti JA, Duncan JR, Nachreiner RF: Alopecia associated with a seminoma. J Am Anim Hosp Assoc 15:33–36, 1979

Boothe HW: Penis. In Slatter DH (ed): Textbook of Small Animal Surgery, pp 1628–1632. Philadelphia, WB Saunders, 1985

Boothe HW: Prepuce. In Slatter DH (ed): Textbook of Small Animal Surgery, pp 1633–1634. Philadelphia, WB Saunders, 1985

Center SA, Randolph JF: Lactation and spontaneous remission of feline mammary hyperplasia following pregnancy. J Am Anim Hosp Assoc 21:56–58, 1985

Greiner TP, Zolton GM: Genital emergencies. In Morrow DA (ed): Current Therapy in Theriogenology, pp 614–618. Philadelphia, WB Saunders, 1980

Hayden DW, Johnston SD, Kiang DT: Feline mammary hypertrophy/fibroadenoma complex: Clinical and hormonal aspects. Am J Vet Res 42:1699–1703, 1981

Herron MA: Tumors of the canine genital system. J Am Anim Hosp Assoc 19:981–994, 1983

Hinton M, Gaskell CJ: Non-neoplastic mammary hypertrophy in the cat associated either with pregnancy or with oral progestagen therapy. Vet Rec 100:277–280, 1977

Ogilvie GK: Feline mammary neoplasia. Compend Cont Ed Pract Vet 5:384–390, 1983

Pearson H, Kelly DF: Testicular torsion in the dog: A review of 13 cases. Vet Rec 97:200–204, 1975

Rhoades JD, Foley CW: Cryptorchidism and intersexuality. Vet Clin North Am 7:789–793, 1977

Stein BS: Tumors of the feline genital tract. J Am Anim Host Assoc 17:1022–1025, 1981

Stone EA: The uterus. In Slatter DH (ed): Testbook of Small Animal Surgery, pp 1661–1671. Philadelphia, WB Saunders, 1985

Wheeler SL, Magne ML, Kaufman J, et al: Postpartum disorders in the bitch. Compend Cont Ed Pract Vet 6:493–501, 1984

Wykes PM, Olson PN: The vulva. In Slatter DH (ed): Textbook of Small Animal Surgery, pp 1678–1680. Philadelphia, WB Saunders, 1985

43

Abortion, Abnormal Estrous Cycle, Infertility

JEANNE A. BARSANTI

This chapter describes two major reproductive problems: abortion and infertility.

ABORTION

Definition

Abortion refers to the expulsion of fetuses prior to term. Abortion is usually accompanied by abdominal contractions and a vaginal discharge. Diagnosis may be made by observing the abortion, by finding aborted material, or by confirming loss of pregnancy. It is possible for dogs and cats to abort some but not all fetuses and to carry the remaining fetuses to term.

Pathophysiology

The causes of abortion include maternal factors such as infection, trauma, and hormonal abnormalities and fetal factors such as chromosomal abnormalities (see list).

Viral, bacterial, and protozoal infections can result in abortion. Viral causes in dogs include canine distemper and, rarely, canine herpesvirus. Other signs of herpesvirus infection include vesicular vaginitis and mild rhinitis. Viral causes in cats include feline leukemia virus, feline panleukopenia, feline rhinotracheitis, feline calicivirus, and feline infectious peritonitis. Of these, feline leukemia and feline panleukopenia virus infections are most important in natural as opposed to experimental infections. Feline leukemia typically causes abortion at 4 to 7 weeks of pregnancy.

Brucella canis is the major bacterial cause of abortion in dogs. Abortion typically occurs at 45 to 55 days of pregnancy. Other bacteria have also been sporadically associated with abortion, including beta-hemolytic streptococci type L, *Escherichia coli,* and *Leptospira* species. *Toxoplasma* is the main protozoal

Causes of Abortion in Dogs and Cats

- Maternal factors
  - Infection
    - Dogs
      - Viral
        - Canine distemper
        - Canine herpesvirus
      - Bacterial
        - *Brucella canis*
        - beta hemolytic streptococci
        - *Escherichia coli*
        - Leptospira
      - Protozoa
        - Toxoplasmosis
    - Cats
      - Viral
        - Feline leukemia
        - Feline panleukopenia
        - Feline rhinotracheitis
        - Feline calicivirus
        - Feline infectious peritonitis
      - Bacterial
  - Trauma
  - Endocrine disease
    - Hypoluteoidism
    - Hypothyroidism
- Fetal factors
  - Chromosomal abnormalities

organism associated with abortion in dogs. Toxoplasmosis is not associated with abortion in cats.

Abortion has been attributed to hypothyroidism in dogs. Hypoluteoidism has also been suspected of causing recurrent abortion in dogs and cats but has not been confirmed. Progesterone from the corpus luteum is essential for maintaining pregnancy to term in dogs but is only required in cats through days 42 to 45. Whether inability to maintain progesterone concentrations is a mechanism for abortion in dogs and cats requires measurement of progesterone concentrations near the time abortion occurs.

Trauma is a potential cause of abortion but is relatively infrequent.

Chromosomal abnormalities have been found in aborted fetuses in cases in which no maternal abnormalities could be identified.

Diagnostic Plan

Dogs

The diagnostic plan in dogs begins with a thorough history and physical examination. The physical examination should include a digital and visual vaginal examination. A complete blood count (CBC), vaginal cytology, brucella titer, and urine analysis should be performed. If the freshly aborted fetus is available, necropsy with histopathology of major body tissues and stomach culture for bacteria should be performed. The abortus can be karyotyped if no maternal causes for abortion are evident. All aborted material and discharges from the vagina should be handled carefully (wearing gloves) since *B. canis* is infectious to humans. If infection with bacteria is suggested by vaginal cytology or urine analysis, bacterial cultures should be performed of urine collected by cystocentesis and of discharge collected from the anterior vagina using a guarded culturette such as a Tiegland swab. If the initial diagnostic tests are negative or normal, paired titers for toxoplasmosis are indicated. If no evidence of toxoplasmosis is found, testing of thyroid function with a thyroid-stimulating hormone (TSH) response test is indicated. If abortion has occurred previously with no apparent cause, serum progesterone concentrations should be monitored during the next pregnancy.

Cats

The diagnostic plan in cats also begins with a thorough history, physical examination, vaginal cytology, histopathology, culture, and possible karyotyping of the abortus. A CBC and feline leukemia virus test are always indicated. If the cause is not determined, paired titers for coronavirus (FIP) should be considered. Since coronavirus titers are not specific for feline infectious peritonitis, a thorough physical examination including fundic examination, a blood chemistry profile, and urine analysis are often required to document this systemic disease. If uterine bacterial infection is suspected, vaginal and urine (cystocentesis sample) cultures are indicated. If the queen has a history of repeated abortion of unknown cause, serum progesterone concentrations should be monitored during the next pregnancy.

Therapeutic Plan

Therapy depends on the cause of abortion. Progesterone should be used to maintain pregnancy only if other causes of abortion have been eliminated and, preferably, if low serum concentrations of progesterone have been confirmed. Progesterone therapy can prolong gestation; therefore, accurate breeding dates are essential so that therapy can be discontinued 7 to 10 days prior to term. High progesterone concentrations have the potential of masculinizing female fetuses.

Prognosis

The prognosis for future successful breeding depends on the cause of the abortion. Rebreeding is not recommended for animals with brucellosis or feline leukemia.

ABNORMAL ESTROUS CYCLES AND INFERTILITY IN THE BITCH

Definition

Normal onset of estrous cycles in the bitch occurs at 4 to 18 months of age. The marked variation in age is in part due to different breed sizes, with smaller breeds cycling earlier and larger breeds later. In general, late onset of estrus is not considered abnormal until the bitch is 2 years old or until 6 months after growth plateau occurs. The normal interestrous interval is 5 to 8 months, but individual variation is marked and a range of 4 to 14 months is considered acceptable. Variation does not seem to be related to breed size. Interestrous intervals normally increase in bitches over 8 years of age. The normal duration of standing estrus is 9 days, with a range of 3 to 21 days. Acceptance of a male for over 21 days is considered abnormal.

Estrous cycle abnormalities associated with infertility include absence of estrous cycles in bitches 2 to 8 years of age; prolonged standing estrus; short, "split," or "false" heats; prolonged proestral bleeding; very short interestral intervals; and very long interestral invervals. Infertility can also occur in bitches with normal-appearing estrous cycles.

Pathophysiology

The diagnostic plan is based on three categories: infertility with a normal estrous cycle, with an abnormal estrous cycle but a normal interestrous interval, and with an abnormal estrous cycle with an abnormal interestrous interval (see Causes of Infertility in the Bitch).

Normal Estrous Cycle

If a bitch is infertile but her estrous cycles are normal, the major possibilities are bacterial uterine infection or reproductive tract obstruction.

One infectious cause of reproductive failure in a bitch with apparent normal cycles is early embryonic death due to *B. canis* infection. Because the normal vaginal flora contains many different potentially pathogenic bacteria, other bacterial causes of chronic bacterial metritis with subfertility are difficult to confirm without uterine biopsy or direct uterine culture. A presumptive diagnosis is usually based on cultures of the anterior vagina collected by a guarded swab (*e.g.*, Tiegland swab) during proestrus, vaginal cytology, and response to antibiotic therapy.

Causes of Infertility in the Bitch

- Infertility associated with normal estrus
  - Infection
    - *Brucella canis*
    - Other bacteria
  - Vaginal stricture
  - Uterine tumor
  - Oviduct obstruction
- Abnormal estrus, normal interestrous interval
  - Failure to stand
    - Vaginal/vestibular strictures
    - Inexperience
    - Inaccurate timing of estrus
  - Cystic ovaries
- Abnormal interestrous interval
  - Short intervals
  - Prolonged intervals
    - Endocrine diseases
    - Nutritional problems
    - Cystic endometrial hyperplasia
    - Aging
  - Absence of cycles
    - Endocrine disease
    - Ovarian dysfunction
    - Congenital dysfunction (intersex)
    - Previous ovariohysterectomy
    - Young or old age

A vaginal or vestibular stricture preventing mating may also result in apparent infertility with normal estrous cycles. These strictures may be congenital or acquired as a result of injury, as might occur during a previous whelping. Congenital strictures include persistent imperforate hymen and congenital atresia of the vagina. These abnormalities are identified with carefully performed vaginal examination.

A uterine tumor might result in normal estrous cycles but failure to conceive.

Oviduct obstruction may also result in subfertility or infertility if it is bilateral. Diagnosis requires laparoscopy or celiotomy.

Abnormal Estrous Cycle, Normal Interestrous Interval

Certain causes of abnormal estrous cycles may be associated with a relatively normal interestrous interval. These include failure to stand (acceptance of male for coitus), prolonged standing, and prolonged proestral bleeding.

Failure to stand during estrus may be due to vaginal/vestibular strictures that cause pain during penile penetration, dislike of the male, or inexperience. One must always consider human error in determining standing estrus. Because of individual variation in length of proestrus and estrus, the bitch may be wrongly accused of failure to stand when the timing of breeding was inappropriately determined. Correlation of acceptance behavior with vaginal cytology may detect this problem. Some bitches seem to have prolonged proestral-type bleeding into estrus. If the timing of breeding is based only on disappearance of bleeding, standing heat may be missed. Vaginal cytology and alternate-day exposure to the male after 9 days of proestrus may help detect this variation of normal estrus.

Prolongation of standing heat without conception usually indicates prolonged estrogen secretion with failure of ovulation. The usual cause is cystic ovaries.

Abnormal Interestrous Interval

An abnormal interestrous interval can be too short, too long, or due to absence of the estrus cycle.

A short interestrous interval is defined as one less than 4 months in duration. A "split" heat refers to vulvar swelling and blood-tinged vaginal discharge that stops within a few days without progression to standing estrus. The cycle reverts to anestrus followed by a true, fertile estrus in 4 to 6 weeks. This may be a normal variant in the estrus cycle of some bitches. It may be caused by an increased estrogen level near the end of anestrus due to transient follicular growth. It is documented by measuring weekly estradiol and progesterone concentrations. The bitch should be bred according to her standing behavior and not according to the days from onset of bloody vaginal discharge. Other dogs may have short interestrous intervals without "split" heats. The cause is not known, but infertility may be associated. The infertility may be due to endometrial implantation failure since complete endometrial desquamation and repair have not occurred.

Prolonged interestrous intervals may be associated with hormonal abnormalities such as hypothyroidism and hyperadrenocorticism, cachexia or obesity, and cystic endometrial hyperplasia.

Absence of cycling can be associated with hypothyroidism, primary ovarian or adrenal dysfunction, intersex conditions, previous unreported ovariohysterectomy, and young (<2 years) or old (>8 years) age. Ovarian dysfunction can be congenital (hypoplasia) or acquired (neoplasia). Some bitches have "silent" heats. Only repeated vaginal cytology (or frequent reexposure to a male dog) will detect that these bitches are truly cycling.

Diagnostic Plan

The diagnostic plan must include a thorough history, including a complete breeding record with dates of start of proestrus, time of mating, duration of standing estrus, duration of the interestrus interval, and the breeding record of the males involved. The general medical history, including current health and previous problems and treatments, should be obtained. In addition to a regular physical examination, special attention should be paid to abdominal palpation of the uterus and rectal examination of the pelvis and vagina. The vagina should also be examined digitally and then by vaginoscopy. It may be easier to detect a vaginal stricture by digital examination than by vaginoscopy.

A CBC, urine analysis (cystocentesis sample), and *B. canis* titer should be performed. If these tests are negative, a blood chemistry profile and thyroid response testing should be done. If the cause is still not evident and the dog is cycling, the next estrous cycle should be followed with vaginal cytologic examinations, characteristics of standing behavior, and determination of serum estradiol and progesterone concentrations. If the dog is not cycling, celiotomy for examination of the ovaries and uterus and biopsy and culture of the uterus are indicated. The patency of the oviducts should be tested.

Treatment

Treatment depends on identification and correction of the underlying cause. Attempts to induce estrus in bitches have been reported with varying success. The most recent studies indicate that hormonal therapy to induce a fertile estrus is not effective.

ABNORMAL ESTROUS CYCLES AND INFERTILITY IN QUEENS

Definition

Reproductive cycles in the normal queen begin between 5 months and 1 year of age. Queens cycle every 14 to 21 days when exposed to 14 hours of light per day. Cats kept outdoors are seasonally polyestrus in association with length of daylight. Calling, rolling, rubbing, lordosis, and tredding are the normal behavioral signs of estrus. Novice cat owners may conclude that their cat has developed a serious neurologic problem on first observing this behavior. In contrast to the dog, there is little vulvar swelling and no proestral bleeding. Otherwise, vaginal cytology is similar. The cat ovulates only in response to coitus. If a male is present, receptivity usually lasts 1 to 4 days. If no male is present, the estrous cycle will last 7 to 10 days. A quiescent period will occur for 2 to 3 weeks and then estrus will recur. These cycles will be repeated throughout the breeding season, which seems to be determined largely by day length. An abnormal estrous cycle is failure to show estrus during the breeding season, and infertility is failure of conception in spite of normal estrous behavior and the presence of a male cat. Coitus is rarely observed, because it is rapidly completed in cats. The typical postcoital behavior of the queen (rolling and crying) may be observed by the owner.

Causes of Infertility in Queens

- Absence of estrus
  - "Silent" estrus
  - Drug therapy
  - Ovarian dysfunction
  - Cachexia
  - Endocrine disease
  - Cystic endometrial hyperplasia
  - Environment
  - Previous ovariohysterectomy
- Failure of conception
  - Infertile cycles
    - Cystic ovaries
    - Cystic endometrial hyperplasia
  - Early embryonic death
    - Feline leukemia
    - Cystic endometrial hyperplasia

Pathophysiology and Causes

There are two major categories for abnormal estrous cycles and infertility in cats: lack of apparent estrus and lack of conception despite of apparent normal cycling and presence of male cats (see Causes of Infertility in Queens).

Anestrus

If the cat does not cycle during the usual breeding season, "silent" heats, use of progesterone type drugs for other medical problems, congenital ovarian defects (dysgenesis), debility, endogenous hormonal imbalance, uterine (cystic hyperplasia) or ovarian (neoplasia, cystic change) disease, and environmental factors (lack of at least 12 hours of light per day, lack of exposure to other cats) should be considered. A previous ovariohysterectomy unknown by the current owners should also be considered. Megestrol acetate, commonly used for dermatologic and behavioral problems in cats, can completely suppress estrus when used at 5 mg/day for 3 days and then 2.5 to 5 mg/week. These doses are well within usual therapeutic guidelines for dermatologic and behavioral problems.

Failure of Conception

Failure to conceive in cats that apparently cycle indicates infertile cycles or that early embryonic death has occurred. Lack of fertile cycles can be due to cystic ovarian follicles. These are most commonly reported in older, nulliparous queens and may be associated with cystic uterine hyperplasia. Cystic endometrial hyperplasia has also been associated with poor conception rate. A remnant of ovarian tissue left from a previous ovariohysterectomy may cause estrus, with infertility due to the hysterectomy.

Early embryonic death is most commonly associated with feline leukemia virus infection. Cystic endometrial hyperplasia may also cause early embryonic death.

Diagnostic Plan

As in the bitch, a good history may provide the key to problem resolution. This history should include (1) evidence of reproductive problems in the parents or littermates, (2) all medical problems of the queen, (3) vaccination status of the queen, (4) housing, nutrition, and contact with other cats, (5) the past or present use of hormonal therapy, (6) surgeries performed, (7) the dates and length of estrus cycles, (8) the characteristics of any pregnancy, (9) a description of sexual behavior, (10) the presence of any vaginal discharges, (11) breeding record of the male, and (12) the presence of any environmental stress factors.

A thorough physical examination should be performed, with careful abdominal palpation of the uteus, visual examination of the vulva and vagina, and vaginal cytology. A feline leukemia virus test is essential. If no cause is determined, a CBC, blood chemistry profile, and urine analysis (cystocentesis sample) should be performed. Further tests to be considered include a TSH response test for thyroid function, reproductive hormone assays, and celiotomy with examination of the ovaries and uterine biopsy and culture.

Treatment Plan

Successful treatment depends on identification of the cause of the infertility or abnormal cycle.

INFERTILITY IN THE MALE DOG

Definition

Infertility in the male dog is usually identified by failure of conception in bitches bred to him. Semen analysis is the major diagnostic test used to further characterize the problem. In the normal dog, an ejaculate has three fractions produced in the order of (1) presperm, (2) sperm-rich, and (3) prostatic fluid. The presperm and sperm-rich fractions are often difficult to distinguish, because of the small volume of the presperm fraction. These two fractions are usually considered together. The sperm-rich fraction is normally opalescent and milky white; prostatic fluid is clear. The total volume of an ejaculate can vary from 0.5 to 30 ml, mainly due to the amount of prostatic fluid collected, since prostatic fluid may be released for up to 30 minutes.

Sperm motility, numbers, and morphology are more related to fertility than ejaculate volume. When checked on a warmed microscope slide after dilution with one drop of warmed normal saline, one drop of semen should contain greater than 80% motile sperm. Sperm numbers should be greater than 300×10^6/ml. Sperm numbers less than 100×10^6/ml are consistent with poor fertility. Over 80% of the sperm should be morphologically normal. If there are greater than 20% of sperm with primary (head and midpiece changes) or secondary (tail) abnormalities, disease of the testes or epididymis, respectively, should be suspected. Testicular sperm production is temperature sensitive. Any increase in scrotal temperature can adversely affect sperm production, which is why cryptorchid testes are not fertile.

Physiology and Causes

The major causes of infertility in the male dog can be grouped according to whether the problem is testicular, epididymal, prostatic, or with the penis and prepuce.

Testicular problems associated with decreased fertility can be congenital or acquired. Congenital problems include hypoplasia, cryptorchidism, chromosomal abnormalities in the germ cells, abnormal androgen or pituitary hormone production, and the immotile cilia syndrome. Acquired problems include inguinal hernia, testicular degeneration with aging, neoplasia, sperm granulomas, trauma, infection, toxins, systemic or metabolic disease, use of hormonal therapy for other diseases, sexual overuse, and environmental stress (especially high ambient temperatures). However, a recent study indicated that dogs adapted to tropical climates did not have decreased sperm numbers. Sperm are not recognized as self by the body's immune system. Whenever an inflammatory, traumatic, or neoplastic process disrupts testicular structure and sperm come in contact with the immune system, an antigen/antibody reaction ensues. Sperm granulomas form by this mechanism and have been postulated to result in an autoimmune orchitis with sperm destruction.

Inguinal hernias of intestines and omentum into the scrotal sac have been associated with decreased testicular function due to increased heat and irritation from intestinal motility. Scrotal inflammation or trauma may also decrease testicular sperm production by generation of heat. Seasonal hypospermia is related to decreased semen quality in long-haired dogs in very hot environments. Drugs and toxins associated with decreased sperm production include cadmium, cyclophosphamide, vinblastine, and amphotericin B. In some infertile male dogs, only oligospermia or azoospermia of unknown origin can be documented.

Congenital or acquired epididymal diseases can block the flow of sperm from the testicles. Congenital problems include aplasia of the epididymis. Acquired problems include trauma and infection such as canine brucellosis.

The deferent ducts may be congenitally aplastic or can become obstructed as they pass through a diseased prostate.

Prostatic infections have been suspected to cause subfertility even in the absence of obstruction of the deferent ducts. This association has not been proven in humans or dogs. The prostatic fluid is a transport fluid that is not essential for fertility. Recently in dogs, a role for prostatic fluid in sperm capacitation has been proposed.

Lesions of the penis and prepuce may prevent erection and/or mating (see chapter on abnormalities of the external genitalia).

Diagnostic Plan

The breeding history of the male should include (1) the breeding record of the bitches served, (2) the timing of each breeding, (3) the mating behavior of the male, (4) the number of bitches bred, (5) the number of bitches whelping, (6) the frequency of breeding, (7) housing and handling procedures, (8) all previous and current medical problems, and (9) all previous and current drugs is use. This history will usually determine if the problem is congenital or whether it has been acquired.

A semen evaluation should be performed prior to physical examination to minimize any anxiety or excitement. Behavior during ejaculation, appearance of the penis and prepuce during ejaculation, and semen color and volume should be recorded. Sperm motility, numbers, and morphology should be determined. Numbers of neutrophils should be noted.

Any scrotal, testicular, epididymal, spermatic cord, prostatic, preputial, or penile abnormalities should be detected by physical examination.

This diagnostic plan usually localizes the abnormality and determines the adequacy of sperm production. Further diagnostic tests to consider are CBC, blood chemistry profile, urine analysis, serum testosterone concentrations, thyroid function testing by TSH response, quantitative culture of semen, and biopsy of testicle or prostate. Serum testosterone concentrations have a wide normal range (0.5–5.0 ng/ml), making them difficult to evaluate. Possible contamination of semen samples by the normal bacterial flora of the distal urethra and prepuce during sample collection must be considered when interpreting results of semen culture. Semen cultures should be quantitative, and results should be correlated with the presence of inflammation on semen cytology.

Treatment Plan

Successful treatment depends on identification of the cause and its reversibility.

Prognosis

The prognosis depends on reversibility of the underlying cause. In idiopathic oligospermia or azoospermia, the prognosis is poor.

INFERTILITY IN THE MALE CAT

The causes of infertility in the male cat are similar to those in the dog. This section will discuss the differences between the two species.

Pathophysiology and Causes

The major causes of infertility in the tom are congenital lesions, infection, trauma, and disturbances of territorial behavior. Endocrine diseases such as hypothyroidism are possible but not common. Administration of female reproductive hormones as therapy for other diseases may adversely affect fertility. Nutritional causes such as malnutrition, obesity, and hypervitaminosis A are also possible. Congenital defects described in the tom include testicular hypoplasia, segmental aplasia of the epididymis or deferent ducts, and chromosomal abnormalities. The major chromosomal abnormality described is the XXY trait found in tortoiseshell males. The major infectious causes of infertility in toms are bacterial orchitis as a result of cat bite wounds to the scrotum and feline infectious peritonitis granulomas. A hair ring around the base of the glans penis will inhibit mating. Territorial changes in relation to other toms may also inhibit mating.

Diagnostic Plan

A good history and physical examination, as described for dogs, are mandatory. Collecting semen for examination is difficult in that electroejaculation under anesthesia is required unless the cat has been trained to allow collection in the presence of a queen in estrus. Normal semen volume is very small (0.1–0.7 ml), which further increases the difficulty in collection and analysis. Greater than 60% of the sperm should be motile, and greater than 70% should have normal morphology. The diagnostic plan may also include a CBC, blood chemistry profile, urine analysis, and feline leukemia virus test as well as thyroid function testing in cats in which no etiology can be found.

Treatment Plan

Treatment depends on determination of the cause.

SUGGESTED READINGS

Allen WE, Patel JR: Autoimmune orchitis in two related dogs. J Small Anim Pract 23:713–718, 1982

Cline EM, Jennings LL, Sojka NJ: Feline reproductive failures. Feline Pract 11:10–13, 1981

Colby ED: The estrous cycle and pregnancy. In Morrow DA (ed): Current Therapy in Theriogenology, pp 832–839. Philadelphia, WB Saunders, 1980

Greene CE, Kakuk TJ: Canine herpesvirus infection. In Greene CE (ed): Clinical Microbiology and Infectious Diseases of the Dog and Cat, pp 419–429. Philadelphia, WB Saunders, 1984

Johnston SD: Diagnostic and therapeutic approach to infertility in the bitch. J Am Vet Med Assoc 176:1335–1338, 1980

Johnston SD: Spontaneous abortion. In Morrow DA (ed): Current Therapy in Theriogenology, pp 606–608. Philadelphia, WB Saunders, 1980

Johnston SD: Management of pregnancy disorders in the bitch and queen. In Kirk RW (ed): Current Veterinary Therapy VIII, pp 952–955. Philadelphia, WB Saunders, 1983

Johnston SD: Feline fertility and infertility. Carnation Res Digest 20:1–3, 15, 1984

Larsen RE: Infertility in the male dog. In Morrow DA (ed): Current therapy in Theriogenology, pp 646–654. Philadelphia, WB Saunders, 1980

Lein DH, Concannon PW: Infertility and fertility treatments and management in the queen and tom cat. In Kirk RW (ed): Current Veterinary Therapy VIII, pp 936–942. Philadelphia, WB Saunders, 1983

Olson PN, Nett TM, Soderberg SF: Infertility in the bitch. In Kirk RW (ed): Current Veterinary Therapy VIII, pp 925–931. Philadelphia, WB Saunders, 1983

Phemister RD: Abnormal estrous activity. In Morrow DA (ed): Current Therapy in Theriogenology, pp 620–622. Philadelphia, WB Saunders, 1980

Shille VM, Thatcher MJ, Simmons KJ: Efforts to induce estrus in the bitch, using pituitary gonadotropins. J Am Vet Med Assoc 184:1469–1473, 1984

Smith F, Larsen RE: The infertile stud dog. In Kirk RW (ed): Current Veterinary Therapy VIII, pp 962–964. Philadelphia, WB Saunders, 1983

Wong WT, Dhaliwal GK: Observations on semen quality of dogs in the tropics. Vet Rec 116:313–314, 1985

Part Eleven

MUSCULOSKELETAL PROBLEMS

44

Lameness

JONATHAN N. CHAMBERS

DEFINITION

Lameness is a dysfunction of the limb(s), creating a perceptible variation in movement or gait due to an alteration in one or more of the organs of locomotion.

PATHOPHYSIOLOGY

Lameness can be caused by pain alone, instability in the skeleton, or mechanical abnormalities. Pain is also often encountered in combination with an instability or mechanical problem.

Acute inflammation due to minor trauma, localized infection, or a foreign body (thorn in the foot) is the usual cause of lameness when pain alone is involved. A recent fracture causes instability and pain from inflammation, whereas instability alone is the primary cause of lameness when the acute inflammatory process (pain) regresses and chronic nonunion (pseudarthrosis) of the fracture becomes established. Loss of joint mobility causes marked changes in limb mechanics and may or may not be accompanied by pain. An acute inflammatory process (and pain) of the joint or muscle-tendon unit usually precedes the development of a stiff nonpainful joint. Lameness can also be caused by neurologic dysfunction (discussed elsewhere in this text).

CLASSIFICATION

Once lameness has been identified as the problem, it should be classified as to severity and course of onset, since this is helpful in establishing a list of possible causes, even before the thorough orthopaedic examination. The age, breed, and sex are also important to note. Many puppyhood problems are developmental

(*Text continues on p 394.*)

Table 44-1. Predispositions to Causes of Lameness as Related to Dog Breeds

PREDIS-POSITION	HIP DYS-PLASIA	PAN-OSTEITIS	OSTEO-CHON-DRITIS DIS-SECANS OF SHOULDER	OSTEOCHON-DRITIS DISSECANS OF ELBOW/ FRAGMENTED CORONOID PROCESS	OSTEO-CHON-DRITIS DIS-SECANS OF TARSUS	OSTEO-CHON-DRITIS DIS-SECANS OF THE STIFLE
Sex	–	M	M	M	M	M
Breeds						
Large	+	+	+	+	+	+
Small	–	–	–	–	–	–
Hunting	+	+	+	+	+	+
German shepard	+	+	+	+	–	–
Labrador retriever	+	+	+	+	+	+
Golden retriever	+	+	+	+	+	–
Irish setter	+	+	+	–	+	–
Pointer	–	+	–	–	–	–
St. Bernard	+	+	+	+	–	–
Newfound-land	+	+	+	+	–	–
Irish wolf-hound	–	+	±	–	–	+
Great dane	+	+	+	–	–	–
Doberman pinscher	–	+	–	–	–	–
Rottwieler	±	+	+	+	+	–
Boxer	+	+	+	–	–	–
Basset hound	+	+	–	+	–	–
Toy miniature poodle	–	–	–	–	–	–
Pekingese	–	–	–	–	–	–
Wire haired fox terrier	–	–	–	–	–	–
West highland terrier	–	–	–	–	–	–
Lakeland terrier	–	–	–	–	–	–
Carin terrier	–	–	–	–	–	–
Yorkshire terrier	–	–	–	–	–	–
Boston terrier	–	–	–	–	–	–
Pomeranian	–	–	–	–	–	–
Chihuahua	–	–	–	–	–	–

±, No known report of predisposition, but body size and type are similar to those of breeds with documented predisposition.

UNUNITED ANCONEAL PROCESS	INFRASPI-NATUS CON-TRACTURE	HYPER-TROPHIC OSTEO-DYSTROPHY	LATERAL PATELLAR LUXATION	MEDIAL PATELLAR LUXATION	LEGG-CALVÉ-PERTHES DISEASE	EROSIVE IMMUNE-MEDIATED ARTHROPATHY
–	–	M?	–	F	–	–
+	+	+	+	–	–	–
–	–	–	+	+	+	+
–	+	–	–	–	–	–
+	–	+	–	–	–	–
–	+	+	–	–	–	–
–	–	+	–	–	–	–
–	–	+	–	–	–	–
–	–	+	–	–	–	–
+	–	–	+	–	–	–
+	–	+	+	–	–	–
–	–	–	–	–	–	–
–	–	+	–	–	–	–
–	–	+	–	–	–	–
–	–	–	–	–	–	–
–	–	+	–	–	–	–
+	–	+	–	–	–	–
–	–	–	–	+	+	±
–	–	–	–	+	+	±
–	–	–	–	–	+	±
–	–	–	–	–	+	±
–	–	–	–	–	+	±
–	–	–	–	+	+	±
–	–	–	–	+	±	+
–	–	–	–	+	±	±
–	–	–	–	+	±	±
–	–	–	–	+	±	±

and relatively breed specific. Some of the more common predispositions are given in Table 44-1.

Severity of Lameness

The degree of lameness may not correlate with the seriousness of the disease process, but a rule out list can usually be established from this knowledge alone. For example, a thorn in the foot pad and a bone cancer might both be included in the rule out list for a dog presented for a severe off-weight bearing lameness. A I to IV grade system is suggested:

Grade I—Barely perceptible lameness
Grade II—Noticeable lameness, but weight bearing most of the time. This would be typical of a disease in the developing state, *e.g.*, degenerative joint disease or panosteitis or recovery state, *e.g.*, healing traumatic injury.
Grade III—Severe lameness, with use limited to touching the paw to the ground for balance
Grade IV—No weight bearing; the limb is carried

The more common causes of lameness can be classified by the most typical grade of severity at presentation (see list). Some variation is seen, depending on the stage of a disease and pain tolerance of the individual.

Course of Onset

How quickly a lameness develops is often an indicator of the type of problem. Acute onset lameness is typical of traumatic diseases and infections. These include foot lacerations and foreign bodies, blunt trauma, fractures, muscle strains, and sprains, including the most common sprain, rupture of the cranial cruciate ligament. The history of a patient presenting with chronic lameness must be scrutinized for an acute onset, which may indicate one of the aforementioned problems in a static or resolving stage.

A chronic, insidious onset without an acute initiation is most typical of degenerative problems, especially those involving the joints. These include hip dysplasia, the osteochrondroses, developmental patellar luxation, Legg-Calvé-Perthes disease, or the immune-mediated arthropathies.

Several problems not only present as an insidious lameness but also have a cyclic or shifting nature. Included are panosteitis, infectious polyarthritis, and immune-mediated arthropathy or myopathy. A cyclic course may also indicate differing stages of a single disease. For example, puppies with developing hip dysplasia are often very painful at the age of 6 to 10 months due to stretching and microtrauma of the pliable tissues of the developing joint. The lameness appears to abate as the tissues mature, only to recur a few months later as secondary degenerative joint disease develops.

The more common causes of lameness are listed according to the most typical course of onset.

Typical Severity of Lameness at Initial Presentation

- Grade I
  - Minor trauma, contusion, laceration, strain, etc
  - Osteochrondrosis of the distal femur
  - Biceps brachii tenosynovitis
  - Polymyositis
- Grade II
  - Degenerative joint disease (hip dysplasia)
  - Infraspinatus contracture
  - Panosteitis
  - Avulsion of long digital extensor tendon
  - Immune-mediated arthropathy
  - Legg-Calvé-Perthes disease
  - Osteochondroses of shoulder, elbow, and tarsus
  - Developmental patellar luxation
- Grade III
  - Cranial cruciate rupture
  - Hypertrophic osteodystrophy
  - Infections
  - Bone neoplasia
  - Congenital patellar luxation
- Grade IV
  - Fracture
  - Luxation
  - Foreign body in foot
  - Snake bite

DIAGNOSTIC PLAN

Orthopaedic Examination

After a thorough history (with a special note of the age, breed, and sex) is collected, the clinician will find a properly performed orthopaedic examination to be the most valuable diagnostic tool. Coupled with sound knowledge of normal anatomy, the skill of orthopaedic examination is gained only by examining many normal dogs and watching them gait.

The proper environment for the examination is essential. Grades III and IV lameness can usually be pursued in the standard examination room. Ideally, all examinations for a more subtle lameness should be performed where there is enough space and solid footing to gait the patient at a run and trot. Weather permitting, one should perform the entire examination in a large grassed area. The patient must be comfortable and relaxed about the surroundings and examination; otherwise, erroneous results will ensure.

Typical Clinical Onset of Common Lameness

- Acute
  - Trauma
    - Fracture, luxation, sprain, etc
  - Snakebite
  - Foreign body in foot
  - Panosteitis
  - Hypertrophic osteodystrophy
  - Cranial cruciate rupture
- Cyclic or shifting onset
  - Panosteitis
- Chronic insidious
  - Degenerative joint disease (hip dysplasia)
  - Osteochrondroses
  - Infections
  - Congenital and developmental patellar luxation
  - Bone neoplasms
  - Legg-Calvé-Perthes disease
  - Infraspinatus contracture
  - Biceps brachii tenosynovitis
  - Immune-mediated arthropathy and myopathy
  - Avulsion of long digital extensor muscle

The patient is first walked, trotted, and run; the examiner watches from all angles. The exercise should be strenous if the lameness is historically exercise related. Next, the patient is observed and palpated in a standing position. Weight distribution among the limbs is noted. Start the palpation at the head and proceed caudally, feeling for swelling, atrophy, and pain. The standing palpation of the forelimbs and then the hindlimbs is done simultaneously to check for gross or subtle changes in symmetry. Each limb is raised to check for the animal's willingness or reluctance to distribute the weight to the other three.

The next part of the examination is done with the patient in lateral recumbency. Each limb is thoroughly examined, palpated, and manipulated from the toes proximally. The patient is turned and the procedure repeated on the other side. An equivocal assymetric finding such as subtle pain or instability is repeated as many times as necessary to confirm or refute its presence. Finally, the dog is gaited again. Subtle lameness is often exacerbated by exercise followed by vigorous manipulation of the affected limb.

Physical Signs Related to Lameness

Almost all lameness involves inflammation in one stage or another. Therefore, the clinician is trying to detect the cardinal signs of inflammation (pain, swelling, heat, redness, and loss of function).

Lameness is synonymous with loss of normal limb function, but more specific manifestations are often present. Joints have a normal combination of mobility (range of motion) and stability. Abnormal mobility and stability (restrictive ankylosis) are both manifestations of loss of normal function. Atrophy of muscles is another indication of less than normal use and a valuable localizing sign. Although the atrophy may be somewhat generalized in long-standing lameness, the most severe atrophy is often localized to the muscle group primarily responsible for moving the diseased (painful) joint or part, for example, the shoulder muscles in humeral head osteochondritis dissecans or the gluteal muscles in hip dysplasia.

Radiographic Examination

After the physical (orthopaedic) examination, radiographs are the most common and useful diagnostic aid for lameness. Prior localization of the problem to a specific limb, and optimally a part of the limb, limits the number of radiographs necessary for further definition of the problem. Standard views (craniocaudal and mediolateral) are taken first, followed with special techniques if necessary. The quality of the radiographs must be high because many lesions are quite subtle. Oblique projections may help to delineate some lesions; stress positioning of joints may help in documenting and defining a clinical instability. As with the physical examination, equivocal lesions should be evaluated by radiographing the opposite limb and checking for symmetry.

Special Diagnostic Aids

Diagnostic aids may be required to ultimately define the problem (see list). Common sense must prevail in deciding when a particular test is indicated. For example, fine needle aspiration for cytology and culture is indicated in cases of localized soft tissue swelling, and arthrocentesis is indicated when the cause of a joint problem is not readily apparent. The indications for a more sophisticated test such as a bone scan are less apparent, and the probable value must be decided on a case-by-case basis. There are situations in which the most accurate, expeditious, and cost-effective method of diagnosis is exploratory surgery and biopsy.

SYMPTOMATIC TREATMENT

Control of pain, inflammation, or instability is often indicated in conjunction with or prior to specific diagnosis and treatment of lameness. The unstable limb should be splinted, with the coaptation incooperating the joint above the instability and the entire limb distal to it. This places the limb at rest and prevents further injury. The splint may be bulky and soft or rigid, depending on the degree of instability and soft tissue involvement. A bulky soft wrap is usually better when the soft tissues are highly inflamed and swelling is a prominent sign.

Diagnostic Aids for Lameness

- Serial orthopedic examinations
- Radiography
  - Routine
  - Oblique views
  - Stress view
  - Arthrogram
  - Radionucleotide (bone) scan
- Fine needle aspiration
  - Cytology
  - Culture and sensitivity
- Arthrocentesis
  - Cytology
  - Culture
  - Mucin clot
- Arthroscopy
- Immune profile
  - Lupus erythematosus prep
  - Rheumatoid factor
  - Antinuclear antibody
- Exploratory surgery and biopsy
  - Muscle
  - Joint capsule
  - Other soft tissue
  - Bone

Pain due to inflammation can usually be controlled with the nonsteroidal prostaglandin inhibitors. Aspirin, given to dogs at a dose of 20 mg/kg/day split in three or four equal doses, has been recommended. Enteric-coated tablets are best, but gastric irritation can be a problem in some individuals even at recommended doses. The acetaminophen-codeine combination appears to be a safer alternative with equal or better results. Phenylbutazone and meclofenamic acid are other antiprostaglandin drugs that have been used with varying success. In general, these drugs are highly toxic to cats and should be avoided. Aspirin is the least toxic, but the dose schedule must be greatly modified (10 mg/kg every 52 hours).

45

Bone, Joint, and Periskeletal Swelling or Enlargement

JAMES P. TOOMBS

Swelling is the transient abnormal increase in volume of a body part not caused by proliferation of cells. Swelling may involve joints and periskeletal tissues, but not bone. Increased bony volume depends upon cellular proliferation and is more accurately described as bony enlargement. Enlargement is an increase in the size of an organ or body part attributable to hypertrophic, hyperplastic, metaplastic, or neoplastic processes. Enlargement may involve bone, periskeletal tissues, or joints.

PATHOPHYSIOLOGY

Bone Enlargement

The response of bone to injury or disease is limited to several basic processes: (1) production of new bone—osteogenesis and (2) resorption of existing bone—osteolysis. These processes are generally concurrent, although one or the other may predominate. Bony enlargement occurs when osteogenesis exceeds osteolysis. Osteogenic response to injury or nonneoplastic disease is most pronounced in animals that have not reached skeletal maturity and progressively declines from maturity to old age. Osteogenic response is also dependent upon the region of the bone involved. Regions of bone that are predominently cancellous (long bone epiphyses and metaphyses) are generally capable of greater and more immediate osteogenic response than regions of bone that are entirely cortical (long bone diaphyses). Bone enlargement associated with fracture healing involves periosteal, intercortical, and endosteal surfaces. Bone enlargement associated with disease frequently involves only the periosteal surface.

Joint Swelling or Enlargement

The essential components of synovial joints include articular cartilage, joint capsule, synovial membrane, and synovial fluid. Normal synovial fluid is a dialysate of plasma into which synovial membrane B cells secrete hyaluronate. This fluid is clear, highly viscous, relatively acellular, similar in glucose content to plasma, and slightly lower in protein content than plasma and has an albumin : globulin ratio of approximately 4 : 1. Its volume in normal synovial joints is generally less than 1 ml.

Joint swelling (effusion) occurs when dynamics of the synovial membrane are altered by trauma or disease. It is associated with up to a 20-fold increase in fluid volume and qualitative changes dependent upon the disease process. Joint effusion may be serous, fibrinous, purulent, or hemorrhagic. It most commonly occurs secondary to inflammation of the synovial membrane (synovitis).

Joint swelling is often accompanied by joint enlargement. Joint enlargement involves hyperplasia, metaplasia, or neoplasia of the synovial membrane, joint capsule, articular cartilage, or periarticular bone.

Periskeletal Swelling or Enlargement

Swelling or enlargement of muscular and fascial tissues surrounding bones and joints may occur independently of or concurrently with similar processes involving bones and joints. Swelling may involve hemorrhage, edema, or inflammatory exudate, while enlargement of these tissues generally involves hyperplastic, metaplastic, or neoplastic processes.

For the remainder of this chapter, "swelling" will be used as a synonym for "swelling" or "enlargement."

DIFFERENTIAL DIAGNOSIS OF MUSCULOSKELETAL "SWELLING"

History

Certain aspects of the medical history facilitate diagnosis of musculoskeletal "swelling." Information regarding signalment, previous geographic residence, diet, activities or events preceding onset of "swelling", and duration and progression of swelling are critical to formulating a concise list of rule outs.

Signalment

Breed and sex predispositions to various diseases associated with musculoskeletal "swelling" are catalogued in Tables 45-1 through 45-3. While some diseases are usually confined to immature animals, others rarely occur except in mature, middle-aged, or older animals. In an 8-year-old dog with a swollen, painful lesion involving the distal tibial metaphysis, primary bone neoplasia might head a list of rule outs. Although neoplasia should not be totally discounted in a puppy with the same lesion, hypertrophic osteodystrophy or osteomyelitis would be more likely causes.

(*Text continues on p 404.*)

Table 45-1. Predispositions of Diseases That Cause Bone Enlargement

DISEASE	BREED	SEX	AGE	COMMON ANATOMIC SITES	DISTRIBUTION
Bone cysts	Doberman, LB	M	I	Metaphyses, long bones	F or MC
Cartilage analogue of fibromatosis			A	Skull	F
Craniomandibular osteopathy	Terriers		I	Mandibular rami and tympanic bullae	MC, BS
Enostosis	German shepard		I	Radius and ulna	U
Feline Maroteaux-Lamy syndrome	Siamese Siamese-X		I	Costochondral junction of ribs and ends of long bones	MC
Fractures					F or MC
Fractures (humeral)	Spaniels		A	Distal humerus	F
Fractures (stress)	Italian greyhound		A	Distal radius and ulna	F
Hypertrophic osteodystrophy	LB, GB		I	Distal metaphyses—radius, ulna, and tibia	MC
Hypertrophic osteopathy			A	Distal extremities	MC, BS
Hypervitaminosis A	Cats		A	Cervical vertebrae	F or MC
Ossifying fibroma			A	Maxilla and mandible	F
Osteochondromatosis (canine)			I	Vertebrae, ribs, metaphyses—long bones and pelvis	F or MC
Osteochondromatosis (feline)			A	Ribs, scapulae, vertebrae, skull, and pelvis	F or MC
Osteoma			A	Bones formed by intramembranous ossification, especially skull	F
Osteomyelitis (fungal)				Long bone epiphyses	MC
Osteomyelitis (hematogenous-bacterial)			I	Long bone epiphyses or diaphyses	MC
Osteomyelitis (trauma-associated)					F or MC
Panosteitis	German shepard, LB	M	I	Diaphyses—humerus and ulna	MC
Polyostotic fibrous dysplasia	Doberman		I	Distal metaphyses—radius and ulna	MC, UB
Tumors of bone (malignant primary)	LB, GB		A	Long bone metaphyses, skull, vertebrae, ribs, and pelvis	F
Tumors metastatic to bone			A	Vertebrae, ribs, and long bones, especially humerus and femur	MC

I, immature animals; LB, large breeds; M, Male; F, focal (monostotic); MC, multicentric (polyostotic); A, adult, middle-aged, and older animals; BS, bilaterally symmetric; U, unilateral; GB, giant breeds; UB, unilateral or bilateral

Table 45-2. Predispositions of Diseases That Cause Joint Swelling or Enlargement

DISEASE	BREED	SEX	AGE	ANATOMIC SITES	COMMON FEATURES
Arthritis (feline progressive polyarthritis)		M	YA	Carpus, tarsus	b; E=e,g,h,k; L=n,o
Arthritis (immune-mediated secondary to chronic infectious diseases)				Major weight-bearing joints	b; E=e,g,h,k,m; L=o
Arthritis (infectious)					E=f,g,h,l; L=n,o
Arthritis (lupus)	German shepherd	F	YA	Elbow, carpus, stifle	b; E=e,g,h,k,m; L=o
Arthritis (rheumatoid)			A	Carpus, tarsus	b; E=e,g,h,k,m,n; L=o
Fractures (articular)					a,c; E=f,g,j; L=o,p
Fractures (physeal)			I	Long bone physes	a,c; E=f,g,j; L=o,p
Hemarthrosis					
Hypofibrinogenemia	St. Bernard				
Hemophilia A	*				
von Willebrand's disease	†	M	I	Major weight-bearing joints	b; E=f,g,h; L=k,m,n,o
Hemophilia B	‡				
Thrombasthenia	§				
Hip dysplasia	German Shepherd, St. Bernard, LB			Hip	d; E=e,h,l; L=k,m,o,p
Legg-Calvé-Perthes disease	Terriers, TB		I	Hip	c; E=h,k,n; L=j,k,p
Luxations				Hip, shoulder elbow, hock	a,c; E=f,g,j; L=p
Luxations (lateral patellar associated with genu valgum)	Flat-coated retriever, Great Dane, St. Bernard, Irish wolfhound		I	Stifle	d; L=e,k,p

Luxations (medial patellar)	TB	F	I	Stifle	d; L=e,k,p
Neoplastic joint disease			A	Elbow, stifle	a,c; E=f,g,h; L=i,m,n,o
Osteoarthrosis (primary DJD)	WB		A	Major weight-bearing joints	b,d; E=e,l; L=i,k,m
Osteoarthrosis (secondary DJD)			A	Major weight-bearing joints	E=e,l; L=i,j,k,m,o
Osteochondromatosis (synovial)		M	A	Hip, metacarpus	e,h,i,j
Osteochondrosis	LB, GB	M	I	Shoulder, elbow, stifle, hock	b,d; L=e,h,j,k,n,p
Subluxations				Carpus, tarsus, stifle	a,c; E=e,g,l; L=h,p
Subluxations (carpal)	Irish setter			Carpus	a,c; E=e,g,l; L=h,p

Breed: * Irish setter, German shepherd, collie, vizsla, sheltie, greyhound, poodle, chihuahua, beagle, Labrador retriever, weimaraner, schnauzer

† German shepherd, miniature schnauzer, golden retriever, Scottish terrier, Welsh corgi, doberman

‡ Cocker spaniel, St. Bernard, Cairn terrier, coonhound, Alaskan malamute, French bulldog

§ Otterhound, Basset hound, foxhound, Scottish terrier

LB, large; TB, toy, WB, working; G, giant

Sex: M, male; F, female

Age: YA, young adult; A, adult, middle-aged, and older; I, immature

Common features:

Distribution: a, usually monoarticular; b, usually polyarticular; c, usually unilateral; d, usually bilateral

Progression: E, early changes; L, late changes

Findings: e, mild to moderate joint effusion; f, marked joint effusion; g, extracapsular swelling or edema; h, joint capsule enlargement; i, joint capsule calcification; j, intra-articular radiodensities (chip fractures, Joint mice); k, periarticular osteophytes; l, normal subchondral bone; m, sclerotic subchondral bone; n, destruction (lysis) of subchondral bone; o, bone remodeling–juxta-articular; p, possible progression to secondary degenerative joint disease

DJD, degenerative joint disease

Table 45-3. Predispositions of Periskeletal Enlargements

DISEASE	BREED	SEX	AGE	ANATOMIC SITES	COMMON FEATURES
Aneurysmal bone cyst	*		A	Sacral, iliac wing, and coccygeal regions	b,c,e,j,l
Fibrosarcoma			A	Cutaneous, subcutaneous, or oral	a,i,j,k,o
Granuloma					a,o
Hemangiomatosis				Skull, spine, extremities	b,c,e,f,j,o
Hemangiopericytoma			A	Extremities and chest wall	a,h,j,k,o
Hematoma				Fascial planes	a,d,l
Hematoma (subperiosteal)			I		b,d,l
Hygroma	LB, GB		A	Elbow region	a,e,k,m
Lipoma		OF	A	Subcutaneous tissues of thorax, abdomen, and upper portions of extremities	a,o
Myositis (fibrositis) ossificans				Muscles of gluteal and elbow regions	a,f,g,l
Nutritional myopathy (hypovitaminosis E)			I, YA	Muscles of extremities	a,g,m,n
Polymyositis (acute form)				Muscles of mastication	a,g,m,n
Spurious aneurysm				Extremities	a,e,g,l
Tumoral calcinosis			I, YA	Perispinal muscles of cervical region	a,f,o
Undifferentiated sarcoma			A		a,i,j,k,o

Sex: OF, obese females
Breed: LB, large breeds; GB, giant breeds; *, reported mainly in cats
Age: A, adult, middle-aged, or older; I, immature animals; YA, young adult animals
Common features: a, regional bone tissue generally unaffected; b, reactive periosteal new bone; c, regional bone destruction; d, acute extraosseus swelling; e, chronic extraosseus swelling; f, soft tissue calcification or ossification; g, muscular swelling or enlargement; h, nonmetastatic; i, potentially metastatic; j, locally invasive; k, locally recurrent; l, focal lesion; m, bilateral lesions; n, multicentric lesions; o, focal or multicentric

Geographic Residence

Some diseases that cause musculoskeletal swelling are endemic to specific regions of the United States. In a dog with a sclerotic diaphyseal lesion suspected to be osteomyelitis, coccidoidomycosis would be a likely cause if the dog lived in the southwest, whereas blastomycosis would be suspected in a dog residing in the midwest. In a dog with periskeletal swelling in the distal portion of a hindlimb, thromboembolism might be suspected if the dog was from an area where heartworm disease is endemic.

Diet

In animals maintained on commercially prepared balanced diets, certain diseases are unlikely. In a cat with proliferative bony lesions involving the cervical spine, hypervitaminosis A would be suspected only if the cat was being fed a diet of raw liver or being given vitamin A supplements. In a similar cat with a normal diet, osteochondromatosis would be more likely. Other diseases associated with musculoskeletal swelling in which an abnormal diet has been incriminated include hypertrophic osteodystrophy (hypersupplementation, especially with calcium), nutritional secondary hyperparathyroidism (all meat diet—low calcium, excessive phosphorus), and nutritional myopathy (hypovitaminosis E).

Activity

In animals with known trauma, musculoskeletal swelling is often attributable to fractures, dislocations, ligamentous injuries, and associated hemorrhage and inflammation. In a sedentary house dog with a long bone fracture and no history of trauma, underlying metabolic or neoplastic disease should be considered. A sedentary older dog taken to the mountains for the weekend might present on Monday morning with a swollen painful joint. Exacerbation of chronic degenerative joint disease by overactivity might be a likely explanation of this dog's problem. In contrast, a younger active dog with similar history and signs would more likely have suffered an acute traumatic injury.

Duration and Progression

Fractures and other traumatic injuries are generally associated with extensive swelling of acute onset. Snake and insect bites and some bacterial infections often result in acute focal swelling. Chronic progressive swelling is more commonly associated with neoplastic and certain metabolic and infectious musculoskeletal diseases.

PHYSICAL FINDINGS

Careful palpation may determine whether swelling or enlargement or both are present and whether bones, joints, periskeletal tissues, or some combination of these are involved. Swelling is usually fluctuant, and pitting may be noted following deep palpation. Rule outs and physiologic mechanisms for periskeletal swelling are listed in Table 45-4. Enlargements are firm and may be appreciated as discrete masses or increased thickness of a part. Rule outs for enlargements have been tabulated by location—bone (see Table 45-1), joints (see Table 45-2), and periskeletal tissues (see Table 45-3).

Swelling is often accompanied by other cardinal signs of inflammation (redness, heat, and pain). Crepitance, laxity, and abnormal increases or decreases in range of motion are highly suggestive of fractures, dislocations, or subluxations.

Location and distribution of lesions are highly significant (see Tables 45-1 through 45-3). Some diseases are confined to a single focus, whereas others are almost always multicentric (polyostotic). Involvement of specific bones or joints, symmetry and assymetry, and confinement of lesions to specific regions of bones or joints are hallmarks of certain diseases (Tables 45-1 through 45-3 and Tables 45-5 through 45-9).

(*Text continues on p 408.*)

Table 45-4. Periskeletal Swelling

TYPE	PHYSIOLOGIC MECHANISMS AND CAUSATIVE DISEASES
Hemorrhage	Traumatic vascular disruption
	Vascular disruption secondary to
	Infection
	Neoplasia
	Minor trauma and bleeding disorder
	Congenital clotting factor deficiencies
	Acquired clotting factor deficiencies
	Platelet dysfunction
Edema	Lymphatic disruption or occlusion
	Traumatic lesions
	Inflammatory diseases
	Neoplastic diseases
	Anomaly—congenital primary lymphedema
	Increased capillary hydrostatic pressure
	Cardiac failure
	Thromboembolism
	Allergic reactions
	Increased capillary permeability
	Burns
	Allergic reactions
	Bacterial toxins
	Hypoalbuminemia
	Excessive loss—renal, gastrointestinal, from burns or open wounds, etc.
	Decreased production—hepatic, pancreatic, or intestinal disease or malnutrition
Inflammatory exudate	Reaction of tissues to irritants—dilation and increased permeability of capillaries and release of chemical mediators
	Infectious diseases
	Chemical poisons
	Mechanical and thermal injuries
	Immune reactions

Table 45-5. Rule Outs for Long Bone Lesions by Region

EPIPHYSIS	METAPHYSIS	DIAPHYSIS
Fractures	Bone cysts	Enostosis
Osteomyelitis (hematogenous)	Fractures	Fractures
Joint diseases (see Table 45-6)	Hypertrophic osteodystrophy	Hypertrophic osteopathy
Congenital	Osteochondromatosis	Panosteitis
Infectious	Tumors of bone (primary)	Tumors of bone (metastatic)
Immune-mediated		
Neoplastic		
Degenerative		

For predispositions of a specific disease see Table 45-1.

Table 45-6. Rule Outs for Subchondral Bone Lesions by Changes in Bone Density

PREDOMINANTLY SCLEROTIC	PREDOMINANTLY LYTIC	MIXED PATTERN—SCLEROTIC AND LYTIC
Hip dysplasia Immune-mediated arthritis, polyarthritis secondary to chronic infectious disease Lupus arthropathy Osteoarthrosis Primary DJD Secondary DJD	Feline progressive polyarthritis Infectious arthropathy Legg-Calvé-Perthes disease Osteochondrosis	Hemophilic arthropathy Joint neoplasia Rheumatoid arthritis

For predispositions of a specific disease see Table 45-2.
DJD, degenerative joint disease

Table 45-7. Rule Outs for Bone Lesions of the Axial Skeleton by Region

SKULL OR MANDIBLE	VERTEBRAE	RIBS
Cartilage analogue of fibromatosis Craniomandibular osteopathy Feline osteochondromatosis Fractures Hemangiomatosis Ossifying fibroma Osteoma Osteomyelitis Tumors of bone (primary)	Aneurysmal bone cyst Fractures Hemangiomatosis Hypervitaminosis A Osteochondromatosis Osteomyelitis Tumoral calcinosis Tumors (metastatic to bone) Tumors of bone (primary)	Feline Maroteaux-Lamy syndrome Fractures Osteochondromatosis Osteomyelitis Tumors metastatic to bone Tumors of bone (primary)

For predispositions of a specific disease, see Tables 45-1 and 45-3.

Table 45-8. Rule Outs for Osteoproliferative Lesions by Distribution (Patterns of Increased Bone Density)

POLYOSTOTIC LESIONS	MONOSTOTIC LESIONS
Craniomandibular osteopathy* Feline Maroteaux-Lamy syndrome* Healing fractures*,†,‡,§ Hematogenous osteomyelitis*,†,§ Hypertrophic osteodystrophy* Hypertrophic osteopathy* Osteochondromatosis# Panosteitis*,† Tumors metastatic to bone†,§	Enostosis† Healing fractures*,†,‡,§ Ossifying fibroma*,‖ Osteochondromatosis# Osteoma* Osteomyelitis*,†,§ Subperiosteal hematoma* Traumatic periostitis* Tumors of bone—malignant primary*,§,‖ Tumors metastatic to bone†,§

* Periosteal new bone
† Endosteal new bone
‡ Thickening of cortical bone
§ Thickening and increased number of cancellous trabeculae
‖ Soft tissue ossification
\# Perichondrial new bone and cartilage

Table 45-9. Rule Outs for Osteolytic Lesions and Pathologic Fractures by Distribution

GENERALIZED LOSS OF BONE DENSITY—ENTIRE SKELETON	MULTICENTRIC OR MULTIFOCAL OSTEOLYTIC LESIONS	MONOSTOTIC FOCAL OSTEOLYTIC LESIONS
Hyperadrenocorticism	Bone cysts	Bone cysts
Hyperparathyroidism	Fibrous dysplasia	Fibrous dysplasia
Primary	Hemangiomatosis	Hemangiomatosis
Secondary	Multiple myeloma	Osteomyelitis
	Osteomyelitis	Tumors of bone—primary
	Tumors metastatic to bone	Tumors metastatic to bone

RADIOGRAPHY

Radiographic examination is often the most efficient method of determining the cause of musculoskeletal swelling. Films of the swollen part should be taken in two projections and should include the bones or joints proximal and distal to the area of interest.

If bony lesions are detected, anatomic location and distribution should be initially considered. Rule outs for long bone lesions according to whether they affect the epiphysis, metaphysis, or diaphysis are listed in Table 45-5. If the lesions predominantly affect subchondral bone, rule outs can be established by changes in bone density (see Table 45-6). Rule outs for bony lesions of the axial skeleton are listed in Table 45-7. Focal (monostotic) versus multicentric (polyostotic) distribution of lesions is considered in Tables 45-8 and 45-9.

The second step in condensing the rule out list for bony lesions is identification of the predominant pattern of change in bone density. Subchondral bone lesions are differentiated on the basis of sclerotic, lytic, or mixed patterns of density (see Table 45-6). Bony lesions at other locations that are mainly osteoproliferative are listed in Table 45-8. Those that are mainly osteolytic are listed in Table 45-9. Presentation of an animal with osteolytic lesions is sometimes prompted by acute lameness attributable to pathologic fracture of the involved bone. Chronic pathologic fractures may manifest a mixed pattern of bone density changes—a lytic pattern attributable to the initial disease process and a proliferative pattern attributable to the body's attempt to heal the fracture.

Table 45-10. Common Radiographic Characteristics of Bone Lesions by Rate of Expansion or Change

SLOW EXPANSION OR CHANGE—BENIGN LESIONS	RAPID EXPANSION OR CHANGE—MALIGNANT LESIONS
Well-defined zone of transition	Poorly defined zone of transition
Distinct margin	Indistinct margin
Sclerotic border	Motheaten border
Intact cortex	Broken cortex
Smooth periosteal new bone	Irregular periosteal new bone

Table 45-11. Common Synovial Fluid Findings by Disease

		NONINFLAMMATORY		INFLAMMATORY			
SYNOVIAL FLUID (SF) FINDING	NORMAL JOINT	Degenerative Joint Disease	Hemarthrosis	Rheumatoid Arthritis	Lupus Arthropathy	Neoplastic Joint Disease	Septic Arthritis
Color	C	PY	R	YBT	YBT	YBT	CCS
Turbidity	*	†	‡	§	§	§	‡
Viscosity	Normal	Normal	Reduced	Reduced	Reduced	Reduced	Reduced
Mucin clot	Good	Good	Fair	Poor	Fair	Good	Poor
RBCs	None	Few	Many	Moderate	Moderate	Moderate	Moderate
WBCs $\times 10^3/\mu l$	0.25–3	1–5	3–10	8–38	4.4–371	3–10	40–267
% PMNs	0–6	0–12	60–75	20–80	15–95	15–75	90–99
% Mononuclear cells	94–100	88–100	25–40	20–80	5–85	25–85	1–10
Ragocytes	–	–	–	+	–	–	–
LE cells	–	–	–	–	+	–	–
Neoplastic cells	–	–	–	–	–	+	–
Microorganisms	–	–	–	–	–	–	+
SF glucose (% of blood glucose)	100	80–100	100	50–80	50–80	50–80	<50

C, colorless; PY, pale yellow; R, red; YBT, yellow to blood-tinged; CCS, cream-colored to sanguinous
*, not turbid; †, slight turbidity; ‡, marked turbidity; §, moderate turbidity
–, absent; +, present

Further condensation of the rule out list is benefitted by evaluation of the pattern(s) of increased bone density (see Table 45-8) and the rate of expansion or change of the lesions (Table 45-10). Osteoproliferation may be manifested by cortical thickening, thickening or increase in the number of cancellous trabeculae, periosteal new bone, endosteal new bone, or some combination of these (see Table 45-8). Radiographic appearance of bony lesions is often highly dependent upon their rate of expansion or change. Lesions that develop slowly are usually well defined, have distinct borders, and are associated with smooth periosteal new bone formation. In contrast, rapidly developing lesions are poorly defined, have indistinct borders, often disrupt cortical continuity, and are associated with irregular periosteal new bone formation (see Table 45-10).

DEFINITIVE DIAGNOSIS

In formulating rule out lists for a lesion, the reader is encouraged to (1) evaluate the lesion by physical and radiographic examination, (2) based upon initial findings, consult pertinent areas of Tables 45-4 through 45-9, (3) make an initial rule out list, and (4) consult the appropriate disease catalogue (see Tables 45-1 through 45-3) and consider predispositions of suspected diseases to condense or rank order the rule out list. Final diagnosis may depend upon additional diagnostic aids, including needle aspirates for cytologic, microbiologic, and biochemical evaluation; incisional or trephine biopsies for histopathologic evaluation; skeletal survey radiography or bone scintigraphy to locate occult lesions in polyostotic diseases; and appropriate clinicopathologic testing to confirm or rule out certain systemic or metabolic diseases. Synovial fluid analysis and culture are especially helpful in differentiating various joint diseases. Synovial fluid findings for normal dogs are compared with findings commonly associated with different joint diseases in Table 45-11.

SYMPTOMATIC THERAPY

Definitive therapy of swelling depends upon correction of the underlying disease process when possible. Symptomatic therapy often involves restricted physical activity and application of cold packs or immersion of the swollen part in an ice bath during the acute phase of injury. Hot packs or compresses may be desirable in chronic situations in which healing is in progress and increased perfusion of an area is desirable. In most fractures or ligamentous injuries, application of appropriate support bandages or coaptation splints will limit swelling and prevent further tissue damage until definitive treatment can be attempted. When swelling is attributable to an inflammatory disease process, selected patients benefit from administration of corticosteroids or nonsteroidal antiinflammatory drugs. The severe pain that often accompanies musculoskeletal swelling may be alleviated by administration of narcotics such as oxymorphone or meperidine.

46

Pain

DENNIS N. ARON

PROBLEM DEFINITION AND RECOGNITION

Many diseases and disorders encountered in veterinary medicine cause pain. The ability to facilitate the diagnosis of many different diseases depends greatly on the veterinarian's knowledge of how to identify and localize the painful stimulus, understanding the physiology and disease mechanisms of actual pain (projected pain), awareness that pain can be referred from one part of the body to another (referred pain), and knowledge of the different conditions that lead to pain. The treatment of pain for the relief of suffering is frequently overlooked in veterinary medicine because animals are unable to communicate abstract concepts. The veterinarian must recognize subtle behavioral changes that indicate that an animal has pain and must understand the diagnostic and therapeutic principles that afford pain resolution and control.

Pain is a concept that includes the mechanisms of the nervous system for the transmission and integration of stimuli to the body and a psychologic component, including affect, emotion, and memory. It is difficult to interpret human emotions and even more difficult to transpose these to animals. It is best to assume that animals perceive pain, react to stimuli, and respond to therapy in a manner similar to human beings. Fortunately, much research on pain is in animal models, and the results suggest that these assumptions are correct.[4]

Terminology is not standardized, even in the research literature. The following terms are defined for use in this chapter:

Noxious stimuli—those that threaten or actually produce damage to tissues
Nociceptors—sense organs that primarily respond to noxious stimuli
Pain—the sensation caused by a noxious stimulus
Hyperalgesia—increased sensitivity to noxious stimuli
Hyperesthesia—increased sensitivity to stimulation, even that which is normally not noxious[4]

PATHOPHYSIOLOGY[1]

The pain receptors (nociceptors) are free nerve endings that are especially numerous in superficial layers of the skin, cornea, anus, and internal tissues such as the periosteum, the arterial walls, the joint surfaces, and the falx and tentorium of the cranial vault. Most of the other deep tissues are weakly supplied with pain endings, but widespread tissue damage can cumulatively cause pain in these areas. Three types of pain receptors exist in tissues: those responding to excessive mechanical stress, those responding to extreme heat, and those responding to abnormal chemicals. Different chemicals (*e.g.*, bradykinin, serotonin, histamine, potassium ions, acids, prostaglandins, acetylcholine, and proteolytic enzymes) stimulate the chemosensitive receptors. These chemicals are highly concentrated in inflamed tissue. In contrast to most other sensory receptors of the body, pain receptors do not adapt to the initial stimulus. This mechanism keeps the animal appraised of the damaging stimulus.

The viscera (unlike the skin, periosteum, and joints) contain only pain sensory receptors; localized damage to the viscera rarely causes severe pain. Conversely, any disease that results in diffuse stimulation of pain nerve endings throughout a viscus can result in extreme pain. In addition to true visceral pain, some pain sensations are also transmitted from the viscera through nerve fibers that innervate parietal peritoneum, pleura, or pericardium (parietal pain pathway).

Pain signals are transmitted from the periphery to the spinal cord by small A-delta type fibers at velocities between 6 and 30 meters per second and by type C fibers at velocities between 0.5 and 2 meters per second. In humans, the fast type A pain fibers conduct pain perceived as a pricking sensation, and the slower type C fibers conduct pain impulses perceived as a slow burning sensation. The slow burning sensation tends to become more painful over time, which gives the person the intolerable suffering of long-continued pain.

Pain fibers enter the cord through the dorsal roots and ascend or descend a few segments; the two fiber types terminate on neurons contained in separate sections in the dorsal horns of the cord gray matter. Most of the signals then probably pass through one or more additional short-fibered neurons, the last of which gives rise to long fibers that cross immediately to the opposite side of the cord and appear to pass up the spinal cord in the intermingled spinothalamic and spinoreticular tracts and dorsal column postsynaptic system. There is also a bilateral, multisynaptic, small fiber pathway, possibly in the propriospinal system, that conducts pain. It is difficult to destroy: it survives hemisections of the spinal cord on opposite sides if they are spaced three to five segments apart. Compression lesions, such as disk protrusion, abolish proprioception, descending motor function, and cutaneous (superficial) pain sensation before eliminating all pain sensation. These have been termed the *deep pain pathways,* referring to the severe stimulus to deep structures such as periosteum, which activate the system. The majority of fibers pass to the pontobulbar reticular system with ongoing pathways to the thalamus, hypothalamus, and mesencephalic areas. In humans, stimulation of the higher centers produces feelings of pricking pain, numbness and burning, and intense fear, along with autonomic signs associated with fear such as anguish, anxiety, crying, depression, nausea, and excess muscular excitability. The thalamus reinforces the emotional aspects of pain; the reticular formation is involved in arousal and possibly in the conscious appreciation of pain.

Two related types of compounds with morphine-like actions are the enkephalins and endorphins. The enkephalins are found in areas of the brain associated with pain control, and the endorphins are concentrated in the hypothalamus and pituitary gland. The enkephalins and the endorphins act as excitatory transmitter substances that activate portions of the brain's analgesic system. Stress and fear cause the release of these substances, which act as analgesics. In part, this system works through descending pathways to the neurons in the dorsal horn of the spinal cord. As fear and anxiety subside, pain may increase due to decreased release of these endogenous analgesics.

Stimulation of large sensory fibers from the peripheral tactile receptors depresses the transmissions of further pain signals from the same area of the stimulus or even from areas located several body segments away. The feedback circuits from the large afferents and the descending pathways constitute the gating mechanism in the dorsal horn, which tends to limit the response to noxious stimuli. This response and simultaneous excitation of the central analgesic system are probably the basis for pain relief by acupuncture.

The source of pain may appear at a site considerably removed from the diseased tissues. This is referred pain and it may confuse the localization of the diseased tissue. It is chiefly noted with pain initiated by one of the visceral organs referred to an area of the body surface. Referred pain occurs because sensation from the viscera is conducted through some of the same neurons that conduct pain signals from the surface (excitatory convergence).

SPECIFIC MECHANISMS

Tissue destruction produces pain through stimulation of mechanosensitive, thermosensitive, and chemosensitive pain receptors. The presence and intensity of pain are dependent on several variables. First, it is necessary for the tissue to contain pain receptors; the central nervous system does not. Second, the density of pain receptors varies with the tissue. Skin, joint surfaces, and periosteum contain numerous receptors; hence, focal stimulation of these tissues may cause severe pain. Tissues with less density of receptors, such as the viscera, require diffuse stimulation of tissue and, therefore, nerve endings before the pain becomes severe. Third, even though the lowest intensity of stimulus that will produce the sensation of pain (pain threshold) is constant across species, the tolerance of a painful stimulus varies widely, relative to the situation, within a single species.

Pain emanating from the joints can be an interesting phenomenon, as some conditions cause intense pain while others cause a waxing and waning pain. Stimuli involving the joint capsule, ligaments, and synovium are very painful, because receptors are numerous in these components of the joint. With degenerative joint disease (DJD), pain can be variable and episodic. This is because DJD may not be particularly painful until the condition is exacerbated by stimulus of the joint capsule and ligaments through increased instability, pressure, or stimulus of the synovium through increased inflammation. With DJD, inflammation is created by excessive wearing of the joint surfaces, which leads to matrix degeneration, allowing mucopolysaccharides to leach from the substance of the cartilage, creating a painful chemical synovitis. Prolonged rest can be an effective treatment for painful DJD; rest reduces degeneration of the cartilage matrix, allowing the synovitis to abate.

Ischemia is an important cause of pain to most tissues of the body. The mechanism is through the chemical stimulation of pain receptors. When blood flow to a tissue is disrupted, acidic metabolic end products (lactic acid) or tissue degenerative products (bradykinin, proteolytic enzymes, and others) are generated because of cell death. Both probably stimulate pain nerve endings. Ischemia of the spinal cord and brain does not produce pain because there are no pain receptors in these tissues. In humans, muscle spasm is a very common cause of severe pain and is the basis of many clinical pain syndromes. This pain probably results partially from the direct effect of muscle spasm in stimulating mechanosensitive pain receptors and partially from the indirect effect of muscle spasm in causing ischemia and thereby stimulating chemosensitive pain receptors. Muscle spasm creating pain is uncommonly seen in dogs and cats but has been reported to occur with exertional rhabdomyolysis in racing greyhounds, status epilepticus producing exertional rhabdomyolysis in dogs, and muscle cramping in Scottish terriers during excitement or heavy exercise.

Any stimulus that excites pain nerve endings in diffuse areas of the viscera causes visceral pain. Such stimuli include ischemia of visceral tissue, chemical damage to the surfaces of the viscera, spasm of the smooth muscle in a hollow viscus, distension of a hollow viscus, and stretching of the ligaments. Two sources of pain result from visceral damage. (1) True visceral pain originates from structures in the thoracic and abdominal cavities. (2) Pain sensations are also transmitted from the viscera through nerve fibers that innervate the parietal peritoneum, pleura, or pericardium. The parietal surfaces of the visceral cavities are supplied mainly by spinal nerves that penetrate from the surface of the body inward. A disease that affects a viscus often spreads to the parietal wall of the visceral cavity. The wall is supplied with extensive innervation from spinal nerves, which include the "fast" type A fibers, producing a sharp pain. The kidney and ureters, being retroperitoneally located, are supplied by both visceral and parietal pain fibers and seem to be very painful when affected by abnormalities.

Clinically, certain lesions that involve the spinal column can be very painful (Table 46-1), but others may be nonpainful. Meningitis is usually very painful because of the diffuse involvement of the meninges (similar mechanism as pleuritis or peritonitis). Focal disk disease is severely painful because of the numerous tissues being stimulated. These tissues include the periosteum, which is known to be especially dense with pain receptors, the dorsal nerve root, the

(*Text continues on p 418.*)

Table 46-1. Differential Diagnosis of Diseases That Produce Spinal Column Pain: Predispositions and Clinical Signs

RULE OUT	BREED	PREDOMINANT AGE AND SEX	LOCALIZATION OF PAIN	PREDOMINANT CLINICAL SIGNS
Cervical				
Atlantoaxial instability	Miniature and toy dog breeds	6–18 mo	Cranial	Cervical pain Neurologic deficits are variable.
Cervical malformation, malarticulation (Wobbler)	Great dane, Doberman pinscher (other large dog breeds)	Great dane—young Doberman pinscher—middle age Male	Caudal and middle	Bilateral ataxia and paresis of pelvic limbs, occasionally thoracic limbs Cervical pain not marked
Diskospondylitis	German shepherds, Great danes (large dog breeds)	Middle age Male	Caudal	Anorexia, depression, fever Lameness Stilted gait Paresis Hyperesthesia, abdominal tenseness
Disk disease	Dachshund, beagle, toy poodle (chondrodystrophoid and small breeds, in general) Cat—rare	Middle age Variable	Cranial (can occur at other sites)	Cervical pain
Fractures/luxation	Variable (dog and cat [rare])	Variable Variable	Cranial	Cervical pain Proprioceptive deficits, quadriplegia
Hypervitaminosis A	Cat	Variable Variable	Cranial	Lethargy, anorexia Hyperemia and edema of gums Abdominal distension Cervical pain Lameness Spinal exostosis History of exclusive liver diet or excessive vitamin A concentration

(Continued)

Table 46-1. Differential Diagnosis of Diseases That Produce Spinal Column Pain: Predispositions and Clinical Signs (*Continued*)

RULE OUT	BREED	PREDOMINANT AGE AND SEX	LOCALIZATION OF PAIN	PREDOMINANT CLINICAL SIGNS
Meningitis	Variable (dog and cat)	Variable Variable	Diffuse	Pain ± Neurologic deficits Increased white cell count and protein of CSF
Tumors of spinal cord or vertebrae	Variable (dog and cat)	Middle, old age Variable	Variable	Cervical pain Radicular pain Weight loss, anorexia, lethargy ± Neurologic deficits Usually extramedullary if pain is produced
Back				
Diskospondylitis	Similar to cervical lesion with pain localized to the region involved—midthoracic spine, L2–L4 (plant migration), L7–S1 affected most commonly			
Disk disease	Dachshund, pekingese, beagle, Welsh corgi, lhaso apso, shih tzu, (chondrodystrophoid and small breeds in general but type II disk disease in nonchondrodystrophoid breeds occurs)	Chondrodystrophoid 3–6 yr Nonchondrodystrophoid 6–8 yr Variable	Upper	Neurologic deficits Pain
Fractures/luxations	Variable (dog and cat [rare])	Variable Variable	Upper or lower	Upper Pain ± Paraparesis–paraplegia Lower Pain Proprioceptive deficits in hindlimbs Severe urinary and fecal incontinence

				± Paraparesis ± Perineal and flexor hyporeflexia
Hemivertebrae	English bulldog, Boston terrier, pug ("screwtail" breeds)	Variable Variable	Upper	Usually an incidental finding Pain ± Paraparesis
Lumbosacral stenosis	Toy or miniature poodle (small dog breeds)	Middle age Variable	Lower	Same as lumbosacral malarticulation, malformation Lameness worsens with exercise Paresthesia
Lumbosacral malarticulation, malformation	German shepherds (large dog breeds)	Middle age Male	Lower	Pain Proprioceptive deficits in hind limbs Urinary and fecal incontinence ± Paraparesis ± Perineal and flexor hyporeflexia
Meningitis	Similar to cervical lesion, diffuse pain is most common			
Progressive hemorrhagic myelomalacia	Variable	Variable Variable	Upper Diffuse	Painful, irritable, anxious Pyrexia Dysparity of radiographic focal lesion with diffuse clinical signs No treatment—will die in 1–3 days of respiratory paralysis
Tumors of spinal cord or vertebrae	Similar to cervical lesion with pain localized to the region involved			

±, widely variable; CSF, cerebrospinal fluid

meninges, and the anulus of the disk itself. Diskospondylitis is painful due to the diffuse stimulation of many of the same tissues.

DIAGNOSTIC PLAN

The recognition of pain in animals may be difficult; however, the localization of pain to a region, segment, or part of the body is often necessary for a correct diagnosis. Pain can be inferred from clinical signs such as lameness, dysphagia, and dysuria (see related chapters). However, sometimes there is no functional impairment for only behavioral changes such as depression, lethargy, irritability, reduced playfulness, or changes in eating habits. The emotional responses of increased blood pressure, heart rate, pupillary dilation, and changes in respiratory pattern are also signs of pain. Even though an emotional response is usually associated with perception of pain, the absence of such a response is not an assurance that the animal has not perceived pain.

An algorithm for the localization of pain to a region, segment, or part of the body is given in a separate list. Identification and localization of long bone periosteal or joint pain is usually straightforward, whereas abdominal pain is difficult to localize beyond the cranial or caudal regions. Frequently, pain that seems to be emanating from the abdomen actually has its source referred from the spinal column and vice versa. Signs of abdominal pain include restlessness, panting, abdominal splinting upon gentle palpation, and possibly a "praying" posture.

Thoracic pain is uncommon and is usually associated with pleural diseases. The pain is usually referred directly to the overlying thoracic wall. The discomfort is greatly accentuated by inspiratory movement; this leads to splinting of the affected side of the thorax and rapid, shallow, and grunting respiration.

Pain affecting the appendicular skeleton is common and easily diagnosed because it almost always is reflected as lameness (see chapters 44 and 45). Since any lesion involving the periosteum, ligaments, joint capsule, and synovium will lead to extreme focal pain, palpation of the lame limb usually leads to successful localization of the site of the abnormality.

Generally, pain emanating from facial structures is exhibited by behavioral changes, but functional disturbances also occur. Painful corneal lesions cause the functional disturbances of blepharospasm, epiphora, and photophobia; pain due to glaucoma is usually recognized as behavioral alterations. Painful oral lesions can be exhibited by excessive salivation and dysphagia along with behavioral changes.

Pain is a very useful localizing sign for cervical diseases and syndromes (Table 46-1) and is the most prominent sign in cervical disk protrusions and meningitis. An animal with cervical pain holds its head and neck low and rigid. Cervical muscle spasms and a "walking on eggs" gait are common. Behavioral signs may consist of continuous crying or whining for no apparent reason and a reluctance to eat or drink. The animal may continuously or periodically resist any palpation or movement of the neck. Careful deep palpation of vertebrae may

Localization of Pain by Region of Body

- Appendicular skeleton
  - Long bone (See chapters 44 and 45.)
  - Joint (See chapters 44 and 45.)
  - Muscle
    - Exertional rhabdomyolysis
    - Muscle cramping (Scottish terriers)
    - Myositis ossificans
    - Polymyositis
    - Status epilepticus
  - Other
    - Aortic thromboembolism (saddle thrombus—cat)
    - Sensory polyneuropathy
- Facial
  - Ocular (See chapter 56.)
  - Oral (See chapters 3, 30, and 31.)
  - Bone/muscle
    - Craniomandibular osteopathy
    - Fractures maxilla, mandible, or both
    - Myositis
    - Temporomandibular joint disorders
- Cervical (see Table 46-1)
- Back
  - Actual (see Table 46-1)
  - Referred
    - Acute pancreatitis
    - Cholelithiasis
    - Pyelonephritis
    - Prostatitis
- Thoracic cavity
  - Pleuritis
- Abdominal cavity
  - Actual (See chapter 36.)
  - Referred
    - Back trauma
    - Disk disease
    - Diskospondylitis
    - Meningeal disease
- Perianal
  - Anorectal trauma
  - Anal/rectal cancer
  - Anal sac abscess/impaction
  - Perianal fistulas
  - Rectal strictures

localize the pain to the cranial, middle, or caudal cervical segments. When the lesions involve the spinal cord, neurologic signs will reinforce localization of the lesion (see chapter 47). Even though pain from cervical disk protrusion is a common clinical sign, pain from thoracolumbar (cranial back) disk disease may be transient before profound neurologic deficits of paresis or paralysis occurs. However, with more chronic cranial back syndromes, especially with disk disease, pain may be a constant sign. Terminal thoracic and lumbar spinal lesions (caudal back) may also cause generalized pain and arching of the back. With either cranial or caudal back syndromes, the animal may object to handling, walking up stairs, or jumping into a car. Frequent crying or whining, exaggerated tendon reflexes, and rigid limbs and dorsal musculature are also signs of back pain.

Generally, when evaluating the back for pain, obvious reactions include vocalization and aggressive or fearful behavior upon palpation and manipulation. More subtle responses may include resistance to movement and muscle tensing. By placing one hand on the abdomen and pressing on each vertebrae with the other hand, a tensing of the abdominal muscles can be felt as painful areas are palpated. This palpation is followed by pinching the skin with a hemostat or pricking the skin with an 18-gauge needle. The skin is pinched gently to avoid significant behavioral reaction in normal areas. Stimulating areas of hyperesthesia will evoke an exaggerated skin twitch or behavioral response. This test should be conducted in a caudal to cranial direction, because areas caudal to the lesion will usually have decreased sensation. A level of normal or increased sensation can be determined by this test. If a spinal lesion is present, the sensory area should have the conformation of a dermatome. As further confirmation of the level of thoracolumbar lesions, the cutaneous trunci (panniculus) reflex can be elicited with a needle in the same manner as for detecting hyperesthesia. The panniculus reflex is insufficient for localization of lesions when minor neurologic deficits are present and pain is the primary sign. The motor evaluation of the neurologic examination localizes the lesion to one of six regions of the spinal cord or to the brain, whereas the sensory evaluation should localize the lesion to within three segments of the spinal cord (see chapter 47).

Painful perianal diseases and syndromes are often displayed by the behavioral signs of scooting, dragging, or rubbing the perineum on the floor, coupled with biting or chewing of the painful area. Functional disturbances common to problems of the perianal region include tenesmus, constipation, and dyschezia, along with intermittent diarrhea, constipation, and weight loss as the problem becomes progressive.

SYMPTOMATIC THERAPY[2,3,5]

Analgesic drugs are divided into two broad categories: the potent morphine or morphine-like analgesics and mild analgesics. The mild analgesics are effective in relieving mild to moderate pain and exhibit a "ceiling" effect. Once the ceiling is reached, increasing dosages will not give increased pain relief. The narcotic

(*Text continues on p 424.*)

Table 46-2. Clinical Considerations and Dosages of Potent Narcotic Analgesics and Mild Analgesics

GENERIC NAME (TRADE NAME)	CONSIDERATIONS AND EFFECTS	PRECAUTIONS	DOSAGE	
			Dog	Cat
Morphine or morphine-like analgesics				
Morphine sulfate	Hypothermia, panting Respiratory depression Nausea, emesis Constipation Urethral sphincter spasm, urinary retention Bradycardia Hypotension (large dosages) Spasm of biliary and pancreatic duct (biliary spasm reversed with atropine) Increase intracranial pressure Can be antagonized by naloxone, nalorphine	Head injury Impaired respiratory function Pancreatitis, hepatitis, cholecystitis Hepatopathy	0.25 mg/kg q 4 hr SQ, IM	0.1 mg/kg q 4 hr SQ, IM
Meperidine hydrochloride (Demerol)	Little sedation produced in most animals, except when used for severe pain or after general anesthesia Respiratory depression Abolishes corneal reflex Bradycardia Profound hypotension if given rapidly IV Can be antagonized by naloxone, nalorphine Metabolized more rapidly than in humans; duration, 1–2 hr in dogs	Same as for morphine	5.5 mg/kg q 4 hr IM	5.5 mg/kg q 4 hr IM

(Continued)

Table 46-2. Clinical Considerations and Dosages of Potent Narcotic Analgesics and Mild Analgesics (*Continued*)

GENERIC NAME (TRADE NAME)	CONSIDERATIONS AND EFFECTS	PRECAUTIONS	DOSAGE	
			Dog	Cat
Codeine	Two grains (120 mg) is equivalent to 10 mg of morphine for analgesia Effective when given orally Minimal addiction potential Frequently combined with mild analgesic for an additive effect Can be antagonized by naloxone, nalorphine	Same as for morphine	1.5 mg/kg PO	Not recommended
Oxymorphone hydrochloride (Numorphan)	1 mg is equivalent to 10 mg of morphine for analgesia In dogs, produces more tranquilization and less hypnosis than morphine Respiratory depression is less marked than with morphine Longer duration than morphine Can be antagonized by naloxone, nalorphine	Same as for morphine	0.1–0.2 mg/kg IM (usually combined with acepromazine)	0.05–0.1 mg/kg IM
Narcotic agonists/antagonists				
Pentazocine (Talwin-V)	Clinically, less effective than meperidine for postoperative orthopedic pain No adverse effect on blood pressure Minor respiratory depression Can be antagonized by naloxone but not nalorphine Nonaddicting	None at dosages recommended (much safer than meperidine or oxymorphone when given IV)	3 mg/kg IM (lasts 40 min) 1 mg/kg IV (lasts 30 min)	No experience in cats
Butorphanol tartrate (Stadol, Torbutrol)	Potent analgesic—stronger than pentazocine; in humans, 2 mg butorphenol = 18 mg morphine	Reported to be addictive	0.2–0.4 mg/kg IM 1/2 dose IV	No experience in cats

Mild analgesic				
Salicylates (aspirin)	Ceiling effect—in human dosages above 600 mg q 4 hr, no further analgesic effect Absorption of buffered and nonbuffered is same Buffered does not decrease dyspepsia Analgesia same for buffered and nonbuffered Variable results with enteric-coated products Hepatic metabolism of aspirin is very slow in cats. Both central analgesic activity and peripheral antiinflammatory activity	Be careful of dosages; dyspepsia, gastrointestinal bleeding, or hemorrhage may result, especially in cats. Avoid with surgical candidates	10 mg/kg q 12 hr PO	10 mg/kg every other day
Acetaminophen (Tylenol)	In humans—comparable analgesia to aspirin No gastric irritant effect or gastric hemorrhage	Contraindicated in cats	10 mg/kg q 12 hr PO	Contraindicated
Phenylbutazone (Butazolidin)	In humans—leukopenia, agranulacytosis, thrombocytopenia, aplastic anemia, dyspepsia, peptic ulceration, stomatitis, fluid retention Less toxic in dogs than humans—more rapidly excreted in dogs Plasma half-life is 6 hr in dog vs 72 hr in humans	Coexisting heart disease Renal disease	9 mg/kg q 8 hr PO	5–7 mg/lb q 12 hr
Indomethacin	Not recommended due to extreme gastrointestinal irritation			

SQ, subcutaneously; IM, intramuscularly; IV, intravenously; PO, per os

analgesics are effective against severe pain in relatively small dosages. It has been reported that these agents have no ceiling for pain relief: pain relief increases concurrently with dosage. Research indicates that a ceiling effect may exist with some of the potent agents (meperidine, pentazocine, and butorphanol).[3] Mild analgesics elevate the pain threshold but have minimal effect on the tolerance of pain. Conversely, instead of raising the pain threshold, narcotic analgesics increase the tolerance for pain by creating an emotional indifference to pain. Tranquilizers are useful in reducing the affective response to pain, because some animals need mental modification as well as analgesia to produce a quiet patient. By combining a narcotic analgesic and a tranquilizer (neuroleptanalgesia), one can use a reduced dose of each agent, which will minimize the adverse effects of each agent but still achieve the desired result. Listed in Table 46-2 are the commonly used and recommended potent morphine analgesics and mild analgesics.

REFERENCES

1. Guyton AC: Somatic sensations: II. Pain, visceral pain, headache, and thermal sensations. In Guyton AC (ed): Textbook of Medical Physiology, 6th ed. pp 611–625. Philadelphia, WB Saunders, 1981
2. Kaplan M: Pain. In Ettinger S (ed): Textbook of Veterinary Internal Medicine, pp 39–45. Philadelphia, WB Saunders, 1983
3. Trim C: Personal communication, 1985
4. Wall PD: Pain. In Swash M, Kennard C (eds): Scientific Basis of Clinical Neurology. Edinburgh, Churchill Livingstone, 1985
5. Yoxall AT: Pain in small animals: Its recognition and control. J Small Anim Pract 19:423–438, 1978

Part Twelve

NEUROLOGIC PROBLEMS

47

Paresis or Paralysis

JOHN E. OLIVER

PROBLEM DEFINITION AND RECOGNITION

Paralysis is the loss of motor function in a part, due to dysfunction of neural or muscular systems.[1] Paresis is partial paralysis. The most useful clinical definition of paralysis is loss of *voluntary* motor function. The term *paresis* will be used in this chapter to include both paresis and paralysis. Terms used to define the extent of paresis are monoparesis (one limb), pelvic limb paresis or paraparesis (both pelvic limbs), tetraparesis or quadriparesis (all four limbs), and paresis of specific structures (*e.g.*, facial paresis).[2]

PATHOPHYSIOLOGY

The final common pathway for all motor function is the lower motor neuron (LMN), the efferent neuron connecting the central nervous system to a muscle. All activity of the nervous system is expressed through LMNs located in the ventral and intermediate columns of the gray matter of the spinal cord and in the cranial nerve nuclei in the brain stem. The axons of these neurons form the peripheral spinal and cranial nerves. The LMN includes the nerve cell body, the axon, and the neuromuscular junction.

Dysfunction of a LMN prevents activation of the muscles (paresis), abolishes reflexes (areflexia), eliminates the normal tone in the muscle (flaccidity), and, in a short time, causes the muscle to atrophy. Paresis, areflexia, loss of tone, and early severe atrophy are the signs of LMN lesions.

The nervous system is arranged in a segmented fashion. Each spinal cord segment is demarcated by a pair of spinal nerves. The brain is less orderly in its segmentation, but anatomic and functional regions can be identified. Paresis of a muscle or group of muscles can be traced to a specific peripheral nerve, spinal nerve, or brain stem or spinal cord segment(s). Lesions of peripheral nerves cause severe LMN signs in all the muscles innervated. Peripheral nerves usually originate in several spinal cord segments; therefore, spinal nerve or cord lesions usually affect portions of the muscles rather than entire muscle groups. Brain stem lesions are more likely to affect all of the neurons in a nucleus and appear as complete lesions.

Voluntary movement requires control from the brain. The LMN is under the control of motor pathways from the cerebral cortex and brain stem, the upper motor neuron (UMN). Cortical control is directed primarily through brain stem locomotor centers in the midbrain and pons. The pathways, which extend through the brain stem and spinal cord, are responsible for the initiation and maintenance of normal movements. Pathways from the vestibular nuclei maintain tone in the extensor muscles to support the body against gravity. The UMN includes the nerve cell in the brain and the axon, forming the brain stem and spinal cord pathway.

Dysfunction of the UMN prevents voluntary movement (paresis) and may cause hyperactive reflexes, an increase in muscle tone, and abnormal reflexes (*e.g.*, crossed extensor reflex). Paresis, normal or exaggerated reflexes, normal or increased muscle tone, and abnormal reflexes are the signs of UMN lesions. Table 47-1 summarizes the characteristics of LMN and UMN signs.[2]

DIAGNOSTIC PLAN

The diagnosis includes localization of the lesion, the anatomic diagnosis, and the cause of the lesion (the etiology).

Anatomic Diagnosis

The first step is to determine that the problem is neurologic in origin. Lameness and weakness may be caused by a variety of musculoskeletal and systemic problems. The neurologic examination, especially tests of postural reactions and reflexes, both spinal and cranial nerves, provides the necessary information. Abnormal proprioceptive positioning reactions or depressed reflexes are virtually always the result of neuromuscular disease.

Table 47-1. Summary of LMN and UMN Signs

	LMN SIGN(S)	UMN SIGN(S)
Motor function	Paralysis of muscle or group of muscles	Paralysis or paresis of part of body
Reflexes	Hyporeflexia to areflexia	Normal or hyperreflexia
Muscle tone	Decreased	Normal to increased
Muscle atrophy	Early (weeks) and severe; affects all muscles denervated	Late (months) and mild; affects entire limb
Electromyography	Fibrillation potentials and positive sharp waves after 5–7 days	No change

Localization of peripheral spinal nerve lesions is summarized in Table 47-2. The examination must identify which muscles are paretic. Deficits of cranial nerves with motor function are summarized in Table 47-3, including the appropriate tests. Localization of spinal cord or spinal nerve lesions is outlined in Table 47-4. Postural reactions and spinal reflexes provide the data necessary to recognize LMN and UMN signs. Lesions in the brain stem causing UMN signs in the limbs will usually also cause cranial nerve signs, which are localizing. Lesions in the cerebrum or diencephalon may cause UMN paresis of the limbs without cranial nerve signs. Associated abnormalities of disease in these areas are listed in Table 47-5. (Remember that LMN signs are localizing to a small specific area.) If only UMN signs are present, other findings are needed to accurately localize the lesion. The sensory examination, including hyperesthesia, and the ability to perceive superficial and deep pain are useful to accurately localize the lesion. A single lesion is assumed until the examination clearly demonstrates a multifocal abnormality.

(*Text continues on p. 433.*)

Table 47-2. Spinal Nerves: Distribution and Clinical Signs of Dysfunction

NERVE (SPINAL CORD ORIGIN)	MUSCLES	FUNCTION(S)	SIGNS OF DYSFUNCTION
Brachial plexus—thoracic limb			
Suprascapular (C6–7)	Supraspinatus Infraspinatus	Extends shoulder	Slight loss of shoulder extension Atrophy of muscles with prominent spine of scapula
Axillary (C6,7,8)	Deltoideus Teres major Teres minor	Flexes shoulder	Decreased shoulder flexion
Musculocutaneous (C6,7,8)	Biceps brachii Brachialis Coracobrachialis	Flexes elbow	Decreased elbow flexion at gait and on withdrawal Decreased sensation of medial forearm
Radial (C7–T1)	Triceps brachii Extensor carpi radialis Common and lateral digital extensors Ulnaris lateralis	Extends elbow, carpus, and digits	Loss of extension If triceps is involved, loss of weight bearing Decreased triceps and extensor carpi radialis reflexes Decreased sensation of dorsal forearm and paw
Median (C8–T1)	Flexor carpi radialis Superficial digital flexor	Flexes carpus and digits	Decreased flexion of carpus and digits Decreased flexion of carpus on withdrawal

(*Continued*)

Table 47-2. Spinal Nerves: Distribution and Clinical Signs of Dysfunction (*Continued*)

NERVE (SPINAL CORD ORIGIN)	MUSCLES	FUNCTION(S)	SIGNS OF DYSFUNCTION
Ulnar (C8–T1)	Flexor carpi ulnaris Deep digital flexor	Flexes carpus and digits	Decreased flexion of carpus and digits Decreased flexion of carpus on withdrawal Decreased sensation of caudal forearm and fifth digit
Lumbosacral plexus—pelvic limb			
Femoral (L4–6)	Iliopsoas Quadriceps Sartorius	Flexes hip and extends stifle	Loss of extension of stifle, reduced hip flexion, unable to bear weight Decreased quadriceps (knee-jerk) reflex Decreased sensation on medial surface of leg
Obturator (L4–6)	External obturator Adductor Pectineus Gracilis	Adducts pelvic limb	Limb slides laterally on slick surfaces
Sciatic (L6–S2)	Biceps femoris Semimembranosus Semitendinosus	Extends hip and flexes stifle (see also tibial and peroneal)	Decreased flexion of stifle at gait and on reflex Decreased sensation below stifle
Tibial	Gastrocnemius Popliteus Deep digital flexor Superficial digital flexor	Extends hock and flexes digits	Decreased extension of hock Decreased sensation plantar surface of foot
Peroneal	Cranial tibial Peroneus longus Long and lateral digital extensors	Flexes hock and extends digits	Decreased flexion of hock and extension of digits Foot knuckles over Decreased sensation of dorsocranial surface of foot, hock, and stifle

Table 47-3. Cranial Nerves: Distribution and Signs of Motor Dysfunction

NERVE	ORIGIN	CLINICAL TESTS	SIGNS OF DYSFUNCTION
III Oculomotor	Midbrain	Pupillary light reflex Voluntary and vestibular eye movements	Dilated, unresponsive pupil Ventrolateral strabismus, unable to move eye dorsally or medially
IV Trochlear	Midbrain	Eye movements, difficult to detect	Rotation of eye, minimal deficit
V Trigeminal	Pons Medulla	Jaw strength, palpate temporal and masseter muscles Sensory exam of face	Atrophy of temporal and masseter muscles Decreased jaw tone Loss of sensation on face
VI Abducens	Medulla	Eye movements	Medial strabismus, unable to move eye laterally or to retract the eye
VII Facial	Medulla	Observation of face, palpebral reflex, menace reaction, tone of facial muscles	Unable to move muscles of face Decreased blink reflex Assymetry of lips, eyelids, and ears
IX Glossopharyngeal	Medulla	Gag reflex	Dysphagia, weak gag reflex
X Vagus	Medulla	Gag reflex, examination of larynx	Dysphagia, inspiratory dyspnea, altered vocalization
XI Accessory	Medulla	Palpation of trapezius, sternocephalicus, and brachiocephalicus muscles	Atrophy of trapezius, sternocephalicus, and brachiocephalicus muscles
XII Hypoglossal	Medulla	Examination of tongue	Atrophy of tongue Unable to lick in all directions Tongue deviates to side of lesion

Table 47-4. Signs of Lesions in the Spinal Cord

LOCATION OF LESION	CLINICAL SIGNS
C1–C5	Tetraparesis, UMN all four limbs
C6–T2 (brachial plexus)	Tetraparesis, UMN pelvic limbs, LMN thoracic limbs
T2–L3	UMN pelvic limb paresis, normal thoracic limbs
L4–S2 (lumbosacral plexus)	LMN pelvic limb paresis, normal thoracic limbs
S1–S3 (pelvic plexus)	LMN bladder and sphincters
Cd1–Cd5	LMN paresis of tail

UMN, upper motor neuron; LMN, lower motor neuron

Table 47-5. Signs of Lesions in the Brain

	MENTAL STATUS	POSTURE	MOVEMENT	POSTURAL REACTIONS	CRANIAL NERVES
Cerebral cortex	Abnormal behavior, depression, seizures	Normal	Gait normal to slight hemiparesis (contralateral)	Deficits (contralateral)	Normal (vision may be impaired, contralateral)
Diencephalon (thalamus and hypothalamus)	Abnormal behavior, depression, seizures (endocrine and autonomic)	Normal	Gait normal to slight hemiparesis (contralateral) or tetraparesis	Deficits (contralateral)	II
Brain stem (midbrain, pons, medulla)	Depression, stupor, coma	Normal, turning, falling	Ataxia, hemiparesis, tetraparesis	Deficits (ipsilateral or contralateral)	III–XII
Vestibular central (medulla)	Depression	Head tilt, falling	Ataxia, hemiparesis, tetraparesis	Deficits (ipsilateral or contralateral)	VIII, may also affect V and VII, nystagmus
Vestibular peripheral (labyrinth)	Normal	Head tilt	Normal to ataxia	Normal, although may be awkward	VIII, sometimes VII, Horner's syndrome, nystagmus
Cerebellum	Normal	Normal	Ataxia, tremors, dysmetria	Normal, but dysmetric	Normal, deficit of menace reaction, nystagmus

(Oliver JE, Lorenz MD: Handbook of Veterinary Neurologic Diagnosis, p 69. Philadelphia, WB Saunders, 1983)

Etiologic Diagnosis

The etiology of the disease is derived from information obtained in the signalment and history, the location of the lesion, and ancillary studies such as hematology, serum chemistries, urine analysis, radiology, electrodiagnostic tests, and cerebrospinal fluid analysis.

The history provides data on the rate of onset and progression of the signs. Most diseases can be classified as acute nonprogressive, acute progressive, or chronic progressive. This information, plus the signalment and location of the lesion, will usually narrow the cause of the problem to three to five general categories of disease. The diagnostic plan for most of the specific diseases in a category is usually the same. The major categories of disease are listed with their usual classification in Table 47-6. Those diseases which may be either acute or chronic in onset are listed twice; the order indicates the relative probability of occurrence.

The more common diseases are listed according to this classification in Tables 47-7 through 47-11. Diagnostic plans for the major categories of disease are listed in Table 47-12.[3]

Table 47-6. Characteristics of Major Categories of Disease

DISEASE	AGE	ONSET	COURSE	DISTRIBUTION
Degenerative	Young	Chronic	Progressive	Diffuse
Storage diseases	Young	Chronic	Progressive	Diffuse
Demyelinating diseases	Young	Chronic	Progressive	Diffuse
Neuronopathies	Young	Chronic	Progressive	Diffuse
Abiotrophies	Variable	Chronic	Progressive	Diffuse
Vertebral and disk	Adult	Chronic	Progressive	Focal
Anomalous	Young	Birth	Nonprogressive	Focal
Brain malformations	Young	Birth	Nonprogressive	Focal
Hydrocephalus	Young	Birth	Progressive	Focal
Vertebral malformations	Young	Birth	Nonprogressive	Focal
Myelodysplasia	Young	Birth	Nonprogressive	Focal
Metabolic CNS signs secondary to other disorder (*e.g.*, liver, renal, hypoglycemia)	Variable	Variable	Variable	Diffuse
Neoplastic	Adult	Chronic	Progressive	Focal
Nutritional	Variable	Chronic	Progressive	Diffuse
Thiamine	Variable	Variable	Progressive	Diffuse
Vitamin A	Variable	Chronic	Progressive	Variable
Idiopathic	Variable	Variable	Variable	Variable
Inflammatory	Variable	Variable	Progressive	Diffuse
Viral	Young	Acute	Progressive	Diffuse
	Adult	Chronic	Progressive	Diffuse
Bacterial	Variable	Acute	Progressive	Diffuse
Rickettsial	Variable	Acute	Progressive	Diffuse
Fungal	Variable	Chronic	Progressive	Diffuse
Protozoal	Variable	Chronic	Progressive	Diffuse
Toxic	Variable	Variable	Progressive	Diffuse
Traumatic	Variable	Acute	Nonprogressive	Focal
Vascular	Adult	Acute	Nonprogressive	Focal

Table 47-7. Etiology of Monoparesis

CATEGORY	ACUTE NONPROGRESSIVE	ACUTE PROGRESSIVE	CHRONIC PROGRESSIVE
Degenerative		Disk protrusion	
Neoplastic			Neurofibroma
Immune		Brachial plexus neuritis	
Inflammatory		Rabies	
Traumatic	Nerve injury		
Vascular	Infarction		

SYMPTOMATIC THERAPY

Specific therapy is directed at the cause. Many spinal cord lesions require surgical decompression. Supportive therapy is often necessary until function is restored.

Physical therapy is necessary in many forms of paresis to maintain muscle integrity. Some form of hydrotherapy, either whirlpool or bathtub with massage, is extremely beneficial in animals with paralyzed limbs. Passive and active exer-

(*Text continues on p 437.*)

Table 47-8. Etiology of Pelvic Limb Paresis

CATEGORY	ACUTE NONPROGRESSIVE	ACUTE PROGRESSIVE	CHRONIC PROGRESSIVE
Degenerative		Disk protrusion	Degenerative myelopathy Type II disk Myelopathy of Afghans Neuronopathy Demyelinating disease Lumbosacral malformation
Anomalous	Myelodysplasia		
Neoplastic			Primary Metastatic Vertebral
Nutritional			Hypervitaminosis A (cats)
Inflammatory		Canine distemper Bacterial, fungal, protozoal	Distemper Feline infectious peritonitis Fungal
Traumatic	Spinal cord injury		
Vascular	Fibrocartilaginous or septic emboli Hemorrhage		

(Modified from Oliver JE, Lorenz MD: Handbook of Veterinary Neurologic Diagnosis, p 149. Philadelphia, WB Saunders 1983)

Table 47-9. Etiology of Tetraparesis (Upper Motor Neuron)

CATEGORY	ACUTE NONPROGRESSIVE	ACUTE PROGRESSIVE	CHRONIC PROGRESSIVE
Degenerative		Disk protrusion	Cervical spondylopathy Type II disk Storage diseases Neuronopathy Demyelinating diseases Myelopathy of Afghans
Anomalous	Myelodysplasia	Atlantoaxial luxation	Vertebral malformations Spinal dysraphism
Neoplastic			Primary Metastatic Vertebral
Nutritional			Hypervitaminosis A (cats)
Inflammatory		Canine distemper Bacterial, fungal, protozoal	Distemper Feline infectious peritonitis Fungal
Traumatic	Spinal cord injury		
Vascular	Fibrocartilaginous or septic emboli Hemorrhage		

(Modified from Oliver JE, Lorenz MD: Handbook of Veterinary Neurologic Diagnosis, p 190. Philadelphia, WB Saunders, 1983)

Table 47-10. Etiology of Tetraparesis (Generalized Lower Motor Neuron)

CATEGORY	EPISODIC PROGRESSIVE	ACUTE PROGRESSIVE	CHRONIC PROGRESSIVE
Degenerative			Neuronopathies Myopathies
Anomalous		Myotonia	
Metabolic	Polysystemic disorders Hypoglycemia Hyperkalemia Hypercalcemia Hypocalcemia		Diabetes mellitus Hypothyroidism
Nutritional			Thiamine deficiency
Inflammatory	Polymyositis	Polyneuritis Polyradiculoneuritis Polymyositis	Polyneuritis Polymyositis
Immune	Myasthenia gravis	Polymyositis	
Toxic		Tick paralysis Botulism Aminoglycosides	Lead Organophosphates

(Modified from Oliver JE, Lorenz MD: Handbook of Veterinary Neurologic Diagnosis, p 205. Philadelphia, WB Saunders, 1983)

Table 47-11. Etiology of Cranial Nerve Paresis

CATEGORY	ACUTE NONPROGRESSIVE	ACUTE PROGRESSIVE	CHRONIC PROGRESSIVE
Anomalous		Hydrocephalus (CN III, IV, VI)	Laryngeal paralysis (CN IX, X)
Metabolic			Hypothyroidism (CN V, VII, VIII)
Neoplastic			Brain tumors Direct compression (all CN) or secondary to tentorial herniation (CN III)
Idiopathic		Mandibular paralysis (CN V) Facial paralysis (CN VII)	
Inflammatory		Bacterial (retrobulbar CN III, IV, VI; labyrinth CN VII) Rabies (CN IX, X) Polyneuropathies	Polyneuropathies
Traumatic	Head injury (all CN)		
Vascular	Emboli or hemorrhage in brain stem (all CN)		

CN, cranial nerve

Table 47-12. Selection of Diagnostic Tests

DISEASE CATEGORY	DIAGNOSTIC TESTS	
	Useful	Usually Diagnostic
Degenerative		
Brain	EEG, CSF	Biopsy
Spinal cord	Myelography, CSF	None
Vertebrae	CSF	Radiography, myelography
Demyelinating		
Brain	EEG, CSF	Biopsy
Spinal cord	Myelography, CSF	None
Peripheral nerve	EMG, EDT	Biopsy
Anomalous		
Brain	Examination	Radiography
Spinal cord	Radiography	Myelography
Vertebrae	Examination	Radiography
Metabolic	History	Clinical laboratory profile
Neoplastic		
Brain	EEG, radiography	Arteriography, scans
Spinal cord	CSF, radiography	Myelography
Peripheral nerve	EDT	Biopsy
Nutritional	History	Radiography
Inflammation	History, examination	CSF, serology
Traumatic	History, examination	Radiography
Toxic	History	Clinical laboratory profile

EEG, electroencephalography; CSF, cerebrospinal fluid; EMG, electromyelogram; EDT, electrodiagnostic testing

(Oliver JE, Lorenz MD: Handbook of Veterinary Neurologic Diagnosis, p 119. Philadelphia, WB Saunders, 1983)

cise of the affected parts is imperative. If the urinary bladder is not functioning normally, it must be emptied at least three times daily or more frequently if necessary to prevent overdistention. Aseptic catheterization is preferred unless manual expression is easy and effective. Monitoring for urinary tract infection must be done regularly by urine analysis. Vigorous treatment must be instituted if infection develops (see chapters 38 through 40).

PROGNOSIS

The prognosis primarily depends on the severity and duration of the paresis. Complete LMN lesions usually have a poor prognosis. If the nerve cell in the central nervous system is destroyed, it will not be replaced. peripheral axons regenerate, but with complete lesions, recovery of normal function is unusual. Prognosis of UMN paralysis is based on other findings. In lesions of the spinal cord between T3 and L3 producing pelvic limb paresis, the presence of sensation caudal to the level of the lesion is most important. If there is no response to a strong pinch of the digits of the pelvic limbs using a hemostat, it is assumed that the deep pain pathways are damaged, and the prognosis is grave. If the lack of sensation persists for over 48 hours, there is little hope for functional recovery.

REFERENCES

1. Dorland's Illustrated Medical Dictionary, 26th ed. Philadelphia, WB Saunders, 1981
2. Oliver, JE, Lorenz MD: Handbook of Veterinary Neurologic Diagnosis. Philadelphia, WB Saunders, 1983
3. Oliver JE, Hoerlein BF, Mayhew IG: Veterinary Neurology. Philadelphia, WB Saunders, 1987

48

Ataxia

JOHN E. OLIVER

PROBLEM DEFINITION AND RECOGNITION

Ataxia is incoordination of movements, without spasticity, paresis, or involuntary movements, although each of these may be seen in association with ataxia. The animal usually has a wide-based stance. Limb movements are incoordinated. Truncal ataxia is swaying of the body.[2]

PATHOPHYSIOLOGY

Ataxia is caused by disorders of the conscious or unconscious proprioceptive systems (sensory ataxia), disorders of the cerebellum, or disorders of the vestibular system.

The proprioceptive systems provide information about the location of the parts of the body. Without this information, the movements are poorly coordinated. Receptors are located in the skin, joints, tendons, and muscles. The nerve fibers are large and heavily myelinated. The pathways in the spinal cord are primarily in the dorsal and dorsolateral columns and are also large fibers. The pathways terminate in the cerebellum and cerebral cortex. These large fiber pathways are susceptible to compression, so that compressive lesions of the spinal cord often cause ataxia as the first clinical sign. Paresis commonly follows. Localization is essentially the same as in paresis (see chapter 47). For example, ataxia of the pelvic limbs with normal thoracic limbs indicates a lesion caudal to T3. Ataxia of all four limbs indicates a lesion cranial to T2 (see Table 47-4).

The cerebellum coordinates motor activity by comparing the intended action with the performance. It receives information from spinal pathways and from the cerebral cortex. The output of the cerebellum is to the brain stem and cortex. There are no direct cerebellar pathways to the spinal cord, and paresis is not seen with cerebellar lesions. Cerebellar ataxia has distinctive manifestations that are usually symmetric. Dysmetria is a disorder of the range of movements:

they may be too long (hypermetria) or too short (hypometria). Clinically, hypermetria is easily recognized since it causes a goose-stepping gait. Tremor, small oscillatory movements of the part, is common in cerebellar disease. Typically it is an intention tremor, one that becomes worse as the animal starts a movement and subsides at rest. Cerebellar disease usually causes dysmetria or tremor of the head, which distinguishes it from spinal tract disease (sensory ataxia). Nystagmus in cerebellar disease is usually a fine tremor of the eyes, especially as the animal shifts its gaze. Jerk nystagmus, with a fast and slow component, as seen in vestibular disease, may be seen in lesions of the flocculonodular lobes, which are intimately related to the vestibular system. Generalized cerebellar disease frequently causes a deficit in the menace reaction, although vision and the palpebral reflex are normal.[1]

The vestibular system detects the position and movement of the head, providing the nervous system with information necessary to maintain normal posture. Ataxia associated with vestibular disease is usually asymmetric, with falling or rolling to one side. Head tilt and nystagmus are commonly seen in vestibular disease. Vestibular disease is discussed in chapter 49. The distinguishing characteristics of these three syndromes are listed in Table 48-1.

DIAGNOSTIC PLAN

The diagnosis of ataxia includes lesion localization and finding the cause of the disease.

Ataxia is usually a sign of nervous system disease. Generalized weakness may cause the gait to appear ataxic. Abnormal postural reactions indicate disease of the nervous system. Sensory ataxia is characterized by deficits in postural reactions, especially proprioceptive positioning. Proprioceptive deficits are similar to motor deficits in determining the location of the lesion, as discussed in chapter 47 (see also Table 47-4, substituting ataxia for paresis). Cerebellar disor-

Table 48-1. Localization of Lesion Causing Ataxia

			VESTIBULAR	
CLINICAL SIGN	SENSORY	CEREBELLAR	Central	Peripheral
Asymmetric ataxia	Usually no	No	Yes	Yes
Head tilt	No	No	Yes	Yes
Head tremor	No	Yes	No	No
Intention tremor	No	Yes	No	No
Proprioceptive deficit	Yes	No	Yes	No
Paresis	Often	No	Often	No
Nystagmus	No	Often tremorlike	Yes	Yes
Nystagmus altered in direction with head position	No	No	Yes	No

ders are characterized by dysmetria and intention tremor. Involvement of the head should be present if the cerebellum is involved. This is most obvious when the animal eats or drinks, as the head overshoots or undershoots the container. If paresis is present with cerebellar signs, motor pathways of the brain stem or spinal cord are involved in the disease. The signs of vestibular disease, head tilt, nystagmus, altered eye movements, and asymmetric ataxia are easily recognized. Vestibular disease is discussed in chapter 49.

The general category of the etiologic diagnosis is suggested by the history. The onset, course, and location of the problem should indicate no more than three to five major categories; for example, acute, nonprogressive disorders are almost always traumatic or vascular in origin. Chronic, progressive diseases are usually neoplastic, degenerative, or inflammatory, although some toxic, metabolic, or nutritional diseases may present similarly. Characteristics of the major categories of disease are outlined in Table 48-2. The diagnosis is confirmed by appropriate laboratory, electrophysiologic, or radiographic studies. Tables 47-8 and 47-9 summarize the diseases causing sensory ataxia. Table 48-3 outlines the most important cerebellar diseases according to this scheme. Tables 49-1

Table 48-2. Characteristics of Major Categories of Cerebellar Disease

DISEASE	AGE	ONSET	COURSE	DISTRIBUTION
Degenerative	Young	Chronic	Progressive	Diffuse
Storage diseases	Young	Chronic	Progressive	Diffuse
Demyelinating diseases	Young	Chronic	Progressive	Diffuse
Neuronopathies	Young	Chronic	Progressive	Diffuse
Abiotrophies	Variable	Chronic	Progressive	Diffuse
Anomalous	Young	Birth	Nonprogressive	Focal
Cerebellar malformations	Young	Birth	Nonprogressive	Focal or diffuse
Metabolic	Variable	Variable	Variable	Diffuse
CNS signs secondary to other disorder (*e.g.*, liver, renal, hypoglycemia)				
Neoplastic	Adult	Chronic	Progressive	Focal
Nutritional	Variable	Chronic	Progressive	Diffuse
Thiamine	Variable	Variable	Progressive	Diffuse
Idiopathic	Variable	Variable	Variable	Variable
Idiopathic cerebellitis	Variable	Acute	Variable	Diffuse
Inflammatory	Variable	Variable	Progressive	Diffuse
Viral	Young	Acute	Progressive	Diffuse
	Adult	Chronic	Progressive	Diffuse
Bacterial	Variable	Acute	Progressive	Diffuse
Rickettsial	Variable	Acute	Progressive	Diffuse
Fungal	Variable	Chronic	Progressive	Diffuse
Protozoal	Variable	Chronic	Progressive	Diffuse
Toxic	Variable	Chronic	Progressive	Diffuse
Traumatic	Variable	Acute	Nonprogressive	Focal
Vascular	Adult	Acute	Nonprogressive	Focal

Table 48-3. Etiology of Cerebellar Disease

CATEGORY	ACUTE NONPROGRESSIVE	ACUTE PROGRESSIVE	CHRONIC PROGRESSIVE
Degenerative	Cerebellar hypoplasia (feline panleukopenia)		Storage diseases Neuroaxonal dystrophy Demyelinating diseases Abiotrophies
Anomalous	Malformation Dysmyelinogenesis		
Neoplastic			Primary Medulloblastoma Choroid plexus papilloma Glioma Meningioma
Inflammatory	Idiopathic cerebellitis	Canine distemper Granulomatous meningoencephalitis Bacterial, fungal, protozoal	Distemper Granulomatous meningoencephalitis Feline infectious peritonitis Fungal
Toxic		Heavy metals (lead) Hexachlorophene Organophosphates	Heavy metals (lead) Hexachlorophene
Traumatic	Occipital trauma		Brain herniations
Vascular	Infarction or septic emboli Hemorrhage		

(Modified from Oliver JE, Lorenz MD: Handbook of Veterinary Neurologic Diagnosis, p 233. Philadelphia, WB Saunders, 1983)

and 49-2 list the diseases of the vestibular system. Table 47-12 lists the most useful tests for each category of disease.

SYMPTOMATIC THERAPY

There is no symptomatic therapy for ataxia. Animals with vestibular disease may benefit from tranquilization during the acute phases of the syndrome. Drugs for motion sickness have been of little benefit.

PROGNOSIS

The prognosis depends on the cause, location, and severity of the disease. Sensory ataxia is similar to paresis, except that the lesion is often less severe and has a better prognosis (see chapter 47). Cerebellar diseases are often caused by untreatable diseases and have a poor prognosis. Exceptions include idiopathic cerebellitis and some toxicities. Peripheral vestibular disease often has a good prognosis; central disease usually does not (see chapter 49).

REFERENCES

1. Holliday TA: Clinical signs of acute and chronic experimental lesions of the cerebellum. Vet Sci Comm 3:259, 1979/1980
2. Oliver JE, Lorenz MD: Handbook of Veterinary Neurologic Diagnosis. Philadelphia, WB Saunders, 1983

49

Head Tilt

JOHN E. OLIVER

PROBLEM DEFINITION AND RECOGNITION

Head tilt is a postural abnormality, usually caused by abnormality of the vestibular system. The head is twisted to one side on its long axis, so that one ear is lower than the other. It must be distinguished from turning of the head and neck, with the head still parallel to the ground, which is usually caused by spasms of the cervical muscles. Animals with head tilt frequently have asymmetric ataxia and nystagmus.[4] Animals with acute otitis externa may tilt the head toward the affected side. There are no signs of neurologic disease.

PATHOPHYSIOLOGY

Head tilt is caused by an imbalance of tone in the cervical muscles, which are controlled in part by the vestibular system. The vestibular system includes the receptors in the inner ear, which detect changes in position of the head with respect to gravity and acceleration of the head, the vestibular nerve (cranial nerve VIII), the vestibular nuclei in the brain stem, the flocculonodular lobes of the cerebellum, and ascending and descending pathways. The vestibular system provides information that allows the animal to maintain a normal posture. Part of this is accomplished by the vestibulospinal tract, which provides tonic stimulation of the extensor motor neurons of the ipsilateral limbs. The vestibular system also controls some types of eye movements through connections in the medial longitudinal fasciculus to the nuclei of cranial nerves III, IV, and VI. This is the anatomic basis for physiologic nystagmus, the fast and slow movements of the eyes when the head is turned from side to side.[2]

Lesions of any part of the vestibular system produce one or more of the following signs: head tilt, usually to the side of the lesion; ataxia, which is usually asymmetric; falling or rolling to the side of the lesion; and nystagmus. It is important to differentiate central vestibular disease, which involves the brain stem, from peripheral disease involving only the receptors in the inner ear. Peripheral lesions disrupt normal posture through an imbalance of input to the nervous system. Central lesions may produce the same effect but, in addition, usually damage some of the sensory (spinocerebellar tracts or medial lemniscus) or motor (reticulospinal, corticospinal, or rubrospinal) pathways, causing ipsilateral proprioceptive deficits or paresis (see chapters 47 and 48).[4]

DIAGNOSTIC PLAN

Anatomic Diagnosis

The signs of vestibular disease, head tilt, asymmetric ataxia, falling to one side, and nystagmus are easily recognized. Differentiation of central lesions from peripheral lesions is essential for management. The most useful distinction is the presence of *postural reaction deficits* in central disease. Animals with acute vestibular syndromes may be difficult to test because of their severe disorientation. However, careful testing of the proprioceptive positioning reaction while the animal is supported will usually produce normal responses in peripheral disease and abnormal responses in central disease. The character of the nystagmus may be different also. Nystagmus in peripheral disease is horizontal, with the fast phase away from the side of the lesion, or rotatory. It does not change directions when the head is held in different positions, although the severity of the nystagmus may change. Nystagmus in central disease may be in any direction and frequently will change directions when the head is held in different positions.

Other cranial nerves may be affected in vestibular disease. The facial nerve (cranial nerve VII) may be involved in both central and peripheral lesions. Horner's syndrome (miosis, ptosis, and enophthalmos with prolapse of the third eyelid) is common with peripheral disease, because the sympathetic nerves pass through the middle ear. It is rare in central disease. Involvement of any other cranial nerves usually signifies central disease (*e.g.*, cranial nerves V, VI, IX, or X). Normal physiologic nystagmus is produced when the animal's head is turned from side to side. This is a useful test of vestibular function as well as a test of cranial nerves III, IV, and VI and the connecting pathway in the brain stem. Either central or peripheral vestibular disease may produce a ventral strabismus of the eye on the affected side when the head is elevated.[2] Table 48-1 summarizes the signs of vestibular disease and compares these with cerebellar and proprioceptive ataxias.

Two less common vestibular syndromes are bilateral vestibular disease and "paradoxic vestibular disease." Bilateral disease is characterized by a more symmetric ataxia, with swaying movements of the head. There is no nystagmus, including physiologic nystagmus. Paradoxic vestibular disease is caused by a lesion in the brain stem near the cerebellar peduncles.[3] It is paradoxic in that some of the signs indicate left-sided disease and others indicate right-sided disease. If other cranial nerve deficits are present, they indicate the side of the lesion.

Table 49-1. Etiology of Peripheral Vestibular Disease

CATEGORY	ACUTE NONPROGRESSIVE	ACUTE PROGRESSIVE	CHRONIC PROGRESSIVE
Anomaly	Congenital vestibular defects		
Metabolic			Hypothyroidism
Neoplasia			Neurofibroma or involving labyrinth
Idiopathic	Geriatric—Dogs Feline		
Inflammatory	Otitis interna	Otitis media—interna	Otitis media—interna
Toxic		Drugs—aminoglycosides	Drugs—aminoglycosides
Trauma	Labyrinth injury		
Vascular	Undocumented cause		

Etiologic Diagnosis

Most peripheral vestibular syndromes are caused by inflammation or are idiopathic. Idiopathic vestibular disease is diagnosed by exclusion of other causes. Rarely, neoplasia, drug toxicities, trauma, or congenital anomalies are the cause (Table 49-1).[1,2,4]

Central vestibular syndromes may be caused by a variety of diseases. The history provides information on the rate of onset, course, previous illness, age, and previous medication. A few general categories of disease can be defined from this information (Table 49-2). Confirmation of the diagnosis requires additional tests. Infection of the middle and inner ear can spread to the brain stem via the vestibular nerve; therefore, it is important to exclude peripheral infection

Table 49-2. Etiology of Central Vestibular Disease

CATEGORY	ACUTE NONPROGRESSIVE	ACUTE PROGRESSIVE	CHRONIC PROGRESSIVE
Anomaly			Hydrocephalus
Metabolic			Hypothyroidism
Neoplasia			Neurofibroma or tumors of brain stem
Nutritional		Thiamine	
Idiopathic	Polyneuropathy		
Inflammatory		Viral, bacterial, rickettsial, fungal, protozoal, granulomatous meningoencephalitis, parasite migration	Viral, bacterial, rickettsial, fungal, protozoal, granulomatous meningoencephalitis, parasite migration
Trauma	Brain stem		
Vascular	Infarction of brain stem		

even if there are signs of central disease. A diagnostic plan is outlined in Table 49-3.

SYMPTOMATIC THERAPY

In the acute stages of vestibular disease, the animal may demonstrate severe falling, rolling, and twisting. These episodes are exacerbated by any stimulus. Sedation or tranquilization and confinement are often necessary to prevent injury. Drugs for motion sickness (usually antihistamine compounds) may be tried but are usually of little benefit.

PROGNOSIS

Peripheral vestibular disease usually has a better prognosis than central disease. Labyrinthitis can usually be treated effectively, although there may be a residual deficit. Most animals with idiopathic disease recover fully in several weeks, with

Table 49-3. Plan for Management: Vestibular Signs

Signalment, history, and physical and neurologic examinations

Signs of vestibular disease: ataxia, head tilt, nystagmus, positional strabismus

Otoscopic examination, radiographs of skull, including bulla ossea; if available, tympanometry, auditory evoked potential recording (helps localize central vs peripheral)

SIGNS OF PERIPHERAL DISEASE ONLY		SIGNS OF CENTRAL DISEASE	
No postural reaction deficits, nystagmus in only one direction		Postural reaction deficits, nystagmus changes direction, abnormality of CN V, IX, X	
Otoscopic exam, radiographs		CSF, EEG if available	
Positive:	Negative:	Positive:	Negative:
Otitis media—interna Treatment: Myringotomy with topical and systemic antibiotics	History of ototoxic drugs: Discontinue drugs No history of drugs Idiopathic Otitis interna Hypothyroidism Neuritis (CN VIII) Congenital	Otoscopic (see otitis media—interna.) Radiographs Otitis media Neoplasia Trauma CSF Inflammatory Neoplasia EEG Inflammatory Hydrocephalus Neoplasia	Treat for inflammation and observe for changes.

CN, cranial nerve; CSF, cerebrospinal fluid; EEG, electroencephalogram

or without treatment. Degeneration of the receptors from toxicity is usually irreversible, but function improves through compensation.

Many central diseases are progressive disorders that are unresponsive to treatment. Bacterial infections can be treated effectively if treatment is started early and appropriate antibiotics are used. Some animals with central syndromes with an acute, nonprogressive history recover with little deficit. It is not known whether these are caused by vascular lesions or some other mechanism. The key finding is the lack of progression of the signs.

REFERENCES

1. Chrisman CL: Problems in Small Animal Neurology. Philadelphia, Lea & Febiger, 1982
2. de Lahunta A: Veterinary Neuroanatomy and Clinical Neurology. Philadelphia, WB Saunders, 1983
3. Holliday TA: Clinical signs of acute and chronic experimental lesions of the cerebellum. Vet Sci Comm 3:259, 1979/1980
4. Oliver JE, Lorenz MD: Handbook of Veterinary Neurologic Diagnosis. Philadelphia, WB Saunders, 1983

50

Collapse (Seizures, Syncope, and Narcolepsy)

JOHN E. OLIVER

PROBLEM DEFINITION AND RECOGNITION

There are three major types of sudden collapse: seizures, syncope, and narcolepsy–cataplexy. All are characterized by a sudden onset and usually by loss of consciousness. All of these are clinical syndromes with more than one cause.

Seizure, fit, and *ictus* are terms describing the stereotyped alterations in behavior resulting from paroxysmal abnormal brain function.[16] *Convulsion* usually refers to a seizure with generalized tonic–clonic muscle activity.[10] One or more of the following behavioral changes are present in a seizure: (1) loss or derangement of consciousness, (2) alteration of muscle tone or movement, (3) alteration of sensation, (4) disturbance of autonomic function, and (5) other psychic manifestations.[11] Epilepsy is a brain disorder characterized by recurring seizures.

Syncope is a sudden loss of consciousness caused by inadequate oxygen or glucose concentrations in the brain.[5] The episodes are usually brief but may recur. Severe oxygen or glucose deprivation also can cause convulsions.

Narcolepsy–cataplexy is a syndrome that includes excessive sleep (narcolepsy) and sudden loss of muscle tone (cataplexy).[1] Cataplexy is a prominent sign in affected animals. The animal suddenly drops to the ground and lies immobile for varying periods of time unless disturbed. Touching or calling the animal usually results in an immediate return to normal behavior.

PATHOPHYSIOLOGY

Seizures

The basic cellular event in seizures is paroxysmal discharge of a group of neurons, called the seizure focus. The focus may be single or multiple in any individual. Some neurons are capable of large depolarization of the membrane (20–50 mV) that lasts 50 to 100 msec. The large depolarization may lead to multiple action potentials in a short time. This depolarization is called the paroxysmal depolarizing shift (PDS). Following the PDS, the membrane usually has a prolonged afterhyperpolarization (AHP). The AHP tends to stabilize the population, preventing further discharge for a period. Some neurons have a prolonged after-depolarization (ADP), which may lead to ictal behavior. Apparently, both synaptic and ionic changes contribute to these events. Altered inhibitory neurotransmitters, such as gamma aminobutyric acid (GABA), may be a factor in the seizure mechanism as well.[13,17,18]

Spread of seizure activity from a focus is necessary for a seizure to occur. The activity can spread both locally to adjacent neurons and to other areas by axonal propagation. Eventually, other seizure foci will develop. The reticular activating system (RAS) has a role in the genesis of seizures, although the exact mechanism is not clear. Many seizures occur during sleep, when the RAS is least active. Experimentally, decreasing the output of the RAS increases seizure activity.[17]

Termination of seizure activity is primarily a function of the AHP and inhibitory feedback circuits from the cerebellum, thalamus, caudate nuclei, and possibly other areas of the brain. The concept of "metabolic exhaustion" of the neurons is probably not valid.

There is a variability of susceptibility to seizure activity in various populations of neurons and in various individuals. For example, the neurons of the hippocampus develop ictal activity easily, and individuals within a species vary in their threshold for seizures. A genetic predisposition for seizures may be just a lowered threshold. The threshold also may be lowered by a variety of internal and external factors, such as sleep and increased estrogen levels. Alterations in energy substrates, electrolytes, and many endogenous and exogenous toxins may precipitate seizures.

The occurrence of seizures increases the probability of more seizures. The synaptic changes have been compared with "learning mechanisms" responsible for memory. There is also a pathologic change in neurons after seizures, primarily in the structure of the dendrites. These changes range from minor distortions, to neurons virtually devoid of processes, to eventual death of the neuron. Prevention of these changes is a major consideration in the decision of whether to treat an animal with seizures.[17]

Seizures may be classified according to a modification of the international classification of human epilepsy (Table 50-1).[9] Differentiating partial from generalized seizures is important because partial seizures are caused by a focal brain lesion and therefore are acquired, not idiopathic. Generalized seizures involve the entire body at once. Partial seizures, also called focal seizures, have focal signs. Partial seizures may generalize secondarily, so the seizure must be seen from the onset to ascertain the presence of a focal component. Idiopathic seizures are generalized, but all generalized seizures are not idiopathic. Idiopathic seizures may be inherited. Table 50-2 lists the breeds that have been studied by controlled breeding programs and those reported as frequently having idiopathic seizures.

Table 50-3 lists the major causes of seizure disorders in small animals.

Table 50-1. Classification of Seizures

CLINICAL MANIFESTATION	COMMENTS
Generalized seizures	
Tonic–clonic (grand mal, major motor)	Most common type May be caused by organic brain disease, toxins, or metabolic disorders Idiopathic form may be genetic.
Absences with or without motor phenomena (petit mal)	Rare in animals
Partial seizures	
Partial motor (focal motor)	Focal signs during seizure may generalize to tonic–clonic seizure. Indicates an acquired brain lesion
Psychomotor	Complex behavioral activity that is stereotyped and similar each time. Believed to be lesion of limbic system

Table 50-2. Breed Susceptibility to Collapse

SEIZURES	NARCOLEPSY	SYNCOPE
Inherited	Inherited	Inherited
Beagle	Doberman pinscher	Pugs
Dachshund	Labrador retriever	
German shepherd (Alsatian)		
Keeshond		
Tervuren shepherd (Belgian)		
High incidence	Reported cases	High incidence
Cocker spaniel	Afghan hound	Boxer
Collie	Airedale	Doberman pinscher
Golden retriever	Corgi	Miniature schnauzer
Irish setter	Dachshund	
Labrador retriever	Irish setter	
Miniature schnauzer	Malamute	
Poodle	Poodle	
St. Bernard	Springer spaniel	
Siberian husky	Wire-haired griffon	
Wire-haired fox terrier	Mixed breed	

Inherited: breeding studies indicate genetic trait
High incidence: frequently reported
Reported cases: published reports

Table 50-3. Causes of Seizures

CATEGORY	DISEASES
Degenerative	Storage diseases
Anomalous	Hydrocephalus
	Lissencephaly
	Porencephaly
Metabolic	Hypoglycemia
	Hypocalcemia
	Renal failure
	Hepatic failure
Neoplastic	Brain tumors (primary and metastatic)
Nutritional	Thiamine
	Parasitism (multiple factors)
Idiopathic	Unknown
	Genetic
Inflammatory	Viral: canine distemper, rabies, feline infectious peritonitis
	Bacterial: any
	Mycotic: many
	Protozoon: Toxoplasmosis
Toxic	Heavy metals: lead
	Organophosphates
	Chlorinated hydrocarbons
	Strychnine
	Tetanus
	Many others
Traumatic	Acute head injury
	Posttraumatic: weeks to months after injury
Vascular	Infarctions
	Arrhythmias

Syncope

Transient loss of consciousness is caused by a temporary deprivation of oxygen or glucose supplies to the brain. It is usually of short duration but can lead to sudden death. Syncope is the result of (1) impaired cerebral circulation, (2) a transient decrease in cardiac output, (3) decreased systolic blood pressure, or (4) inadequate energy substrates delivered to the brain.[2,5] The causes of syncope are summarized in Table 50-4. The various causes of syncope are discussed in detail in the chapters listed in that table.

Narcolepsy–Cataplexy

Narcolepsy is a disorder of the sleep mechanism of the brain. The primary complaint in humans, excessive daytime sleepiness, is not usually recognized in animals; however, it has been documented in laboratory studies.[7] Cataplexy is readily recognized in affected animals. The animal has a sudden loss of muscle

Table 50-4. Causes of Syncope

GENERAL CAUSE	PATHOPHYSIOLOGY	DISEASE OR PROBLEM
Decreased cerebral circulation	Vascular obstruction or insufficiency	Thrombus, embolus, atherosclerosis, neoplasia, trauma
Decreased cardiac output	Abnormal heart rate or rhythm (See chapter 21.)	Dysrhythmias Impulse conduction Impulse formation
	Destruction (See chapters 21 and 22.)	Congenital heart diseases Acquired heart diseases
Decreased blood pressure	Decreased blood volume (See chapter 23.)	Blood loss
	Increased vascular resistance (See chapter 23.)	Postural, drugs, hyperventilation, carotid sinus
Metabolic	Decreased oxygen (See chapters 23, 24, 26, 60, and 63.)	Cardiopulmonary dysfunction, abnormal hemoglobin, anemia
	Decreased glucose (See chapter 61.)	Insulin-secreting tumors, insulin overdose, glycogen storage disease, inadequate nutrition (mostly toy breeds, young animals)

tone, causing complete collapse. Usually, consciousness is maintained and the animal is easily aroused by touch or noise.

The physiology of sleep is poorly understood, so the pathophysiology of sleep disorders is still largely unknown. Normal sleep has two distinct stages: random eye movement (REM) sleep and nonrandom eye movement sleep (NREM). REM sleep is characterized by atonic muscles, occasional fasciculation of distal and facial muscles, and rapid eye movements. An electroencephalogram (EEG) shows low voltage with mixed frequency. NREM sleep has two components: Light, slow-wave sleep is characterized on the EEG by higher voltage slow waves, with at least one 10-Hz to 14-Hz spindle per 30 seconds. Deep, slow-wave sleep has even higher voltage slow waves (<4 Hz) with spindles. REM sleep normally occurs after about 90 minutes of NREM sleep and recurs intermittently thereafter. It accounts for 11% to 13% of the sleep cycle.[1]

Narcoleptic dogs have significantly less REM sleep than normal dogs but have episodes of cataplexy, which has some of the features of REM sleep. There are other changes in the pattern of sleep, suggesting that narcoleptic dogs have a disruption of the sleep–wake cycle rather than hypersomnia.[1]

Most cases of narcolepsy are idiopathic. Inheritance has been established in Doberman pinschers and Labrador retrievers.[7] A variety of other breeds of dogs and horses and ponies have been recognized to have narcolepsy (Table 50-2).

DIAGNOSTIC PLAN

A data base for animals with collapse (see list) should be adequate to differentiate syncope and narcolepsy from seizures.[13] The plan is based on the assumption that seizures are caused by three major categories of disease: (1) extracranial abnormalities, such as metabolic and toxic disorders, (2) intracranial disease, such as encephalitis, brain tumors, or trauma, and (3) idiopathic or primary generalized epilepsy.[14–16] The causes of syncope are extracranial, either cardiovascular, pulmonary, or metabolic (hypoglycemia). Narcolepsy is considered idiopathic, although it may occur subsequent to a primary brain disorder.

The minimum data base should identify most extracranial causes of collapse. Some findings may be suggestive, requiring other specific tests to make a definitive diagnosis. Abnormal findings on the neurologic examination may require the tests listed in the "more complete data base" or "focal brain disease suspected" sections.

SYMPTOMATIC THERAPY

If a specific cause is identified, it is treated appropriately. The cause of syncope should be readily determined in most cases, although some of the cardiac arrhythmias may be difficult to document without long-term monitoring.[3] Symptomatic therapy is indicated in animals with seizures or narcolepsy if no treatable disease is identified.

Seizures

Anticonvulsant therapy is indicated in animals with frequent, severe seizures. It is not recommended if the animal has had one brief seizure. Continuous anticonvulsant medication may be impractical if the animal has only two to three seizures a year. However, the knowledge that seizures cause brain damage, and increase the probability of more frequent seizures, should make therapy preferable in most situations. Table 50-5 outlines the primary anticonvulsants, dosages, and recommended serum levels.

Table 50-5. Anticonvulsant Drugs

DRUG	DOSAGE (mg/kg)	SERUM CONCENTRATION (μg/ml)
Phenobarbital	1.5–5 b.i.d.	15–30
Primidone	10–15 t.i.d.	15–30 (phenobarbital)
Phenytoin	35 t.i.d.	10–20
Na valproate*	10–60 t.i.d.	40–100 (human)

* In combination with phenobarbital

Data Base for Collapse

- Minimum data base: One or more episodes
  - Signalment
    - Species, breed, age, sex
  - History
    - Environment
    - Immunizations
    - Previous illness or injury
    - Description of collapse
      - Age of onset
      - Frequency
      - Precipitating factors
        - Exercise
        - Time of meals
      - Behavioral changes
      - Conscious?
  - Physical examination
    - Special attention to cardiovascular and nervous systems
    - Fundoscopic examination
  - Neurologic examination
    - If collapse was within 24–48 hr and neurologic examination is abnormal, repeat in 24 hr.
  - Laboratory tests
    - Complete blood count
    - Urine analysis
    - Chemistries (at least)
      - Blood urea nitrogen
      - ALT (serum glutamic-pyruvic transaminase)
      - Alkaline phosphatase
      - Calcium
      - Fasting blood glucose
  - Others
    - Electrocardiogram (ECG)
    - Blood lead
- More complete data base
  - Seizures not controlled or evidence of central nervous system disease
    - Cerebrospinal fluid analysis: cell count, total and differential; protein
    - Electroencephalogram
    - Skull radiographs
  - Syncope suspected, but cause not found
    - Monitoring of ECG
  - Narcolepsy suspected but not demonstrated
    - Provocation test[9]
- Focal brain disease suspected
  - Contrast radiography
  - Brain scan: computed axial tomography, nuclear

Phenobarbital is the preferred anticonvulsant for dogs and cats. It is relatively safe and effective, has few undesirable side effects, and is economical. Primidone is largely metabolized to phenobarbital; a small amount metabolizes to phenylethylmalonamide (PEMA). Primidone and PEMA have very short half-lives. There is no documented evidence that primidone is any more effective than phenobarbital, although many clinicians believe it is. Primidone is more toxic than phenobarbital. One study found no advantage to primidone in dogs unresponsive to phenobarbital.[6] Phenytoin is widely used in humans but is relatively ineffective in dogs. It is poorly absorbed and rapidly metabolized; therefore, large doses at frequent intervals must be used if it is to be effective. Primidone and phenytoin are not recommended for cats. All of the anticonvulsants have some degree of toxicity for the liver in all species. Increased liver enzymes in the serum are common in animals on any anticonvulsant therapy. Primidone has been shown to cause more severe liver damage in dogs, including cirrhosis and hepatic failure in a few animals.[4,13]

Sodium valproate is a relatively new anticonvulsant with some promise. There is inadequate information to clearly establish its efficacy or safety. It has been shown to be effective in some animals refractory to phenobarbital.[12] It is generally used in conjunction with phenobarbital because of its short half-life.

The benzodiazepines, including diazepam, clonazepam, and lorazepam, have been used, but little controlled data is available. Diazepam is recommended for treatment of status epilepticus. Clonazepam and lorazepam have longer half-lives and may find a place in treatment of epilepsy. However, there is evidence that clonazepam will lose effectiveness in a relatively short time.[8] Diazepam is useful for tranquilization of epileptic animals who should not be given phenothiazine tranquilizers.[8,13]

Client education about the treatment of epilepsy is as important as the selection of drugs. The primary reasons for treatment failure are (1) progressive disease, (2) unresponsiveness to medication, and (3) failure to follow an appropriate plan of medication. Progressive disease will be detected by the diagnostic plan. Refractory seizures may occur in any animal but are most common in the large breed dogs, such as German shepherds, St. Bernards, and Irish setters. Client education is important to avoid misunderstanding.

Some important principles for clients to understand are the following:

1. Successful treatment is a reduction in severity, frequency, and duration of seizures. Only in ideal circumstances are seizures completely eliminated.
2. Medication must be given continuously, on a regular schedule, for a long time. Seizures can not be treated intermittently.
3. The dose and schedule vary considerably between individuals; therefore, the initial plan may be changed several times before success is achieved. Metabolism of the anticonvulsant drugs is extremely variable by different individuals. The treatment regimen must be tailored to the individual. Efficacy should not be judged until the drug has achieved a steady state and serum levels are appropriate.

4. Medication should not be changed or discontinued suddenly, even if it is not adequately controlling the seizures. Suddenly lowering the blood levels of a drug may cause status epilepticus.
5. Phenothiazine tranquilizers are contraindicated in epileptics. They reduce the threshold for seizures.
6. Epilepsy may be an inherited problem. If no cause can be determined, neutering should be considered. It is recommended in females because estrogens lower the threshold for seizures.
7. Care of the animal during a seizure should be discussed. Most animals will not hurt themselves during the episode. Intervention to prevent events such as "swallowing the tongue" is more likely to result in injury to the person. Preventing the animal from hitting furniture or falling down stairs should be the primary concern. If the seizure lasts longer than 3 minutes, medical help should be sought immediately.[16]

Narcolepsy

The cataplectic episodes seen in canine narcolepsy are not inherently dangerous, but the animal should be in a protected environment. Episodes occurring on a busy street certainly could be dangerous. Successful long-term treatment has not been reported. Short-term improvement is possible, and some animals have fewer episodes as they mature.

General stimulants, such as methylphenidate at a dose of 0.25 mg/kg, reduce excessive somnolence and may reduce cataplectic episodes. It is effective for a time but appears to lose its effect over time. Tricyclic antidepressants such as imipramine and protryptyline may also be effective. Imipramine is given at a dose of 0.05 to 1.0 mg/kg three times daily. Imipramine is reported to cause impotency in the human male.[1]

Monoamine oxidase inhibitors such as pargyline and phenelzine should not be used because of the potential for serious cardiovascular effects.[1]

As in the treatment of seizures, the goal should be to reduce the frequency and severity of the episodes. Complete abolition of cataplectic attacks requires dangerously high doses of the drugs.

REFERENCES

1. Baker TL, Mitler MM, Foutz AS, Dement WC: Diagnosis and treatment of narcolepsy in animals. In Kirk RW (ed): Current Veterinary Therapy VIII: Small Animal Practice. Philadelphia, WB Saunders, 1983
2. Beckett SD, Branch CE, Robertson BT: Syncopal attacks and sudden death in dogs: Mechanisms and etiologies. J Am Anim Hosp Assoc 14:378–386, 1978
3. Branch CE, Beckett SD, Robertson BT: Spontaneous syncopal attacks in dogs: A method of documentation. J Am Anim Hosp Assoc 13:673–679, 1977
4. Bunch SE, Castleman WL, Baldwin BH, Hornbuckle, WE, Tennant BC: Effects of long-term primidone and phenytoin administration on canine hepatic function and morphology. Am J Vet Res 46:105–115, 1985

5. Ettinger SJ: Weakness and syncope. In Ettinger SJ (ed): Textbook of Veterinary Internal Medicine. Philadelphia, WB Saunders, 1983
6. Farnbach GC: Efficacy of primidone in dogs with seizures unresponsive to phenobarbital. J Am Vet Med Assoc 185:867–868, 1984
7. Foutz AS, Mitler MM, Dement WC: Narcolepsy. Vet Clin North Am 10:65–80, 1980
8. Frey HH, Loscher W: Pharmacokinetics of anti-epileptic drugs in the dog: A review. J Vet Pharmacol Ther 8:219–233, 1985
9. Gastaut H: Clinical and electroencephalographic classification of epileptic seizures. Epilepsia 10(suppl):512–513, 1969
10. Holliday TA: Seizure disorders. Vet Clin North Am 10:3–29, 1980
11. Lennox WG: Epilepsy and Related Disorders. Boston, Little, Brown & Co, 1960
12. Nafe LA, Parker A, Kay WJ: Sodium valproate: A preliminary clinical trial in epileptic dogs. J Am Anim Hosp Assoc 17:131–133, 1981
13. Oliver JE, Jr: Seizure disorders and narcolepsy. In Oliver JE, Jr, Hoerlein BF, Mayhew IG (eds): Veterinary Neurology. Philadelphia, WB Saunders, 1987
14. Oliver JE, Jr: Protocol for the diagnosis of seizure disorders in companion animals. J Am Vet Med Assoc 172:822–824, 1978
15. Oliver JE, Jr: Seizure disorders in companion animals. Comp Cont Ed Pract Vet 2:77–85, 1980
16. Oliver JE, Jr, Lorenz M: Handbook of Veterinary Neurologic Diagnosis. Philadelphia, WB Saunders, 1983
17. Pedley TA, Traub RD: Physiology of epilepsy. In Swash M, Kennard C (eds): Scientific Basis of Clinical Neurology. Edinburgh, Churchill Livingstone, 1985
18. Russo ME: The pathophysiology of epilepsy. Cornell Vet 71:221–247, 1981

51

Coma

JOHN E. OLIVER

PROBLEM DEFINITION AND RECOGNITION

Altered states of consciousness vary from depression to coma. The following definitions will be used in this chapter:

Depression—The animal is lethargic and less responsive to its environment but still has the capability to respond in a normal manner.
Disorientation, confusion—Responses are inappropriate.
Stupor—The animal is asleep when undisturbed but can be aroused with strong stimulation.
Coma—The animal is unconscious and does not respond to any stimulus except by reflex activity.
Vegetative state—The animal lacks awareness of the environment but can be aroused.[2]

Depression has many causes, including systemic illness. Confusion, stupor, coma, and the vegetative state are always signs of abnormal brain function.[6]

PATHOPHYSIOLOGY

Consciousness is maintained by sensory stimuli acting through the reticular activating system (RAS). The reticular formation of the rostral brain stem receives input from most of the sensory systems of the body, including somatosensory (*e.g.*, touch, temperature, and pain), visual, auditory, and olfactory pathways. The reticular formation projects diffusely to the cerebral cortex, by way of the intralaminar nuclei of the thalamus, maintaining a background of activity through cholinergic synapses on cortical neurons. A second pathway projects to the hypothalamus and basal forebrain.[7] This activity is balanced by an adrenergic system from brain stem and diencephalic nuclei, which influence sleep (see chapter 50).

Anything that alters the activity of the RAS or interferes with its connections to the cortex can cause a change in the level of consciousness. Coma is usually the result of one of four major categories of abnormality: (1) diffuse, bilateral cerebral diseases, (2) metabolic or toxic encephalopathies, (3) compression of the midbrain or pons, or (4) destructive lesions of the midbrain or pons.[6]

Diffuse, bilateral cerebral hemisphere disease usually causes signs of depression or stupor and, only rarely, coma. The vegetative state is seen in animals with severe cerebral disease. The animal will arouse, vocalize, and have brain stem reflex activity, including paddling movements of the limbs. However, there are no purposeful actions indicating cortical function. This state is most common after severe hypoxic episodes or cortical trauma. Metabolic disease, such as hepatic failure, may cause stupor or coma with preservation of brain stem function.

Lesions of the brain stem in the region of the midbrain or pons frequently cause coma. Head trauma often causes hemorrhage in this area. Typically, the animal is unconscious from the time of the injury and never regains consciousness. Other signs of brain stem dysfunction are present, including abnormal pupillary light reflexes, abnormal eye movements, other cranial nerve deficits, and postural abnormality. Brain stem function can also be compromised by compression either directly from mass lesions or secondarily by tentorial herniation. The brain is enclosed in an inelastic case, the skull. Any increase in volume in the skull must displace part of the contents. Increased pressure causes displacement of the cerebral hemisphere under the tentorium cerebelli, resulting in compression of the brain stem. Unilateral masses produce a herniation on the same side, whereas generalized pressure increases, such as in hydrocephalus or cerebral edema, cause central or bilateral herniation.[5]

DIAGNOSTIC PLAN

Anatomic Diagnosis

Coma always indicates severe brain dysfunction. Structural damage to the brain stem has a grave prognosis, so the neurologic examination should be directed toward evaluating brain stem function. Motor function, pupil function, and eye movements are important parameters to assess. Table 51-1 outlines the findings in the most common syndromes. See chapters 52 through 54 for details on assessing the pupils and eye movements.

Diffuse cerebral disease with normal brain stem function rarely causes coma. When it does, the animal is blind, but the pupils are either normal or constricted. Vestibular eye movements may be present. Extensor hypertonus is not present, as it is frequently in brain stem disease. Walking or paddling movements are often present. When this syndrome persists, it is called the vegetative state, and is seen most often after severe hypoxia. Signs of diffuse cerebral disease are likely to be symmetric.

Metabolic or toxic encephalopathies may cause coma, which is similar to

Table 51-1. Clinical Signs in Coma

LOCATION OF LESION	MOTOR FUNCTION	PUPILLARY LIGHT REFLEX	EYE MOVEMENTS
Diffuse cerebral disease	Tetraparesis; may have locomotor movements, but postural reactions are abnormal	Normal	Normal, but no visual following
Metabolic or toxic encephalopathy	Tetraparesis; reflexes may be depressed	Normal or abnormal, depending on the cause	Normal or abnormal, depending on the cause
Bilateral tentorial herniation	Tetraparesis, increased extensor tone (decerebrate rigidity)	Dilated or midposition, unresponsive	Bilateral ventrolateral strabismus, poor to absent vestibular eye movements
Unilateral tentorial herniation	Hemiparesis or tetraparesis, increased extensor tone on affected side	Dilated ipsilateral	Ipsilateral ventrolateral strabismus, poor vestibular eye movements
Brain stem hemorrhage	Tetraparesis, increased extensor tone (decerebrate rigidity)	Midposition bilateral	No vestibular eye movements; may have bilateral ventrolateral strabismus

the diffuse cerebral syndrome. However, many agents also affect the function of the brain stem even though there is no structural damage. Barbiturates are an example. The animal has no voluntary activity, and reflex activity is depressed (in contrast to most of the other syndromes in which spinal reflexes are present). Signs are usually symmetric. An adequate history is critical for ascertaining the cause in these cases.

Brain stem lesions may be from compression or direct injury. The onset and course of the syndrome provide the key to differentiating the two. Most brain stem hemorrhages or contusions are the result of trauma, with primary vascular disease a relatively rare cause. The animal is usually comatose from the time of the injury and does not change. Herniations secondary to increased pressure develop more slowly. There may be a sudden onset, but there is a definite progression of signs. An early warning sign of tentorial herniation is one dilated pupil. The oculomotor nerve is vulnerable to compression by the herniating cerebrum as it crosses the petrosal bone. Tentorial herniation is likely to produce assymetric signs, whereas brain stem hemorrhage is more likely to be symmetric.

Etiologic Diagnosis

The history and neurologic examination provide information to establish a small number of probable causes of coma. The onset and course of the syndrome are obtained from the history. Focal or diffuse signs are assessed from the neurologic examination. Signs of meningeal irritation, including hyperesthesia on deep

Table 51-2. Etiology of Coma

	ACUTE NONPROGRESSIVE	ACUTE PROGRESSIVE	CHRONIC PROGRESSIVE
Focal or lateralizing signs			
Neoplastic		Metastatic	Primary
Traumatic	Parenchymal hemorrhage	Epidural, subdural hemorrhage	Subdural hematoma (rare)
Vascular	Infarction, hemorrhage		
No focal or lateralizing signs, but evidence of meningeal irritation			
Inflammatory		Meningoencephalitis	
Traumatic	Subarachnoid hemorrhage		
No focal, lateralizing or meningeal signs			
Degenerative			Storage diseases
Anomalous	Brain malformations		Hydrocephalus
Metabolic		Hypoglycemia, hepatic encephalopathy, heat stroke, hypoxia, diabetic coma, uremic encephalopathy	
Nutritional		Thiamine deficiency	
Inflammatory		Encephalitis	Encephalitis
Toxic		Heavy metals (lead), barbiturates, narcotics, carbon monoxide	Heavy metals
Traumatic		Cerebral edema	

(Modified from Oliver JE, Lorenz MD: Handbook of Veterinary Neurologic Diagnosis, p 271. Philadelphia, WB Saunders, 1983)

palpation of the vertebral column, are also significant. Table 51-2 categorizes the most common causes of coma using these findings.

SYMPTOMATIC THERAPY

Two stages of treatment of coma will be discussed: early management after acute head injury and chronic management of the unconscious patient. Specific therapy of the causes of coma will not be discussed.

Acute head injury severe enough to cause loss of consciousness is always potentially life-threatening. Management decisions must be made rapidly and correctly. Priorities for treatment are (1) ventilation, (2) shock, (3) hemorrhage, and (4) cerebral edema. The first three are essential to preserve life and are discussed in numerous texts (see also chapters 23 and 24). Control of cerebral edema is necessary to preserve brain function. There are three major components in the treatment of cerebral edema: ventilation, hyperosmotic agents, and glucocorticosteroids.

Ventilation is essential for prevention and reduction of cerebral edema. Increased pCO_2 and decreased pO_2 are major factors in the evolution of edema in the brain. Because pCO_2 is the more important of the two, simple administration of oxygen may not be adequate. Controlled ventilation is better, with slight hyperventilation preferred. An adequate tidal volume to keep CO_2 levels at or below normal range is necessary (see chapter 63).

Reduction of edema once it has occurred is difficult. Hyperosmotic agents are at least partially effective. The preferred agent is mannitol (20% or 25%) given slowly intravenously. Recommendations on dosage vary from 0.5 mg to 2.0 mg/kg. The lower dose is preferred. It should be repeated at 4- to 6-hour intervals for three doses. Mannitol should not be given if the animal is hypovolemic.

Glucocorticosteroids are somewhat controversial in the treatment of head injury, but the bulk of the evidence supports their use. To be effective, they must be given early after the trauma, preferably within the first hour, and at high doses. The soluble preparations, such as methylprednisolone sodium succinate, should be given at a dose of 30 mg/kg intravenously. A second dose of 15 mg/kg should be given in 2 hours, followed by maintenance doses of 15 mg/kg at 6-hour intervals.[1,4] Dexamethasone may be substituted for the maintenance doses at a level of 6 to 15 mg/kg, but its efficacy is not as clearly documented. These extremely high doses are apparently necessary to have an effect on the CNS.[1,3,4] Therapy should be maintained for 24 hours in most cases. Prolonged treatment can lead to side effects, especially gastrointestinal hemorrhage and ulceration.[8]

Normal fluid and electrolyte balance must be maintained. The hyperosmotic fluids and glucocorticosteroids can cause severe fluctuations in hydration and electrolytes, necessitating careful monitoring and replacement therapy. Although the objective of the hyperosmotic fluids is to remove excess fluid from the brain, it is not necessary to dehydrate the animal. See chapters 61 and 63 for details.

Management of the patient that remains unconscious for more than 24 hours includes maintenance of normal hydration and electrolytes, adequate ventilation, normal body temperature, frequent turning to prevent pulmonary congestion and pressure sores, and monitoring urinary output and preventing urine scalds by cleansing the skin. If the animal is unconscious for a prolonged period, it must be supplied with a source of calories. Intravenous alimentation is possible but expensive. Tube feeding may be tried, but monitoring for regurgitation or vomiting is essential to prevent aspiration pneumonia. Decubital ulcers are a common complication. Bedding, such as fleece or a water bed, are useful adjuncts to frequent turning, baths, and massage of the skin.

PROGNOSIS

The prognosis depends on the cause and the extent of brain damage. In head trauma, animals that are unconscious from the time of injury and remain unconscious for more than 24 hours usually have brain stem hemorrhage with irreversible damage. Some will regain consciousness, but they usually have severe deficits. If the onset is slower and progression can be reversed, the prognosis is more favorable. Management of a comatose patient requires full-time nursing care. It is a major medical challenge.

REFERENCES

1. Braughler JM, Hall ED: Current application of "high-dose" steroid therapy for CNS injury. J Neurosurg 62:806–810, 1985
2. Cartlidge NEF: States of altered consciousness. In Swash M, Kennard C (eds): Scientific Basis of Clinical Neurology. Edinburgh, Churchill Livingstone, 1985
3. Hall ED: High-dose glucocorticoid treatment improves neurological recovery in head-injured mice. J Neurosurg 62:882–887, 1985
4. Hoerlein BF, Redding RW, Hoff EJ Jr, McGuire JA: Evaluation of naloxone, crocetin, thyrotropin releasing hormone, methylprednisolone, partial myelotomy, and hemilaminectomy in the treatment of acute spinal cord trauma. J Am Anim Hosp Assoc 21:67–77, 1985
5. Kornegay JN, Oliver JE, Jr, Gorgacz EJ: Clinicopathologic features of brain herniation in animals. J Am Vet Med Assoc 182:1111–1116, 1983
6. Oliver JE, Jr, Lorenz M: Handbook of Veterinary Neurologic Diagnosis. Philadelphia, WB Saunders, 1983
7. Saper CB: Hypothalamus and brainstem. In Pearlman AL, Collins RC (eds): Neurological Pathophysiology, 3rd ed. New York, Oxford University Press, 1984
8. Toombs JP, Caywood DD, Lipowitz AJ, Stevens JB: Colonic perforation following neurosurgical procedures and corticosteroid therapy in four dogs. J Am Vet Med Assoc 177:68, 1980

Part Thirteen

SPECIAL SENSATION PROBLEMS

52

Blindness

CHARLES L. MARTIN

PROBLEM DEFINITION AND RECOGNITION

Blindness, for purposes of this chapter, is defined as loss of vision in both eyes. The clinical tests that attempt to measure vision in veterinary medicine are crude, nonquantitative, and nonstandardized. They include navigation of an obstacle course in a strange environment, reacting to a menacing gesture, detection of movement such as a falling cotton ball, or optokinetic nystagmus and preferential vision testing. These tests are not specific, and lesions remote from the visual system may create deficits. Objective measurements such as visual evoked responses in the occipital cortex determine the integrity of the visual system but are not quantitative or widely available. The electroretinogram measures the function of the outer half of the retina and cannot be used as a quantitative test for visual function. Pupillary light reflexes (PLR) are not a visual function test but, when critically performed, they are of benefit in localizing lesions that affect vision.

When considering the problem of blindness, one has to consider the possibility of sequential events, for example, dissimilar lesions in each eye, culminating in blindness, as well as simultaneous events. Similarly, an apparent acute blindness may only reflect a change in environment, acute injury to one eye when the opposite eye has been chronicly blind, or the final insult to a chronic minimally functional eye.

PATHOPHYSIOLOGY

Blindness can be produced by bilateral lesions in four general ways: (1) lesions that produce opacification of the clear ocular media, (2) failure of the retina to process the image, (3) failure to transmit or relay the message, and (4) failure in the final processing of the image.

The pathways for vision and the PLR are presented in Figure 53-1 (consult chapter 53 for detailed interpretation). The two pathways are similar until just before the lateral geniculate body, where they diverge. These similarities and differences can be useful for lesion localization, but there are pitfalls. Although the pathways are initially similar, it must be remembered that vision is dependent on not only the quantity but also the quality of light reaching the retina, whereas the PLR is dependent on quantity. Therefore, a lesion that causes a great deal of scattering of light (such as a cataract or any lesion of the clear media) may degrade the retinal image to the point of producing blindness but not be so obstructive to light as to interfere with the pupillary light reflex. The pupillomotor fibers may be spared with some forms of retinal and optic nerve disease. The efferent arm of the PLR is independent of vision and must be considered as the cause for pupillomotor dysfunction before utilizing the afferent arm of the reflex for lesion localization. Finally, the interpretation of a normal or abnormal response is subjective in most testing situations and dependent on the examiner's experience, anxiety of the patient, brightness of the stimulus, contrast of the ambient light to the stimulus, and adaptation of the retina.

RULE OUTS

Blindness From Lesions of the Clear Ocular Media

As a group, these are the easiest to diagnose. Any opacity of the cornea, aqueous humor, lens, or vitreous or combinations of these opacities that are severe enough to block out the light reflex from the tapetum can be interpreted to be severe enough to produce blindness, although the patient may be sensitive to light (see Etiologies of Bilateral Blindness). Patients with a tapetal reflex and blurred fundus detail on ophthalmoscopy are usually functional; consequently, additional lesions should be suspected in the blindness evaluation. Lesions of the clear ocular media can be detected with only a penlight and the patient will have a normal PLR unless there is a concurrent lesion in the efferent arm of the pupillary light reflex.

Blindness From Retinal Lesions

Diffuse bilateral lesions of the retina resulting in blindness also produce dilated pupils under room light conditions. In dogs blind from retinal disease, testing the PLR with a strong light will often produce pupillary constriction, but the amount and speed of constriction are subnormal. The majority of blind patients from retinal causes will have obvious abnormalities on ophthalmoscopy, but important exceptions exist (see list of etiologies). The obvious assumption is that the observer can make an accurate assessment as to the normalcy of the ocular fundus. It is common for lesions of the clear media (*i.e.*, cataracts or asteroid hyalosis) to coexist with advanced retinal lesions. This must always be evaluated, particularly if cataract surgery is being considered as a cure for the blind-

Etiologies of Bilateral Blindness

- Opacification of the ocular media
  - Keratitis: keratoconjunctivitis sicca, immune mediated, multiple ulcerative insults with scarring
  - Keratopathy: lipid dystrophy, endothelial dystrophy
  - Aqueous turbidity: fibrin (anterior uveitis), lipid, hemorrhage from trauma or blood dyscrasia
  - Cataracts: genetic, metabolic, toxic, nutritional
  - Vitreous hemorrhage: blood dyscrasia, trauma, retinal disease
- Diseases of the retina
  - Retinopathy
    - Genetic: progressive retinal atropy in dogs and cats, retinal pigment epitheliopathy (central retinal atrophy)
    - Nutritional: taurine deficiency in cats, vitamin E deficiency, vitamin A deficiency
    - Glaucoma
    - Inborn errors of metabolism
    - Silent retina syndrome (unknown cause for photoreceptor degeneration in dogs)
  - Retinal detachment syndromes
    - Genetic: collie eye anomaly, retinal dysplasia
    - Exudative: systemic mycoses, protothecosis, ehrlichiosis, toxoplasmosis, feline infectious peritonitis, feline leukemia associated
    - Transudative: hypertension, intravenous fluid overloading
    - Neoplastic: reticulosis, metastatic
    - Chorioretinitis: distemper, systemic mycoses, brucellosis, feline infectious peritonitis, toxoplasmosis
- Lesions of the conducting mechanism (optic nerve or tracts)
  - Hypoplasia of the optic nerves
  - Reticulosis or granulomatous encephalomyelitis
  - Distemper encephalitis
  - Feline infectious peritonitis meningoencephalitis
  - Systemic mycoses
  - Neoplasms involving the chiasm
  - Traumatic avulsion
- Lesions of the occipital cortex
  - Hydrocephalus
  - Cerebral malformations (lissencephaly)
  - Distemper encephalomyelitis
  - Feline meningoencephalitis
  - Systemic mycoses
  - Reticulosis (granulomatous meningoencephalitis)
  - Hepatoencephalopathy
  - Inborn metabolic errors
  - Hypoxia
  - Vascular infarcts
  - Traumatic edema or hemorrhage

ness. Ophthalmoscopic lesions that are typical of advanced retinal disease are retinal detachment, attenuation in size and a decrease in number of retinal vessels, diffuse increases or decreases in tapetal reflectivity, marked pigmentary disruptions, and accumulations in the nontapetum or tapetum.

Blindness From Lesions in the Conducting System up to the Lateral Geniculate Body

With the exception of the optic disc, the conducting system cannot be directly observed without special radiographic techniques. Diagnosis is often by exclusion unless sophisticated electronics are available to perform electroretinograms and visual evoked responses. A lesion of the chiasm or bilateral lesions of the optic nerve or optic tracts will interfere with vision as well as the pupillary light reflex. If the process extends to the optic disc, changes in color and elevation of the disc may be observed. Atropy of the disc may be recognized in dogs by the pallor, loss of myelin with scalloping of the disc border, and a decrease in elevation. Elevation of the disc may indicate papilledema or papillitis, clues as to retrobulbar involvement of the conducting system. Papillitis is accompanied by congestion of the retinal vessels, often with hemorrages, peripapillary edema, and vitreous haze. Papilledema is quieter in appearance, with less congestion, fewer hemorrhages, and mild peripapillary edema. Papilledema *per se* does not produce blindness, although the process responsible for the edema may result in blindness.

Bilateral involvement of the conducting system below the lateral geniculate body will produce blindness with loss of the PLR. With the exception of the optic chiasm, these pathways are distant from one another, and bilateral involvement is usually produced by multifocal or diffuse lesions, which often produce accompanying neurologic signs (see list of etiologies).

Cortical Blindness

Lesions of the lateral geniculate body, optic radiations, and occipital cortex will produce blindness with normal PLR and are usually consolidated under cortical blindness. The role of the occipital cortex in vision is "form recognition," whereas the dorsal colliculus in the midbrain is important in "pursuit" or "body orientation" to an object. Bilateral involvement of the occipital cortex may be produced by lesions such as encephalitis, hydrocephalus, or a metabolic or toxic encephalopathy (see list of etiologies) and are usually not selective; thus, a thorough neurologic examination is indicated.

DIAGNOSTIC PLAN

See Figure 52-1 for a diagnostic plan to evaluate the blind patient.

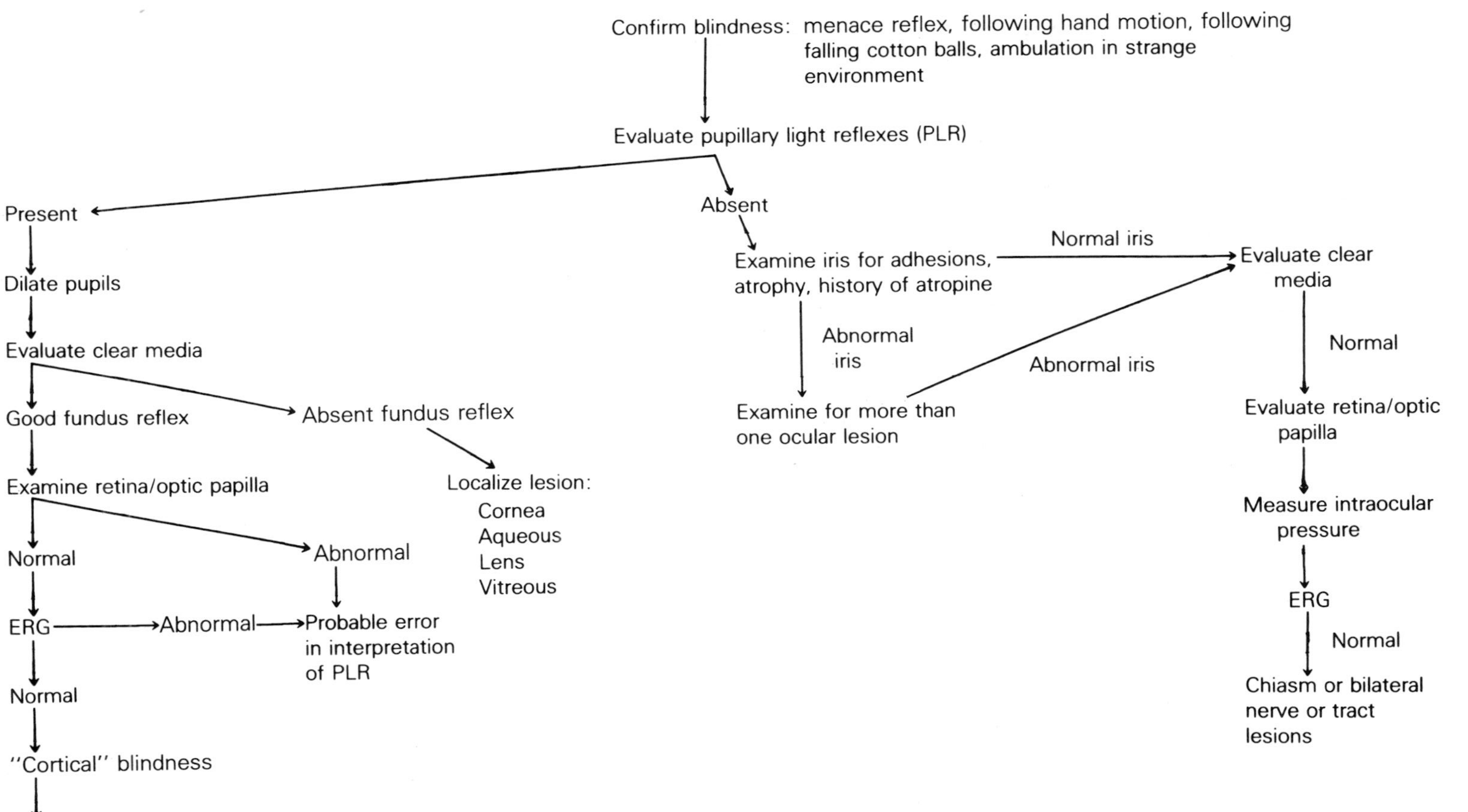

Fig. 52-1. Diagnostic plan for evaluation of a blind patient.

SYMPTOMATIC THERAPY

Symptomatic therapy for blindness of the clear ocular media consists of removing the opacity surgically or using corticosteroids if the lesion is inflammatory. Inflammatory corneal lesions often respond dramatically to topical or subconjunctival corticosteroids but should *not* be used when corneal ulceration or active infection is present. Tear deficiencies can be treated medically or surgically with a parotid duct transplant. Surgical lens extraction, waiting for spontaneous lens resorption (juvenile cataracts), or dilating the pupil to overcome a central opacity are the only therapies for cataracts. In young puppies, if the cataracts are not progressive, they will become smaller in relationship to the total lens, due to growth of the lens. Hyphema is usually treated conservatively with restriction of activity. Fibrin and lipids in the anterior chamber are associated with an anterior uveitis that is treated for the specific infectious agent or with topical and perhaps systemic corticosteroids if nonseptic. Opacities in the vitreous are not treated unless they are thought to be infectious in origin. Hemorrhage and fibrous bands are often treated in humans with vitreous excision, but this procedure is not practiced routinely in veterinary ophthalmology. Refer to chapters 55, 56, and 57 for a more detailed discussion on treatment of diseases of the clear ocular media and anterior uveitis.

Most retinal causes of blindness are not treatable. Nutritional causes for retinal degeneration (if diagnosed before blindness) might be arrested, but once the animal is blind, the process is usually irreversible. Glaucoma-induced retinal/optic nerve blindness can be wholly or partially reversed if the intraocular pressure is lowered, but the duration of the tolerated elevated pressures is inversely related to the degree of elevation. Intraocular pressures between 60 and 80 mm Hg may produce permanent blindness after only a few days. Emergency therapy for glaucoma consists of osmotic diuretics and carbonic-anhydrase-inhibiting diuretics (see chapter 55).

Retinal detachments that produce blindness are usually complete. Detachments due to large peripheral tears, such as in the genetic syndromes, are some of the most difficult to surgically reattach and are rarely attempted by veterinary ophthalmologists. Exudative detachments may reattach if the subretinal exudate is reabsorbed, but most of the infectious agents that produce these syndromes also produce massive disruption of the retina itself; thus, it rarely returns to function. Animals with transudative detachments are the most likely to retain some vision after reabsorption of the subretinal fluid. If the cause is hypertension, the retina will reattach when the hypertension is controlled. Numerous antihypertensive agents are available for humans but veterinarians have minimal experience with them.

Very little symptomatic therapy is available for blindness of neurologic origin. Patients with acute optic nerve blindness should have a trial of antiinflammatory doses of prednisolone if there is no evidence of systemic infection. Acute idiopathic optic neuritis and reticulosis are often steroid responsive; when treated early, a dramatic return of vision may occur. Cortical blindness from hepatoencephalopathy is transient; treatment is directed at lowering the dietary protein and correcting the vascular anomaly (if present). Cortical blindness from hypoxia improves spontaneously after a 2- to 4-week delay. Many animals with hypoxia also have lower lesions, as evidenced by dilated pupils, and do not improve spontaneously.

53

Anisocoria

CHARLES L. MARTIN

PROBLEM DEFINITION AND RECOGNITION

Anisocoria, or unequal pupils, can be divided anatomically into ocular and neurologic causes. Because the ocular causes can often be directly observed, it is usually expedient to eliminate ocular etiologies of anisocoria before proceeding to a neurologic explanation. If vision is impaired, the reader is referred also to chapter 53 (blindness). Determining which of the two pupils is abnormal may be difficult. If a pupil is immobile to either light or dark stimulation or both, it is obviously abnormal. Normalcy of pupils that are not completely immobile must be judged by evaluating the range of their excursions, the briskness of the constriction, the size of the pupil expected at a given ambient light, and response to the swinging light test. Anatomic abnormalities such as an irregularity that may indicate synechiae or atrophy of the sphincter may provide additional clues to pupil abnormality.

PATHOPHYSIOLOGY

The pathways for the pupillomotor fibers and vision are illustrated in Figure 53-1.

The afferent arm of the pupillary light reflex (PLR) consists of three neurons: bipolar cells, ganglion cells, and neurons in the pretectal nucleus. The afferent arm of the pupillomotor fibers course with the visual fibers until just before the lateral geniculate body. Seventy-five percent and 65% of the dog and cat, respectively, visual and pupillomotor fibers decussate (cross) at the optic chiasm.[3] The majority of pupillomotor fibers then cross again in the pretectum to the original side.[7]

The efferent arm of the PLR consists of two neurons: the first originates in the parasympathetic nucleus of the oculomotor nerve (cranial nerve III) and remains ipsilateral to synapse in the ciliary ganglion; the second neuron passes

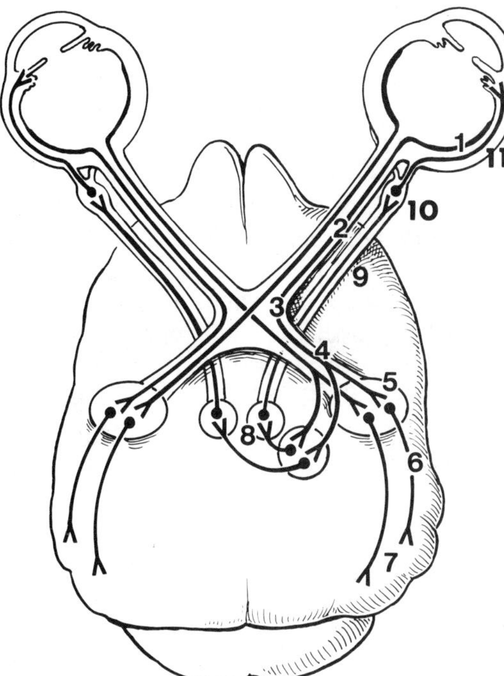

Fig. 53-1. Pupillary light reflex and vision pathways. The two types of fibers have similar pathways until point 4, where they diverge. *1,* retina; *2,* optic nerve; *3,* chiasm; *4,* optic tract; *5,* lateral geniculate body; *6,* optic radiation; *7,* occipital cortex; *8,* parasympathetic nuclei of oculomotor nerve; *9,* oculomotor nerve; *10,* ciliary ganglion; *11,* short ciliary nerve. (Modified from Oliver JE, Lorenz MD: Handbook of Veterinary Neurologic Diagnosis, p 255. Philadelphia, WB Saunders, 1983)

from the ciliary ganglion in the short ciliary nerves to the iris sphincter muscle. The short ciliary nerves differ in the dog and cat. In the dog, multiple branches supply the globe; in the cat, only two branches are present.[7]

Evaluation of PLR and dynamic anisocorias requires an appreciation of the differences in the proportion of optic nerve fibers that cross at the chiasm, and subsequently the midbrain, in the particular species examined. This lack of equal input to both eyes when stimulating the PLR in one eye explains the dynamic anisocoria in the normal dog; that is, the consensual reflex is not as strong or complete as the direct PLR. Data extrapolated from humans and primates, in which 50% of the fibers cross, are not completely applicable.

Sympathetic innervation to the iris provides the stimulation for dilation by relaxing the sphincter muscle and contracting the dilator muscle. The sympathetic chain is long and consists of three neurons. The first neuron originates in the hypothalamus, passing with some decussation down the brain stem and cervical spinal cord to synapse at the level of thoracic segments 1, 2, and 3. The second neuron passes through the rostral chest and up the neck in the vagosympathetic trunk to synapse in the cranial cervical ganglion. The third neuron traverses the tympanic bulla and joins the ophthalmic division of the fifth cranial nerve in the cranial vault to reach the globe via the long ciliary nerve.

Anisocoria can be classified as a static or dynamic inequality of pupils. Static anisocoria is manifested without stimulation of the PLR and is constant, whereas dynamic anisocorias manifest during or immediately after stimulation of the pupillary light reflex.[4]

TESTING THE PUPILLARY LIGHT REFLEXES

Direct and consensual reflexes are best determined by utilizing a strong stimulating light in a room with dim ambient light. The direct response is determined and the consensual response is evaluated while alternately directing the light quickly from one eye to the other at 2- to 4-second intervals (swinging light test). The pupils will normally have minimal excursions during the swinging light test. An afferent defect in the pupillary light reflex can be detected even if an efferent arm lesion such as synechiae or oculomotor paralysis is present. Afferent arm lesions are detected in the presence of efferent lesions with the swinging light test by the detection of further constriction of the opposite normal eye when the light is swung over to it. This is not as sensitive in animals as in humans, due to the normal dynamic anisocoria that is present with the unequal decussation of the optic nerve. Afferent arm lesions are normally determined by pupil dilation when the light is shown in the abnormal eye on the swinging light test (Marcus Gunn pupil).

ANISOCORIAS INDUCED BY OCULAR DISEASE

When evaluating an eye with anisocoria, one must note whether the pupil is capable of movement with either the direct or consensual PLR, whether vision is present, and the size of the immobile or relatively immobile pupil. An animal that has an immobile pupil creating anisocoria has a problem with the efferent arm of the reflex arc (oculomotor parasympathetic nucleus or nerve) or the target organ (iris).

Diseases of the Iris

Anisocorias associated with iris disease constitute an efferent arm defect. Several relatively common conditions involving the iris will produce static anisocorias: anterior uveitis, glaucoma, sphincter iris atropy, iris hypoplasia, and pharmacologic blockade. Anterior uveitis (iritis) typically produces a miotic pupil that is relatively resistant to mydriatic drugs (atropine or tropicamide). Additional signs of anterior chamber flare, iris color changes, iris texture changes, and hypotony are usually present. Posterior synechiae frequently develop and are an additional cause for static anisocoria with anterior uveitis. Posterior synechiae are recognized by irregular pupil margins and pigment debris on the anterior lens capsule.

Iris atrophy near the pupil weakens the sphincter muscle function, resulting in a dilated pupil that is resistant to pharmacologic constriction. Sphincter atropy may occur in otherwise normal eyes, but when it occurs with cataracts, it makes evaluation of the preoperative cataract patient difficult. Miniature and toy poodles frequently develop atrophy of the pupillary margin of the iris. The condition is usually bilateral; however, if severity is asymmetric, a static anisocoria results. Atrophy of the sphincter is most reliably recognized by observing a scalloped pupillary margin, often with patches of iris that transilluminate against the tapetal reflex. Although the pupillary margin is irregular, as with posterior synechiae, it is not adhered with pigmented extensions of iris onto the anterior lens capsule.

A "normal" mild anisocoria can be discerned in animals with heterochromia. The blue iris will be mildly dilated in relation to the darker iris.

Intraocular Pressure Elevation

Primary glaucoma usually manifests with a static anisocoria produced by a dilated pupil that is unresponsive to light. When the intraocular pressure exceeds the intraocular diastolic blood pressure (about 50 mm Hg), the pupil becomes dilated if it is not adherent and is unresponsive to light or pharmacologic stimulation. Additional signs of increased firmness and globe size are typical of glaucoma. Anterior uveitis and glaucoma share the signs of conjunctival and episcleral injection and corneal edema. Secondary glaucoma from pupil occlusion and seclusion usually leaves the pupil immobile in midposition.

Drug-Induced Anisocoria

Topical application of belladona alkaloids will produce a static anisocoria that may last for 4 to 5 days or longer after the last application. If the application was accidental, the history may not be helpful and the cause can only be diagnosed by the lack of ocular signs such as synechiae, increased pressure, or iris atrophy and the lack of response to direct-acting miotic drugs (pilocarpine). Improvement after several days aids in retrospectively diagnosing drug-induced mydriasis. Similarly, unilateral application of miotic agents may complicate the diagnosis, although those compounds have a shorter duration of action.

Anisocoria Induced by Corneal Disease

The pain of superficial corneal ulceration may produce a very strong miosis and static anisocoria. The miosis is atropine resistant and mediated by antidromic impulses via the ophthalmic nerve (see chapter 56).

Anisocoria Induced by Lenticular Disease

Mild anisocorias, either dynamic or static, may occur with lens subluxations, luxations, and hypermature cataracts that interfere with pupil mobility. Dyscoria, or a misshapened pupil, is often present with the latter conditions.

Anisocoria Induced by Retinal Blindness

Unilateral retinal and optic nerve blindness will produce a mild static anisocoria with pupillary dilation in the involved eye in the dog and cat, due to the weaker consensual input to the blind eye. The blind eye will exhibit a pupillary escape phenomenon or dilate when the light is moved from the visual eye to the blind eye during the swinging light test. This is termed a *Marcus Gunn reaction.*

ANISCORIA ASSOCIATED WITH NEUROLOGIC DISEASE

Afferent Arm Lesions

Unilateral lesions of the afferent arm of the pupillary light reflex will produce mild static anisocorias, due to the unequal distribution of crossed and uncrossed fibers in the dog. These will become more manifest with dynamic anisocorias upon PLR testing.

Optic Nerve Lesions

Unilateral lesions of the optic nerve produce a more dilated pupil ipsilaterally, which reacts consensually and exhibits a Marcus Gunn pupil or redilates on direct stimulation in the swinging light test. Unilateral optic nerve lesions manifest similarly to retinal lesions and are differentiated by ophthalmoscopy and electroretinography. Eyes with afferent arm lesions will dilate in the dark to equal pupil size.

Optic Tract Lesions

Unilateral lesions of the optic tract are harder to localize with the PLR, because they contain a mixture of crossed and uncrossed fibers and because the lesions may not be complete. Complete lesions manifest with a mild static anisocoria, with the lesion being contralateral to the more dilated (abnormal) pupil. They may be differentiated from optic nerve and retinal lesions with the swinging light test by the lack of a Marcus Gunn response, due to the intact uncrossed fibers.[7] Both pupils will dilate and be equal in darkness.

Efferent Arm Lesions

Lesions of the parasympathetic nuclei, oculomotor nerve, and ciliary ganglion produce an ipsilateral dilated pupil and static anisocoria. The anisocoria with efferent arm lesions is more marked than that with afferent arm lesions. Lesions that involve the parasympathetic nuclei usually also involve the motor nuclei and are often bilateral. Most oculomotor nerve lesions involve both the parasympathetic and motor fibers, creating an ocular deviation that, when acute, is lateral-ventral. The globe is immobile except for lateral and intorsional movements (lateral rectus muscle is innervated by cranial nerve VI; dorsal oblique muscle is innervated by cranial nerve IV).[3] Oculomotor nerve involvement may arise intracranially, in the orbital fissure, or intraorbitally. In dogs, orbital lesions may involve both the oculomotor nerve and ciliary ganglion. In the latter instance, both the ocular parasympathetics and sympathetic fibers are damaged, producing a fixed-midpoint pupil that does not constrict to light or dilate with darkness. Cats may have an isolated palsy of one of the two short ciliary nerves (postganglionic parasympathetic fibers), which produces a D- or reversed-D–shaped pupil due to the hemidilation.[7]

Feline Dysautonomia (Key-Gaskell Syndrome)

A syndrome of generalized dysautonomia with ocular manifestations of dilated pupils has been described in Great Britain. The etiology is unknown, but it does not appear to be related to the feline leukemia virus, as does the alternating anisocoria syndrome. Cats with dysautonomia may have an initial anisocoria that subsequently dilates; the eyes are visual, the third eyelid is prolapsed, and tear secretions are decreased. The lesion is characterized as an efferent arm parasympathetic lesion. Additional signs of dysautonomia are constipation, regurgitation, dry mucous membranes, bradycardia, and urinary incontinence.[6,8]

Paradoxic Anisocoria in Cats

In cats, a startling syndrome is observed, in which a marked anisocoria develops and may alternate between eyes at irregular intervals of hours or days. The abnormal pupil may be dilated or constricted, or both pupils may be dilated or constricted. On ocular examination the eyes are normal; although urinary incontinence may be a complaint, most cats are systemically normal.[1,5] Most affected cats are positive on feline leukemia testing and die within the following 6 months. Scagliotti has demonstrated the leukemia virus in the ciliary nerves and ganglion of involved cats.[7] The pupils do not respond predictably to pharmacologic testing.

Efferent Sympathetic Lesions

Interruption of the sympathetic fibers of the dog and cat produce a cluster of signs ipsilaterally known as Horner's syndrome. The signs of Horner's syndrome vary between species but, in the dog and cat, consist of ptosis, miosis, prolapsed third eyelid, and enophthalmos or apparent enophthalmos. The anisocoria of Horner's syndrome is characterized by a miosis that will not dilate to be equal with the normal pupil. The anisocoria is most evident in dim light.

The ocular sympathetic neuron chain is long and the location and type of lesion can be quite varied. Lesion localization is determined by association with other neurologic or systemic signs, pharmacologic testing, chest and tympanic bulla radiographs, ear examination, and palpation of the cervical region. Horner's cases of central nervous system origin usually have other neurologic complaints or deficits, which aid in lesion localization. Occasionally, Horner's syndrome of central nervous system origin is prodromal to other neurologic signs that manifest in days to a few weeks. Preganglionic lesions from the thoracic segments 1, 2, and 3 to the cranial cervical ganglion are common and may be detected by chest radiographs and palpation. The postganglionic chain is often affected by disorders of the middle ear such as otitis media and interna. Associated signs of ipsilateral peripheral vestibular disease and, perhaps, facial nerve paralysis are frequent with Horner's syndrome of otitis origin.

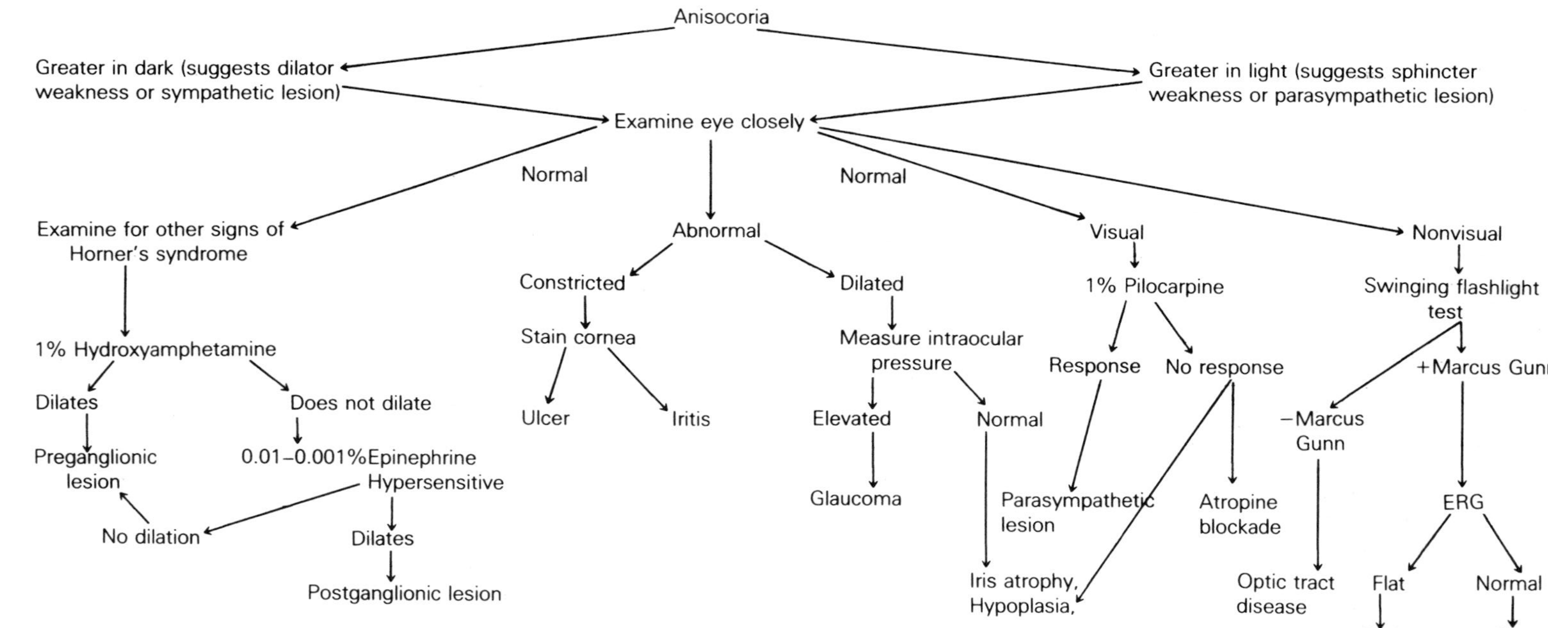

Fig. 53-2. Algorithm for the diagnosis of anisocoria.

DIAGNOSTIC PLAN

Figure 53-2 outlines a diagnostic plan for anisocoria. Pharmacologic testing can be utilized, but because responses can vary, a control eye, preferably the normal eye, should also be monitored. Pharmacologic testing employs the phenomenon of denervation hypersensitivity to the missing neurotransmitter if the third neuron is involved and the intact response when stimulated with indirect-acting drugs when the first and second neurons are destroyed. Third neuron disease of either the parasympathetic or sympathetic chain induces an exaggerated response to acetylcholine (or other direct-acting parasympathomimetics) or epinephrine/norepinephrine (or other direct-acting sympathomimetics) due to the lack of uptake and neutralization of the neurotransmitters by the missing third neuron.[2] Indirect-acting parasympathetics and sympathetics act by stimulating the release of neurotransmitters or interfering with the neutralization of the neurotransmitters and thus require an intact third neuron to release the neurotransmitter. Tables 53-1 and 53-2 lists the results of pharmacologic testing and lesion localization. Preganglionic lesions require a thorough neurologic evaluation. The prognosis is usually worse with either sympathetic or parasympathetic lesions.

Table 53-1. Pharmacologic Lesion Localization in Horner's Syndrome

DRUG	NORMAL	CENTRAL LESION	PREGANGLIONIC LESION	POSTGANGLIONIC LESION
1% Hydroxamphetamine	+	+	+	0
1% Phenylephrine	0	0	0	+
0.001% Epinephrine	0	0	Mild +	+

+, dilates; 0,

Table 53-2. Pharmacologic Lesion Localization With a Dilated Pupil

DRUG	NORMAL	CENTRAL PARASYMPATHETIC LESION	PERIPHERAL PARASYMPATHETIC LESION	IRIS ATROPHY	GLAUCOMA	ATROPINE BLOCKADE
1% Pilocarpine	+	+	+ (hypersensitive)	0	0	0
0.01% Phospholine iodide	+	+	0	0	0	0

+, constriction; 0,

THERAPY

Anisocoria associated with Horner's syndrome may be treated with a direct-acting sympathomimetic such as topical 2% epinephrine or 10% phenylephrine. The cosmetic improvement has to be weighed against the ocular discomfort of these drops, and the cost and bother to the owner must be considered. Anisocoria is a sign rather than a disease. Therapy is directed at the etiology rather than the anisocoria.

REFERENCES

1. Barsanti J, Downey R: Urinary incontinence in cats. J Am Anim Hosp Assoc 20:979, 1984
2. Bistner S, Rubin L, Cox T, Condon W: Pharmacologic diagnosis of Horner's syndrome in the dog. J Am Vet Med Assoc 157:1220, 1970
3. de Lahunta A: Visual system—special somatic afferent system. In Veterinary Neuroanatomy and Clinical Neurology, p 266. Philadelphia, WB Saunders, 1977
4. Duke-Elder S, Scott GI: The pupillary and ciliary systems. In System of Ophthalmology, Vol XII, p 613. London, Henry Kimpton, 1971
5. Martin C: Ocular signs of systemic disease, part I. Mod Vet Pract 1982, p 639
6. Rochlitz I: Feline dysautonomia (the Key-Gaskell or dilated pupil syndrome): A preliminary review. J Small Anim Pract 25:587, 1984
7. Scagliotti R: Neuro-Ophthalmology. In Kirk R (ed): Current Veterinary Therapy VII, p 510. Philadelphia, WB Saunders, 1980
8. Sharp N, Nash A, Griffiths I: Feline dysautonomia (the Key-Gaskell syndrome): A clinical and pathological study of forty cases. J Small Anim Pract 25:599, 1985

54

Abnormal Ocular Movement and Position

CHARLES L. MARTIN

PROBLEM DEFINITION AND RECOGNITION

Abnormal ocular movements can be divided into ocular deviations (strabismus), paralysis of gaze, and nystagmus.[3] Nystagmus is defined as an rhythmic involuntary movement of the eye(s) and may be in a horizontal, vertical, or rotary direction. The eye(s) may be in an abnormal position due to movement around its center of rotation or by displacement of the globe within the orbit.[4] The latter movement is termed *translational* and may be active in domestic animals as a result of disorders of the retractor bulbi muscle or passive such as from a space-occupying lesion of the orbit.

The term *duction* refers to movement of only one eye and is modified by a prefix to indicate the direction of movement: adduction is movement of the eye medially in a horizontal plane, abduction is lateral movement, supraduction is dorsal movement, and infraduction is ventral movement. Torsional ductions include intorsion (incycloduction), in which the dorsal pupil rotates medially, and extorsion (excyloduction), in which the dorsal pupil rotates laterally (Fig. 54-1).[5]

Versions are the simultaneous movement of both eyes in the same direction (conjugate movement), *e.g.*, horizontal versions of dextroversion and levoversion and the vertical versions of supraversion and infraversion. Vergence is the simultaneous and equal movement of the eyes in opposite directions, *i.e.*, convergence and divergence (Fig. 54-2).[5]

The position of the frontally placed eyes when normally fixating on a distant object that is straight ahead is the primary position of the eyes. Eyes that have a manifest deviation are said to have a tropia (*e.g.*, exotropia, esotropia). Eyes with a latent deviation that is manifested when shielded from fixation have a phoria (*e.g.*, exophoria, esophoria). A comitant trophia is constant in all directions of gaze; a noncomitant deviation varies with the direction of gaze.[5]

(Text continues on p 486.)

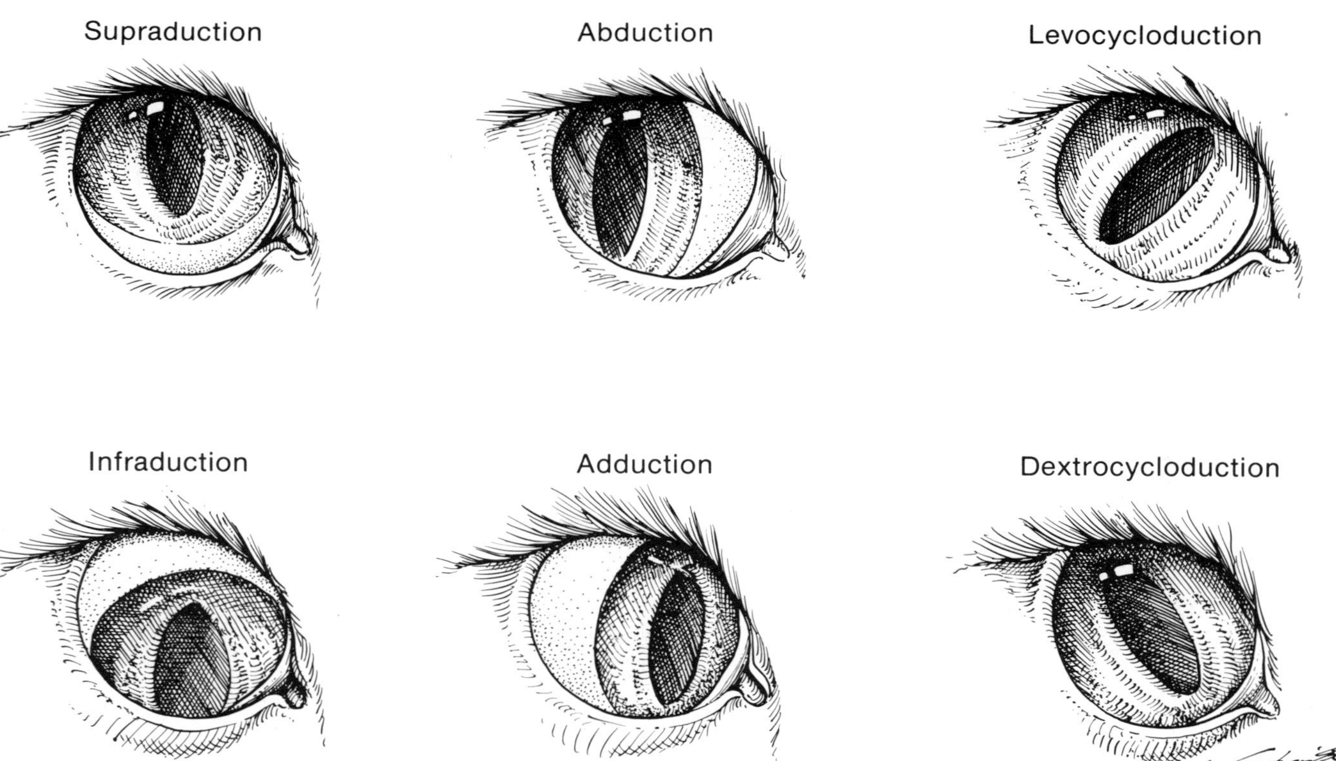

Fig. 54-1. Ductional movements in a cat eye.

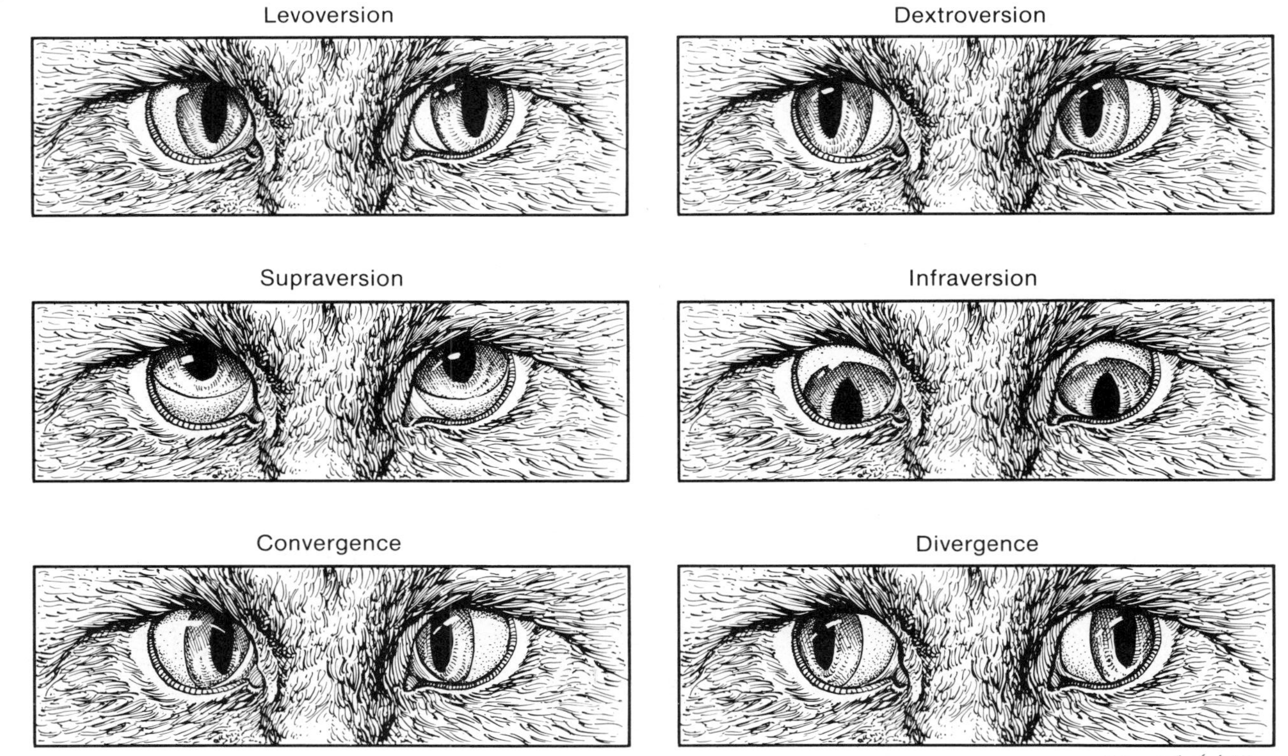

Fig. 54-2. Version and vergence eye movements in a cat.

PATHOPHYSIOLOGY

The extraocular muscles in mammals are skeletal muscle, but differ from other skeletal muscle in having at least two fiber systems. One type of muscle fiber usually found in skeletal muscle is composed of well organized myofibrils, innervated with thick myelinated nerves, and is responsible for the rapid eye movements, or saccades. The second type of fiber is not composed of definite myofibrils and is innervated by small myelinated nerves. These fibers are responsible for the smooth, slow contractions that hold the eyes in position or are used in following. The extraocular muscles are much more richly innervated than other skeletal muscle, which reflects their function of rapid and fine adjustment in eye position.[4,8] Domestic animals generally have relatively limited ocular motility compared with humans. In general, the amount of exposed sclera in the palpebral fissure is directly related to the ocular motility in the species. The lack of ocular motility is compensated by either the lateral positioning of the eyes or the increased ability to swivel the head, *i.e.*, as in the owl.[7] The actions of the individual extraocular muscles varies between species, due to variable insertion sites. The main actions of the extraocular muscles are presented in Table 54-1. The resultant deviations that would result from acute muscle or nerve function are given in Table 54-2. In animals with a retractor bulbi muscle, compensation apparently occurs and the acute ocular deviations are less apparent with time.

Figures 54-3 and 54-4 illustrate the extraocular muscles of the cat. The lateral rectus muscle and retractor bulbi muscle are innervated by cranial nerve VI; the dorsal oblique by cranial nerve IV; and the medial, ventral, and dorsal rectus and ventral oblique muscle by cranial nerve III. The pathways and control of ocular movements are complex and incompletely understood. Supranuclear pathways (above the cranial nerve nuclei) are involved with movement of the eyes in a coordinated manner, rather than contraction of an individual muscle.[6]

Cortical Centers for Ocular Movement

The frontal cortex serves voluntary control of the ocular movements, and the occipital cortex serves movement of the eye in response to visual stimuli (opto-

Table 54-1. Action and Innervation of Extraocular Muscles

MUSCLE	ACTION	INNERVATION
Dorsal rectus	Supraduction, adduction	CN III
Medial rectus	Adduction	CN III
Ventral rectus	Infraduction, adduction	CN III
Ventral oblique	Extorsion, adduction	CN III
Dorsal oblique	Intorsion, adduction	CN IV
Lateral rectus	Abduction	CN VI
Retractor bulbi	Retraction of globe	CN VI

CN, cranial nerve

Table 54-2. Acute Signs of Dysfunction of Extraocular Muscles and Cranial Nerves

MUSCLE/NERVE	SIGN	TEST
Dorsal rectus	Infratropia, inability to supraduct	Move head downward
Medial rectus	Exotropia, inability to adduct	Move head horizontally, visual following
Ventral rectus	Supratropia, inability to infraduct	Move head upward
Ventral oblique	Inability to extort eye	Rotate head
Dorsal oblique	Inability to intort eye	Rotate head
Lateral rectus	Esotropia, inability to abduct	Move head horizontally, visual following
Retractor bulbi	Inability to retract globe	Touch cornea
CN III	Extropia, infratropia, pupil dilated ±	
CN IV	No obvious signs (See dorsal oblique.)	
CN VI	Esotropia (See lateral rectus.)	

CN, cranial nerve; ±, may or may not be present

motor). The optomotor stimuli produce slow, smooth, following movements of the eye; the voluntary movements produce rapid, jerky jumps, or saccades. Stimulation of the frontal cortex unilaterally produces lateral conjugate movements to the opposite side; thus, unilateral lesions of the frontal cortex produce transient paresis of conjugate gaze until the opposite cortex assumes bilateral control (in a few weeks).[6]

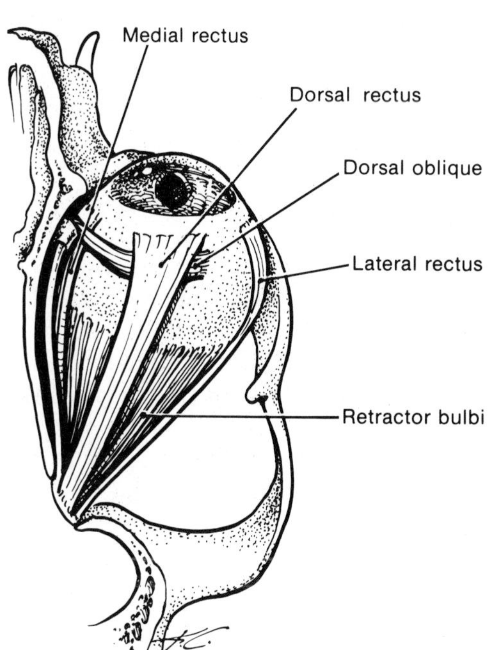

Fig. 54-3. Dorsal view of the extraocular muscles of the cat.

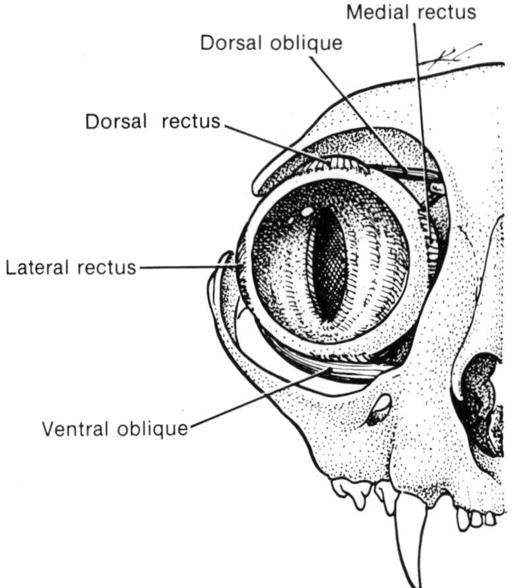

Fig. 54-4. Anterior view of the cat eye and the extraocular muscles.

The occipital cortex optomotor fibers pass down to the superior colliculus and serve the functions of keeping a moving target on the macula and orienting the body to a moving object. Connections between the frontal and occipital cortex are present, but the frontal eye reflexes predominate. Optokinetic nystagmus is the ocular movement produced by following a moving target going in one direction. The smooth following movement of the optomotor movements (occipital lobe) is followed by the rapid, jerky recovery saccade from the frontal cortex. A bilateral disease of the frontal cortex or a lesion interfering with the interconnection of the two cortices will produce a slow movement of the eyes without the rapid recovery phase.[6]

Vestibular (Labyrinth) Ocular Movements

Vestibular reflex tonus coordinates changes in posture with movements of the eyes. These reflexes can be categorized into (1) static reflexes that respond to the head's position or gravitational changes and (2) kinetic reflexes that respond to movement such as acceleration or deceleration. Vestibular reflexes produce only conjugate movements (both eyes moving in the same direction). Each labyrinth exerts tone on the opposite lateral rectus and ipsilateral medial rectus via connections through the medial longitudinal fasciculus from the vestibular nucleus (Fig. 54-5). With a balanced input from both sides, the eyes are kept straight. Stimulation of one labyrinth produces a slow movement to the opposite side, followed by a rapid saccadic movement that is a corrective movement from the frontal cortex. The direction of the nystagmus is named according to the rapid or cortical phase. Destruction of a labyrinth produces a slow drift to the affected side due to the imbalanced input from the intact side. The fast-phase movement

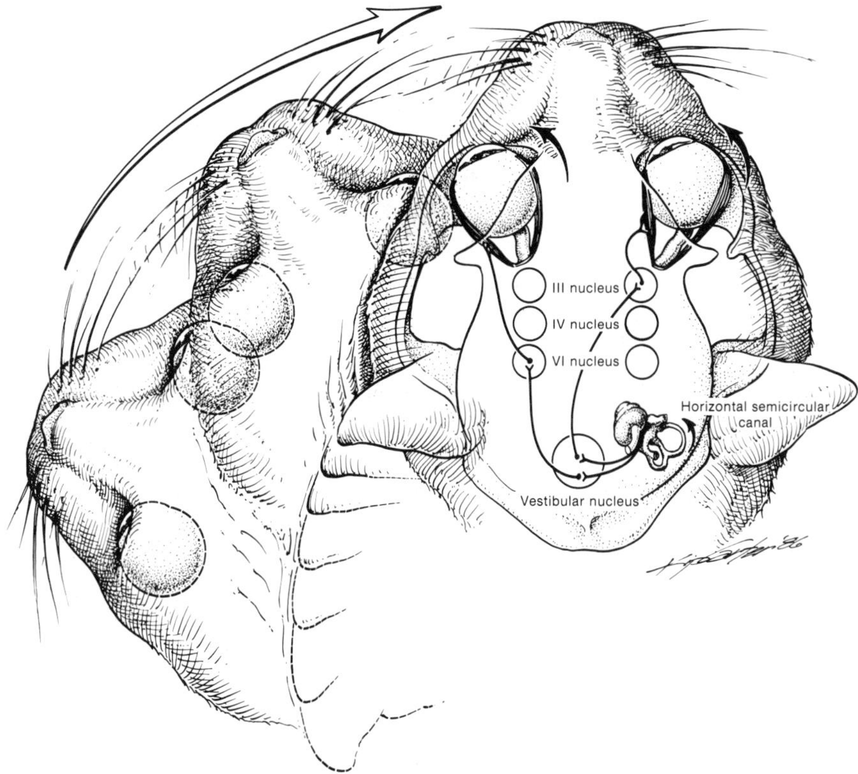

Fig. 54-5. Connections of the horizontal labyrinth with the extraocular muscles and the stimulation of vestibular induced eye movements by movement of the head.

(nystagmus) is to the contralateral side. The direction of the nystagmus with a unilateral lesion will depend on whether the lesion is irritative (stimulating) or destructive.[6,8]

The otolith of the utriculus produces tonic sustained contractions of the extraocular muscles, which are designed to keep the eyes fixed in position despite changes in the head position. They keep the eyes in a vertical position with tilting of the head to the side and looking at the horizon when tilting the head ventral or dorsal.[6]

Nystagmus

Nystagmus may be characterized by the rate (rapid or slow), amplitude (coarse or fine), direction (horizontal, vertical, or rotary), and type of movement (pendular or jerk). The jerk nystagmus, such as vestibular nystagmus, has a fast and slow component, whereas with pendular nystagmus the eye movements in each direction are equal. The direction of the jerk nystagmus is, by convention, named after the fast component. Most cases of nystagmus are conjugate, with both eyes beating in the same direction. A few examples of nystagmus are relatively specific for lesion localization; however, many neurologic forms of nystagmus are nonspecific for lesion localization. Some forms of jerk nystagmus can be overridden by moving the head, which is indicative of peripheral vestibular disease.[3]

A congenital horizontal pendular nystagmus, or flutter, may be present with cerebellar disease (cerebellar flocculi) or with congenital ocular anomalies such as microphthalmia.[1,2,3,6]

DIAGNOSTIC PLAN

The evaluation of ocular position with the eyes in the primary position (straight ahead) is performed by using a light on the midline about 2 feet from the eyes and determining where the specular light reflex from the corneal surface lies in relationship to each respective pupil. With normal alignment (orthophoria), the light reflex falls in the center of the pupil or just medial to the center. Constriction of the pupil allows for more critical evaluation of the location of the corneal reflex in relationship to the pupil. Dissimilar positions of the light reflex in relationship to the pupil are indicative of strabismus and can be utilized for evaluating horizontal or vertical misalignments. Misalignment in positions of gaze other than the primary position is determined by eliciting following eye movements in attentive animals. Paresis of muscle action is determined by utilizing the vestibular ocular reflex and observing for deficits in horizontal, vertical, and torsional movement. Torsional deficits are most readily determined in species with an elongated pupil. In dogs, finding a landmark on the ocular surface and observing the fundus vessels or tapetal-nontapetal junction are means of determining torsional movements.

Determining whether the deviation is similar in different planes of eye movement is an attempt to differentiate comitant from noncomitant strabismus. Comitant strabismus is constant through movement of the eyes in all planes of movement. Noncomitant strabismus is also termed *paretic strabismus* and varies on whether the gaze is directed in the direction of the parentic muscle or nerve. Two separate phenomena occur to create paretic strabismus: (1) lag due to weakness and (2) overreaction due to increased neural impulses going to the yoke muscle. The amount of deviation varies with which eye is fixating in paretic strabismus.

Translational movement of the globe is determined by observing the animal from the dorsal view and determining whether the corneal apices are equal in their prominence. The result of this observation is combined with retropulsion of the globe in the orbit to determine the presence of an orbital space-occupying lesion. The two orbits are compared as to how easily the eye can be pushed into the orbit. Acquired exophthalmos must be differentiated from buphthalmos (enlarged globe) and shallow orbits (in brachycephalic breeds). Translational movement of the eye forward in the orbit is often combined with strabismus when it is due to space-occupying masses outside the extraocular muscle cone. The direction of deviation is typically away from the location of the space-occupying lesion. Examination of the oral cavity for pain on opening the mouth, tooth root abscessation, and swelling or fistulas behind the last molar is indicated in animals with orbital space-occupying lesions. Additional evaluation of the orbit with radiographs, ultrasound, and fine needle aspiration of localized lesions is indicated. Positive and negative contrast studies of the orbital spaces may provide additional information to characterize the noninflammatory lesions, but most require surgical exploration and biopsy for definitive diagnosis. Bony orbital involvement radiographically is typical of secondary orbital tumors that have invaded from the frontal sinus or nasal cavity.

Nystagmus is evaluated as to whether it is directional and, if so, what direction and whether it can be overridden by closing the eyes. The presence of accompanying neurologic signs or ear pathology is determined. Jerk nystagmus that is horizontal or rotary and cannot be overridden is indicative of peripheral vestibular disease; the fast phase is toward the normal side (assuming that a destructive lesion is present).[3]

SYMPTOMATIC THERAPY

The most important causes of ocular deviation in the dog and cat are traumatic injury to the extraocular muscles or nerves (postproptosis), space-occupying masses in the orbit (neoplastic or inflammatory), and neurologic lesions producing cranial nerve deficits. Many individuals in the brachycephalic breeds have a noncomitant form of strabismus without signs and require no therapy.

Strabismus postproptosis is very common and often quite severe. It typically is directed out and upward. The degree of strabismus improves over a 2-month period and does not require surgical correction in most instances. The strabismus, combined with lagophthalmos and a dry eye, produces an exposure keratoconjunctivitis that may need surgical aid. Attempts to bring the eye into primary position with sutures from the orbital rim to the globe or trying to replace torn muscles have been made, but an easier functional and cosmetic solution has been to perform a medial tarsorrhaphy. This procedure offers protection to the exposed medial cornea and gives the impression that the eye is straight.

Symptomatic therapy directed against translational movement producing proptosis is to protect the cornea from an exposure keratitis with liberal topical lubricants or to surgically protect it with a third eyelid flap or tarsorrhaphy. Specific therapy directed at the etiology of the space-occupying lesion is necessary.

REFERENCES

1. Cogan DG, Chu FC, Reingold DB: Ocular signs of cerebellar disease. Arch Ophthalmol 100:755, 1982
2. de Lahunta A: Cranial nerve—lower motor neuron: General somatic efferent system, special

visceral efferent system. In Veterinary Neuroanatomy and Clinical Neurology, p 89. Philadelphia, WB Saunders, 1977

3. Oliver JE, Lorenz MD: Handbook of Veterinary Neurologic Diagnosis. Philadelphia, WB Saunders, 1983
4. Parks MM: Extraocular muscles. In Duane TD, Jaeger EA (eds): Clinical Ophthalmology. Philadelphia, Harper & Row, 1986
5. Parks MM: Eye movement and positions. In Duane TD, Jaeger EA (eds): Clinical Ophthalmology. Philadelphia, Harper & Row, 1986
6. Parks MM: Supranuclear centers and pathways of eye movements. In Duane TD, Jaeger EA (eds): Clinical Ophthalmology. Philadelphia, Harper & Row, 1986
7. Prince JH, Diesem DC, Eglitis I, Ruskell GL: Anatomy and Histology of the Eye and Orbit in Domestic Animals. Springfield, IL, Thomas, 1960
8. Scott AB: Ocular motility. In Records RE (ed): Physiology of the Human Visual System, p 577. Philadelphia, Harper & Row, 1979

55

Red Watery Eyes

CHARLES L. MARTIN

PROBLEM DEFINITION AND RECOGNITION

"Red eye" may be discriptive of intraocular, corneal, episcleral or conjunctival redness. Since most conditions that initiate redness produce irritation or pain, it is common to have reflex lacrimation and concurrent problem of a watery eye.

PATHOPHYSIOLOGY

To understand the genesis of bulbar hyperemia or congestion, the anatomy of the vascular system of the eye and conjunctiva should be reviewed. The iris and ciliary body (anterior uvea) and the choroid (posterior uvea) form the vasular tunic of the eye. The posterior uveal arteries enter the eye around the optic nerve and consist of numerous short posterior ciliary arteries and two long posterior ciliary arteries. The latter course forward from the optic nerve to supply the anterior uvea. The retinal arterioles are branches of the short posterior ciliary arteries. The anterior uvea is also nourished by arterial branches from the rectus muscles, which form the anterior ciliary arteries and penetrate the anterior sclera to supply the episcleral, limbal, and anterior uvea (Fig. 55-1). The bulbar conjunctival arteries originate as branches from the rectus muscles arteries and the palpebral conjunctival archades from arteries supplying the eyelids.[5,10]

The venous returns from the anterior and posterior uvea and sclera freely communicate. The anterior uvea drains anteriorly into the scleral venous plexus and posteriorly into the vortex veins. The choroid drains into the vortex veins, which freely communicate with the scleral venous plexus. The scleral venous plexus not only drains the anterior uvea but also communicates with the bulbar conjunctiva, episclera, and limbus.[4,5,8–10]

The selective conjunctival congestion in glaucoma is due in part to stretching of the thin equatorial sclera and resultant collapse of the posterior communicating intrascleral channels; thus, more drainage is directed into the anterior

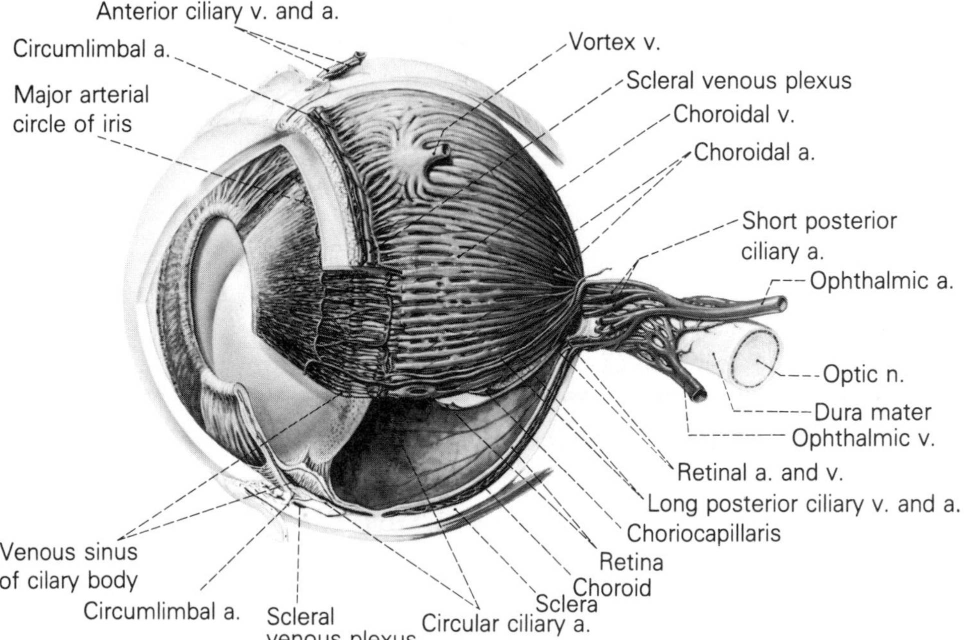

Fig. 55-1. Vascular system of the dog and cat.

venous system. Anterior uveitis produces prostaglandin-induced conjunctival hyperemia.

RULE OUTS

Initially, the redness should be differentiated as being intravascular congestion or extravascular (hemorrhage) and intraocular or on the ocular surface. The rule outs for red eyes, based on an anatomic diagnosis, are listed separately.

Intraocular Redness

Localization of intraocular redness requires differentiation of vitreal from aqueous hemorrhage, intraocular hemorrhage from intense corneal vascularization, and a normal nonpigmented atapetal fundus with a red reflection from hemorrhage. Vitreal hemorrhage is located behind the plane of the pupil, and all three of the Purkinje-Sanson images (cornea, anterior lens capsule, posterior lens capsule) will be present. If the vitreous is liquified (syneresis), the blood will be diffuse; however, if it is a gel, the hemorrhage will be confined into discrete clots.

Hyphema, or hemorrhage into the aqueous, may be partial or complete, clotted or liquified. Hyphema will obscure the iris to a variable degree. As the hemorrhage ages, it becomes darker (eight-ball hemorrhage) and may cause

Rule Outs for Red Eyes

- Intraocular redness
  - Hyphema
  - Vitreous hemorrhage
  - Normal albinotic fundus reflex
- Ocular surface redness
  - Conjunctivitis
  - Subconjunctival hemorrhage
  - Episcleritis
  - Prolapse of the third eyelid or its gland
  - Corneal granulation/neovascularization
  - Superfical keratitis such as pannus
  - Corneal ulceration produced by conjunctival hyperemia and corneal neovascularization
  - Corneal neoplasia
  - Anterior uveitis
  - Glaucoma

blood staining of the cornea, particularly when associated with increased intraocular pressure. Severe blood staining of the inner cornea may be difficult to differentiate from simple hyphema without the aid of a slit lamp.

Determination of the etiology of intraocular hemorrhage is based on history, ocular examination (both eyes), physical examination, and laboratory evaluation. A diagnosis of trauma-induced hemorrhage requires a *definite* history of trauma, choking, or other evidence of trauma to the head (such as skin abrasions).

Congenital anomalies such as the collie eye anomaly, persistent hyperplastic primary vitreous, or vascular anomalies may cause spontaneous intraocular hemorrhage. When the underlying lesion is obscured by hemorrhage in the involved eye, its role is presumed by finding the anomalies in the opposite eye.

Ocular neovascularization is fragile and may hemorrhage spontaneously. Uveitis and neoplasia-induced neovascularization should be ruled out as causes of spontaneous ocular hemorrhage. Primary ocular neoplasia is unilateral, whereas secondary neoplasa is frequently bilateral. Ocular neoplasia is frequently masked by hemorrhage, inflammation, and glaucoma late in the course. Previous degenerative conditions such as absolute glaucoma may lead to spontaneous intraocular hemorrhage, as may treatment of glaucoma (intravitreal injections of gentamicin or cyclocryotherapy).

A physical examination should detect additional evidence of trauma, bleeding, or clotting disorders, systemic infections, and conditions associated with hypertension, hypervolemia, or hyperviscosity syndromes. Multiple hemorrhages or those without an obvious cause should prompt laboratory evaluation for a blood dyscrasia or clotting disorder.

Ocular Surface Redness

Redness on or around the eye is the most common cause of the red eye problem. Exophthalmic breeds have more exposed conjunctiva to observe, and individuals in all breeds may lack pigmentation of the third eyelid and conjunctiva, giving the impression of increased redness. The three most common rule outs for bulbar conjunctival congestion are conjunctivitis, anterior uveitis (iritis, iridocyclitis), and glaucoma. A fourth, less common, but sometimes difficult rule out is episcleritis.

Bulbar conjunctival vascular injection can be either diffuse, with capillary and large vessel injection, or selective, with only large vessel injection. Intraocular diseases such as uncomplicated glaucoma and anterior uveitis characteristically involve injection of the large conjunctival vessels as well as deep episcleral injection (Fig. 55-2). Conjunctivitis typically has a diffuse engorgement due to dilation of capillaries between the larger vessels. Episcleritis is often focal or sectorial and nodular or elevated and produces conjunctival and deep episcleral injection similar to intraocular disease. Tables 55-1 through 55-3 list etiologic rule outs for the anatomic diagnosis of conjunctivitis, anterior uveitis, and glaucoma, respectively.

The causes of bulbar conjunctival and episcleral injection must be differentiated to avoid undertreatment. Anterior uveitis and glaucoma often result in blindness, and misdiagnosing and treating as a conjunctivitis might be catastrophic for vision. The therapies for glaucoma and anterior uveitis are diametrically opposite, so an accurate diagnosis is critical.

Glaucoma and anterior uveitis, being intraocular diseases, are rarely presented only with a problem of ocular redness. Additional problems of corneal

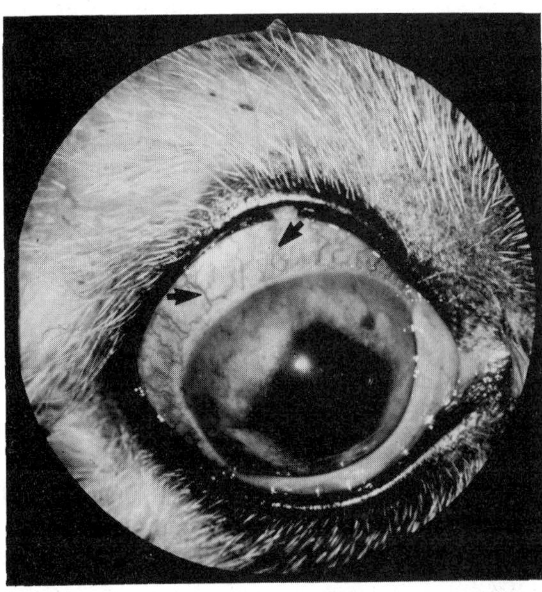

Fig. 55-2. Selective bulbar conjunctival congestion (*arrows*) typical of anterior uveitis and glaucoma. The eye has a secondary glaucoma and an iris bombe associated with lymphosarcoma.

Table 55-1. Etiologies of Conjunctivitis and Diagnostic Testing

ETIOLOGY	DIAGNOSTIC TEST(S)
Bacterial	Culture, cytology
Viral	Cytology, FA testing, systemic signs
Chlamydia	Cytology, response to tetracyclines
Tear deficiency	Schirmer tear test, rose bengal staining
Mechanical irritation	Examination with magnification, eversion of lids, history
Chemical irritation	History
Allergic	History, cytology, physical examination

FA, fluorescent antibody

Table 55-2. Etiologies for Anterior Uveitis

ETIOLOGY	DIAGNOSTIC TEST(S)
Trauma	
Blunt	History, contusions
Perforating	Examine for full-thickness injury to cornea or sclera.
Sterile or septic	Aqueous centesis—cytology, culture
Systemic infectious agents	
Dog	
Ehrlichia canis	Titers, blood smear
Rocky Mountain spotted fever	Titers, FA on skin biopsy
Infectious hepatitis	CBC, liver enzymes, history
Systemic mycoses	Titers, chest x-rays, needle biopsy, vitreous centesis
Aberrant parasites	Observation, removal and identification
Bacterial septicemia	Blood culture
Brucella canis	Titer, aqueous and blood culture
Leishmaniasis	Cytology, bone marrow
Cat	
Feline leukemia virus	FeLV testing
Infectious peritonitis	FIP titers, systemic signs, serum proteins
Systemic mycoses	Titers, ocular centesis with cytology, bone marrow
Toxoplasmosis	Titer, biopsy
Sterile immune-mediated	
Phacoanaphylaxis	Aqueous cytology, history of injury
Phacogenic	Mature to hypermature cataract
VKH syndrome	Dermal depigmentation
Idiopathic	Exclusion of other etiologies Sterile ocular fluid, cytology
Neoplasia	
Primary	Unilateral, observe mass, ultrasound, cytology, biopsy
Secondary	Often bilateral, observe mass, cytology, physical exam, and history

FA, fluorescent antibody; CBC, complete blood count; FeLV, feline leukemia virus; FIP, feline infectious peritonitis

Table 55-3. Etiologies of Glaucoma

ETIOLOGY	DIAGNOSTIC TEST(S)
Primary closed angle	Gonioscopy of both eyes
Primary open angle	Gonioscopy
Lens displacement	Lens in anterior chamber, aphakic crescent, gonioscopy
Inflammation	Observe synechia, iris bombé, gonioscopy, flare, keratic precipitates
Neoplasia	Observe mass or infiltration, aqueous cytology, biopsy
Hyphema	Anterior chamber ¾ full of blood

clarity, changes in pupil size and function, ocular enlargement, and changes in ocular pressure are usually present, whereas they are absent with conjunctivitis. Some forms of episcleritis are very invasive and may result in intraocular signs, but a proliferative lesion on the scleral surface is usually present.

Subconjunctival hemorrhage presents as a red eye, but the blood is extravascular rather than intravascular. A simple subconjunctival hemorrhage should be differentiated from a more serious retrobulbar hemorrhage that has migrated forward. The latter will exhibit proptosis and decreased orbital compressibility on retropulsion of the eye.

DIAGNOSTIC PLAN

Determining the source of the redness, e.g., conjunctiva, cornea, intraocular, is the initial step. A diagnostic plan for conjunctival redness is given in Table 55-4. If one investigates beyond the redness for intraocular signs, the risk of "underdiagnosing" a conjunctivitis when glaucoma or anterior uveitis is present should be minimal. Because anterior uveitis frequently precipitates or results in glaucoma, the diagnosis may be a complex of anterior uveitis and glaucoma.

SYMPTOMATIC THERAPY

It is questionable whether symptomatic therapy for conjunctival redness should be given. Symptomatic therapy for conjunctival redness consists of topical corticosteroids and vasoconstrictive agents. Examples of the latter are phenylephrine and naphazoline and are mainly for cosmetic purposes.

Corneal granulation and superficial keratitis are usually responsive to corticosteroids, however, those agents should *not* be administered in most instances of concurrent *corneal ulceration*. Episcleritis is usually corticosteroid responsive, although a drug such as azathioprine may be required.

Corticosteroids administered by one or more routes are indicated in sterile anterior uveitis. Controlling the inflammation and the usual attendant hypotony may normalize aqueous production, and adhesions of the pupil or angle may

Table 55-4. Diagnostic Plan for Red Eye

	ANATOMIC DIAGNOSIS				
DIAGNOSTIC PLAN	Conjunctivitis	Glaucoma	Anterior Uveitis	Episcleritis	Keratitis
Conjunctival injection ↓					
Examine for diffuse or selective large vessel injection. ↓	Diffuse	Usually selective	Usually selective	Selective	Usually diffuse
Examine intraocular structures, pupil size and symmetry, iris color and texture, and aqueous flare. ↓	Normal	Anisocoria, dilated, fixed flare ±	Anisocoria, constricted, irregular, darker flare ±	Normal	May be miotic if ulcerative
Schirmer tear test ↓ Topical anesthesia	↑ or ↓	Normal or ↑	Normal or ↑	Normal or ↑	↑ or ↓
Fluorescein stain ↓	N	N	N	N	+ If ulcer
Measure IOP ↓	N	↑	↓	N or ↓	N
Conjunctival cytology	Neutrophils, lymphocytes, inclusions ±	N	N	±	±

±, may or may not be present; ↑, increase; ↓, decrease; IOP, intraocular pressure.

Table 55-5. Carbonic-Anhydrase-Inhibiting Diuretics

DRUG	DOSE
Acetazolamide	11 mg/kg b.i.d.–t.i.d.
Diamox	
Vetamox	
Dichlorphenamide	2.2 mg/kg b.i.d.–t.i.d.
Oratrol	
Daranide	
Methazolamide	5 mg/kg b.i.d.–t.i.d.
Naptazine	

become manifest with glaucoma. Atropine (1%) is indicated with anterior uveitis to minimize extensive pupil adhesions and relieve ciliary spasms. Prostaglandin inhibitors such as aspirin (10 mg/kg twice daily) are indicated (many of the signs of inflammation are thought to be prostaglandin mediated). Patching the eye or keeping the animal in a dark environment will minimize the discomfort of photophobia.

Glaucoma is treated symptomatically by decreasing aqueous production with carbonic-anhydrase-inhibiting diuretics (Table 55-5). When rapid reductions of intraocular pressures are required, an osmotic diuretic such as mannitol (1 to 2 g/kg intravenously) is indicated in addition to the carbonic anhydrase inhibitors. Topical therapy with pilocarpine, timolol, and epinephrine, either individually or in combination, may be of benefit, but their effects are not consistent or dramatic.

Cage rest and, if necessary, sedation are the only proven therapies for hyphema.[7] If secondary glaucoma develops, a carbonic anhydrase inhibitor is indicated. Subconjunctival administration of repositol steroid early in the course may minimize clotting and thus facilitate reabsorption.[6] Antifibrinolytic agents such as aminocaproic acid have been recommended to minimize recurrent bleeding, but their use is controversial.[1,3,7] Trauma-induced hyphema is treated with corticosteroids and atropine for the secondary anterior uveitis. Aspirin should not be used in the treatment of traumatic uveitis with hyphema, because of the increased risk of additional bleeding.[2]

REFERENCES

1. Crouch E, Frenkel M: Aminocaproic acid in the treatment of traumatic hyphema. Am J Ophthalmol 81:355, 1976
2. Ganley S, Geiger M, Clement J, Rigby P, Levy G; Aspirin and recurrent hyphema after blunt ocular trauma. Am J Ophthalmol 96:797, 1983
3. Fiscella R: Aminocaproic acid decreases secondary hemorrhage after traumatic hyphema. Arch Ophthalmol 101:1031, 1983
4. Martin C: Gonioscopy and anatomical correlations of the drainage angle of the dog. J Small Anim Pract 10:171, 1969

5. Martin C, Anderson B: Ocular anatomy. In Gelatt K (ed): Veterinary Ophthalmology. Philadelphia, Lea & Febiger, 1981
6. Masket S, Best M, Fisher L, Kronenberg S, Galin M: Therapy in experimental hyphema. Arch Ophthalmol 85:329, 1971
7. Pandolf M: Intraocular hemorrhages: A hemostatic therapeutic approach. Surv Ophthalmol 22:322, 1978
8. Troncosco MU: The intrascleral vascular plexus and its relations to the aqueous outflow. Am J Ophthalmol 25:1153, 1942
9. Van Buskirk M: The canine eye: The vessels of aqueous drainage. Invest Ophthalmol Vis Sci 18:223, 1979
10. Wong V, Macri F: Vasculature of the cat eye. Arch Ophthalmol 72:351, 1964

56

Ocular Pain and Blepharospasm

CHARLES L. MARTIN

PROBLEM DEFINITION AND RECOGNITION

The manifestation of ocular pain is variable. Blepharospasm is the obvious manifestation of pain that brings immediate attention to the eye, but behavioral alterations distant from the eye are frequently not appreciated as having any causal relationship with the eye. Behavior alterations of sleeping excessively, hiding, decreased appetite, loss of playfulness, and worsening of disposition are often more subtle manifestations of ocular discomfort. The correlation of these subtle manifestations to ocular disease is often only retrospective, after the animal has returned to its "normal" behavior.

PATHOPHYSIOLOGY

The sensory innervation to the cornea, conjunctiva, and uveal tract is the ophthalmic division of the fifth cranial nerve (trigeminal). The cornea and the anus contain the most pain fibers of any areas of the body. The iris, ocular muscles, and optic nerve sheaths have marked pain sensation, whereas the retina, lens, and optic nerve have no pain sensation and the sclera has very minimal amounts. Pain from corneal and conjunctival stimulation is sharp and localized and described as a foreign body sensation; pain from the iris and ciliary body is deep seated and throbbing and often radiates over the head to other regions innervated by the fifth cranial nerve.[3]

The innervation of the cornea is from the two long posterior ciliary nerves that arborize in the anterior one third of the cornea. The nerves lose their myelin sheath after entering the cornea and branch extensively, ending as single axons between the superficial epithelial cells. In comparison, the posterior cornea is poorly innervated. The clinical correlation is that the superficial corneal abrasion is typically more painful than the deep ulcer or descemetocele. The severe pain of a superficial ulcer may initiate an antidromic reflex manifested as a strong miosis and hyperemia of the conjunctiva and anterior uvea. This results in additional pain from vasodilation-induced ciliary muscle spasm. Topical atropine counteracts the ciliary muscle spasm of the antidromic reflex and thus decreases some of the discomfort associated with a corneal ulcer. The mediator(s) of the antidromic reflex is unknown, but atropine, prostaglandin inhibitors, and sympathetic denervation do not block the reflex. Adenosine triphosphate (ATP) injected into the eye does not produce the reflex, although it is present in increased amounts in the aqueous after trigeminal stimulation.[2]

Ocular pain can be aggravated by bright light. Photophobia may be present with corneal ulcers and anterior uveitis and results in additional ciliary muscle spasms. Different breeds and individuals may vary as to their corneal sensitivity. "Old world breeds" such as chows, Siberian huskies, and samoyeds are quite "eye conscious" and readily develop blepharospasm with ocular pain. The triad of blepharospasm, prolapsed third eyelid, and retraction of the globe into the orbit can make ocular examination extremely difficult. Topical anesthesia facilitates examination in an animal with blepharospasm, but extreme examples may require regional anesthesia of the palpebral branch of the facial nerve or, occasionally, general anesthesia.

RULE OUTS

Corneal Pain

All animals with blepharospasm should have fluorescein stain applied to the cornea to rule out corneal ulcers or abrasions. Only after eliminating corneal ulceration as the cause of the blepharospasm should the examiner feel confident in diagnosing other sources of ocular pain. If corneal ulceration, abrasions, erosions, or lacerations are present, the subsequent step is to search for a physical cause. These may vary from conformational faults to foreign bodies and may be obvious or very difficult to detect. Certain aspects of the ocular examination should be emphasized when searching for a physical irritant: examine the unrestrained head, examine before and after topical anesthesia (ocasionally after palpebral nerve block), examine with high magnification (5× or more), and evert the lids and third eyelid to visualize all conjunctival surfaces and cul-de-sacs. If these guidelines are followed, the possibility of overlooking a physical cause for corneal pain should be minimal.

Keratitis that is not associated with corneal ulcerations or anterior uveitis does not usually manifest with blepharospasm. Stromal keratitis is usually an extension of anterior uveitis, and discomfort is probably due to ciliary spasm.

Conjunctival Pain

The degree of discomfort manifested with conjunctivitis varies between individuals, species, and cause. Cats manifest blepharospasm more consistently with conjunctivitis than dogs. In general, marked blepharospasm should not be attributed to conjunctivitis.

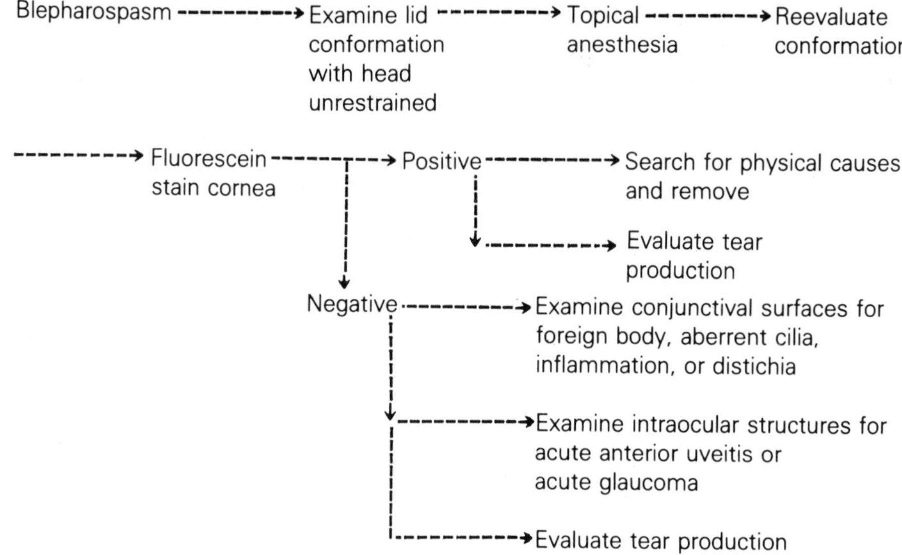

Fig. 56-1. Diagnostic plan for blepharospasm.

Intraocular Pain

Animals with acute anterior uveitis and glaucoma are more likely to have blepharospasm and photophobia than their counterparts with chronic forms of the disorders. Chronic anterior uveitis and glaucoma can be assumed to produce a deep-seated discomfort, because of the typical improvement in mental status and activity when the conditions are corrected. The owners rarely appreciate the behavioral manifestations of pain.

Pure posterior ocular segment disease does not usually create pain. Inflammatory disease of the posterior uvea may cause discomfort, but, because some degree of anterior uveal involvement is usually present, it is difficult to identify the origin of the pain. Patients with optic neuritis seem to be photophobic to a strong examination light, although they are clinically blind. Ocular movements that stretch the inflamed nerve and meningeal sheaths produce discomfort. Some patients with optic neuritis also have other neurologic lesions, so it may be difficult to attribute mental depression and other problems to ocular pain. Figure 56-1 presents a diagnostic flow chart that may be used in evaluating ocular pain.

SYMPTOMATIC THERAPY

If any physical irritant is present (e.g., distichiasis, trichiasis, aberrent cilia, foreign body, etc.), its removal is obviously the primary goal of therapy. Corneal ulcerations should be treated with topical antibiotics to prevent infection and with topical atropine to block ciliary muscle spasms. Topical anesthetics appear to be the therapy of choice for corneal pain, but they are *deliterious to epithelial healing* as they exist in commercial preparations and are short acting (15 minutes). Recent evidence indicates that dilute solutions of anesthetics may retain their analgesic properties but lose their toxicity. Proparacaine (0.05%, or 10% of the strength of commercial solutions) does not have any corneal toxicity. The disadvantage of the short duration (15 minutes) of action remains.[1]

The standard drug used in veterinary medicine to treat ocular pain is 1% atropine ointment or solution. Atropine is not an anesthetic, but is a cycloplegic (paralyzes the ciliary muscle) and thus counteracts the discomfort of ciliary muscle spasm. In the treatment of patients with uveitis, it has the advantage of dilating the pupil, but mydriasis is usually contraindicated in glaucoma. Atropine therapy for ciliary spasm is only needed once or twice per day. Excessive therapy may decreased tear production and interfere with corneal healing.

Systemic analgesics that have antiprostaglandin activity are indicated, particularly with intraocular inflammation-induced pain. Acetylsalicylic acid (10 mg/kg twice daily), phenylbutazone (40 mg/kg three times per day), and flunixin meglumine (0.125 mg/kg once a day) are effective. Side effects limit the duration of use, particularly with flunixin, the renal and intestinal effects of which should limit its use to 1 to 2 days of therapy.

Covering the eye with a bandage will make a painful eye more comfortable, but it limits the frequency of topical therapy. Tarsorrhapy and third eyelid flaps are alternative methods of covering the eye and are indicated when spastic entropion secondary to the severe blepharospasm is aggravating the corneal pain. Confinement away from bright light will prevent further pain from photophobia.

REFERENCES

1. Maul E, Sears M: ATP is released into the rabbit eye by antidromic stimulation of the trigeminal nerve. Invest Ophthalmol Vis Sci 18:256, 1979
2. Maurice DM, Singh T: The absence of corneal toxicity with low-level topical anesthesia. Am J Ophthalmol 99:691, 1985
3. Waltman SR: The cornea. In Moses RA (ed): Adler's Physiology of the Eye: Clinical Application, 7th ed. St Louis, CV Mosby, 1981

57

Abnormal Cornea and Lens

CHARLES L. MARTIN

PROBLEM DEFINITION AND RECOGNITION

Corneal abnormalities are common, easily visible to the owner, and often secondary to lid conformational defects in many breeds. Similarly, problems of the lens are common, since several popular breeds have inherited cataracts that lead to blindness and obvious lenticular opacification. Because both tissues are unique in their transparency, the most common sign of disease is opacification.

PATHOPHYSIOLOGY

Corneal Abnormalities

The most common problems of the cornea are changes in clarity or color, changes in smoothness or regularity, or combinations of the two.

Corneal clarity/color may be altered by edema, vascularization, pigmentation, and lack of smoothness. The normal cornea remains clear due to a combination of unique anatomic and physiologic features. The cornea is normally lacking in blood vessels and pigment (their presence would obviously hinder transparency). The collagen lamella of the stroma are arranged in a uniform parallel fashion and the fibrils at such a distance as to produce mutual interference of light rays; consequently, light rays are not scattered.[16] The corneal stroma has a high water content (78%) that is attributed to glycosaminoglycans surrounding the collagen fibrils. The 78% stromal water is a state of relative dehydration produced by the corneal endothelium through an ATPase-activated Na/Cl pump that removes water from the stroma. On exposure to air, the tear film becomes hypertonic, creating an osmotic gradient across the epithelium that draws water out of the cornea.[19] Loss of either the endothelium or epithelium results in increased stromal water, or edema. Corneal edema results in disruption of the normal lamellar collagen arrangement and scattering of light, with opacification. Corneal edema is most marked with endothelial loss; because of the endothelium's limited regenerative capabilities, edema may be permanent.

The lack of corneal blood vessels or, conversely, the stimulus for neovascularization is incompletely understood. Morphologic features such as tissue compactness are probably of minor importance. Chemical mediators are thought to be important in determining corneal angiogenesis.[6] Corneal pigmentation usually results from the migration of limbal melanocytes with corneal blood vessels.[1]

The smooth corneal surface is produced by the tear film filling in any small surface epithelial irregularities. The epithelial surface is hydrophobic, requiring a mucin layer on the surface for the aqueous phase of the tears to form a film over the corneal surface. A lack of mucin results in the break-up of the aqueous phase and a dry irregular cornea.[12]

Breaks in the corneal epithelium are usually painful because of the concentration of nerve endings in the superficial cornea. Defects in the epithelium are detected by the presence of retained fluorescein stain. Fluorescein is an aqueous solution and will not be retained by the lipophilic, hydrophobic epithelium; however, if a defect in the epithelium is present, fluorescein diffuses into the hydrophilic stroma, where it becomes bright green.

Lens Changes

The lens has the highest protein content of any tissue in the body (33%).[10] The proteins consist of water-soluble proteins (crystallins) and water-insoluble albuminoids. The young lens is predominantly composed of crystallins, which gradually shift with age to increasing amounts of albuminoids. Other unique properties of the lens are its lack of vascularity, glycolytic energy metabolism, and high glutathione levels.[3] Lens growth occurs from the epithelium that lines the anterior capsule, resulting in the newest fibers being present in the outer or superficial layers (cortex). Lens fibers are formed by the epithelium at the equator of the lens, with successive new fibers pushing and condensing the older fibers toward the middle (nucleus). The lens grows most rapidly in young dogs, in which it increases in size. New fiber formation persists throughout most of an animal's life, resulting in an increase in density from compacting with age rather than dramatically increasing in size. The increase in density is responsible for the gray haze or nuclear sclerosis that becomes manifest in dogs by 7 to 8 years of age. Nuclear sclerosis does not significantly impair vision, and it should be distinguished from pathologic senile cataracts.

Many cataracts such as sugar cataracts are initiated by a metabolic imbalance that produces an osmotic accumulation of water in the lens and subsequent scattering of light.[9] These initial vacuolar changes may be reversible, but, if left unchecked, they result in protein aggregation, which is not considered reversible.

Cataracts secondary to inflammation are thought to originate from a breakdown of the blood–aqueous barrier, which allows increased levels of plasma phospholipids such as lysophosphatidyl choline into the aqueous. Lysophosphatidyl choline then diffuses into the lens and lyses membranes of lens fibers.[4]

Many of the cataracts in dogs have a genetic origin, but their mechanism of formation is not known.

The classificaton of cataracts can be based on age of onset, etiology, degree of opacification, location within the lens, description of the opacity, or combinations of two or more of these categories. Cataracts described by age are termed *congenital, neonatal, juvenile,* or *developmental* (up to 5 to 6 years) and *senile* or *degenerative.* Cataracts described by degree of opacity are termed *incipient* (small, not outwardly visible), *immature* (severe, but incomplete opacity with fundus reflex still visible), *mature* (swollen lens with complete opacification), and *hypermature* (late stages with shrinkage due to reabsorption of water). Cataracts described by anatomic location may be anterior or posterior, cortical or nuclear, capsular, equatorial, and fetal nuclear.[18] The location of the opacity may be important in determining a prognosis for progression and dating the onset of the injury when considered in lieu of the mechanism of lens growth (Table 57-1).

The etiologies of cataract formation are broadly categorized into genetic, metabolic (*i.e.,* diabetic or nutritional), traumatic, inflammatory, toxic, and radiation induced. All are relatively common causes for cataracts in dogs, except for toxic and radiation origins. A great deal of species variation exists in the relative importance of the etiologies. Cats have comparatively few genetic cataracts and are resistant to diabetes mellitus–induced cataracts.[17] Intraocular inflammation is the most common cause of lenticular opacities in the cat.

Lens dislocations may occur from familial zonular defects, zonular degenerative changes, zonular ruptures from stretching with buphthalmos, and traumatic rupture. The latter is the least common etiology for lens dislocation. Zonular defects are most common in terrier breeds but have been observed in a wide variety of breeds, in which they manifest as eventual bilateral spontaneous displacement in a previously healthy eye.[5] A biochemical defect has not been defined in the dog with spontaneous lens displacements. Advancing cataracts may spontaneously dislocate due to concurrent degenerative changes in the capsular-zonular attachments or may be associated with inflammatory cells digesting the zonules.[8,15] The increased globe circumference with buphthalmos is

Table 57-1. Prognosis for Cataracts Based on Anatomic Site of Involvement

SITE	PROGNOSIS
Anterior and posterior capsule	Usually nonprogressive
Fetal nuclear	Nonprogressive
Nuclear	Often static, may reduce in size with age
Sutures	Usually nonprogressive
Anterior and posterior cortex	Variable, most will progress
Equator	Usually progressive
Posterior axial subcapsule	Usually nonprogressive

(Modified from Gelatt K: Lens and cataract formation in the dog. Comp Cont Ed)

usually accompanied by a partial rupture of the zonules and some degree of lens displacement. While explosive traumatic ruptures of the globe frequently dislocate or completely expel the lens from the eye, trauma without loss of the integrity of the fibrous ocular tunic is an uncommon cause of lens dislocation.

The lens may partially dislocate (subluxate) to either side or up and down, fall posteriorly into the ventral vitreous (posterior luxation), or move through the pupil into the anterior chamber (anterior luxation).[7] Anterior luxations are most consistently symptomatic with a secondary glaucoma and corneal edema from touching the endothelium.

RULE OUTS

Corneal Disease

Corneal disease is frequently part of an intraocular process, and the latter should be ruled out for accurate treatment and prognosis. Chronic anterior uveitis eventually induces a deep stromal keratitis; anterior chamber fibrin, keratic precipitates, anterior luxated lenses, and glaucoma often compromise the corneal endothelium, resulting in corneal edema. A variety of causes of white corneal opacifications are listed separately. Subtle corneal opacities are commonly observed, and their histopathologic correlate is usually unknown. Corneal edema is a common cause of white opacification (see Rule Outs for Causes of Corneal Edema).

Corneal pigmentation is stimulated by chronic keratitis with neovascularization. Keratitis due to a focal irritant such as trichiasis is limited to the area of corneal contact by the irritant, whereas that associated with diffuse keratitis from immune-mediated causes or keratoconjunctivitis sicca is progressive and diffuse. A second source of corneal pigment is the anterior uvea, which may leave deposits on the endothelial surface from anterior synechia (congenital or acquired), ruptured iris cysts, and pigment dispersion with anterior uveitis.

Rules Outs for White Corneal Opacities

- Stromal scar
- Lipid accumulation—may be associated with stromal scar
- Calcium—may be associated with stromal scar
- Mucopolysaccaridosis—rare
- Edema
- Leukocyte infiltrates
- Mycotic plaques
- Descemet's membrane abnormalities—persistent pupillary membrane syndrome, anterior synechia
- Inclusion cyst—rare

Rule Outs for Causes of Corneal Edema

- Epithelial ulceration
- Endothelilal dysfunction
  - Anterior luxated lens
  - Glaucoma
  - Endothelial dystrophy—congenital (persistent pupillary membrane syndrome), senile
  - Trauma
  - Anterior uveitis
    - Keratic precipitates
    - Fibrin
    - Anterior synechia

Rule Outs for Proliferative Red Corneal Lesions

- Superficial keratitis (pannus)
- Corneal granulation in a healing ulcer
- Fibrous histiocytoma—often in collies
- Intense neovascularization
- Hemangiosarcoma
- Squamous cell carcinoma

Rule outs for a red proliferation on the cornea are listed separately. The most common causes of corneal irregularities are extraneous mucous or hair on the surface or an ulcer. Proliferative lesions produce irregularities that are elevated rather than depressed (as the ulcer). The reader is referred to the list of rule outs for corneal ulceration.

Lens Abnormalities

Opacities on either side of the lens in the aqueous or vitreous may be confused with a cataract. Lipids and fibrin in the aqueous may simulate a cataract or an anterior luxated cataract on cursory examination. Congenital hyperplastic primary vitreal remnants, inflammatory clots, or fibrous proliferations in the anterior vitreous may be difficult to distinguish from a posterior cortical cataract. Quivering or movement of the opacity with ocular movement usually indicates it is loose in the vitreous, but a subluxated lens will exhibit phakodonesis (tremors of the lens).

The level of involvement of the opacity within the eye and lens is most accurately determined with a slit-lamp (biomicroscope). A focal beam of light passing through the eye and observed from the side may suffice for lesion local-

Rule Outs for Corneal Ulceration

- Mechanical irritation
  Distichia, trichiasis, aberrant cilia, entropion, foreign body, dermoid
- Trauma
- Keratoconjunctivitis sicca
- Epithelial bulla rupturing from corneal edema
- Lagophthalmos
  Results in trauma and focal keratoconjunctivitis sicca
  Shallow orbits
  Seventh cranial nerve paralysis
- Neurotrophic—fifth cranial nerve paralysis
- Chemical injury—soaps, acids, alkalies
- Viral—herpes in cats
- Basal lamina defects—slowly healing epithelial erosions

ization by determining where the opacity intercepts the light. The Purkinji-Sanson images will aid gross lesion localization. The Purkinji-Sanson images are three reflections from the optical interfaces that are observed when a light is projected into the eye. The first reflection is bright and arises from the anterior cornea; the second reflection is less bright and arises from the anterior lens capsule; and the third is dimmest and arises from the posterior lens capsule. Opacities can be localized by noting which of the images are obscured by the opacity.

The genetic etiology of cataracts is frequently presumed from observing a certain type of lenticular opacity in a purebred breed with a known defect. Genetic cataracts are, in most instances, eventually bilateral, but they are not symmetric as to time and degree of involvement of each eye. Trauma should be ruled out as an etiology with unilateral cataracts, but the relationship may be nebulous except with penetrating injuries. Cataracts of sudden onset with rapid progression should alert the examiner to consider diabetes mellitus as an etiology, but this progression is not unusual with the more common genetic cataracts. Many diabetic patients are also ketotic: smelling the breath may be a rapid means of making a presumptive diagnosis. Large breeds of dogs, particularly hunting breeds, with extensive cataracts usually have either diabetes mellitus, retinal atrophy, or intraocular inflammation rather than simple genetic cataracts. A blood glucose determination and electroretinogram are routine preoperative screening tests to rule out complicating factors in a blind patient with mature cataracts.

Cataracts may stimulate inflammation (phakogenic uveitis) or be caused by intraocular inflammation (secondary cataract). The anatomic location of the cataract and the opposite eye may help in the differentiation. Phakogenic uveitis is associated with advancing cataracts in the mature to hypermature stages. Anterior uveitis with an advanced cataract in one eye and the presence of a cataract with no inflammation in the opposite eye is presumptive evidence of phakogenic uveitis. A cataract secondary to uveitis is typically capsular and posterior subcapsular in its involvement.

SYMPTOMATIC THERAPY

Corneal Disease

Topical steroids are invaluable in symptomatic therapy for inflammatory corneal disease if ulceration and infection are not present. Corticosteroids minimize corneal scarring but increase the risk of progressive ulceration by activation of collagenase if ulceration is present.[2,13] Corticosteroids may potentiate bacterial, viral, and mycotic infections. The administration of prednisolone acetate, 1% suspension, is the preferred treatment due to that agent's superior corneal absorption.[11]

Corneal pain is minimized with topical 1% atropine applied twice daily and patching, tarsorrhapy, a third eyelid flap, or soft contact lenses to produce a corneal bandage.

Topical broad-spectrum antibiotics are indicated for prophylactic therapy when ulceration is present. Topical lubricants are used with lagophthalmos, exophthalmos, and keratoconjunctivitis sicca to protect the cornea. Hyperosmotic solutions or ointments may be used to reduce corneal edema, but their effect is transient and they often produce a stinging sensation.

Diseases of the Lens

There is no proven medical therapy for cataracts in the advanced stages. Treatment of metabolic, toxic, or nutritional cataracts involves restricting the offending agent or supplying the deficient agent. Early cataracts in a vacuolar stage with fluid imbibition may be arrested or reversed by corrective measures.[9,14] Animals with immature, nuclear, or reabsorbing cataracts often will see better after pupillary dilation that allows light to pass through the clearer peripheral lens. Corticosteroids are frequently needed to treat the phakogenic uveitis.

Posterior lens luxations are usually not surgically treated, and medical therapy consists of controlling any phakogenic uveitis or associated glaucoma. Acute anterior lens luxations are usually treated by lens removal, but an alternative approach is retropulsion of the lens through the pupil by pushing on the cornea. Pilocarpine is used to keep the lens trapped in the posterior chamber after it is pushed through the pupil.

REFERENCES

1. Bellhorn R, Henkind P: Superficial pigmentary keratitis in the dog. J Am Vet Med Assoc 149:173, 1966
2. Brown S, Weller C, Vidrich A: Effect of corticosteroid on corneal collagenase of rabbits. Am J Ophthalmol 70:744, 1970

3. Cotlier E: The lens. In Moses R (ed): Adler's Physiology of the Eye: Clinical Application, 7th ed. St Louis, CV Mosby, 1981
4. Cotlier E, et al: Lysophosphatidyl choline and cataracts in uveitis., Arch Ophthalmol 94:1159, 1976
5. Curtis R, Barnett K: Primary lens luxation in the dog. J Small Anim Pract 21:657, 1980
6. Ezra DB: Neovasculogenesis: Triggering factors and possible mechanisms. Survey Ophthalmol 24:167, 1979
7. Formston C: Observations on subluxation and luxation of the crystalline lens in the dog. J Comp Pathol 55:168, 1945
8. Gwin R, Samuelson D, Powell G, Gelatt K, Wolf D, Merideth R: Primary lens luxation in the dog associated with lenticular zonule degeneration and its relationship to glaucoma. J Am Anim Hosp Assoc 18:485, 1982
9. Kinoshita JH: Mechanisms initiating cataract formation. Invest Ophthalmol Vis Sci 13:713, 1974
10. Kirsch R: The lens. Arch Ophthalmol 93:284, 1975
11. Leibowitz H, Kupferman A: Anti-inflammatory effectiveness in the cornea of topically administered prednisolone. Invest Ophthalmol Vis Sci 13:756, 1974
12. Lemp M, Holly F, Iwata S, Dohlman C: The precorneal tear film: I. The factors in spreading and maintaining a continuous tear film over the corneal surface. Arch Ophthalmol 83:89, 1970
13. Martin C: The effect of topical vitamin A, antibiotic, mineral oil, and subconjunctival steroid on corneal epithelial wound healing in the dog. J Am Vet Med Assoc 159:1392, 1971
14. Martin C: The formation of cataracts with disophenol: Age susceptibility and production with chemical grade 2,6-diiodo-4-nitrophenol. Can Vet J 16:228, 1975
15. Martin C: Zonular defects in the dog: A clinical and scanning electron microscopic study. J Am Anim Hosp Assoc 14:571, 1978
16. Maurice DM: The structure and transparency of the cornea. J Physiol 136:263, 1957
17. Schaer M: A clinical survey of thirty cats with diabetes melliltus. J Am Anim Hosp Assoc 13:23, 1977
18. Slatter D: Lens in Fundamentals of Veterinary Ophthalmology. Philadelphia, WB Saunders, 1981
19. Waltman SR: The cornea. In Moses R (ed): Adler's Physiology of the Eye, Clinical Application, 7th ed. St Louis, CV Mosby, 1981

58

Loss of Sense of Smell

JOHN E. OLIVER

PROBLEM DEFINITION AND RECOGNITION

The sense of smell (olfaction) is highly developed in dogs and cats. Dogs can detect some odors at 1/100 the concentration detectable by humans.[5] The use of dogs for hunting, tracking, and seeking out drugs and explosives exploits this natural ability. Loss of the sense of smell (anosmia) is an uncommon complaint, although it probably occurs frequently. Unless the animal is used in one of the ways mentioned, the owner is unlikely to know. Cats commonly quit eating when they have an upper respiratory infection, which may be in part from anosmia. The most frequent clinical patient is the hunting or tracking dog.[4]

PATHOPHYSIOLOGY

The primary olfactory receptors are in the olfactory epithelium in the nasal mucosa at the caudal part of the nasal cavity.[2] The receptor cell is a bipolar neuron that acts as a chemoreceptor. Cilia projecting from the receptor cell are covered with secretion. Chemical substances (olfactants) dissolved in the secretion stimulate the cell. The axons of the olfactory neurons penetrate the cribriform plate of the ethmoid bone and form the olfactory nerve (cranial nerve I), which synapses on cells in the olfactory bulbs. Axons project from the olfactory bulbs to the cortex of the pyriform lobe. Connections are also made to parts of the limbic system for behavioral reactions.[2]

A second olfactory system originates in the vomeronasal organ on the floor of the nasal cavity. It communicates with the oral cavity by the incisive duct.[3] The vomeronasal organ varies in size and function between species, but it is relatively well developed in dogs and cats. The vomeronasal nerves extend caudally to penetrate the cribriform plate and synapse on the accessory olfactory bulb. This system senses chemical stimuli important for sexual behavior in many species.[1,7]

A third system, through the trigeminal nerve (cranial nerve V), originates from the nasal mucosa. It is probably more sensitive to irritating substances. Although each of these systems is most sensitive to specific substances, it is probably impossible to stimulate only one system.[8]

Lesions of the epithelium, olfactory bulbs, or central pathways can affect the sense of smell. Diseases in the nasal cavity that affect the olfactory receptors in the epithelium are most common.[4,9] Receptor cells can regenerate from other receptor cells, which can be important in the prognosis of diseases that destroy part, but not all, of the receptor cells.[8]

DIAGNOSTIC PLAN

Proving that an animal has anosmia can be difficult. Simple tests involve presenting a noxious or rewarding odor and observing for a behavioral response. Food under a cover may be tried, preferably at home when the animal is more likely to respond normally. Noxious odors that are recommended include cloves, alcohol, garlic, perfume, and a variety of chemicals. Eugenol is reported to be relatively specific for the olfactory receptors.[11] Newer tests using electrophysiologic techniques look promising for providing objective evidence of the function of the olfactory receptors.[9–11]

Functional anosmia can occur after exposure to some substances. Hunting dogs carried in the trunk of a car may have temporary anosmia, presumably from exposure to exhaust fumes.[4]

Anosmia can be caused by lesions of the nasal cavity or the brain (Table 58-1). The history, physical examination, and neurologic examination should identify one of these two sources. Nasal lesions usually cause sneezing, nasal discharge, difficult and noisy respiration, pawing at the nose, or deformity of the nasal or paranasal structures.[12] Lesions of the brain that affect the sense of smell

Table 58-1. Etiology of Anosmia

CATEGORY	NASAL CAVITY	NERVOUS SYSTEM
Metabolic		Diabetes mellitus[9] Hypoadrenocorticism[9] Hypothyroidism[9]
Inflammatory	Viral, bacterial, and fungal infections	Viral, bacterial, and fungal infections
Neoplastic	Adenocarcinomas Other tumors	Tumors near olfactory bulbs, usually meningiomas
Traumatic	Obstruction of air flow	Minor trauma: shearing of olfactory nerve Major trauma: direct damage to olfactory nerve, tracts, or cortex
Functional	Saturation of olfactory epithelium, temporary	

will usually cause behavioral abnormality, depression, seizures, compulsive pacing, or visual deficits.[4,6,13] Tumors or chronic infections can extend from the nasal cavity through the cribriform plate into the brain. Head trauma can cause shearing of the olfactory nerve, even when the trauma is not severe.

Supportive information on nasal lesions is obtained from hematology and serum chemistries, radiographs of the nose, cytologic and microbiologic examination of nasal secretions, and rhinoscopy. Both the rostral and caudal portions of the nasal cavity can be examined with fiberoptic endoscopes.[12] Brain lesions may require contrast radiography, nuclear scans, or computed tomography for confirmation.[13]

SYMPTOMATIC THERAPY

There is no treatment for destruction of the olfactory receptors. If anosmia is secondary to a treatable condition, the receptors may regenerate.

REFERENCES

1. Beaver B: Veterinary Aspects of Feline Behavior. St Louis, CV Mosby, 1980
2. De Lahunta A: Veterinary Neuroanatomy and Clinical Neurology, 2nd ed. Philadelphia, WB Saunders, 1983
3. Evans HE, Christensen GC: Miller's Anatomy of the Dog. Philadelphia, WB Saunders, 1979
4. Holloway CL: Loss of olfactory acuity in hunting animals. Auburn Vet 18:25–28, 1961
5. Houpt KA, Wolski TR: Domestic Animal Behavior for Veterinarians and Animal Scientists. Ames, IA, Iowa State University Press, 1982
6. Hutchinson CP, Buxton DF, Garrett PD: Anatomic basis for the examination of olfactory and visual cranial nerve function in dogs. Comp Cont Ed Pract Vet 6:751–765, 1984
7. Ladewig J, Hart BL: Flehmen and vomeronasal organ function in male goats. Physiolo Behav 24:1067–1071, 1980
8. Moulton DG, Beidler LM: Structure and function in the peripheral olfactory system. Physiol Rev 47:1–52, 1967
9. Myers LJ: Methods of diagnosis of disorders of special senses. I. The sense of smell. Auburn Vet 40:12–14, 1985
10. Myers LJ, Nash R, Elledge HS: Electroolfactography: A technique with potential for diagnosis of anosmia in the dog. Am J Vet Res 45:2296–2298, 1984
11. Myers LJ, Pugh R: Thresholds of the dog for detection of inhaled eugenol and benzaldehyde determined by electroencephalographic and behavioral olfactometry. Am J Vet Res 46:2409–2412, 1985
12. O'Brien JA, Harvey CE: Diseases of the upper airway. In Ettinger SJ (ed): Textbook of Veterinary Internal Medicine, 2nd ed. Philadelphia, WB Saunders, 1983
13. Oliver JE, Jr, Lorenz M: Handbook of Veterinary Neurologic Diagnosis. Philadelphia, WB Saunders, 1983

59

Deafness

JOHN E. OLIVER

PROBLEM DEFINITION AND RECOGNITION

Loss of hearing is difficult to detect in companion animals, except in dogs trained to respond to verbal commands. Unilateral deafness is almost never recognized, except in working dogs, which may have difficulty orienting to the direction of the sound.

PATHOPHYSIOLOGY

The tympanic membrane separates the external ear canal from the middle ear. The middle ear includes the tympanic bulla; the auditory ossicles; the auditory tube to the nasal pharynx; and sympathetic nerve fibers, which innervate the dilator muscles of the pupil. The inner ear is in the petrosal bone and includes the vestibular receptor organs and the cochlea, the coiled portion of the bony labyrinth containing perilymph, which is the receptor organ for hearing. Sound waves move the tympanic membrane, which moves the ossicles. The movement of the last ossicle, the stapes, moves the oval window, imparting the wave form to the perilymph. The wave flow in the perilymph moves the basilar membrane, causing movement of the hair cells of the spiral organ. Movement of the hair cells causes depolarization, which probably causes release of neurotransmitter, activating the fibers of the cochlear nerve.[7,13,35] The cochlear nerve joins the vestibular nerve to form the vestibulocochlear nerve. The cochlear division synapses in the cochlear nuclei in the medulla oblongata. Axons from the cochlear nuclei have two pathways into the medulla: ventrally through the trapezoid body and dorsally over the caudal cerebellar peduncle in the acoustic stria. The pathways proceed rostrally bilaterally, with several synapses and projections to the contralateral side. Nuclei involved in the auditory pathway include the nuclei of the trapezoid body, nucleus of the lateral lemniscus, caudal colliculi, and the medial geniculate nucleus of the thalamus. Axons from the geniculate nucleus project to the temporal lobe of the cerebral cortex. Although the pathway is bilateral, the majority of the projection to the cortex is from the contralateral side.[13]

Total loss of hearing is rarely caused by lesions of the central nervous system. The auditory pathways are bilateral and multisynaptic in the brain, so lesions destroying them produce severe neurologic signs that would remove any concern for hearing loss. Peripheral hearing loss can be of two types: conduction (nonneural) and nerve deafness. Conduction deafness involves an abnormality of the transduction apparatus, including the tympanic membrane, middle ear cavity, or auditory ossicles. Punctures of the tympanic membrane, effusions in the tympanic bulla, or abnormalities of the auditory ossicles do not usually cause complete hearing loss. Acuity is decreased, but this is rarely recognized. Reduction in motion of the ossicles, a common change with aging in humans, may account for the decrease in acuity in some older animals. Complete hearing loss, either unilateral or bilateral, is usually a sign of damage to the receptor in the inner ear or to the cochlear nerve. In acquired disease of these structures, abnormal vestibular function is common and is usually of more concern to the owner (see chapter 49). Congenital deafness is usually a result of abnormal development or degeneration of the spiral organ, the receptor in the cochlea.[2,4,6,23,26] At least one report suggests that the defect is primarily in central structures, with the peripheral changes being secondary.[16] The cochlea is sensitive to damage by various drugs and toxins, the most important being the aminoglycoside antibiotics.[30] Hypothyroidism also causes degeneration of the cochlea as well as some neurologic abnormalities, including vestibular and facial nerve dysfunction.[11,20,28,29,45,46]

DIAGNOSTIC PLAN

One of the most difficult tasks confronting clinicians is establishing the presence of deafness in an animal. Simple tests such as making noises to alert the animal or having the owner give commands are frequently equivocal. One of the best methods is making a loud noise while the animal is asleep.[13] An animal will usually stop panting briefly when alerted, the basis for a behavioral test that can be effective.[47] Other tests involving electrophysiologic techniques will be discussed later. The owner's history may be the most reliable data available.

It is useful clinically to determine if the deafness is congenital or acquired. Congenital deafness is present from birth, although it is usually unrecognized until the animal is old enough to respond to sounds. Hearing is present in dogs by 10 to 11 days of age and in cats by 5 days.[13]

Most congenital deafness is associated with a white or merle hair coat. Cats with a white coat and blue eyes are usually deaf.[2,4,10,15,36–38,48] If the cat has one blue eye, it may be deaf only on the side of the blue eye.[9] The gene for white coat is autosomal dominant in cats but is incompletely penetrant for inner ear degeneration. Deafness shows high penetrance in the homozygote but less in the heterozygote. Total deafness is more often associated with long hair in white cats.[12] Dogs with a white or merle hair coat are at risk for congenital deafness (Table 59-1).[1,6,8,19,24,42] The highest incidence is in Dalmatians.[19,23] Hearing loss may be bilateral or unilateral in these dogs. For this reason, it is important to screen at-risk puppies for hearing, using electrophysiologic tests that can detect unilateral deafness.[1,8,13,33,42]

A complete physical and neurologic examination should be completed on animals presented for deafness. Special attention should be given to the ears, including a thorough otoscopic examination. The tympanic membrane should be intact, not inflamed, and translucent. Normally, it has a ground-glass appearance and the promontory of the petrosal bone can be recognized in the middle ear. Effusions of the middle ear will cause the tympanic membrane to be opaque, discolored, and, in many cases, bulging into the external ear canal. Radiographs of the tympanic bullae are useful as supportive evidence of middle ear disease but are not as reliable as the otoscopic examination.[32] Other neurologic signs associated with middle and inner ear infections are Horner's syndrome, facial nerve paralysis, and vestibular disorders (see chapter 49). The causes of hearing loss are listed under Etiology of Deafness. Infection of the external, middle, or inner ear is the most common acquired problem.[14,18,43,44] Geriatric hearing loss is also fairly common but is usually not total. Hearing loss, sometimes associated with other neural deficits, occurs in animals with hypothyroidism. Some have responded to replacement thyroid hormone therapy.[11,20,28,29,45,46]

Several electrophysiologic tests for hearing are available at referral centers. The best test is the brain stem auditory evoked response (BAER). A computer

Table 59-1. Hereditary Deafness—Additional Information Sources

CANINE*	REFERENCE(S)	FELINE	REFERENCE(S)
Australian heeler	13, 19, 33, 42	White, blue eye	2, 4, 12, 15, 36–38, 48
Australian shepherd	13, 19, 33, 42		
Beagle	13		
Border collies	1, 42		
Boston terrier	13, 19, 33, 42		
Boxer	19		
Bullterrier	1, 13, 33		
Cocker spaniel	33		
Collie	13, 33, 42		
Dalmatian	1, 13, 19, 33, 42		
English bulldog	13, 19, 33		
English setter	13, 19, 33, 42		
Fox terrier	1		
Norwegian dunkerhound	1, 13, 33		
Old English sheepdog	13, 19, 33		
Scottish terrier	1		
Sealyham	1		
Shetland sheepdog	19		
Shropshire terrier	42		
Walker foxhound	1		

* Associated with white or merle color gene

Etiology of Deafness

Acquired

- Degenerative—geriatric
- Metabolic—hypothyroidism
- Neoplastic—tumors of inner ear or CN VIII
- Idiopathic—unknown
- Inflammatory—otitis media or interna
- Toxic—aminoglycoside antibiotics
- Traumatic—head injury

Congenital

- Anomaly—hereditary aplasia, hypoplasia, or degeneration of receptor. See Table 59-1.

signal averager is necessary to perform the test. Tone or click signals are introduced to each ear independently, and responses are recorded from scalp electrodes. The test is noninvasive, safe, and reliable; can be used on immature animals; tests each ear independently; and does not require anesthesia. Function of the peripheral receptors and the brain stem pathway can be assessed.[3,8,21,25,27,31,40,41] The intensity of the stimulus can be varied to estimate hearing acuity.

Tympanometry assesses the integrity of the middle ear system.[17,34] The volume of the external ear canal is estimated by an acoustic impedance bridge. The change in volume with changing pressure measures the compliance of the tympanum. A reflex contraction of the stapedius muscle can be induced by a tone and causes a change in the compliance of the tympanic membrane, the acoustic or stapedial reflex. The combination of these two tests (tympanometry and acoustic reflex) assesses the integrity of the middle ear, hearing, and the facial nerve, which innervates the stapedius muscle.

Electroencephalographic (EEG) audiometry is performed on a conscious animal that is calm enough to obtain slow waves on the EEG or is asleep. A sound is introduced, which will alert the animal, causing a change in the EEG. Use of calibrated tone generators allows quantitation of hearing.[39] Respiratory audiometry is based on the principle that animals change their respiratory pattern when alerted. It can be quantified and made more sensitive by recording respiratory patterns with a strain gauge around the abdomen or thorax.[5] These tests assess hearing but do not provide any information on the source of the problem.

The signalment, history, physical examination, and neurologic examination should differentiate congenital from acquired deafness. An otoscopic examination will confirm infection in all but pure inner ear disease. If infection of the middle ear is found, a tympanotomy should be performed to obtain material for culture and to establish drainage. This can be done by aspirating material from the middle ear with a 22-gauge spinal needle and syringe. If the contents are too thick to aspirate, 0.25 ml to 0.5 ml of saline can be injected into the middle ear and withdrawn. A larger opening can be made with a small intramedullary pin or an ear curette. Culture and assessment of sensitivity of exudate in the middle ear are recommended because many of these infections are resistant to commonly used antibiotics. Radiographs are of less benefit in most cases but are recommended because of secondary changes such as lysis of the bulla, which can affect the prognosis. Radiographs may detect fluid in the middle ear and tumors of the ear or surrounding structures, which are occasionally responsible for hearing loss.[18,43,44]

SYMPTOMATIC THERAPY

There is no treatment for deafness unless the primary disease is treated successfully before permanent damage to the receptors or nerve occurs. Congenital deafness is irreversible. Animals with partial deafness may get worse with time.

Treatment of infections is discussed in several of the references.[14,18,22,43,44] In general, chronic bacterial infection of the middle ear is resistant to many of the commonly used antibiotics. Specific therapy should be predicated from the results of bacterial culture and antibiotic sensitivity tests. Only those antibiotics that penetrate the middle and inner ear tissues in sufficient concentration to inhibit or destroy the causative bacteria are used. The cephalosporins, chloramphenicol, and trimethoprim–sulfa combinations are usually effective. The aminoglycosides should not be used, since they may not penetrate the target tissues and may cause ototoxicity and deafness, even when applied topically.

REFERENCES

1. Adams EW: Hereditary deafness in a family of foxhounds. J Am Vet Med Assoc 128:302–303, 1956
2. Bergsma DR, Brown KS: White fur, blue eyes, and deafness in the domestic cat. J Hered 62:171–185, 1971
3. Bodenhamer RD, Hunter JF, Luttgen PJ: Brain stem auditory-evoked responses in the dog. Am J Vet Res 46:1787–1792, 1985
4. Bosher SK, Hallpike CS: Observations on the histologic features, development, and pathogenesis of the inner ear degeneration of the deaf white cat. Proc R Soc Lond [Biol] 162:147–170, 1965
5. Bradford LJ, McKinley JH, Rousey CL, Klein DE: Measurement of hearing in dogs by respiration audiometry. Am J Vet Res 34:1183–1187, 1973
6. Branis M, Burda H: Inner ear structure in the deaf and normally hearing Dalmation dog. J Comp Pathol 95:295–299, 1985
7. Chrisman CL: Problems in Small Animal Neurology. Philadelphia, Lea & Febiger, 1982
8. Coulter DB: A dog with a partial merle coat, white iris, and bilaterally impaired hearing. Calif Vet 12:9–11, 1982
9. Coulter DB, Martin CL, Alvarado TP: A cat with white fur and one blue eye. Calif Vet 34:11–14, 1980

10. Creel D, Conlee JW, Parks TN: Auditory brainstem anomalies in albino cats. I. Evoked potential studies. Brain Res 260:1–9, 1983
11. Crifo S, Lazzari R, Salabe GB, Arnaldi D, Gagliardi M, Maragoni F: A retrospective study of audiological function in a group of congenital hypothyroid patients. Int J Pediatr Otorhinolaryngol 2:347–355, 1980
12. Delack JB: Hereditary deafness in the white cat. Comp Cont Ed Pract Vet 6:609–616, 1984
13. de Lahunta A: Veterinary Neuroanatomy and Clinical Neurology, 2nd ed. Philadelphia, WB Saunders, 1983
14. Denny HR: The results of surgical treatment of otitis media and interna in the dog. J Small Anim Pract 14:585–600, 1973
15. Faith RE, Woodard JC: Waardenburg's syndrome. Comp Pathol Bull 5:3–4, 1973
16. Ferrara ML, Halnan CRE: Congenital brain defects in the deaf Dalmatian. Vet Rec 112:344–346, 1983
17. Forsythe WB: Tympanographic volume measurements of the canine ear. Am J Vet Res 46:1351–1353, 1985
18. Fraser G, Gregor WW, Mackenzie CP, Spreull JSA, Withers AR: Canine ear disease. J Small Anim Pract 10:725–754, 1970
19. Hayes HM, Wilson GP, Fenner WR, Wyman M: Canine congenital deafness: Epidemiologic study of 272 cases. J Am Anim Hosp Assoc 17:473, 1981
20. Hebert R, Langlois JM, Dussault JH: Effect of graded periods of congenital hypothyroidism on the peripheral auditory evoked activity of rats. Electroencephalogr Clin Neurophys 62:381–387, 1985
21. Holliday TA, Te Selle ME: Brain stem auditory-evoked potentials of dogs: Wave forms and effects of recording electrode positions. Am J Vet Res 46:845–851, 1985
22. Howard PE, Neer TM, Miller JS: Otitis media. II. Surgical considerations. Comp Cont Ed Pract Vet 5:18–24, 1983
23. Hudson WR, Ruben RJ: Hereditary deafness in the dalmatian dog. Arch Otolaryngol 75:213–219, 1962
24. Igarashi M, Alford BR, Cohn AM, Saito R, Watanabe T: Inner ear anomalies in dogs. Ann Otol Rhinol Laryngol 81:249–255, 1972
25. Kay R, Palmer AC, Taylor PM: Hearing in the dog as assessed by auditory brainstem evoked potentials. Vet Rec 114:81–84, 1984
26. Lurie MH: The membranous labyrinth in the congenitally deaf collie and Dalmatian dog. Laryngoscope 58:279–287, 1948
27. Marshall AE: Brain stem auditory-evoked response of the nonanesthetized dog. Am J Vet Res 46:966–973, 1985
28. Mendel D, Robinson M: Electrocochleography in congenital hypothyroidism. Dev Med Child Neurol 20:664–667, 1978
29. Meyerhoff WL: The thyroid and audition. Laryngoscope 86:483–489, 1976
30. Morgan JL, Coulter DB, Marshall AE, Goetsch DD: Effects of neomycin on the waveform of auditory-evoked brain stem potentials in dogs. Am J Vet Res 41:1077–1081, 1980
31. Myers LJ, Redding RW, Wilson S: Reference values of the brainstem auditory evoked response of methoxyflurane anesthetized and unanesthetized dogs. Vet Res Comm 9:289–294, 1985
32. Oliver JE, Jr, Lorenz M: Handbook of Veterinary Neurologic Diagnosis. Philadelphia, WB Saunders, 1983
33. Oliver JE, Hoerlein BF, Mayhew IG: Veterinary Neurology. Philadelphia, WB Saunders (in press)
34. Penrod JP, Coulter DB: The diagnostic uses of impedance audiometry in the dog. J Am Anim Hosp Assoc 16:941–948, 1980
35. Pickles JO: Hearing and listening. In Swash M, Kennard C (ed): Scientific Basis of Clinical Neurology. Edinburgh, Churchill Livingstone, 1985
36. Rebillard G, Rebillard M, Carlier E, Pujol R: Histo-physiological relationships in the deaf white cat auditory system. Acta Otolaryngol 82:48–56, 1976
37. Rebillard M, Pujol R, Rebillard G: Variability of the hereditary deafness in the white cat. II. Histology. Hear Res 5:189–200, 1981

38. Rebillard M, Rebillard G, Pujol R: Variability of the hereditary deafness in the white cat. I. Physiology. Hear Res 5:179–187, 1981

39. Redding RW: Electroencephalography. In Oliver JE, Hoerlein BF, Mayhew IG (eds): Veterinary Neurology. Philadelphia, WB Saunders (in press)

40. Sims MH, Moore RE: Auditory-evoked response in the clinically normal dog: Early latency components. Am J Vet Res 45:2019–2027, 1984

41. Sims MH, Moore RE: Auditory-evoked response in the clinically normal dog: Middle latency components. Am J Vet Res 45:2028–2033, 1984

42. Sims MH, Shull-Selcer E: Electrodiagnostic evaluation of deafness in two English setter littermates. J Am Vet Med Assoc 187:398–404, 1985

43. Spreull JSA: Treatment of otitis media in the dog. J Small Anim Pract 5:107–122, 1964

44. Spreull JSA: Otitis media. Anim Hosp 2:89–99, 1966

45. Uziel A, Legrand C, Rabie A: Corrective effects of thyroxine on cochlear abnormalities induced by congenital hypothyroidism in the rat. I. Morphological study. Dev Brain Res 19:111–122, 1985

46. Uziel A, Marot M, Rabie A: Corrective effects of thyroxine on cochlear abnormalities induced by congenital hypothyroidism in the rat. II. Electrophysiological study. Dev Brain Res 19:123–127, 1985

47. Van Der Velden NA, Rijkse C: A practicable method of making audiograms in dogs. Appl Anim Ethol 2:371–377, 1976

48. Wolff D: Three generations of deaf white cats. J Hered 33:39–43, 1942

Part Fourteen

LABORATORY-DEFINED PROBLEMS

60

Hematologic Problems

CRAIG E. GREENE

ANEMIA

Anemia is a decrease in the hematocrit (<37 in dogs; <27 in cats) and has many causes. Diagnostic and therapeutic plans for anemia are predicted on the basis of the presence or absence of red blood cell (RBC) regeneration (Table 60-1). Nonregenerative anemias are caused by decreased bone marrow production of erythrocytes; regenerative anemias are caused by increased erythrocyte destruction (hemolysis) and blood loss (hemorrhage). Regeneration is best detected by examining blood films for the presence of reticulocytosis (by methylene blue stain), polychromasia (by Wright's stain), or both. Only large aggregate (not punctate) reticulocytes should be used to assess the degree of reticulocytosis in cats. Other findings such as anisocytosis, Howell-Jolly bodies, and nucleated erythrocytes are not specific indicators of adequate RBC regeneration in dogs and cats. The reticulocyte count is normally expressed as a relative percentage of circulating erythrocytes and must be corrected to accurately assess the degree of regenerative response. For instance, a 2% reticulocyte count with a hematocrit of 10 is less impressive than the same count with a hematocrit of 20. A simple correction for relative reticulocyte count is given in Table 60-2.

The clinical signs associated with anemia depend on the degree of anemia, rapidity of development, associated plasma volume loss, and cardiovascular dysfunction. The clinical signs of anemia are described in chapter 23.

The diagnostic plan for regenerative anemia should differentiate blood loss from blood lysis. Plasma protein concentration should be determined. Plasma protein concentrations are normal with most hemolytic disorders and are decreased with hemorrhage. Body excretions (urine, feces, and vomitus) and body cavities should be examined for the presence of blood. Serum icterus, increased bilirubinuria, and hemoglobinuria (if present) are associated with hemolytic disorders. When hemolysis is suspected, additional diagnostic tests should include examination of blood films for the presence of Heinz bodies, stomatocytes, spherocytes, or blood parasites. These tests not only help confirm the presence of

Table 60-1. Causes of Anemia

REGENERATIVE	NONREGENERATIVE
Blood loss	Decreased erythropoietin
Surgery	Endocrine dysfunction
Trauma	Hypothyroidism
Gastrointestinal	Hypoadrenocorticism
Ulceration	Chronic disease
Parasites	Inflammation
Hemostatic disorders	Neoplasia
Urinary tract disorders	Cytotoxic marrow damage
Blood lysis	Chemical agents
Parasites	Cytotoxic drugs
Osmotic changes	Fungal toxins
Membrane	Physical agents
Malamutes—stomatocytes	Irradiation
Basenji—pyruvate kinase deficiency	Immune-mediated cytotoxicity
Cats—porphyria	Pure red blood cell aplasia
Hepatic dysfunction	Myelophthistic diseases
Immune/infectious causes	Lymphocytic, granulocytic, or plasmacytic leukemias
Trauma	Nuclear division dysfunction
Chemicals/toxins	Sulfonamide drugs
Onions, acetaminophen, phenol, methylene blue, topical anesthetics, nitrates	Methotrexate therapy
	Folic acid deficiency
	B_{12} deficiency
	Abnormal erythroid maturation
	Erythroleukemia
	Feline leukemia virus infection
	Heme synthesis interference
	Lead poisoning
	Chloramphenicol
	Microcytic iron deficiency

Table 60-2. Simple Corrected Reticulocyte Response

	DOG	CAT
Normal (%)	≤1	≤0.4
Slight (%)	1–4	0.5–2
Large (%)	5–20	3–4

Normal packed cell volume (PCV) for dogs is 45%; for cats, 35%.
Simple corrected response =

$$\frac{\text{Actual PCV}}{\text{Normal PCV}} \times \text{reticulocyte count (\%)}$$

hemolysis but also always provide valuable clues to the etiology of the hemolytic process. Urine that contains intact RBCs, myoglobin, or hemoglobin will be positive on the urine occult blood test. Urine sediment should also be evaluated. The absence of erythrocytes or blood ghosts (also called phantom corpuscles) in the urine sediment of an anemic animal with a positive urine occult blood suggests hemoglobinuria from intravascular hemolysis or, rarely, myoglobinuria due to severe muscle necrosis. When hemolysis has been proven, definitive tests to establish the etiology are indicated, including Coombs' test, feline leukemia virus (FeLV) test, heartworm test, and chest radiography. When hemorrhage has been proven, coagulation tests and platelet counts are needed to eliminate hemostatic disorders (see chapter 23).

The diagnostic plan for nonregenerative anemia includes evaluation of the erythrocyte indices to determine red cell size (see Causes of Nonregenerative Anemia Based on Erythrocyte Size and Figs. 60-1 and 60-2). Macrocytic anemias are seen with diseases that inhibit nuclear division (B_{12} and folic acid deficiencies). Microcytosis occurs with disorders that inhibit heme synthesis (iron deficiency states). The relative numbers of leukocytes and platelets should be assessed, since certain diseases affect bone marrow elements in addition to the erythrocyte series. FeLV testing is very important, since this disease is a common cause of nonregenerative anemia in cats. In dogs, serologic tests for ehrlichiosis may be necessary. The plasma protein concentration should be evaluated, since hypoproteinemia may suggest chronic blood loss associated with iron deficiency.

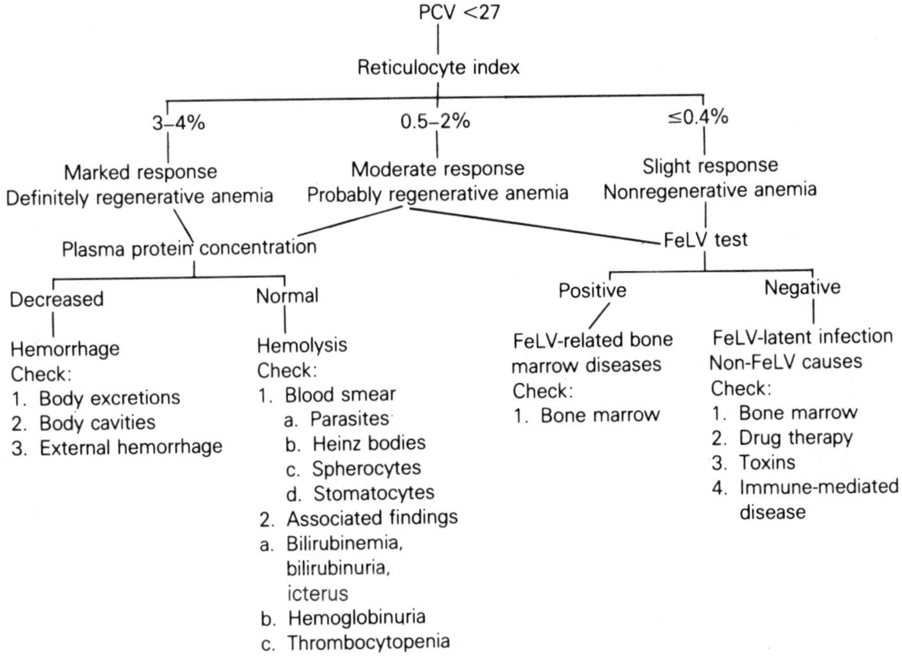

Fig. 60-1. Diagnostic plan for feline anemia.

Causes of Nonregenerative Anemia Based on Erythrocyte Size

- MCV <60—Microcytic anemia
  - Iron deficiency
    - Deficient diet
    - Chronic blood loss
      - Gastrointestinal
      - Reproductive
      - Urinary
  - Pulmonary iron sequestration
  - Chronic intravascular hemolysis
  - Gastrointestinal malabsorption
- MCV 60–77—Normocytic anemia
  - Inadequate diet
  - Body protein loss
  - Decreased hormonal influence
    - Hypothyroidism
    - Hypoadrenocorticism
    - Chronic renal failure
  - Bone marrow intoxication
    - Chloramphenicol
    - Lead poisoning
    - Cancer chemotherapy
    - Estrogens
  - Chronic inflammatory diseases
  - Chronic infectious diseases
    - Feline leukemia virus infection
    - Myeloproliferative disease
    - Chronic ehrlichiosis
  - Pure erythrocyte aplasia
- MCV >77—Macrocytic anemia
  - Folic acid deficiency
    - Sulfonamides
    - Methotrexate
  - B_{12} deficiency

MCV, mean corpuscular volume

Feces should be examined for blood and the presence of helminth eggs or protozoal organisms that cause chronic gastrointestinal blood loss. Many endocrinologic and metabolic diseases (*e.g.,* chronic renal failure) cause nonregenerative anemias of the normocytic normochromic type. Biochemical tests and urinalysis are indicated, since they may reveal the presence of these disorders. Bone marrow examination is indicated when hematologic, biochemical, urinalysis, and FeLV tests fail to establish the diagnosis. Bone marrow examinations are extremely useful in the diagnosis and prognosis of cytotoxic damage,

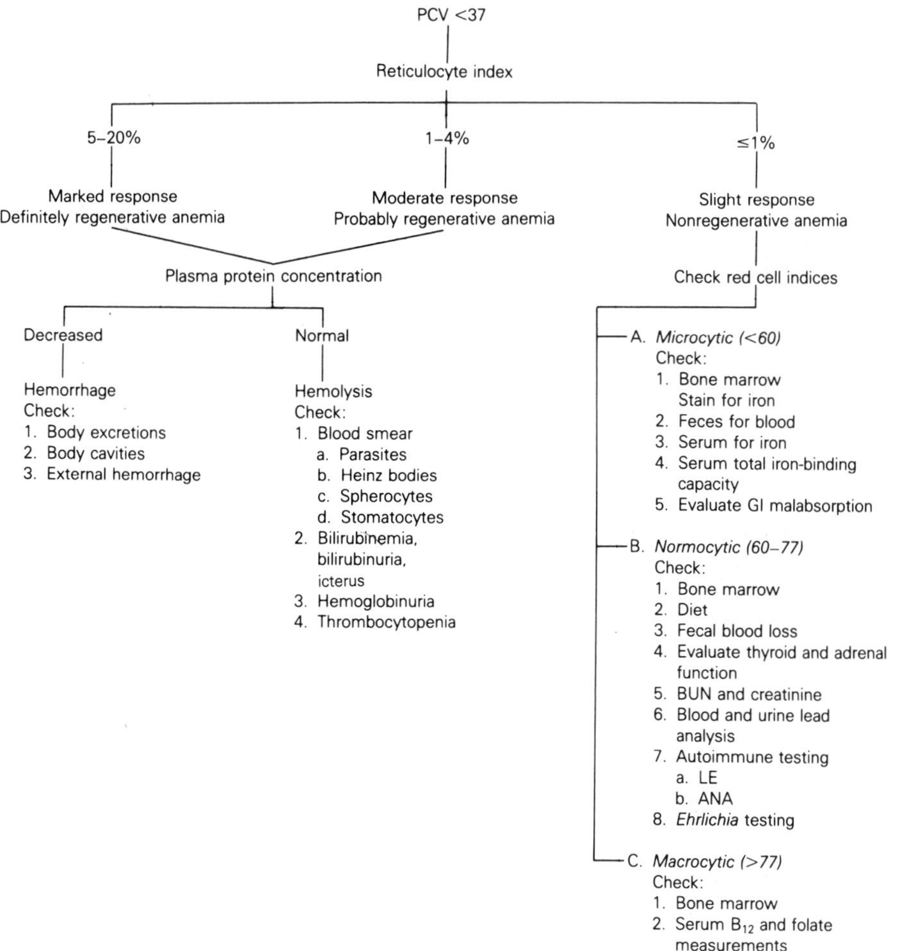

Fig. 60-2. Diagnostic plan for canine anemia.

myelophthistic disease, abnormal erythroid maturation, and interference with heme synthesis (see Table 60-1).

LEUKOPENIA

Leukopenia (panleukopenia) involves a decrease in all leukocytes and is generally associated with severe white blood cell destruction, an overwhelming demand for leukocytes, or decreased bone marrow and lymphoid cell production. The usual causes of panleukopenia are listed in Table 60-3. In severe leukopenia, a second hemogram should be taken within 48 hours for comparison. If leukopenia persists, examination of the bone marrow is needed. Animals with persistent leukopenia are immunodeficient and frequently develop secondary

Table 60-3. Leukocyte Abnormalities

LEUKOPENIA	LEUKOCYTOSIS	NEUTROPENIA	NEUTROPHILIA*
Toxins	Physiologic	Increased usage	Physiologic
Irradiation	(epinephrine)	Peracute overwhelming infection	Increased muscular activity
Fungal (T-2)	Stress	Cellulitis	Increased blood pressure
Infections	(glucocorticoids)	Aspiration pneumonia	Stress
Ehrlichiosis	Inflammation/infection	Endotoxemia	Glucocorticoid therapy
Feline leukemia	(chronic)	Peritonitis	Cushing's disease
Feline panleukopenia		Acute viral infections	Pathologic
Overwhelming sepsis		Decreased production	Inflammation (especially local or chronic)
		Infectious	Neoplastic
		Panleukopenia	Myeloproliferative diseases
		Feline leukemia	Granulomatous and lymphocytic leukemias
		Ehrlichiosis	
		Canine parvovirus infection	
		Chemical	
		Fungal toxin	
		Estrogen	
		Anticonvulsants	
		Cytotoxic drugs	
		Genetic	
		Cyclic hematopoiesis	
		Myelophthistic disorders	
		Myeloproliferative diseases	

* >11,500 in dogs; >12,500 in cats

bacterial infections. When hospitalized, they should be separated from other animals and should receive antimicrobial therapy if infectious complications develop. Bactericidal antibiotics are preferable to bacteriostatic antibiotics when severe leukopenia is present.

LEUKOCYTOSIS

Physiologic increases in leukocyte cell numbers are caused by epinephrine release from excitement, which is more common in cats than dogs (Table 60-3). Diseases associated with endogenous glucocorticoid release can also cause leukocytosis, but lymphopenia and eosinopenia also occur. Chronic localized inflammatory or infectious processes are associated with an increase of all leukocyte types. In these cases, the body often controls the inflammatory process, and bone marrow production of leukocytes meets the demand.

NEUTROPENIA

Because neutrophils comprise a majority of leukocytes, neutropenia usually is associated with leukopenia and can be caused by increased utilization or decreased production of neutrophils. These causes can be distinguished in many cases, because increased utilization is associated with a shift to immature forms. Excessive utilization of neutrophils is associated with overwhelming tissue demand, as with multisystemic or severe inflammatory or infectious processes (Table 60-3). Decreased production of neutrophils is associated with many processes previously discussed under leukopenia; however, many of these can be selective for the neutrophil series.

NEUTROPHILIA

Increased neutrophil counts are commonly associated with an infectious process. However, neutrophilia alone does not confirm the presence of infection, since noninfectious processes such as acute pancreatitis or extravascular hemolysis or hemorrhage show similar increases (Table 60-3). Stress (glucocorticoid release) associated with many systemic disease processes is accompanied by neutrophilia in venous blood, resulting from decreased margination and emigration of the neutrophils. A left shift (increase in immature neutrophils) is usually absent in stress neutrophilia, unless the effect of endogenous glucocorticoids is superimposed on an existing inflammatory process. The degree of shift toward immature band forms correlates reasonably well with the severity of the infection or inflammatory process.

Neutrophilia without a shift may not always indicate that an animal is adequately coping with infection, although the highest counts and mature shifts usually correlate with abscess formation, or walling off of an infectious process.

Defects in neutrophil function are commonly associated with a normal to increased neutrophil count without a shift in the presence of infection, because neutrophils are not effectively consumed in the inflammatory process.

MONOCYTOSIS

Increases in absolute monocyte counts are commonly found in conjunction with neutrophilia, eosinopenia, and lymphopenia in increased endogenous (stress) or exogenous glucocorticoid concentrations. Monocytosis is usually an indicator of granulomatous diseases in which neutrophils have been unsuccessful in eliminating persistent intracellular infectious agents. Monocyte numbers are also increased in cases of neutrophilic defects or persistent neutropenia, when monocytes must perform primary phagocytic functions. A summary of the causes of monocytosis is presented in Table 60-4.

LYMPHOPENIA

Decreased circulating lymphocyte counts are associated with acute infectious or inflammatory processes as well as with stress or Cushing's disease (Table 60-4). Selective lymphopenia is a feature of the viremic period of many acute systemic viral infections. Chronic persistent lymphopenia is a poor prognostic sign in any illness and usually indicates the body's inability to respond to the disease insult. Of the total number of body lymphocytes, only 10% are circulating. These are primarily T cells; therefore, absolute lymphocyte counts cannot always be correlated with the immunocompetency of the host.

LYMPHOCYTOSIS

Lymphocytosis, a common feature of chronic inflammatory diseases, occurs with neutrophilia and monocytosis (Table 60-4). Chronic antigenic stimulation leads to proliferation of lymphoid precursors and, hence, circulating lymphocytes. Lymphocytosis may be found in cats infected with FeLV or in dogs with lymphosarcoma or lymphocytic leukemia. Atypical lymphocytes may also be seen. Cats, unlike dogs, have proportionally more lymphocytes than neutrophils in their peripheral circulation, so, on a percentage basis, many cats appear to have a lymphocytosis.

EOSINOPENIA

Eosinopenia occurs during the acute stress of many disease states associated with endogenous glucocorticoid release, as with canine Cushing's syndrome (Table 60-4). Exogenous glucocorticoid therapy also results in eosinopenia, the duration of which varies with the dosage and drug administered.

Table 60-4. Leukocyte Abnormalities

LYMPHOPENIA	EOSINOPENIA	MONOCYTOSIS	LYMPHOCYTOSIS	EOSINOPHILIA	BASOPHILIA
Glucocorticoids	Exogenous glucocorticoids	Stress (glucocorticoid)	Physiologic (especially cats)	Acute hypersensitivity	Chronic inflammation of mucosal and skin surfaces
Endogenous (Cushing's disease)	Endogenous glucocorticoids	Chronic inflammation	Chronic inflammation	Parasitism	Chronic fasting lipemia
Exogenous (drug therapy)	Stress	Internal hemorrhage/hemolysis	Lymphocytic leukemia	Gastrointestinal (hookworms, roundworms, whipworms)	Cushing's disease
Debilitating disorders	Cushing's disease	Persistent neutropenia	Lymphosarcoma	Pulmonary (lungworms)	Hypothyroidism
Chronic infections		Neutrophil function defect		Vascular (heartworms)	Eosinophilia
Metastatic neoplasia		Granulomatous diseases		Skin (fleas, *Demodex*)	Mastocytoma (especially pulmonary and systemic)
Renal failure				Specific syndromes	
Amyloidosis				Gastrointestinal (eosinophilic infiltrates)	
Loss of lymphocytes				Lung (pulmonary infiltrates)	
Repeated chylocentesis				Muscle (polymyositis)	
Intestinal lymphangiectasia				Skin (miliary dermatitis, eosinophilic granuloma)	
Impaired lymphopoiesis				Soft tissues (eosinophilic infiltrates in dogs)	
Cancer chemotherapy				Neoplasia	
Prolonged use of glucocorticoids				Lymphosarcoma	
Irradiation				Mastocytoma	
Congenital T-cell immunodeficiency				Metastatic types	
				Others	
				Estrus	
				Eosinophilic leukemia	
				Autoimmune disease	

EOSINOPHILIA

In contrast to acute diseases, chronic infectious or inflammatory diseases result in an eosinophilia rather than eosinopenia (Table 60-4). The major tissues in which chronic inflammation results in eosinophil increases (e.g., skin and respiratory, gastrointestinal, and genital mucosae) are those laden with tissue mast cells. Eosinophilia also may be noted with chronic fungal or protozoal infections, but it occurs more consistently in infections caused by metazoal parasites such as fleas, roundworms, hookworms, heartworms, and lungworms.

BASOPHILIA

Chronic antigenic stimulation of skin or mucosal surfaces causes an increase in IgE-mediated inflammatory processes. Basophils, the circulating equivalent of tissue mast cells, are increased in these processes, and their increase is usually associated with eosinophilia (Table 60-4). Conditions associated with fasting hyperlipemia are also associated with basophilia, because basophils contain heparin, an activator of lipoprotein lipase. The basophilia may aid in the clearance of circulating lipids from the blood.

THROMBOCYTOPENIA

Platelets are produced by bone marrow elements, and any process that interferes with marrow production will lead to thrombocytopenia. Various causes of decreased platelet production are listed in Table 60-5 and are discussed further in chapter 23. Increased platelet removal and thrombocytopenia can occur as a result of immune or coagulatory consumption of platelets. Platelets also can be sequestered with splenomegaly from conditions such as portal hypertension, lymphosarcoma, and splenic torsion.

THROMBOCYTOSIS

Thrombocytes increase in the circulation whenever splenic contraction or splenectomy occurs, because the spleen is the major site of platelet storage in the body. Chronic iron deficiencies probably result in thrombocytosis because the marrow is stimulated by myelopoietic hormones to increased the production of erythrocytes. Diseases commonly associated with thrombocytosis are listed in Table 60-5.

HYPERLIPEMIA

Hyperlipemia, an increase in the amount of circulating lipid in the blood, may reflect a variety of diseases associated with altered fat metabolism (see Causes of Fasting Hyperlipemia). Care must be taken to distinguish visible from invisible

Table 60-5. Abnormalities in Platelet Numbers

THROMBOCYTOPENIA	THROMBOCYTOSIS
Decreased production	Reactive
Drugs	Splenectomy
Estrogens	Acute hemorrhage
Cancer chemotherapy	Trauma
Myelophthistic diseases	Fractures
Infections	Infections (chronic)
Ehrlichiosis	Malignancies
Physiologic causes	Iron deficiencies
Estrus	Vincristine
Sertoli tumors	Diabetes mellitus
Increased destruction	Autonomous
Immune	Myeloproliferative disease
Drugs	
Infectious	
Idiopathic	
Coagulatory	
Disseminated intravascular coagulation	
Endotoxin	
Sequestration	
Splenomegaly	
Portal hypertension	

hyperlipemia when determining the cause of this syndrome. Visible hyperlipemia is caused by increased amounts of circulating chylomicrons derived from the digestive process. This normally occurs 1 to 3 hours postprandially. Delays of lipid clearance greater than 3 hours after eating usually reflect deranged lipid clearance and may indicate an increase in circulating invisible lipids. Invisible hyperlipemia, which can be assumed indirectly from the presence of visible hyperlipemia, must be substantiated by lipoprotein electrophoresis. Invisible hyperlipemia also can occur in the absence of fasting hyperchylomicronemia and, in such cases, will only be detected if lipoprotein electrophoresis is performed.

Causes of Fasting Hyperlipemia

- Hypothyroidism
- Hyperadrenocorticism
- Nephrotic syndrome
- Acute pancreatitis
- Steatitis
- Postprandial
- Idiopathic (familial)
  - Schnausers
  - Dachshunds

Serum sample analysis that involves colorimetric procedures is invalidated by the presence of visible lipemia. In some cases, lipemic samples may be cleared by high-speed ultracentrifugation following refrigeration or by administration of heparin to the patient. A more accurate way to assess the lipemic state is to use noncolorimetric procedures (e.g., enzymatic glucose test sticks) or to not feed the animal for 48 to 72 hours and repeat the analysis on the sample after the plasma has cleared.

61

Abnormalities of the Standard Biochemical Profile

LARRY M. CORNELIUS

DECREASED BLOOD UREA NITROGEN

Definition

A decreased blood urea nitrogen (BUN) level is defined as a BUN of <10 mg/dl.

Pathophysiology

Urea is produced in the liver from nitrogenous precursors such as ammonia and amino acids in portal blood. Dietary protein and blood in the intestinal tract are major sources of ammonia and protein. After entering the systemic circulation from the liver, urea is filtered through the glomeruli and excreted into the urine. Urea also enters the intestinal lumen, and a portion is converted to ammonia by bacterial ureases. Most of this ammonia is absorbed into the portal circulation and returned to the liver for resynthesis into urea.

A low BUN can occur because of decreased urea production or increased urea excretion (Fig. 61-1). Decreased production is most common with chronic hepatic dysfunction or long-term consumption of severely restricted protein diets. Increased urea excretion causing a low BUN is often observed in animals with significant polyuria.

Diagnostic Plan

History and Physical Examination

A history of the patient being on a severely restricted protein diet, such as Prescription Diet S-D (Hill's Pet Products, Topeka, KS), for several months or a history of chronic polyuria should alert the clinician to the possibility of a decreased BUN.

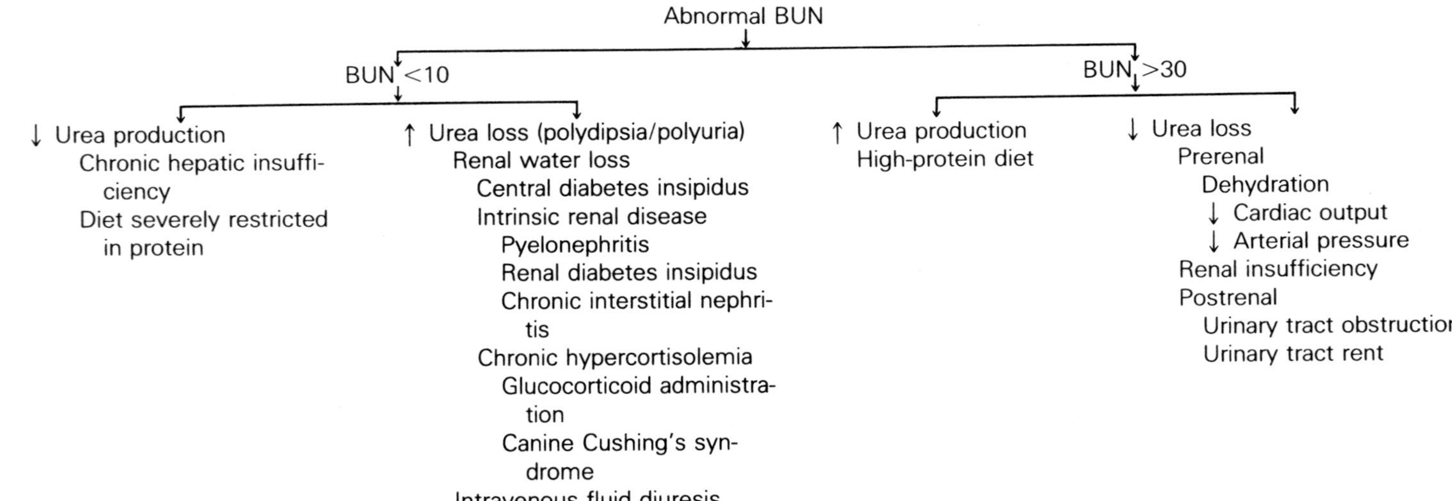

Fig. 61-1. Selected causes of abnormal BUN.

Laboratory Evaluation

BUN is often determined as a part of a standard biochemical profile, which should include a serum creatinine. A urine specimen, preferably obtained prior to therapy and by cystocentesis should be submitted for a complete urine analysis (including sediment examination). Follow-up laboratory procedures, including radiology, will be determined by rule outs being considered after initial results are obtained.

Symptomatic Therapy

Symptomatic therapy of a decreased BUN is not necessary. The etiology should be determined and treated appropriately.

INCREASED BLOOD UREA NITROGEN

Definition

An increased BUN level (azotemia) is defined as a BUN of >30 mg/dl.

Pathophysiology

An increased BUN can be caused by increased urea production in the liver, intestinal tract, or both or by decreased urea excretion by the kidneys (Fig. 61-1). Decreased renal excretion of urea is the most common cause of an increased BUN and may be due to decreased renal blood flow (prerenal), kidney failure (renal), or urinary tract obstruction or rent (post-renal). Signs of uremia are seen more often when the BUN exceeds 100 mg/dl. The more sudden the increase in BUN, generally the lower the BUN concentration required to cause signs of uremia. Most reports indicate that urea is relatively nontoxic, but other wastes that always accompany increased BUN cause signs of uremia.

Diagnostic Plan

History and Physical Examination

As noted above, clinical signs of uremia (anorexia, lethargy, vomiting, melena, dehydration, and oral ulcers) are usually not observed until the BUN exceeds 100 mg/dl. With an increased BUN of 30 to 100 mg/dl (azotemia), dehydration or other signs caused by the primary disorder are usually observed.

Laboratory Evaluation

See Laboratory Evaluation of Decreased BUN.

Symptomatic Therapy

The two methods used most commonly to lower BUN are intravenous fluid therapy and peritoneal dialysis. Fluid diuresis is usually accomplished with lactated Ringer's solution and osmotic diuresis with 10% to 20% dextrose solutions. The symptomatic treatment protocol used depends on the cause of the increased BUN. Specific therapy of the inciting cause should be started as soon as possible.

DECREASED CREATININE

There is no reported clinical significance of a decreased serum creatinine.

INCREASED CREATININE

Definition

Reported normal serum creatinine values vary depending on the particular laboratory procedure used. The upper range of normal is generally considered to be from 1.0 to 2.0 mg/dl.

Pathophysiology

Creatinine is formed largely in muscle, and its production is not significantly affected by dietary protein or blood in the gastrointestinal tract. Renal excretion of creatinine is affected by similar factors as renal urea excretion (see Pathophysiology of Decreased and Increased BUN). As is the case with urea, creatinine is not believed to be toxic but is accompanied by toxic waste products in conditions in which there is decreased renal excretion of creatinine (azotemia or uremia).

Diagnostic Plan

History and Physical Examination

Clinical signs are either those of uremia (see History and Physical Examination of Increased BUN) or of the primary disorder.

Laboratory Evaluation

See Laboratory Evaluation of Decreased BUN.

Symptomatic Therapy

Symptomatic treatment of an increased serum creatinine is the same as that for an increased BUN (see earlier discussion). Patients with chronic renal insufficiency can usually be stabilized on symptomatic therapy (*e.g.*, low-protein diet) if the serum creatinine concentration can be lowered to less than 5.0 mg/dl.

HYPOALBUMINEMIA

Definition

Hypoalbuminemia is defined as a serum albumin concentration of less than 2.5 g/dl. Most normal adult dogs and cats have a serum albumin concentration of around 3.0 g/dl, whereas puppies and kittens have a slightly lower serum albumin level.

Pathophysiology

Albumin is synthesized in the liver from dietary amino acids. The normal half-life of serum albumin is about 7 to 10 days. Small amounts of albumin are normally lost in the urine and feces, but most albumin turnover is due to use in various metabolic processes such as tissue healing and repair. Albumin is not normally catabolized as a source of calories, but with chronic starvation, sepsis, trauma, and hepatic failure, albumin may be utilized for energy.

The primary functions of serum albumin are to maintain colloid osmotic pressure of plasma and serve as a carrier for various compounds, both endogenous (hormones, bilirubin, calcium, and others), and exogenous (drugs, toxins, and others). With significant hypoalbuminemia, there is a decrease in plasma colloid osmotic pressure and an increased tendency for the formation of edema and body cavity effusions. Serum albumin must be severely decreased (<0.8 g/dl) before hypoalbuminemia alone will cause fluid accumulation. However, less marked hypoalbuminemia may contribute to the formation of edema and effusions whenever other potential causes of edema are present (vascular damage, increased blood pressure, lymphatic blockage, and increased sodium and water retention).

Causes of hypoalbuminemia may be classified as being due to decreased production, increased loss, sequestration, and dilutional. It is helpful in the assessment of hypoalbuminemia to also consider the serum globulin level (Table 61-1).

Diagnostic Plan

History and Physical Examination

A variety of clinical disorders may cause hypoalbuminemia; therefore, the history and physical examination findings are variable. With severe hypoalbuminemia, evidence of peripheral edema, ascites, and pleural effusion may be observed. While it would be expected that peripheral edema would be diffuse and symmetric, this is not always the case. In the early stages of edema due to hypoalbuminemia, only one leg may be involved. The exact reasons for this

Table 61-1. Causes of Hypoalbuminemia

GLOBULIN DECREASED	GLOBULIN NORMAL OR INCREASED
DECREASED PRODUCTION	
	Chronic hepatic insufficiency
	Chronic starvation
INCREASED LOSS	
Protein-losing enteropathies	Renal loss
Hemorrhage	Glomerulonephritis
	Amyloidosis
SEQUESTRATION	
	Body cavity effusions
	Ascites
	Pleural effusion
	Vasculopathies
	Immune-mediated (lupus)
	Infectious
	Endotoxemia/bacteremia
	Rickettsial diseases (*Ehrlichia;* Rocky Mountain spotted fever)
DILUTIONAL	
Fluid therapy	

observation are not clear but may relate to other factors affecting circulation such as the effects of gravity on the dependent limb.

Laboratory Evaluation

Serum albumin is usually determined as a part of a biochemical profile that includes measurement of serum total protein. Globulin is then determined by subtracting the albumin concentration from the total protein concentration. Albumin and globulin should each be interpreted independently. The albumin/globulin ratio is of little or no value in the assessment of clinical disorders. Follow-up laboratory procedures will be determined by rule outs being considered after initial results are obtained.

Symptomatic Therapy

Effective symptomatic treatment of hypoalbuminemia is difficult unless the primary cause can be corrected. Diuretics such as furosemide can be used to reduce accumulated fluid (pleural effusion, ascites, and edema). Removal of large quantities of pleural or ascitic fluid by centesis should be avoided, unless the accumulated fluid is restricting respiration and causing dyspnea. Fluid removal will worsen the hypoalbuminemia.

Plasma transfusion can be tried in order to increase serum albumin. About 20 ml of plasma per kilogram of body weight is infused intravenously over 1 to 2 hours. Pretreatment with antihistamines is recommended to prevent plasma transfusion reactions (urticaria or facial swelling). Clinical experience indicates that serum albumin levels are increased only slightly by this procedure. It is possible that albumin loss continues at a rapid rate due to the uncorrected primary cause of hypoalbuminemia and that much larger amounts of plasma are actually needed. Unfortunately, it is difficult to maintain adequate supplies of canine plasma to use in most practice situations.

INCREASED SERUM ALBUMIN

Definition

An increased serum albumin is defined as an albumin concentration of greater than 3.8 g/dl.

Pathophysiology

See the section on Pathophysiology of Hypoalbuminemia above. The only recognized cause of hyperalbuminemia is dehydration. The serum globulin concentration will also be increased in dehydration (see Hyperglobulinemia).

Diagnostic Plan

See Hypoalbuminemia.

Symptomatic Therapy

It is not necessary to specifically treat an animal for increased serum albumin, but associated dehydration should be corrected with appropriate fluid therapy.

HYPOGLOBULINEMIA

Definition

Hypoglobulinemia is defined as a serum globulin concentration of less than 2.0 g/dl.

Pathophysiology

Most globulin is synthesized in plasma cells and lymphocytes as a part of the immunoglobulins, but the liver also makes globulin. The major functions of globulin are to act as antibodies in the humoral immune response and to bind certain compounds in the body, such as hormones, and aid in their transport through the bloodstream to their sites of action. With severe hypoglobulinemia, the animal may become more susceptible to various infections.

Causes of decreased serum globulin may be grouped into those due to decreased globulin production, increased globulin loss, or dilutional causes. One should always also consider the serum albumin in the assessment of the serum globulin concentration (Table 61-1).

Diagnostic Plan

History and Physical Examination

The history and physical examination findings associated with severe hypoglobulinemia, when present, are those that are the result of infection. Depression, fever, lymphadenopathy, and a variety of other signs may be observed.

Laboratory Evaluation

Serum globulin is usually determined indirectly by subtracting the serum albumin concentration from the total protein concentration. It is usually assessed as a part of a standard biochemical profile. Follow-up plans will be determined by the particular diagnoses being considered.

Symptomatic Therapy

Symptomatic treatment of hypoglobulinemia is seldom necessary. Concentrated globulin solutions are sometimes used to provide temporary increases in circulating antibodies for animals that have been exposed to infectious diseases.

HYPERGLOBULINEMIA

Definition

Hyperglobulinemia is defined as a serum globulin of greater than 3.8 g/dl.

Pathophysiology

Hyperglobulinemia may result from either increased globulin production or dehydration. Increased globulin production is usually the result of chronic antigenic stimulation such as may occur with chronic inflammatory conditions, either infectious or noninfectious, or neoplastic disorders associated with tissue necrosis. Some tumors involving cells of the humoral immune system (some lymphosarcomas and plasma cell myelomas) may also produce large amounts of globulin and cause hyperglobulinemia.

Diagnostic Plan

History and Physical Examination

A variety of disorders may be associated with increased globulin production, dehydration, or both; therefore, the history and physical examination findings are variable.

Laboratory Evaluation

See Hypoglobulinemia.

Symptomatic Therapy

Symptomatic treatment of hyperglobulinemia is generally not necessary. The etiology of the disorder causing the increased serum globulin should be determined and treated appropriately. If dehydration is present, fluid therapy may be necessary.

DECREASED SERUM ALANINE AMINOTRANSFERASE

There is no known significance of a decreased serum alanine aminotransferase (S-ALT) level.

INCREASED SERUM ALANINE AMINOTRANSFERASE

Definition

An increased S-ALT level is defined as an S-ALT above the normal species reference range for the particular laboratory procedure being used.

Pathophysiology

Increased serum activity of the commonly determined enzymes is due to either increased cellular release or increased cellular production.[8] ALT is located in the cytosol of hepatocytes and is released whenever there is hepatocellular membrane injury or hepatic necrosis. ALT is liver specific in dogs and cats. Other "release" enzymes, including aspartate aminotransferase (formerly glutamic-oxaloacetic transaminase [SGOT]) and lactate dehydrogenase (LDH), are found in other tissues besides liver and are not as useful for the evaluation of hepatic disease.

The magnitude of the increase in serum enzyme activity parallels the number of hepatocytes damaged but provides no information regarding the reversibility of the injury at the cellular level, the regenerative capacity on the tissue level, nor the status of function on the organ level.[8] Neither S-ALT nor serum alkaline phosphatase determinations (see below) are liver *function* tests.

The duration of increased serum enzyme activity depends not only on leakage from hepatocytes but also on the rate of plasma disappearance. Inactivation of plasma enzymes involves stereochemical denaturation and subsequent loss of the enzyme's catalytic capabilities. The plasma half-life of most enzymes is 2 to 4 days; however, the half-life of ALT injected into dogs is 2.5 hours. Renal excretion of hepatic enzymes is normally insignificant due to their large molecular size, which precludes glomerular filtration.

The magnitude of serum enzyme activity cannot be equated with reversibility of the hepatic injury. Any condition causing diffuse hepatocellular injury, such as hypoxia associated with shock, may result in markedly increased serum enzyme activity; however, all hepatocytes would be expected to recover. Organ function may remain near normal despite greatly increased serum enzyme values. On the other hand, hepatic failure may exist with normal serum enzyme levels. Causes of an increased S-ALT are listed in Figure 61-2.

Diagnostic Plan

History and Physical Examination

There are no historical or physical examination findings attributable to an increased S-ALT. However, signs of hepatic disease, such as icterus or ascites, are often associated with an increased S-ALT.

Laboratory Evaluation

S-ALT should be determined as part of a biochemical profile. The initial laboratory work-up should include a complete blood count (CBC) and urine analysis. Follow-up laboratory evaluation will be determined by the diagnoses being considered after assessment of the initial test results.

Symptomatic Therapy

Symptomatic treatment of an increased S-ALT is not necessary.

DECREASED SERUM ALKALINE PHOSPHATASE

There is no known significance to decreased serum alkaline phosphatase (SAP) activity.

INCREASED SERUM ALKALINE PHOSPHATASE

Definition

An increased SAP level is defined as an alkaline phosphatase above the normal species reference range for the particular laboratory procedure being used.

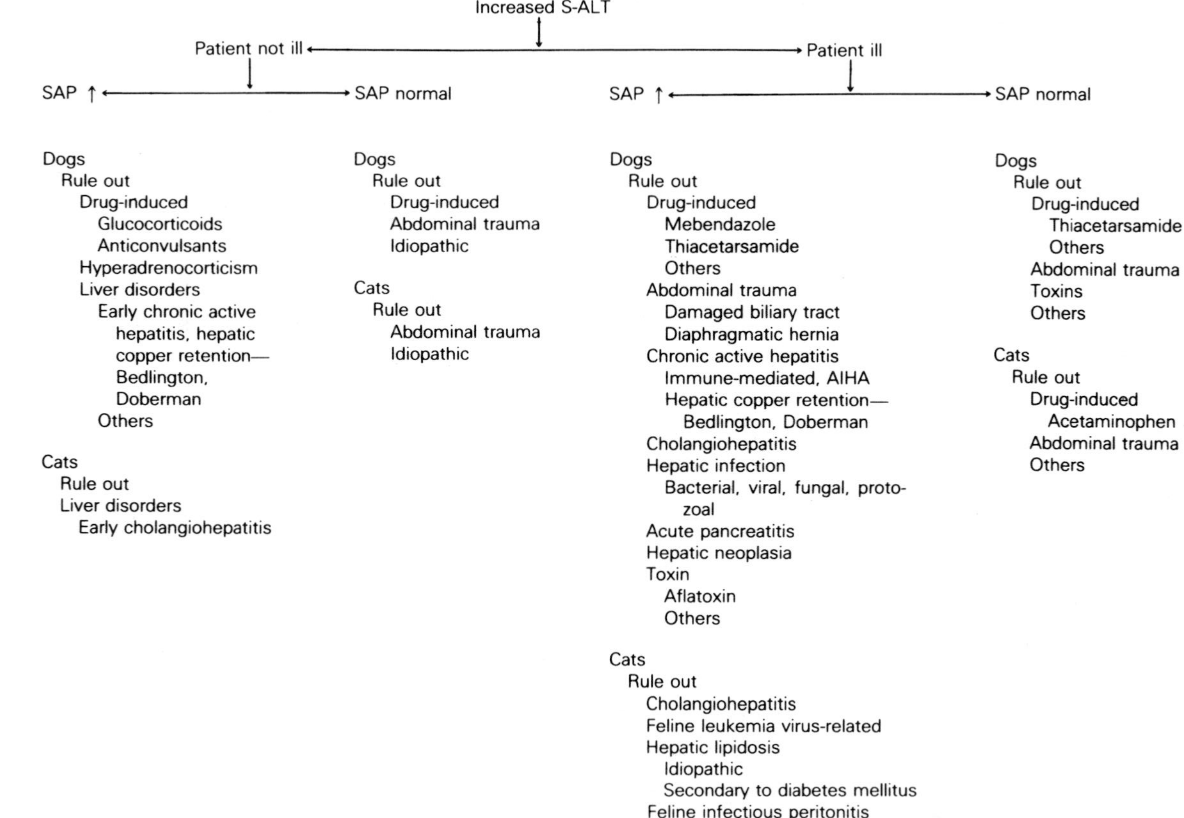

Fig. 61-2. Selected causes of increased S-ALT.

Pathophysiology

Certain enzymes can gain access to the extracellular fluid and blood without necrosis or damage to the membranes of the cells that produce the enzymes.[8] Alkaline phosphatase and gamma glutamyl transpeptidase (GGT) are two such enzymes. Significant increases in SAP are caused by increased cell production of alkaline phosphatase and not usually by cell injury or necrosis.

Total SAP activity is comprised of the action of all the isoenzymes of alkaline phosphatase. Tissues and cells known to produce these isoenzymes include osteoblasts, hepatocytes, biliary epithelial cells, intestine, placenta, and some neoplasms. Increased cellular production by any of these tissues may cause increased SAP activity.

Drug-induced increases must always be considered in the interpretation of serum enzyme activity. In dogs, excessive glucocorticoids are the most common cause of an increased SAP (Fig. 61-3 and Table 61-2). Although the precise mechanisms are unknown, it has been reported that glucocorticoids induce synthesis of an hepatic isoenzyme of alkaline phosphatase. Glucocorticoids cause accumulation of glycogen and water in hepatocytes, which may cause intrahepatic cholestasis, resulting in further induction of alkaline phosphatase synthesis (see below). Increased SAP activity is commonly observed following glucocorticoid therapy and in Cushing's syndrome (hyperadrenocorticism) in dogs. The duration of the glucocorticoid-induced increase in SAP is unpredictable, but it can take several months for the SAP to normalize. Cats are much more resistant to the hepatic effects of glucocorticoids, and there is usually no change in SAP following glucocorticoid treatment.

Cholestasis, either intrahepatic or extrahepatic, is associated with increased alkaline phosphatase production by biliary epithelial cells and hepatocytes. Although neither the mechanism nor the reason for the increased production is known, the result is an increased SAP activity. This increased activity may be detected prior to the onset and in the absence of hyperbilirubinemia. The magnitude of the increased SAP activity varies between 1.5 and 150 times normal. The magnitude of SAP increase in cats with cholestasis is less, probably due to the shorter half-life of feline SAP (Table 61-2). Normal feline SAP values are about

Table 61-2. Comparison of Causes of Increased Serum Alkaline Phosphatase

	MAGNITUDE OF INCREASE (× NORMAL)	
DISORDER	Dogs	Cats
Hypercortisolemia	1.5–200	Normal
Cholestasis	1.5–150	1.5–15
Anticonvulsants	1.5–5	Normal (?)
Bacteremia/endotoxemia	1.5–5	1.5–3
Osteoblastic activity	1.5–3	Normal
Neoplasia	Normal–100 (?)	Normal–10 (?)

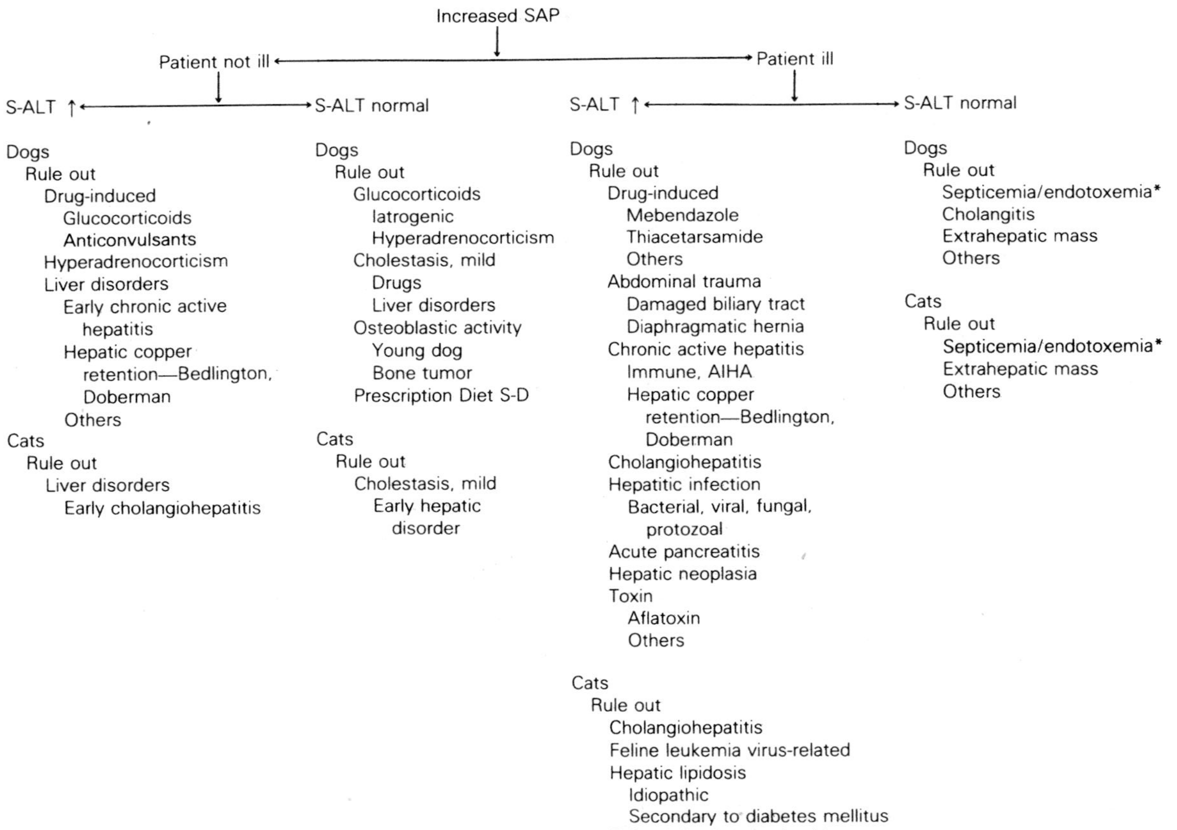

* Toxic neutrophils, thrombocytopenia, increased SAP, hypoalbuminemia, and hypoglycemia are often present.

Fig. 61-3. Selected causes of increased SAP.

one third of normal canine values; therefore, even minor increases in SAP in cats (1.5–2 times normal) are significant.

Some neoplasms reportedly may cause marked increases in SAP. In dogs, adrenal cortical adenocarcinomas, mixed mammary tumors, hemangiosarcomas, lymphomas, and oral carcinomas have been associated with increased SAP activity. Neoplasms are far more likely to cause an increased SAP when they involve the hepatobiliary system and cause cholestasis.

Increased osteoblastic activity and associated increases in SAP activity characterize normal bone growth of puppies as well as pathologic causes of increased osteoblastic activity such as canine panosteitis. The magnitude of the increase in SAP activity associated with either physiologic or pathologic increase in osteoblastic activity is usually moderate or on the order of 1.5 to 3.5 times normal SAP activity (Table 61-2).

Diagnostic Plan

History and Physical Examination

There are no historical or physical examination findings attributable to an increased SAP. However, a history of administration of glucocorticoids or anticonvulsants to dogs is often associated with an increased SAP. Evidence of cholestasis, such as icterus, often will be found in dogs and cats with an increased SAP.

Laboratory Evaluation

SAP should be determined as a part of a serum biochemical panel. In addition, a CBC and urine analysis will usually be helpful in the assessment of problems causing an increased SAP. Follow-up laboratory evaluation will be determined by the rule outs being considered after assessment of the initial data.

Symptomatic Therapy

Symptomatic therapy of an increased SAP is not necessary. The etiology should be determined and treated appropriately.

HYPOGLYCEMIA

Definition

Hypoglycemia is a decrease in blood glucose concentration below 70 mg/dl.

Pathophysiology

Blood glucose concentration is a net result of glucose production and utilization in the body. Sources of blood glucose are exogenous (food intake) and endogenous (glycogenolysis and gluconeogenesis). When food is not available, continuing tissue glucose utilization necessitates endogenous glucose production. The liver, under hormonal influences, is the fulcrum of glucose homeostasis (glycogenolysis and gluconeogenesis), although the kidneys may synthesize significant amounts of glucose (renal gluconeogenesis) during prolonged fasting.[12]

During fasting, glycogenolysis in the liver maintains blood glucose for about 24 hours, after which hepatic glycogen is depleted. Thereafter, body proteins (mainly muscle) are the main sources of endogenous glucose via hepatic and renal gluconeogenesis. Glycerol derived from body fat breakdown is also utilized for gluconeogenesis.[12]

Several hormones increase blood glucose by promoting gluconeogenesis or glycogenolysis or inhibiting cellular utilization of glucose. These include glucagon, glucocorticoids, catecholamines such as epinephrine, growth hormone, and progesterone. Insulin lowers blood glucose by inhibiting gluconeogenesis and causing uptake of glucose by insulin-dependent cells, primarily muscle and fat. Other cells, such as those in the central nervous system and kidneys, do not require insulin for glucose uptake.

Minute-to-minute regulation of blood glucose concentration is maintained quite efficiently by glucagon and insulin. Whenever blood glucose decreases, glucagon output from alpha cells in the pancreatic islets increases and insulin secretion from pancreatic beta cells is suppressed. Hyperglucagonemia promotes glycogenolysis, gluconeogenesis, or both, resulting in increased blood glucose, which in turn suppresses glucagon secretion and enhances insulin output.

Hypoglycemia can result from decreased glucose production or increased glucose utilization (Fig. 61-4). Decreased glucose production occurs because of decreased food intake or decreased endogenous glycogenolysis, gluconeogenesis, or both. Unlike people, normal dogs and cats do not become significantly hypoglycemic for days or weeks during fasting because of endogenous glucose production. This ability is probably necessary for survival in the wild, where food intake may not occur for many days. Exceptions are often encountered in puppies and toy breeds of dogs, in which hypoglycemia may occur within a few hours of fasting. Increased glucose utilization occurs *in vitro* (delay in separating erythrocytes from serum) or *in vivo* due to hyperinsulinemia or increased uptake of glucose by various tissues.

Diagnostic Plan

History and Physical Examination

The history and physical examination will help rule out certain causes of hypoglycemia (Table 61-3). Short-term (24 to 48 hours) fasting in puppies and toy breeds of dogs often results in hypoglycemia. Endogenous glucose production is inadequate for unknown reasons. Chronic starvation results in cachexia and malabsorption and is characterized by diarrhea, steatorrhea, and weight loss. Hypoglycemia may be observed. Hepatic insufficiency severe enough to cause hypoglycemia is usually accompanied by other signs of hepatic failure such as icterus, ascites, melena, and central nervous system (CNS) disturbances (hepatoencephalopathy). Polydipsia and polyuria are sometimes observed in

(Text continues on p 557.)

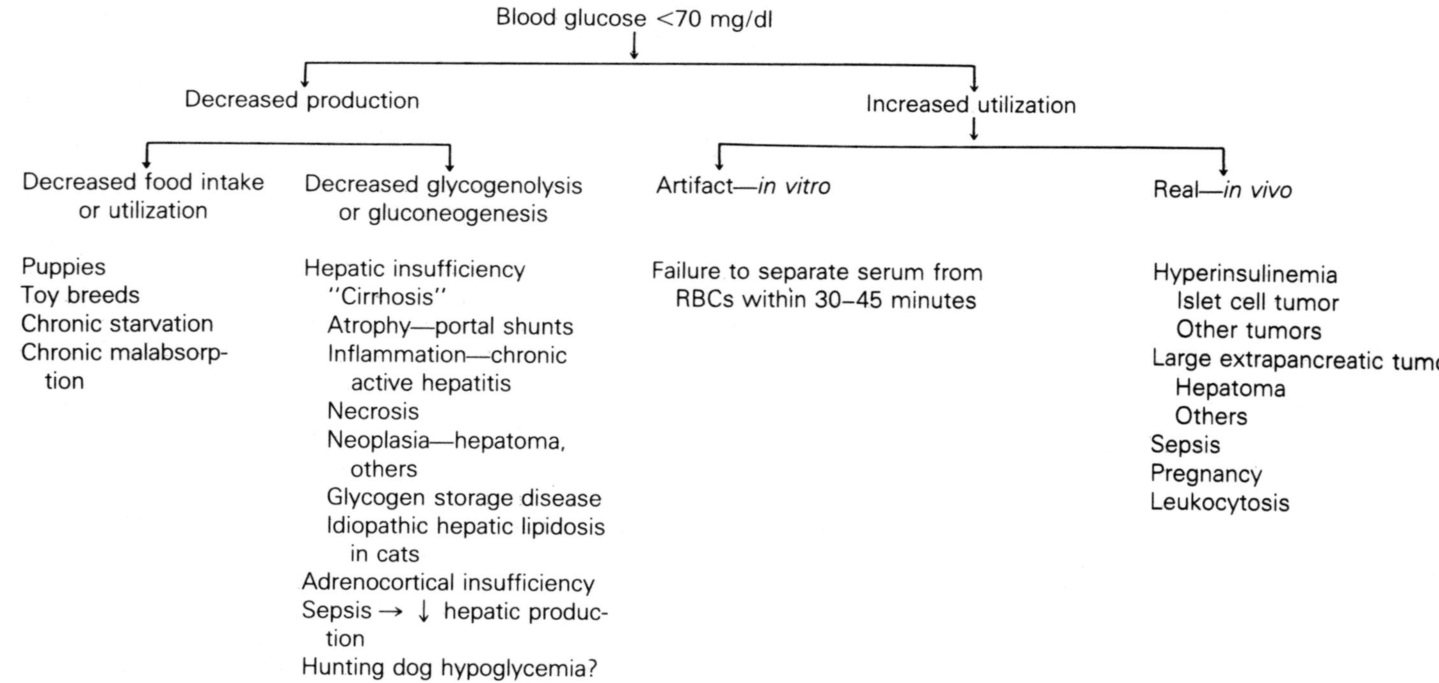

Fig. 61-4. Causes of hypoglycemia.

Table 61-3. Characteristic Findings of Common Disorders Causing Hypoglycemia

DISORDER	CLINICAL SIGNS OTHER THAN THOSE OF HYPOGLYCEMIA*	HEMATOLOGY	URINE ANALYSIS	BIOCHEMISTRY OTHER THAN HYPOGLYCEMIA	SPECIAL TESTS
Decreased production					
Decreased food intake or utilization					
Puppies	No other signs History of being off food >24–48 hr	Normal	Normal	Serum glucose <50 mg/dl	None; usually respond to intravenous glucose and feeding
Toy breeds	Same as for puppies	Normal	Normal	Serum glucose <50 mg/dl	Same as for puppies
Chronic starvation	Weight loss	Normal or mild nonregenerative anemia	Normal	$\downarrow$ Albumin ±	None; respond to feeding
Chronic malabsorption	Diarrhea Steatorrhea Cachexia	Mild to moderate nonregenerative anemia $\downarrow$ Plasma protein	Normal	$\downarrow$ Albumin $\downarrow$ Ca^{++}	See chronic small bowel diarrhea (chapter 33)
Decreased glycogenolysis/gluconeogenesis					
Hepatic insufficiency	Signs of hepatic failure Icterus Hepatoencephalopathy—stupor, coma, seizures, excessive salivation, head-pressing Ascites Melena Young dog or cat with hepatic atrophy due to congenital portal shunt Palpably enlarged liver with hepatic neoplasia	Anemia, regeneration variable Stomatocytosis ± $\uparrow$ Target cells in portal shunt cases $\downarrow$ Plasma protein WBC variable	Hyposthenuria ± Ammonium biurate crystals ±	$\downarrow$ Albumin $\uparrow$ Globulin ± $\downarrow$ BUN ± Serum glucose <70 mg/dl $\uparrow$ ALT and SAP ± $\uparrow$ Bilirubin ±	BSP retention $\uparrow$ Blood NH_3 $\uparrow$ or abnormal NH_3 tolerance Abnormal coagulogram ± Abnormal portal venography in portal shunt cases Abnormal liver biopsy
Adrenocortical insufficiency	Anorexia and lethargy Sporadic vomiting and diarrhea Bradycardia Dehydration Collapse—signs of shock	$\uparrow$ PCV and total protein Eosinophilia and lymphocytosis ±	Usually normal Sometimes $\downarrow$ specific gravity	$\uparrow$ Albumin and globulin (dehydration) Mild $\uparrow$ BUN $\downarrow$ Na, $\uparrow$ K (Na : K ratio <23)† $\downarrow$ TCO_2	ECG—signs of hyperkalemia Plasma cortisols—low baseline and little or no response to ACTH

(Continued)

Table 61-3. Characteristic Findings of Common Disorders Causing Hypoglycemia *(Continued)*

DISORDER	CLINICAL SIGNS OTHER THAN THOSE OF HYPOGLYCEMIA*	HEMATOLOGY	URINE ANALYSIS	BIOCHEMISTRY OTHER THAN HYPOGLYCEMIA	SPECIAL TESTS
Sepsis	Depression progressing to signs of shock Fever progressing to hypothermia Vomiting Diarrhea-melena	↑ PCV and plasma protein ± Neutrophilic leukocytosis with left shift progressing to leukopenia with inappropriate left shift Toxic neutrophils Thrombocytopenia	↑ Bilirubin ±	↓ Albumin ± (vasculitis → albumin leakage) ↑ Globulin ± ↑ SAP ± Mild ↑ bilirubin ±	Blood cultures × 3 at hourly intervals during febrile episode and when off antibiotics >48 hr
Large extra pancreatic tumors, *e.g.*, hepatoma	See section under Increased Utilization later in this table.				
Hunting dog hypoglycemia	Weakness and collapse during hunting	Normal	Normal	Normal; hypoglycemia difficult to document	None; usually responds to frequent high-protein feedings
Increased utilization					
Artifact—*in vitro*					
Failure to separate serum from RBCs within 30–45 minutes	No signs of hypoglycemia	Normal	Normal	Normal	Repeat biochemistry with proper handling of sample.
Real—*in vivo*					
Hyperinsulinemia; islet cell tumor	Mostly in dogs >7 yr old	Normal	Normal	Usually normal	High plasma insulin on a sample with a blood glucose <60
Large extrapancreatic tumors, *e.g.*, hepatoma	Mostly in dogs >7 yr old Decreased appetite Weight loss Sporadic vomiting and diarrhea Palpable inraabdominal mass Others depending on organ involved	Mild to moderate nonregenerative anemia WBC variable	Normal or Bilirubinuria	↓ Albumin ± ↑ Globulin ± ↑ ALT and SAP ± ↑ Bilirubin ±	BSP retention ↑ Blood NH_3 ↑ or abnormal NH_3 tolerance Abnormal liver biopsy: neoplasia
Sepsis	See section under Decreased Production earlier in this table.				

↓, decreased; ±, present or absent; ↑, increased; WBC, white blood cells; BUN, blood urea nitrogen; ALT, alanine aminotransferase; SAP, serum alkaline phosphatase; BSP, bromosulfophthalein; PCV, packed cell volume; TCO_2, total CO_2; ECG, electrocardiogram; ACTH, adrenocorticotropic hormone

* Common signs of hypoglycemia include weakness, ataxia, collapse, hypothermia, and seizures.

† In rare cases, only glucocorticoids are deficient and serum Na and K are normal.

both adrenocortical insufficiency and hepatic failure. Whenever sepsis is the cause of hypoglycemia, other signs are generally obvious and may include depression, fever, "muddy" mucous membranes, "injected" sclera, dyspnea, and signs of shock. Extrapancreatic tumors causing hypoglycemia may be palpable and may cause other signs of organ dysfunction such as weight loss, vomiting, diarrhea, and icterus. Islet cell tumors are small and generally cause few signs other than intermittent weakness, collapse, or seizures associated with hypoglycemia. Signs may occur during fasting, after exercise, or occasionally from 2 to 8 hours after eating, due to excessive insulin output (insulin "overshoot") from the beta cell tumor.

Laboratory Evaluation

The laboratory work-up of a hypoglycemic dog or cat will depend on associated clinical signs. A hemogram, serum biochemical profile, and urine analysis are indicated for each animal. Follow-up diagnostic plans will depend on the assessment of results obtained (Table 61-3). In suspected cases of hyperinsulinism, plasma insulin concentration should be measured on a sample from which the blood glucose concentration is less than 60 mg/dl. In a normal patient with a low blood glucose, the plasma insulin will be decreased below the normal range, whereas in an animal with an insulin-secreting tumor, the plasma insulin will be high or, occasionally, in the high normal range. Plasma insulin should be determined in a laboratory where the procedure has been validated for dogs and cats.

Symptomatic Therapy

Decreased blood glucose concentration should stimulate output of counterregulatory hormones (glucagon, cortisol, epinephrine, and growth hormone) to stabilize blood glucose. With multiple episodes of acute hypoglycemia, or with chronic hypoglycemia, these counterresponse mechanisms may be exhausted and the blood glucose level will decrease markedly. The severity of clinical manifestations of hypoglycemia is better correlated with the rate of decline of blood glucose than with the blood glucose concentration itself. A rapid decline in blood glucose concentration is more likely to result in clinical signs of hypoglycemia than is a gradual decrease in blood glucose.

Many cells, including neurons in the brain, are dependent on glucose as an energy source for vital metabolic functions. Sustained hypoglycemic coma for more than a few hours (6 to 8 hours?) may cause irreversible brain damage. Other cells normally impermeable to glucose may take up glucose, thus preventing a significant increase in blood glucose following intravenous glucose administration and further depriving the brain of glucose. For these reasons, symptomatic therapy should be administered without delay whenever signs of hypoglycemia are observed.

Over the phone, owners are instructed to rub Karo syrup into the buccal mucosa and immediately seek veterinary care. Glucose is administered slowly intravenously as a 50% solution to effect (usually 1 to 2 g of glucose/kg). Intravenous dexamethasone (2 mg/kg) may also be given to animals having prolonged hypoglycemia to help increase blood glucose (increased gluconeogenesis), stabilize cell membranes injured as a result of hypoglycemia, and reduce cerebral edema. A favorable response to glucose infusion is usually observed within minutes. At that time, the animal should be fed a high-protein meal, unless otherwise contraindicated. Lack of a clinical response and little change in blood glucose concentration despite repeated administration of glucose intravenously suggest that irreversible changes have occurred and that the prognosis is extremely poor.

Efforts to establish a definitive diagnosis should proceed without delay. During the diagnostic work-up, the diet will depend on the suspected etiology of hypoglycemia. In suspected hyperinsulinemia caused by islet cell tumors, multiple daily feedings of a high-protein diet are recommended. Diazoxide can be used to help maintain blood glucose concentration. In most cases, surgical exploration is indicated to attempt tumor removal. With hepatic insufficiency, the composition of the diet depends on whether or not signs of hepatoencephalopathy are present. CNS signs suggestive of hepatoencephalopathy (stupor, coma, head-pressing, salivation, blindness, and seizures) necessitate a protein-restricted (1 g of protein/20 calories/day), high-carbohydrate diet. The protein source should be high in biologic value (*e.g.*, eggs and cottage cheese) and include proteins with a high branched-chain to aromatic amino acid ratio (*e.g.*, milk proteins). Meat proteins should be avoided. If no abnormal CNS signs are present, a high-quantity, good-quality protein diet is recommended to aid in hepatic regeneration.

HYPERGLYCEMIA

Definition

Hyperglycemia is an increase in blood glucose concentration above 120 mg/dl. Mild hyperglycemia is frequently observed in dogs and cats, probably due to the effects of fear and struggling during blood collection.

Pathophysiology

Normal regulation of blood glucose concentration was discussed in the section on hypoglycemia. Hyperglycemia results from similar pathophysiologic mechanisms as were discussed for hypoglycemia, except in reverse (*i.e.*, increased glucose production or decreased glucose utilization) (Fig. 61-5).

Diagnostic Plan

Blood glucose levels should always be evaluated on blood samples obtained after a 12-hour fast. Although the blood glucose concentration after a meal should not exceed the renal threshold value (about 180 mg/dl) in a normal animal, postprandial hyperlipemia (due to circulating chylomicrons) may cause a signifi-

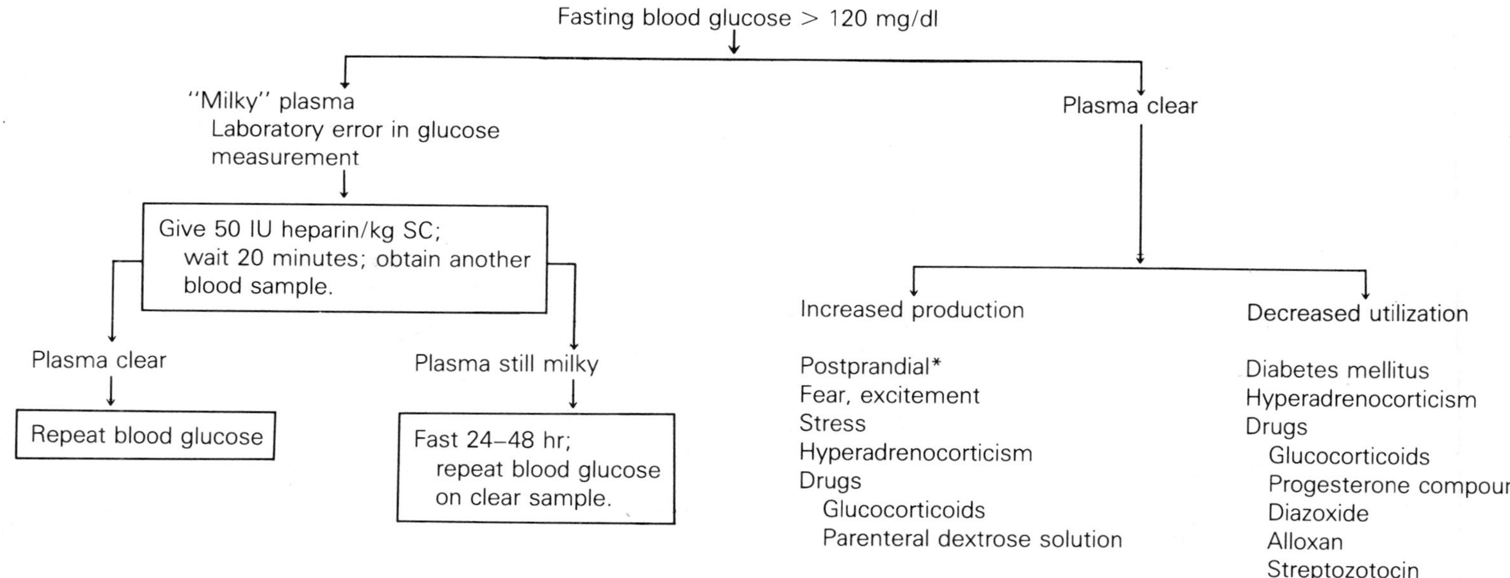

* Blood glucose does not exceed renal threshold in normal animal.

Fig. 61-5. Causes of hyperglycemia.

cant error in some laboratory methods of measuring blood glucose, resulting in markedly increased glucose readings. If it is necessary to measure blood glucose from an animal with lipemia, subcutaneous administration of heparin (50 IU/kg) will sometimes cause clearing of lipemia in about 20 minutes (by activating lipoprotein lipase, which breaks down chylomicrons). Some dogs, especially miniature schnauzers, may require 24 to 96 hours of fasting to clear chylomicronemia.

History and Physical Examination

The most common causes of mild to moderate hyperglycemia in dogs and cats are fear, excitement, and struggling associated with blood sample procurement and stress caused by a variety of medical and surgical disorders (Table 61-4). Fear and excitement cause catecholamine release, which results in hepatic glycogenolysis. Stress causes glucocorticoid secretion by the adrenal glands, which results in hepatic gluconeogenesis. Effects of stress on blood glucose are more dramatic in cats than in dogs. Blood glucose values from stressed cats may be as high as 300 mg/dl and be associated with moderate to marked glucosuria. In dogs, stress hyperglycemia seldom exceeds 150 mg/dl, and glucosuria is not present. History is usually sufficient to rule out these causes of hyperglycemia. It may be more difficult to decide whether marked hyperglycemia and glucosuria in a cat are due to stress or diabetes mellitus. Ketonuria may be present in either condition. Diabetes mellitus usually occurs in obese or formerly obese cats with a history of marked polydipsia and polyuria. Similar signs are usually present in diabetic dogs. Concurrent disorders in a diabetic patient may cause other signs such as anorexia, depression, vomiting, and diarrhea. In diabetic dogs, acute pancreatitis, hyperadrenocorticism, ketoacidosis, and various infections are common. Ketoacidosis, hepatic insufficiency due to hepatic lipidosis, and infection are common in diabetic cats.

Hyperadrenocorticism (canine Cushing's syndrome), either naturally occurring or iatrogenic, may cause mild hyperglycemia due to glucocorticoid-induced gluconeogenesis and inhibition of insulin action. Other signs of Cushing's syndrome, such as polydipsia, polyuria, alopecia, thin skin, abdominal distention, and hepatomegaly, may be present. Signs of hyperadrenocorticism may be easily overlooked in a diabetic dog. Large amounts of insulin (>2.0 units/kg) may be necessary to normalize blood glucose in a diabetic with concurrent Cushing's syndrome, and blood glucose values may fluctuate markedly from day to day, even though insulin dosage, diet, and exercise are kept reasonably constant. Plasma cortisol values before and after adrenocorticotropic hormone (ACTH) stimulation and dexamethasone suppression are necessary to diagnose hyperadrenocorticism.

Laboratory Evaluation

The laboratory evaluation of a dog or cat with hyperglycemia will depend on associated clinical signs. A hemogram, serum biochemical profile, and urine analysis are usually indicated. Follow-up diagnostic plans will depend upon the assessment of results obtained. It is seldom necessary to do glucose tolerance testing to evaluate hyperglycemia in dogs and cats. Patients with diabetes mellitus usually have a blood glucose concentration greater than 250 mg/dl. With lesser degrees of hyperglycemia (blood glucose of 120 to 200 mg/dl), the cause of the increased blood glucose concentration can usually be determined without glucose tolerance testing.

Symptomatic Therapy

It is not usually necessary to treat hyperglycemia symptomatically except in the specific instance of diabetes mellitus. Insulin therapy is necessary in the management of diabetic dogs and cats.

HYPONATREMIA

Definition

Hyponatremia, defined as a decrease in serum sodium concentration below 141 mEq/liter, may occur with an increased, decreased, or normal extracellular fluid volume.

Pathophysiology

Sodium salts are primarily responsible for the osmolality of extracellular fluid and are the major determinants of extracellular fluid volume and distribution of water between extracellular and intracellular fluid.[12] Signs associated with deficit and excess states of sodium reflect its role in the regulation of extracellular fluid volume. Cell membranes are relatively impermeable to sodium but are freely permeable to water. Sodium ions that gain access to the cell interior are actively extruded back into the extracellular fluid by energy-requiring enzymatic "pumps" in the cell membrane. The sodium pump is coupled with potassium ions, and as sodium is extruded from cells, potassium is "pumped" into cells.[1] Potassium salts are mainly responsible for intracellular osmotic pressure. Since water rapidly equilibrates between extracellular and intracellular fluid, osmotic concentrations of both these major fluids is always the same.

Thirst receptors in the hypothalamus respond to increases in plasma osmolality to initiate water consumption, thereby helping maintain body water. Supraoptic nuclei in the hypothalamus respond to increased plasma osmolality to cause secretion of antidiuretic hormone (ADH) from the posterior pituitary. ADH increases the permeability to water of the collecting ducts in the kidneys, causing reabsorption of water.

Sodium balance is closely regulated and maintained within narrow limits despite large variations in dietary intake of sodium. Although sodium is excreted from both the gastrointestinal tract and kidneys, day-to-day regulation of sodium balance occurs primarily in the renal tubules. Several factors influence handling of sodium by the kidneys, including aldosterone secretion by the adre-

(Text continues on p 564.)

Table 61-4. Characteristic Findings of Common Disorders Causing Hyperglycemia

DISORDER	CLINICAL SIGNS	HEMATOLOGY	URINE ANALYSIS	BIOCHEMISTRY OTHER THAN HYPERGLYCEMIA	SPECIAL TESTS
Artifact					
Hyperlipemia	Usually normal or Obesity Abdominal pain, vomiting ± (acute pancreatitis) Seizures?	Hemolysis and lipemia of sample ↑ Plasma protein by refractometry (artifactual) Neutrophilic leukocytosis with left shift ± (acute pancreatitis)	Normal	May interfere with other tests: consult clinical pathology text ↑ Serum lipase ±, mild hypocalcemia ± (acute pancreatitis)	Usually none Serum triglyceride and lipoprotein electrophoresis, if available
Increased production					
Postprandial	Normal	Mild to marked lipemia ↑ Plasma protein by refractometry (artifactual)	Normal	Lipemia may interfere with other tests: consult clinical pathology text	None
Fear, excitement, stress	Fear, nervousness, struggling during blood sampling Other signs associated with a variety of diseases leading to stress	Stress leukogram	Normal	↓ TCO_2 ± (↑ lactic acid due to struggling)	None
Hyperadrenocorticism	Polydipsia and polyuria Alopecia Thin skin "Pot-belly" Hepatomegaly Others	Stress leukogram	↓ Specific gravity Bacteriuria ±	↑ SAP ↑ ALT	Plasma cortisols before and after ACTH stimulation and dexamethasone suppression

Drugs					
Glucocorticoids	See Hyperadrenocorticism.				
Parenteral dextrose solutions	Usually normal Polyuria ±	Normal	Glucosuria	Normal	Normal
Decreased utilization					
Diabetes mellitus	Polydipsia and polyuria Obesity or weight loss Hepatomegaly Cataracts ± Others depending on complications Vomiting Abdominal pain Coma Others	Variable depending on complications	Glucosuria Ketonuria ± ↑ WBC and bacteriuria ±	Variable depending on complications	None for diabetes mellitus Depends on complications
Drugs					
Progesterone-like compounds (megesterol acetate [Ovaban, Megase], medroxyprogesterone acetate [Depo-Provera])	See Diabetes mellitus.				
Others (diazoxide, alloxan, streptozotocin)	See Diabetes mellitus.				
Diestrus—progesterone	Older unspayed female dogs See Diabetes mellitus.	See Diabetes mellitus.			

±, present or absent; ↑, increased; ↓, decreased; TCO_2, total CO_2; SAP, serum alkaline phosphatase; ALT, alanine aminotransferase; ACTH, adrenocorticotropic hormone; WBC, white blood cells

nal cortex. Decreased plasma sodium concentration causes decreased blood volume and blood flow to the kidneys. Renin is secreted by the renal juxtaglomerular cells, which stimulates aldosterone release. Aldosterone causes sodium and water reabsorption and potassium excretion in the renal tubules. The opposite changes occur whenever sodium intake is increased.

Hyponatremia can be due to decreased intake or increased excretion of sodium, as well as overhydration (Table 61-5). It is unusual for decreased sodium intake alone to cause hyponatremia, because of the ability of the kidneys to reabsorb sodium so completely and to excrete free water. Hyponatremia is commonly due to combinations of the above mechanisms.[11]

Any decrease in plasma sodium concentration following sodium loss is initially corrected by inhibition of both thirst and ADH secretion. Initially, plasma sodium concentration is preserved—but at the expense of extracellular fluid volume. With progressive sodium loss, extracellular fluid volume contracts and, at a critical point, vascular volume receptors stimulate ADH production and thirst, causing a gain in water and a decrease in plasma sodium concentration. Thus, sodium loss may be characterized by signs of volume depletion (decreased skin pliability, weak pulse, or shock) and, unless sodium loss is abrupt, by hyponatremia.

On the other hand, hyponatremia is associated frequently with sodium gain and relative water excess.[11] This occurs most commonly with conditions characterized by a decrease in effective circulating blood volume such as congestive heart failure and hypoalbuminemic disorders (*e.g.*, cirrhosis and nephrotic syndrome). The kidneys respond to decreased perfusion by secreting renin, which causes aldosterone secretion, resulting in retention of sodium and water. Hyponatremia is worsened by stimulation of thirst and ADH output, due to low effective circulating blood volume. Thus, hyponatremia may reflect sodium loss or sodium gain with water excess.

Pseudohyponatremia may occur due to the presence of hyperlipemia or marked hyperproteinemia. Excessive lipids or proteins cause hyponatremia because sodium is present only in the water portion of plasma; the laboratory measurement is done on the lipid, protein, and water phases.

Osmotically active substances such as glucose and mannitol in plasma attract water from cells into the extracellular fluid, resulting in dilution of plasma sodium. Despite the fall in serum sodium concentration, plasma osmolality is normal or slightly increased.

Diagnostic Plan

It is helpful to categorize causes of hyponatremia into five general areas: (1) factitious, (2) redistribution of body water, (3) dehydrated, (4) overhydrated, and (5) normally hydrated.

History and Physical Examination

A history of administration of glucose solution or a history of disorders causing dehydration (*e.g.*, anorexia, vomiting, or diarrhea) may help initially

(Text continues on p 568.)

Table 61-5. Characteristic Findings of Common Disorders Causing Hyponatremia

DISORDER	CLINICAL SIGNS	HEMATOLOGY	URINE ANALYSIS	BIOCHEMISTRY OTHER THAN HYPONATREMIA	SPECIAL TESTS
Artifact					
Hyperlipemia	Usually normal Signs of acute pancreatitis ± Seizures?	Lipemia Hemolysis ± Inflammatory leukogram ±	Normal	Usually normal ↑ Amylase and lipase ±	None
Redistribution of fluid into extracellular compartment					
Hyperglycemia	See Table 61-4.				
Hyperproteinemia	Dehydration Depression Other CNS signs and hemorrhagic tendencies associated with hyperviscosity	Nonregenerative anemia ± Malignant cells in circulation ± (multiple myeloma)	Proteinuria ± in myeloma	↑ Albumin and globulin Others depending on site of tumor involvement	Skeletal radiographs for myeloma Others depending on sites of tumor involvement
Dehydration					
Vomiting, diarrhea	See chapters 32 and 33.				
Adrenocortical insufficiency	Anorexia and lethargy Sporadic vomiting and diarrhea Bradycardia Dehydration Collapse—signs of shock	↑ PCV and plasma protein ± Eosinophilia and lymphocytosis ±	Usually normal—sometimes ↓ specific gravity	↑ Albumin and globulin (dehydration) Mildly ↑ BUN ↓ Na, ↑ K (Na : K ratio <23) ↓ TCO_2	ECG—signs of hyperkalemia See Table 61-10. Plasma, cortisols—low baseline and little or no response to ACTH
Renal loss of Na					
Diuretic use	Polydipsia/polyuria Dehydration	↑ PCV and plasma protein	Low specific gravity	↑ Albumin and globulin ↑ BUN (prerenal) ↓ Na and K	High urine Na
Renal failure	Polydipsia/polyuria Dehydration Vomiting Depression	Variable	Low urine specific gravity Rest of urine analysis variable	↑ BUN ↑ P Rest of biochemistry variable	Abdominal radiographs or ultrasound Rest of work-up variable, including renal biopsy

Table 61-5. Characteristic Findings of Common Disorders Causing Hyponatremia *(Continued)*

DISORDER	CLINICAL SIGNS	HEMATOLOGY	URINE ANALYSIS	BIOCHEMISTRY OTHER THAN HYPONATREMIA	SPECIAL TESTS
Overhydration					
Congestive heart failure	Coughing Dyspnea Cyanosis Ascites-modified transudate Peripheral edema—rare Tachycardia Heart murmur	Normal	Normal	Normal or Mildly ↑ ALT and SAP	Thoracic radiographs ECG Low urine Na
"Cirrhosis"	Ascites—transudate Icterus CNS signs (hepatoencephalopathy) Stupor Coma Head-pressing Others Melena Vomiting Polydipsia/polyuria Hemorrhagic tendencies	Anemia—regeneration variable Stomatocytosis ± ↓ Plasma protein WBC variable ↓ Platelets ±	Hyposthenuria ±	↓ Albumin ↑ Globulin ± ↓ BUN ± Mildly ↑ ALT and SAP ↓ Glucose ± ↑ Bilirubin ±	↑ BSP retention ↑ Blood NH_3 or abnormal ammonia tolerance Abnormal coagulogram ± Small liver on abdominal radiographs Low urine Na Abnormal liver biopsy
Nephrotic syndrome	Ascites Peripheral edema Lethargy Signs of renal failure ± Anorexia and vomiting Polyuria/polydipsia Others Hypercoagulation tendencies with thromboses Dyspnea, coughing (pulmonary thrombosis) Others	Nonregenerative anemia ±	↓ Specific gravity ± Proteinuria	↓ Albumin ↑ Cholesterol ↑ BUN ±	Quantitate urine protein (24-hr collection) Coagulogram Abdominal radiographs Renal biopsy

Iatrogenic water-loading (5% dextrose therapy), especially for oliguric renal failure	Polyuria or Oliguria with renal failure	↓ PCV and plasma protein	Decreased specific gravity Glucosuria except in oliguric renal failure	↓ Albumin and globulin Slightly ↑ blood glucose ↑ BUN, ↑ K in oliguric renal failure	Abdominal radiographs—renal size
Compulsive water drinking	Polydipsia/polyuria	Normal or ↓ PCV and plasma protein ±	Hyposthenuria	Normal or ↓ Albumin and globulin	Water deprivation test; urine specific gravity >1.035 Low urine Na
Inappropriate ADH secretion	Signs of water intoxication—CNS Depression Weakness Confusion Focal, neurologic signs Convulsions Coma Signs of primary disease (example: heartworms) Coughing Dyspnea Exercise intolerance Others	Normal or Changes due to the primary disease	Inappropriately hypertonic—see Special Tests	Normal or Changes due to the primary disease	Urine osmolality may exceed serum osmolality Water intake $>$ urine output High urine Na Normal plasma cortisols pre and post ACTH Water restriction and normal sodium diet correct hyponatremia

±, present or absent; ↑, increased; CNS, central nervous system; ↓, decreased; BUN, blood urea nitrogen; TCO_2, total CO_2; ECG, electrocardiogram; ACTH, adrenocorticotropic hormone; PCV, packed cell volume; ALT, alanine aminotransferase; SAP, serum alkaline phosphatase; WBC, white blood cells; BSP, bromosulfophthalein

categorize hyponatremia. Dehydration is usually associated with decreased skin pliability, dry mucous membranes, and decreased capillary refilling time (Table 61-6). Hyponatremic dehydration predisposes to early, severe vascular volume depletion and vascular collapse (shock). Overhydration may be difficult to distinguish clinically from normal hydration. Generalized edema and ascites are sometimes present (Table 61-6). Signs of water intoxication may be observed (CNS signs such as depression, weakness, confusion, focal neurologic signs, convulsions, and coma). Other signs depend on the specific disorder causing hyponatremia.

Laboratory Evaluation

Serum sodium levels should be evaluated on blood samples obtained after a 12-hour fast, because hyperlipemia may cause pseudohyponatremia. The initial laboratory work-up of a dog or cat with hyponatremia should include a hemogram, microfilariae check, biochemical profile, and urine analysis. Dehydration frequently causes increased packed cell volume (PCV), total plasma protein, urine specific gravity, and sometimes BUN (prerenal). Depending on initial laboratory results, follow-up diagnostic procedures will vary (Table 61-5). Measurement of urine sodium concentration sometimes helps differentiate causes of hyponatremia. Plasma aldosterone determination may be warranted in more difficult cases.

Symptomatic Therapy

Before initiating symptomatic treatment for hyponatremia, one must determine whether the patient is dehydrated, overhydrated, or euhydrated (Tables 61-5 and 61-6), because appropriate treatment is different.

Hyponatremia With Dehydration

The initial treatment of hyponatremia associated with dehydration is rehydration with a fluid containing sodium in a similar concentration as normal plasma. Isotonic (0.9%) sodium chloride solution or lactated Ringer's solution

Table 61-6. Helpful Signs in the Assessment of Hyponatremia

ASSESSMENT	DEHYDRATION	OVERHYDRATION
Skin pliability	Decreased	Normal
Peripheral edema or ascites	Absent	Present
Capillary refilling time	Prolonged	Normal
Peripheral veins	Normal or collapsed	Normal or distended
Others	Tachycardia and weak pulse	Signs of congestive heart failure Pulmonary edema Ascites

with added sodium bicarbonate may be used. The cause of the hyponatremic dehydration should be appropriately treated.

Hyponatremia With Overhydration

The treatment of hyponatremia associated with overhydration depends on the cause. Water restriction is indicated for all animals in this category. Restriction of sodium is warranted in those disorders characterized by excessive sodium retention (congestive heart failure, "cirrhosis," or nephrotic syndrome). The syndrome of inappropriate ADH secretion is characterized by water overload and renal sodium excretion; therefore, sodium chloride should be added to the diet while water is restricted. In hypoalbuminemic disorders, attempts should be made to minimize albumin loss and stimulate albumin synthesis (with a high-quality protein diet). If congestive heart failure or hypoalbuminemia cannot be corrected, correction of the serum sodium concentration will have little effect on the long-term clinical course of the patient.

Hyponatremia With Normal Hydration

Human patients with a variety of chronic debilitating diseases reportedly have hyponatremia due to resetting of the hypothalamic osmostat. No adverse signs are noted and the hyponatremia is reversible with correction of the primary disorder. This form of hyponatremia has not been reported in dogs and cats.

HYPERNATREMIA

Definition

Hypernatremia is defined as an increase in serum sodium above 155 mEq/liter.

Pathophysiology

As was discussed in the section on hyponatremia, sodium salts are primarily responsible for tonicity of extracellular fluid.[12] Therefore, hypertonicity may result from absolute or relative excess of sodium (as well as glucose). Urea freely diffuses across cell membranes and does not contribute to effective plasma osmotic pressure (tonicity), although it does affect measured osmolality. Effective plasma osmolality can be estimated from the following formula:

$$\text{Effective plasma osmolality} = 2(\text{Na} + \text{K}) + \frac{\text{Glucose}}{18}$$

Signs of CNS depression or coma may be observed when effective plasma osmolality is greater than 375 mOsm/liter.

Theoretically, hypernatremia can occur as the result of excessive sodium intake, with or without excessive water loss, inadequate water intake, excessive water loss (usually with inadequate water intake), and losses of both water and sodium, with water loss predominating (Fig. 61-6 and Table 61-7).

Diagnostic Plan

Causes of hypernatremia are shown in Figure 61-6 and Table 61-7. It is very important to assess whether or not dehydration is present (as indicated by decreased skin pliability, dry mucous membranes, increased urine specific gravity, and increased BUN).

History and Physical Examination

Most patients with hypernatremia will also be dehydrated. Therefore, a careful history regarding water intake and conditions causing fluid loss (*e.g.*, vomiting, diarrhea, or polyuria) is warranted. Severe hypernatremia causes hypertonicity of extracellular fluid, which causes transfer of water out of brain cells (CNS desiccation). Severe weakness, depression, coma (hyperosmolal syndrome) and seizures may be observed.[11] Other signs depend on the primary disorder present (Table 61-7). Severe hyperthermia and excessive panting typify heat stroke. A history of polydipsia and polyuria is usually present with diabetes insipidus and renal failure. Signs of uremia, including anorexia and vomiting, may also be present in patients with renal failure.

Laboratory Evaluation

The laboratory work-up for hypernatremia is similar to that previously discussed for hyponatremia.

Symptomatic Therapy

Appropriate treatment for hypernatremia depends on the presence or absence of dehydration.

Hypernatremia due to Excessive Sodium Intake

If hypernatremia resulted from excessive sodium intake (little or no dehydration), cessation of sodium intake should suffice if cardiovascular and renal functions are intact. Providing water for drinking in gradually increasing quantities over a 4- to 6-hour period is indicated.

Hypernatremia Associated With Dehydration

Appropriate therapy for hypernatremic dehydration depends on the severity of hypernatremia and the underlying disorder. If too little water has been provided or the animal has been too debilitated to drink, simply making sure the patient drinks water may be adequate. In the rare case of a defective CNS thirst center, adding water to the patient's food is necessary.[2,6]

(Text continues on p 575.)

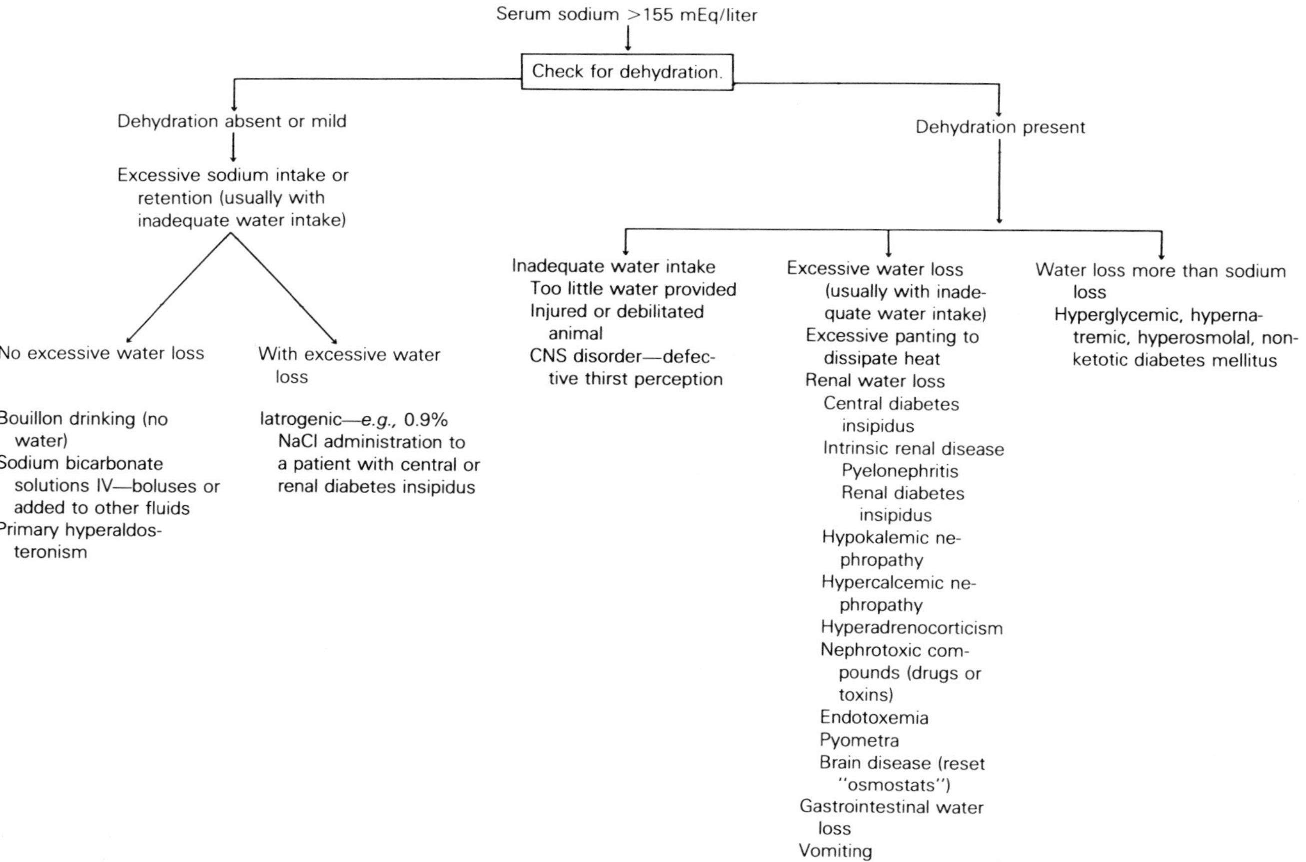

Fig. 61-6. Causes of hypernatremia.

Table 61-7. Characteristic Findings of Common Disorders Causing Hypernatremia

DISORDER	CLINICAL SIGNS	HEMATOLOGY	URINE ANALYSIS	BIOCHEMISTRY OTHER THAN HYPERNATREMIA	SPECIAL TESTS
Excessive sodium intake					
No excessive H_2O loss					
Bouillon drinking (no water)	CNS Depression Confusion Weakness Seizures Coma Mild dehydration	Mild ↑ PCV and total protein	Specific gravity >1.040	Mild ↑ albumin and globulin ↑ Cl	Urine Na ↑
Sodium bicarbonate solutions IV	See Bouillion drinking (above).	Normal	Normal or Urine pH >7.5	↑ TCO_2	Urine Na ↑
Primary hyperaldosteronism	See Bouillon drinking (above).	Variable	Variable	↓ K ↑ Cl ↑ TCO_2	↓ Urine Na ↑ Plasma aldosterone
With excessive water loss					
Iatrogenic, *e.g.*, 0.9% NaCl administration to a patient with central or renal diabetes insipidus	Same as in No excessive H_2O loss (above)	Same as in No excessive H_2O loss (above)	Specific gravity >1.030	Same as in No excessive H_2O loss (above)	Urine Na normal to slightly ↑
Inadequate H_2O intake					
Too little water provided	Dehydration Thirst Later—depression, weakness	↑ PCV and total protein	Specific gravity >1.040	↑ Albumin and globulin ↑ Cl	Urine Na ↓
Injured or debilitated animal	Same as above and Signs of the primary injury or illness	Variable depending on injury or illness	Same as above	Variable	Urine Na ↓
CNS disorder—defective thirst perception	Depression, lethargy Decreased water intake Dehydration	Same as above	Same as in above	Same as above	Urine osmolality: plasma osmolality ratio >4 No change in urine osmolality after ADH administration

Excessive water loss with inadequate water intake					
Increased insensible losses					
Excessive panting	Excessive panting to dissipate heat ↑ Body temperature ↑ Thirst Signs of heat stroke ±	↑ PCV and total protein Stress leukogram ±	Specific gravity >1.040	↑ Albumin and globulin Others if heat stroke is present	None
Renal H_2O loss					
Central diabetes insipidus	Polyuria/polydipsia Rapid dehydration when water is denied Signs of hypertonicity when water is denied Depression, lethargy Weakness Stupor, coma, death	Normal or ↑ PCV and total protein	Specific gravity <1.005	Normal or ↑ Albumin and globulin ↑ Cl	Water deprivation test → little change in urine specific gravity ADH response test → urine specific gravity >1.030 Urine Na ↓
Intrinsic renal disease					
Pyelonephritis	Lethargy, depression Fever ± Abdominal pain Vomiting ±	Normal or Neutrophilic leukocytosis with left shift	↓ Urine specific gravity Pyuria and bacteriuria Hematuria, proteinuria, casts ±	BUN ↑ ± If septic: ↓ Albumin ↑ SAP ↓ Glucose	Urine culture Excretory urogram Renal biopsy
Renal diabetes insipidus	See Central diabetes insipidus. Signs of renal failure ±	Variable	Specific gravity <1.012	BUN ↑ ±	Water deprivation test → little change in urine specific gravity ADH response test → little change in urine specific gravity
Hypokalemic nephropathy	Polyuria/polydipsia Weakness Ileus ± Dehydration ±	Mild ↑ PCV and total protein ±	↓ Urine specific gravity	K <3.7 Others depending on cause of ↓ K	None
Hypercalcemic nephropathy	Polydipsia/polyuria Signs of renal failure ± Others variable	Variable	↓ Urine specific gravity	↑ BUN ± ↑ Ca Others variable	Variable depending on suspected cause
Hyperadrenocorticism	Polydipsia/polyuria Thin skin Bilaterally symmetric alopecia	Stress leukogram	↓ Urine specific gravity Pyuria and bacteriuria ±	↑ SAP ↑ ALT ± ↓ K ± ↑ TCO_2 ±	Plasma, cortisol panel—ACTH stimulation and dexamethasone suppression

(Continued)

Table 61-7. Characteristic Findings of Common Disorders Causing Hypernatremia *(Continued)*

DISORDER	CLINICAL SIGNS	HEMATOLOGY	URINE ANALYSIS	BIOCHEMISTRY OTHER THAN HYPERNATREMIA	SPECIAL TESTS
Nephrotoxic drugs or toxins	Urine output variable Signs of renal failure ±	Variable	↓ Urine specific gravity Proteinuria ± Glucosuria ± Casts ±	↑ BUN Others variable	Usually none
Endotoxemia	Temperature variable Scleral injection Dehydration Signs of shock Others variable	WBC variable ↓ Platelets ±	↓ Urine specific gravity Others variable	↑ SAP ↓ Albumin ↓ Glucose	Blood cultures Others variable
Pyometra	Polydipsia/polyuria Enlarged uterus Vaginal discharge Depression and dehydration	Leukocytosis with neutrophilia and left shift Others variable	↓ Urine specific gravity Pyuria and bacteriuria ±	See Endotoxemia (above).	Abdominal radiographs
Gastrointestinal H_2O loss					
Vomiting	See chapter 32.				
Diarrhea	See chapter 33.				
Water loss more than sodium loss					
Hyperglycemic, hyperosmolal, nonketotic diabetes mellitus	Stupor or coma Dehydration Signs of shock History of polyuria and polydipsia	↑ PCV and total protein Stress leukogram	Glucosuria Specific gravity variable	↑ Albumin and globulin Marked hyperglycemia ↑ Cl Others depending on complications	Plasma osmolality >375 Others variable

CNS, central nervous system; ↑, increased; PCV, packed cell volume; IV, intravenously; TCO_2, total CO_2; ↓, decreased; ADH, antidiuretic hormone; ±, present or absent; BUN, blood urea nitrogen; SAP, serum alkaline phosphatase; ALT, alanine aminotransferase; ACTH, adrenocorticotropic hormone; WBC, white blood cells

If dehydration associated with hypernatremia is moderate to severe, parenteral fluid therapy is indicated. Whenever serum sodium is less than 180 mEq/liter and, especially whenever estimated effective plasma osmolality (2[Na + K] + [glucose/18]) is less than 375 mOsm/liter, correction of water loss can be accomplished with 5% dextrose solution administered intravenously over a 6- to 12-hour period. If electrolytes have been lost along with water (in various renal and gastrointestinal disorders), it is better to use a polyionic solution similar to plasma such as lactated Ringer's solution or half-strength lactated Ringer's solution with 2.5% dextrose.

In the management of severe hypernatremia (serum sodium >180 mEq/liter, estimated effective plasma osmolality >375 mOsm/liter), caution must be used in the rate of reduction of plasma osmotic pressure. Lowering serum sodium too rapidly can cause "rebound" cerebral edema, whereas reduction too slowly can cause death due to CNS dehydration. Clinical experience in dogs and cats with hypernatremia indicates that increased serum sodium is difficult to lower and that aggressive treatment is warranted. If dehydration is severe, treatment must first be directed at expanding the extracellular fluid volume and increasing blood pressure. This should be done by administering isotonic lactated Ringer's solution intravenously alone or with whole blood if the PCV is decreased. The rate of administration should be about 90 ml/kg/hr until capillary refilling time and pulse are improved. For correction of hypertonicity, either half-strength lactated Ringer's and 2.5% dextrose solution or 0.45% saline solution by a slow, intravenous drip should be used. Plasma osmolality should be steadily lowered over a 24- to 48-hour period. It is imperative that the animal's neurologic status be closely observed, that serum sodium and estimated plasma osmolality values be frequently determined (preferably every 6 hours), and that adjustments in therapy be made as needed. If a significant decrease in serum sodium is not observed within 6 hours and the animal's neurologic status does not improve, the intravenous fluid should be changed to either 2.5 or 5% dextrose solution and intravenous furosemide (1 to 2 mg/kg three or four times daily) should be administered. Spironolactone, an aldosterone-inhibiting diuretic, is sometimes more effective than furosemide in lowering the serum sodium concentration.

HYPOKALEMIA

Definition

Hypokalemia, as defined by a serum potassium concentration of less than 3.6 mEq/liter, may occur with an increased, normal, or decreased total body potassium.

Pathophysiology

Of the approximate 50 mEq of potassium per kilogram of body weight, almost 98% is located intracellularly at a concentration of about 150 mEq/liter. The remaining 2% that is in the extracellular fluid is closely maintained at a normal concentration of 3.6 to 5.6 mEq/liter. Thus, a large concentration gradient normally favors the transfer of potassium from cells into the extracellular fluid.[12] This situation is opposite to that which exists for sodium. The maintenance of high intracellular potassium and high extracellular sodium concentrations is accomplished with sodium-potassium "pumps" located in cell membranes (see Hyponatremia).

Maintenance of the normal high intracellular and low extracellular potassium concentration is critical. Cellular potassium depletion may cause abnormalities in many biologic processes, including cell volume; acid-base status; electrophysiologic properties of cells; and synthesis of RNA, protein, and glycogen.[9] Abnormal extracellular potassium concentration can cause derangements in acid-base status and electrophysiologic properties of cells.

The normal total body potassium content is determined by the balance between potassium intake and excretion (external potassium balance). Equally important is the distribution of potassium between extracellular and intracellular fluid (internal potassium balance).

External Potassium Balance

Daily ingestion of potassium in the diet equals or exceeds the amount of potassium in extracellular fluid. If potassium intake were not matched by excretion, fatal hyperkalemia would soon result. Since normal skin, salivary, and gastrointestinal potassium losses are minor, renal excretion of potassium is vital. Conversely, daily glomerular filtrate normally contains much more potassium than is present in extracellular fluid. Therefore, tubular reabsorption of potassium is critical to normal potassium balance. In health, the kidney efficiently maintains plasma potassium within a narrow range. However, in contrast to the kidney's ability to completely reabsorb sodium in hypovolemic conditions, small but significant amounts of potassium continue to be excreted despite severe extrarenal potassium depletion.

Factors known to affect renal handling of potassium include (1) potassium intake, (2) renal tubular cell potassium concentration, (3) delivery of sodium and fluid to the distal tubule, (4) anions accompanying sodium to the distal tubule, (5) mineralocorticoid (mainly aldosterone) effects, and (6) functional integrity of the distal tubular cells.[10] Increases in potassium intake, delivery of sodium and fluid to the distal tubule, and relatively impermeable anions (such as bicarbonate) accompanying sodium to the distal tubule all cause renal potassium excretion. Aldosterone is secreted in response to extracellular fluid volume reduction (increased adrenal output) and increased extracellular fluid potassium concentration. Aldosterone causes sodium reabsorption and potassium excretion in the distal tubules. The colon also responds to aldosterone by reabsorbing sodium and excreting potassium. Finally, distal tubular cell dysfunction can cause potassium retention, especially in oligoanuric renal failure. However, hyperkalemia is usually not observed in polyuric renal failure until the terminal stages of the disorder.

In disorders characterized by diarrhea or vomiting, potassium losses may be significant. With diarrhea, loss of large quantities of potassium in feces may occur. Gastric juice contains small amounts of potassium, but metabolic alkalosis and extracellular fluid volume depletion due to gastric juice hydrochloric acid loss induce loss of large amounts of potassium in the urine.

Internal Potassium Balance

Internal balance of potassium refers to the distribution of potassium between extracellular and intracellular fluid and is critically important in the control of plasma potassium concentration. As previously discussed, membrane-situated ion exchange pumps normally maintain extracellular-intracellular potassium distribution. When potassium intake temporarily exceeds renal excretory capacity, cellular potassium uptake prevents the accumulation of excess potassium in extracellular fluid. When renal or gastrointestinal potassium losses exceed potassium intake, transfer of potassium from cells into extracellular fluid helps delay hypokalemia.

The most important factors modifying distribution of potassium between extracellular and intracellular fluid are (1) cellular integrity, (2) hormonal effects (mainly insulin and aldosterone), and (3) acid–base status. Severe tissue trauma, such as in crush injuries, may cause significant cellular release of potassium and hyperkalemia. Good renal function generally prevents marked hyperkalemia in the latter condition.

Evidence suggests that plasma potassium concentration influences secretion of both insulin and aldosterone and that feedback control exists for both hormones.[5] It appears that these two hormones are released in response to a potassium-rich meal. Insulin promotes cellular uptake of potassium, and aldosterone causes renal potassium excretion, thereby preventing large diet-induced changes in plasma potassium concentration. Reduced plasma potassium inhibits insulin and aldosterone release, although other factors (*i.e.*, plasma glucose concentration and extracellular fluid volume) take precedence in determining insulin and aldosterone release.

Accumulation of hydrogen ions in extracellular fluid (acidosis) causes transfer of hydrogen ions from extracellular to intracellular fluid. To maintain electroneutrality, potassium ions shift from intracellular to extracellular fluid. Acidosis also favors renal retention of potassium ions because less bicarbonate is presented to the distal tubules (see External Potassium Balance); thus, acidosis increases serum potassium concentration. Hydrochloric and carbonic acids (as in respiratory acidosis), but not organic acids (*e.g.*, lactic acid and ketoacids), displace potassium ions from cells, thereby causing hyperkalemia. Hypokalemia is induced by metabolic and respiratory alkaloses.

Hypokalemia can occur because of decreased potassium intake, redistribution of potassium from extracellular to intracellular fluid, and loss of potassium from the body (mainly renal and gastrointestinal losses).

Diagnostic Plan

Causes of hypokalemia are shown in Figure 61-7 and Table 61-8. A thorough history is extremely important in the assessment of decreased potassium.

(*Text continues on p 581.*)

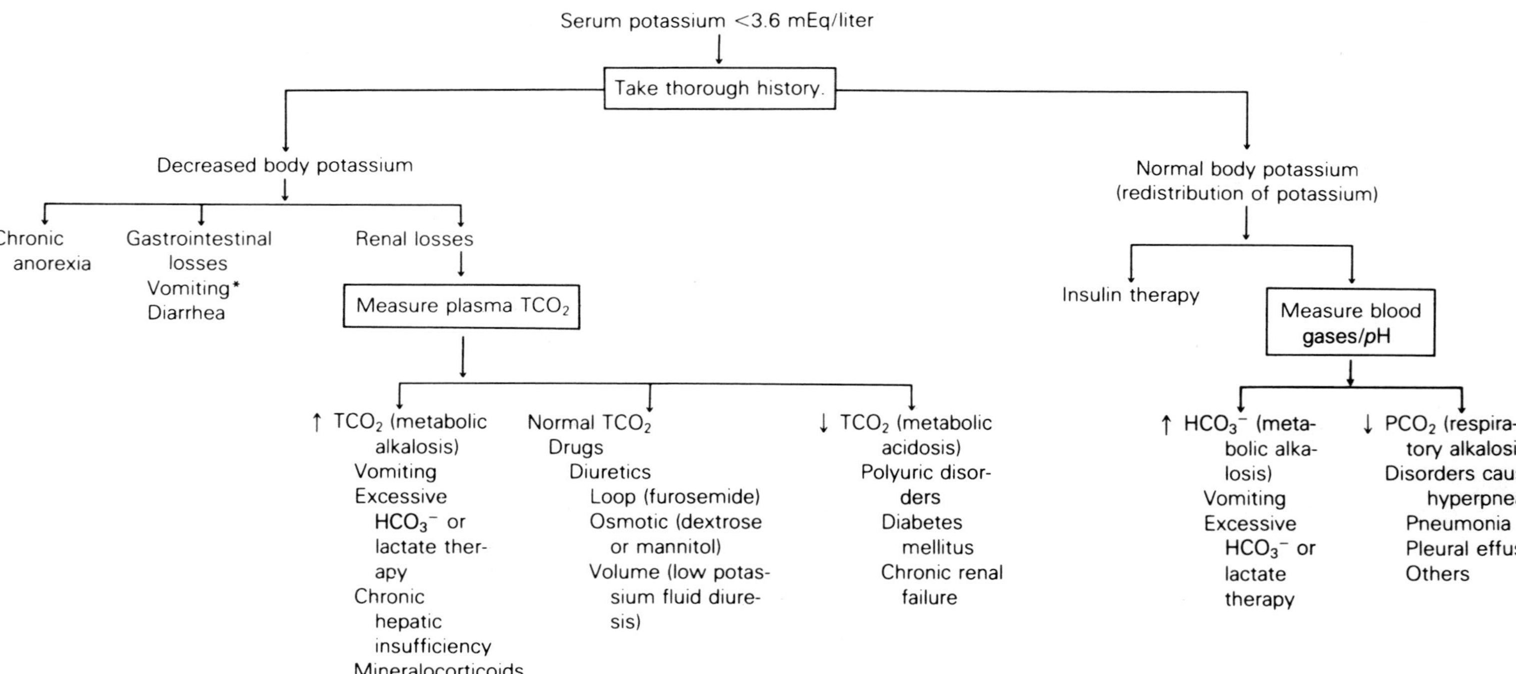

* Metabolic alkalosis causes renal potassium losses and redistribution of potassium from extracellular to intracellular fluid.

Fig. 61-7. Causes of hypokalemia.

Table 61-8. Characteristic Findings of Common Disorders Causing Hypokalemia

DISORDER	CLINICAL SIGNS	HEMATOLOGY	URINE ANALYSIS	BIOCHEMISTRY OTHER THAN HYPOKALEMIA	SPECIAL TESTS
Decreased body potassium					
Chronic anorexia	Poor appetite Weakness Weight loss Others depending on cause	Mild to moderate nonregenerative anemia ± ↓ Plasma protein ±	Normal	↓ Serum albumin ±	None
Gastrointestinal losses					
Vomiting	Vomiting Anorexia, depression Weakness Dehydration Others depending on cause	↑ PCV and plasma protein ± Others depending on cause	Variable	Variable ↑ TCO_2	Depends on cause (See chapter 32.)
Diarrhea	Diarrhea Dehydration Weakness Others depending on cause	↑ PCV and plasma protein Others depending on cause	Variable	Variable	Depends on cause (See chapter 33.)
Renal losses					
Vomiting	See chapter 32.				
Excessive HCO_3^- or lactate therapy	Weakness ± CNS depression ± (paradoxic CSF acidosis)	Normal	Urine *p*H >7.5	↑ TCO_2 ↑ Serum Na ±	None
Chronic hepatic insufficiency	Signs of hepatic failure Icterus Hepatoencephalopathy—stupor, coma, seizures, excessive salivation, head-pressing Ascites Melena	Anemia—regeneration variable Stomatocytosis ± ↓ Plasma protein WBC variable	Hyposthenuria ± Ammonium biurate crystals ±	↓ Albumin ↑ Globulin ± ↓ BUN ± Serum glucose <70 ↑ ALT and SAP ± ↑ Bilirubin ± ↑ TCO_2	↑ BSP retention ↑ Blood NH_3 or ↓ NH_3 tolerance Abnormal coagulogram ± Abnormal liver biopsy

(Continued)

Table 61-8. Characteristic Findings of Common Disorders Causing Hypokalemia *(Continued)*

DISORDER	CLINICAL SIGNS	HEMATOLOGY	URINE ANALYSIS	BIOCHEMISTRY OTHER THAN HYPOKALEMIA	SPECIAL TESTS
Drugs					
Diuretics	Polyuria Dehydration ± Weakness ±	↑ PCV and plasma protein ±	↓ Urine specific gravity Glucosuria if dextrose is being used	↑ Albumin and globulin ↑ Glucose if dextrose is being used ↑ BUN ±	None
Mineralocorticoids	Weakness ±	Normal	Normal	↑ Na ± ↑ TCO_2 ±	None
Polyuric disorders					
Diabetes mellitus	Polydipsia/polyuria Obesity or weight loss Hepatomegaly Cataracts ± Others depending on complications	Variable depending on complications	Glucosuria Ketonuria ± ↑ WBC and bacteriuria ±	Glucose >200 mg/dl Others depending on complications	Depends on complications
Chronic renal failure	Polydipsia and polyuria Signs of uremia ± Depression, anorexia Dehydration Vomiting	Nonregenerative anemia ± ↑ Plasma protein ±	Specific gravity <1.025	↑ BUN ↑ Albumin and globulin ±	Small kidneys on abdominal radiographs ±
Normal body potassium (redistribution)					
Insulin therapy	Weakness Cardiac arrhythmias	Normal	Normal	Normal	None
Metabolic alkalosis					
Vomiting	See chapter 32.				
Excessive HCO_3 or lactate therapy	See section under renal losses (above).				
Respiratory alkalosis (*e.g.*, pneumonia, pleural effusion)	Hypernea Others depending on cause	Depends on cause	Normal	↓ TCO_2 Others depending on cause	Blood gases/*p*H show respiratory alkalosis and usually ↑ arterial PO_2

↓, decreased; ±, present or absent; ↑, increased; PCV, packed cell volume; TCO_2, total CO_2; CNS, central nervous system; CSF, cerebrospinal fluid; WBC, white blood cells; BUN, blood urea nitrogen; ALT, alanine aminotransferase; SAP, serum alkaline phosphatase; PO_2, partial pressure of oxygen

History and Physical Examination

Anorexia, vomiting, and diarrhea cause depletion of body potassium and account for most cases of hypokalemia in dogs and cats. History and physical examination findings depend on the specific cause, but severe potassium depletion may cause muscular weakness, ileus, and polydipsia-polyuria due to a defect in renal concentrating ability. Hypokalemia and potassium depletion predispose the animal to digitalis intoxication, and cardiac arrhythmias are common. A history of use of diuretics (loop, osmotic, or volume) may be noted in hypokalemic patients. Finally, polyuric disorders such as diabetes mellitus and chronic renal insufficiency may cause hypokalemia. History and physical examination findings will be typical of these two disorders.

Laboratory Evaluation

The laboratory work-up of a hypokalemic patient usually depends on the cause of the disorder. A hemogram, serum biochemical profile, and urine analysis are indicated. As previously mentioned, acid-base status affects extracellular potassium concentration. Measurement of blood gases and *p*H, or plasma total CO_2, may help in the interpretation of hypokalemia. Alkalosis causes reduction of serum potassium, and acidosis increases serum potassium. Measurement of total body potassium is impractical. Therefore, frequent measurement of serum potassium is necessary to assess response to treatment.

Symptomatic Therapy[4]

Correction of hypokalemia depends on whether body potassium is decreased or normal (redistribution of potassium). Since 98% of body potassium is located intracellularly and is not practically available for measurement, determining whether or not potassium deficit is present in an indirect process. The serum potassium concentration can be measured and then must be correlated with cellular potassium content. Although mild cellular potassium depletion can occur with a normal serum potassium concentration, especially in acidotic animals, most patients with significant body potassium depletion will be hypokalemic. Hypokalemia usually indicates cellular potassium depletion but can also be caused by redistribution of potassium from extracellular to intracellular fluid (as seen in alkalosis and insulin therapy).

The rate and route of potassium replacement will depend on the severity of clinical signs and cause of potassium loss. Before administering potassium, one should make certain that urine production is adequate. It may be safer to rehydrate the patient with low potassium fluids prior to administering potassium-enriched solutions. Life-threatening hypokalemia is rare; therefore, intravenous potassium replacement is usually not necessary and is potentially dangerous (it can lead to hyperkalemic cardiotoxicity). Potassium given intravenously should be administered at a rate not exceeding about 0.5 mEq potassium/kg/hr. Oral potassium replacement is preferred whenever vomiting is not a problem. Most

Table 61-9. Guidelines for Potassium Administration in Dogs and Cats[3]

SERUM POTASSIUM (mEq/liter)	SEVERITY OF POTASSIUM DEPLETION*	DAILY POTASSIUM DOSE (mEq/kg)
3.0–3.7	Mild	1–3
2.5–3.0	Moderate	4–6
<2.5	Severe	7–9

* Accompanying alkalosis indicates less severe potassium depletion, whereas coexistent acidosis indicates more severe potassium depletion.

commercial dog and cat foods contain sufficient potassium to correct mild potassium deficiencies. For moderate and severe potassium depletion, potassium chloride tablets and potassium gluconate liquids for oral use are commercially available. Liquids are preferred over tablets because of more dependable absorption. Subcutaneous administration of polyionic, isotonic fluids, such as Ringer's or lactated Ringer's solutions enriched with 30 mEq of potassium chloride per liter, is a safe method of potassium replacement. Total daily potassium dosage is estimated based upon the suspected severity of potassium depletion (Table 61-9). Acid–base disturbances should be corrected, and the primary disorder should be treated appropriately.

Hypokalemia due to redistribution of potassium may be corrected by appropriate treatment of the cause (*e.g.*, correction of alkalosis or reduction of insulin dosage).

HYPERKALEMIA

Definition

Hyperkalemia is defined as a serum potassium concentration of greater than 5.6 mEq/liter.

Pathophysiology

Like the hypokalemic syndromes, those of hyperkalemia may occur with normal or altered total body potassium. However, since the electrophysiologic manifestations of severe hyperkalemia are potentially lethal (cardiotoxicity), only extracellular potassium concentration is considered to be clinically important. Theoretically, hyperkalemia may be caused by increased intake, decreased excretion (mainly renal), or redistribution of potassium from cells into the extracellular fluid. Clinically, important hyperkalemia is almost always associated with decreased urinary excretion (Fig. 61-8 and Table 61-10).

Decreased urinary excretion of potassium can be due to (1) urinary tract obstruction or tear, (2) decreased delivery of sodium and fluid to the distal nephron, (3) acidosis, (4) severe distal tubule damage, (5) deficiency of aldosterone (Addison's disease), and (6) use of aldosterone–inhibiting diuretics (spironolactone).

(Text continues on p 586.)

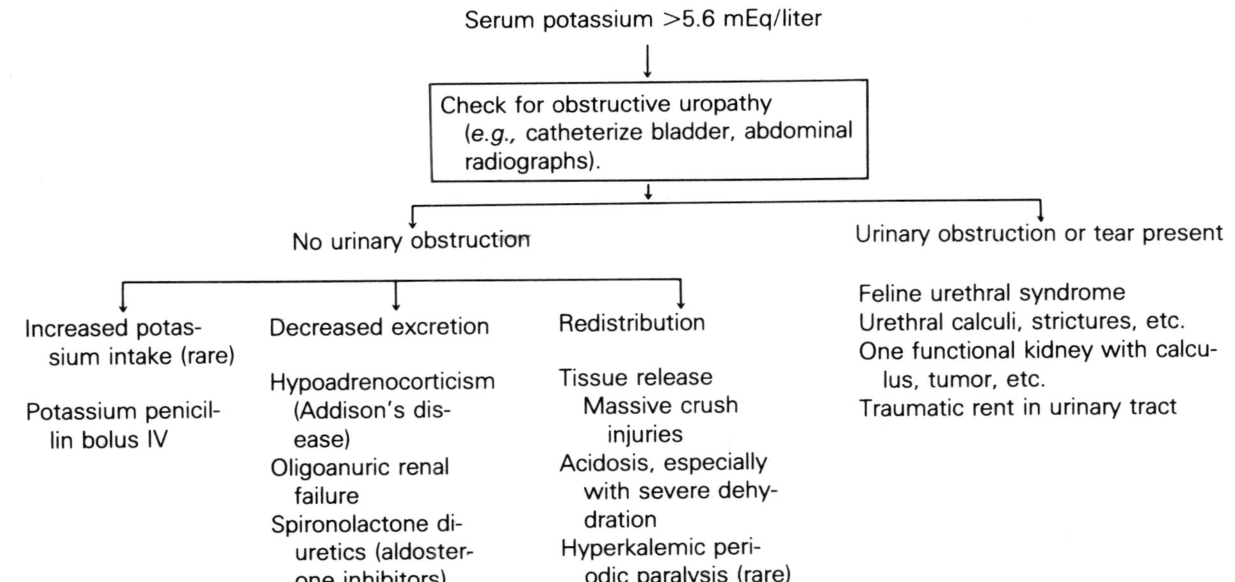

Fig. 61-8. Causes of hyperkalemia.

Table 61-10. Characteristic Findings of Common Disorders Causing Hyperkalemia

DISORDER	CLINICAL SIGNS	HEMATOLOGY	URINE ANALYSIS	BIOCHEMISTRY OTHER THAN HYPERKALEMIA	SPECIAL TESTS
No urinary obstruction					
Increased potassium intake					
Potassium penicillin bolus IV	Bradycardia Acute death	Normal	Normal	Normal	ECG shows: Tall, peaked T waves Bradycardia, Flattened P waves Atrial standstill Cardiac arrest
Decreased potassium excretion					
Hypoadrenocorticism (Addison's disease)	Chronic lethargy and anorexia Sporadic vomiting and diarrhea Weakness Dehydration Bradycardia Collapse, shock, death	↑ PCV and plasma protein Eosinophilia and lymphocytosis ±	Low specific gravity ±	↓ Na Na : K ratio <23 to 1 ↑ BUN ↓ Glucose ± ↑ Albumin and globulin (dehydration) ↓ TCO_2	ECG (See above) Plasma cortisols—low baseline and little or no response to ACTH
Oligoanuric renal failure	Depression, anorexia Vomiting Dehydration	↑ PCV and plasma protein Stress leukogram ±	May be anuric Variable depending on cause	↑ BUN ↑ Phosphorus ↑ Albumin and globulin ↓ TCO_2	Consider urine culture. Abdominal radiographs ±
Spironolactone diuretics (aldosterone inhibitors)	Polyuria Dehydration ±	↑ PCV and plasma protein ±	↓ Specific gravity	↓ Na ↑ BUN	None

Redistribution of potassium					
Tissue release, as with crush injuries	Signs associated with trauma	Associated with trauma Regenerative anemia Stress leukogram	Normal	Depends on injuries	Depends on injuries
Acidosis, especially with severe dehydration	Depends on specific cause Depression Dehydration Cardiac arrhythmia	Depends on specific cause ↑ PCV and plasma protein	Depends on specific cause Specific gravity >1.035 pH <6.0	Depends on specific cause ↑ Albumin and globulin	Depends on specific cause ECG may show arrhythmia or other signs of hyperkalemia (See Increased potassium intake [above])
Urinary obstruction					
Feline urethral syndrome	Depression Vomiting Dehydration Grossly distended bladder Dysuria Later—collapse, bradycardia, shock, death	↑ PCV and plasma protein Stress leukogram	Gross hematuria Triple phosphate crystals	↑ BUN ↑ Phosphorus ↓ TCO_2 ↑ Albumin and globulin	None
Urethral calculi, strictures, and others	Similar to Feline urethral syndrome (above)				Abdominal radiographs—survey and contrast urethrography
One functional kidney with ureteral calculus, tumor, etc. causing obstruction	Similar to Feline urethral syndrome (above)				Abdominal radiographs Excretory urogram

ECG, electrocardiogram; ↑, increased; PCV, packed cell volume; ↓, decreased; BUN, blood urea nitrogen; TCO_2, total CO_2, ACTH, adrenocorticotropic hormone

Diagnostic Plan

Causes of hyperkalemia are shown in Figure 61-8 and Table 61-10. Whenever serum potassium exceeds 8.0 mEq/liter, primary attention should be devoted to quickly reducing serum potassium or antagonizing its electrophysiologic effects and diagnostic procedures should be temporarily delayed.

History and Physical Examination

Urinary tract obstruction should be excluded initially. A history of dysuria with little or no urine being passed is suggestive. In most cases of urinary tract obstruction, the blockage is located from the neck of the bladder distally to the external urethral orifice. A distended bladder is palpable on physical examination. Occasionally, hyperkalemia caused by urinary tract obstruction is due to unilateral ureteral obstruction with only one functional kidney. In this situation, the bladder contains little or no urine, and dysuria is unlikely. Depending on the duration of urinary tract obstruction, signs of uremia (depression, dehydration, and vomiting) or hyperkalemia (bradycardia, cardiac arrhythmia, and collapse) may be observed.

With adrenocortical insufficiency (Addison's disease), a history of anorexia, lethargy, weakness, and sporadic vomiting and diarrhea followed by collapse is typical. Bradycardia, dehydration, and signs of shock may be observed. Similar history and physical examination findings may be present with oligoanuric renal failure.

Laboratory Evaluation

The initial laboratory work-up for hyperkalemia is similar to that previously discussed for hypokalemia, except that electrocardiographic monitoring may be important. Radiographs of the abdomen may be needed to help assess the urinary system for an obstruction or a rent.

Symptomatic Therapy

Hyperkalemia may be life-threatening, and therapy should not be delayed. Treatment of hyperkalemia can be directed at antagonizing effects of potassium on the heart by giving calcium, causing urinary excretion of potassium by administering low-potassium fluids, or at redistributing potassium into the cell by administering an alkalinizing solution (sodium bicarbonate or lactated Ringer's solutions) or insulin and glucose. The use of exchange resins and dialysis to reduce body potassium is not usually practical in dogs and cats.

The particular treatment used should probably depend on the cause and severity of hyperkalemia. If urinary tract obstruction is present, it should be promptly relieved. Fluid volume replacement with an alkalinizing solution such as lactated Ringer's may be sufficient. Increased delivery of sodium, bicarbonate, and water to the distal nephron will increase renal potassium excretion. Alkalinization of extracellular fluid causes redistribution of potassium into cells.

For extreme hyperkalemia (serum potassium >8.0 to 8.5 mEq/liter and severe electrocardiographic abnormalities), intravenous administration of regular insulin and 5% glucose (1 unit of insulin per 4 to 5 g of glucose) may be necessary. Cellular uptake of potassium temporarily decreases the plasma potassium concentration while the underlying problem is being corrected. Calcium will directly counteract the cardiotoxic effects of hyperkalemia and can be administered intravenously as 10% calcium gluconate solution. Since the effective dosage of calcium gluconate is variable (usually 0.5 ml/kg), the heart rate or electrocardiogram (ECG) should be carefully monitored while slowly injecting calcium gluconate: the infusion should be stopped when the heart rate increases or the ECG becomes more normal.

Appropriate treatment of the underlying cause of hyperkalemia must be initiated without delay. Frequent measurement of serum potassium and electrocardiographic monitoring are helpful.

HYPOCALCEMIA

Definition

Hypocalcemia is defined as a total serum calcium concentration of less than 9.0 mg/dl.

Pathophysiology

Calcium has several important functions in both intracellular and extracellular fluid. In addition to its structural role in bone, intracellular calcium is critical for muscle contraction, nerve impulse transmission, and release of neurotransmitters. Calcium also serves as an intracellular messenger for a variety of metabolic functions. Extracellular calcium concentration is important for the intracellular functions mentioned above, because of its influence on calcium pumps in cell membranes and its effects on cell membrane permeability to other ions.[7]

Calcium is present in extracellular fluid in three forms: (1) ionized, (2) protein bound (mainly albumin), and (3) chelated with anions. Only ionized calcium is biologically active. Most laboratory methods for measuring serum calcium determine the sum of the three forms of calcium mentioned above (total serum calcium). Special equipment is needed to measure ionized calcium separately. Although the determination of total serum calcium may provide helpful information, it must be remembered that altered values, especially hypocalcemia, may be due to changes in the biologically inactive portions and therefore not dangerous to the patient. Examples include hypoalbuminemia and changes in blood *p*H. Decreased serum albumin causes hypocalcemia. The following formulas may be used to correct the hypoalbuminemia for calcium:[7]

1. Adjusted Ca (mg/dl) = Ca (mg/dl) − albumin (g/dl) + 3.5

2. Adjusted Ca (mg/dl) = Ca (mg/dl) − [0.4 × total serum protein (g/dl)] + 3.3

Causes of Decreased Total Serum Calcium in Dogs and Cats

- Hypoalbuminemia (see Table 61-1)
- Renal failure
- Eclampsia
- Acute pancreatitis
- Antifreeze (ethylene glycol) poisoning
- Dietary deficiency
- Malabsorption of calcium, vitamin D, or both
- Hypoparathyroidism
- Bone calcium uptake
    - Adenoma removal
    - Osteoblastic tumor
- Hyperphosphatemia
    - Phosphate-containing enema
- Hypomagnesemia
- Inappropriate sample-handling
    - Calcium-binding anticoagulant

These correction formulas do not account for the effects of blood pH on serum calcium. Alkalosis decreases ionized serum calcium, and acidosis has the opposite effect.

Causes of hypocalcemia in dogs and cats are listed separately. The previously listed correction formulas should always be used before assessing a decreased serum calcium. Total serum calcium values above 5.0 mg/dl are usually not associated with clinical signs unless the ionized serum calcium is disproportionately low. Even though the animal is not showing clinical signs of hypocalcemia, the reduced serum calcium may be helpful in determining which clinical disorder is present in the patient.

Diagnostic Plan

History and Physical Examination

The classic clinical signs in a patient with hypocalcemia are muscle tremors and fasciculations, panting, nervousness, restlessness, seizures, and increased body temperature. Anorexia, depression, listlessness, aggressive behavior, and sensory abnormalities may be observed. These signs may sometimes be sporadic instead of constant.

Laboratory Evaluation

Serum calcium should be determined as a part of a standard biochemical panel, which should include measurement of serum phosphorus. As previously mentioned, most laboratories measure total serum calcium. Since there is some variation from one laboratory to another, normal serum calcium values for dogs and cats should be determined in the particular laboratory being used for patients.

Symptomatic Therapy

Symptomatic hypocalcemia is potentially life-threatening and should be treated without delay. Calcium gluconate (10% solution) should be administered slowly to effect (usually about 0.5 ml/kg) intravenously while the animal's heart rate and rhythm are monitored. The infusion should be stopped when the abnormal clinical signs are corrected or when there is a significant increase in the heart rate or the occurrence of an arrhythmia. The underlying cause of the decreased serum calcium should be determined and treated appropriately as soon as possible.

HYPERCALCEMIA

Definition

Hypercalcemia is defined as a total serum calcium concentration of greater than 12.0 mg/dl.

Pathophysiology

Most of the abnormalities caused by hypercalcemia are attributable to its physiologic functions previously mentioned (see Hypocalcemia, Pathophysiology). Because of calcium's role in muscle contraction and neuromuscular transmission, severe hypercalcemia (serum calcium >16.0 mg/dl) may be fatal. Concomitant elevations in serum calcium and phosphorus with a calcium × phosphorus product of greater than 60 are more likely to cause soft tissue mineralization.[7] Severe renal damage is a likely consequence of renal calcification (see Causes of Hypercalcemia in Dogs and Cats).

Causes of Hypercalcemia in Dogs and Cats

- Pseudohyperparathyroidism
  - Lymphosarcoma
  - Perianal carcinoma
- Renal failure
- Primary hyperparathyroidism
- Hypervitaminosis D
- Osteolytic lesions
- Hypoadrenocorticism
- Hemoconcentration/hyperproteinemia
- Immobilization

Diagnostic Plan

History and Physical Examination

Clinical signs of hypercalcemia may vary depending on the cause. Depression, anorexia, vomiting, constipation, weakness, polyuria, polydipsia, and arrythmias may be observed.

Laboratory Evaluation

See Hypocalcemia. Follow-up diagnostic plans will depend on the rule outs being considered after the initial results are assessed. In dogs, pseudohyperparathyroidism caused by lymphosarcoma is the most common cause of hypercalcemia. A careful search for enlarged lymph nodes or organomegaly, including abdominal and thoracic radiography, is warranted. Fine needle aspirates of enlarged structures should be obtained for cytology. In some cases, the diagnosis must be established by excisional biopsy.

Symptomatic Therapy

Severe hypercalcemia (>16.0 mg/dl) may require emergency treatment. As previously mentioned, soft tissue mineralization is more likely when the serum phosphorus is also increased (calcium × phosphorus > 60). The following steps are recommended for the emergency treatment of hypercalcemia:

1. Promote diuresis by the intravenous administration of 0.9% saline solution at a daily dosage of 80 ml/kg. Approximately half of this infusion should be given during the first 6 hours.
2. After hydration is established, administer furosemide intravenously at an initial dosage of 5 mg/kg followed by a maintenance infusion of 5 mg/kg/hr until the serum calcium is less than 12 mg/dl. Hydration must be maintained during administration of furosemide.
3. Consider administering prednisone or prednisolone at a dosage of 1 mg/kg in two daily divided doses. Glucocorticoids are more effective in decreasing an elevated serum calcium caused by lymphosarcoma than for other causes.
4. Mithramycin has been reported to be effective in reducing an elevated serum calcium but has the disadvantages of being potentially toxic and expensive.

The underlying cause of the hypercalcemia should be corrected as soon as possible.

REFERENCES

1. Burke MD: Electrolyte studies: 1. Sodium and water. Postgrad Med 64:147–153, 1978
2. Conley SB, et al: Recurrent hypernatremia: A proposed mechanism in a patient with absence of thirst and abnormal excretion of water. J Pediatr 89:898–903, 1976
3. Cornelius LM: Principles of fluid therapy (small animal). In Anderson NV (ed): Veterinary Gastroenterology, 2nd ed. Philadelphia, Lea & Febiger (in press)

4. Cornelius LM: Fluid, electrolyte, acid-base, and nutritional management. In Bojrab MJ (ed): Pathophysiology in Small Animal Surgery, pp 12–32. Philadelphia, Lea & Febiger, 1981
5. Cox M, Sterns RH, Singer I: The defense against hyperkalemia: The roles of insulin and aldosterone. N Engl J Med 299:525–532, 1978
6. Crawford MA, Kittleson MD, Fink GD: Hypernatremia and adipsia in a Miniature Schnauzer. J Am Vet Med Assoc 184:818–821, 1984
7. Finco DR: Interpretations of serum calcium concentration in the dog. Compend Cont Ed 5:778–788, 1983
8. Moss DW, Butterworth PJ: Enzymology and Medicine. London, Pitman Medical Co, 1974
9. Nardone DA, McDonald WJ, Giard DE: Mechanisms in hypokalemia: Clinical correlation. Medicine (Baltimore) 57:435–446, 1978
10. Narins RG, et al: Diagnostic strategies in disorders of fluid, electrolyte, and acid–base homeostasis. Am J Med 72:496–520, 1982
11. Taclob LT, Needle MA: Hyponatremic syndromes. Med Clin North Am 57:1425–1433, 1973
12. Thier SO: The kidney. In Smith LH, Thier SO (eds): Pathophysiology—The Biological Principles of Disease, pp 799–920. Philadelphia, WB Saunders, 1981

62

Urine Analysis

JEANNE A. BARSANTI

This chapter will review each component of the urine analysis and its correct interpretation.

SAMPLE COLLECTION

Correct interpretation of a urine analysis is based on knowledge of methods of sample collection. The method of collection should *always* be recorded. Samples collected by cystocentesis are usually preferred, since these avoid contamination from the urethra and external genitalia. The only disadvantage of cystocentesis is that some blood may be introduced into urine during collection. For this reason, if the animal's problem is possible hematuria, a voided urine sample is taken first to confirm the presence of blood. The only contraindication to cystocentesis is a markedly distended bladder with a potentially ischemic or otherwise abnormal wall. Cystocentesis is usually still safe if the distention is relieved immediately thereafter. In fact, cystocentesis is often recommended just prior to the relief of a urethral obstruction to remove the back pressure from a full bladder.

If cystocentesis is unsuccessful, a catheterized sample is preferred in male dogs, since preputial contamination is avoided. Catheterization should always involve a sterile catheter and aseptic technique. Voided or expressed samples can be used in female dogs and cats when cystocentesis is unsuccessful, since catheterization is often difficult and can be associated with induction of infection in female dogs, even when careful technique is utilized. This does not imply that catheterization should never be used to obtain a urine sample in female dogs. The information to be gained from the urine analysis may warrant risk of infection. For example, in a dehydrated female dog, urine specific gravity must be obtained prior to fluid therapy to correctly assess renal ability to respond to dehydration. This information is *vital* to determine the cause of dehydration; if catheterization is necessary to obtain the sample, it should be performed.

COMPONENTS OF THE COMPLETE URINALYSIS

There is a strong tendency among veterinarians to consider a dipstick analysis as a complete urine analysis. In doing so, very important parts of a urine analysis are omitted: determination of specific gravity and sediment examination. Without knowledge of the urine specific gravity, neither renal function nor the dipstick analysis for protein or bilirubin can be accurately assessed. Many cases of urinary tract disease will be missed if the urine sediment is not examined. A prime example is urinary tract infection in association with canine Cushing's disease or steroid therapy. In these cases, hematuria is usually absent (negative occult blood), yet bacteriuria may be marked. The essential components of a urine analysis are listed on page 594.

After urine has been collected, it should be examined as soon as possible. If it is not examined within 30 minutes, the sample should be refrigerated and examined within a few hours. Bacterial culture should be performed within 8 hours to avoid significant changes in bacterial numbers. Changes in *p*H, cellular deterioration, fragmentation and dissolution of casts, and precipitation of crystals can also occur during storage.

INTERPRETATION OF THE COMPONENTS OF URINE ANALYSIS

Urine Specific Gravity

In dogs and cats, any urine specific gravity may be normal. Because the kidneys maintain water balance, urine specific gravity will vary with water and solute intake and body needs. In dehydrated dogs and cats, urine should be concentrated to a specific gravity greater than 1.035. Thus, specific gravity should always be interpreted in light of the animal's hydration status. Urine specific gravity is also greatly affected by administration of diuretics, corticosteroids, radiographic contrast agents, and fluid therapy. These treatments reduce the usefulness of specific gravity as an indicator of renal function. Thus, it is *essential* to collect urine prior to any treatment. Large amounts of protein or glucose also increase specific gravity approximately 0.001 for each 0.3 g/dl glucose and 0.4 g/dl protein.

Specific Gravity >1.045

A specific gravity of this magnitude in the dog indicates normal urine concentrating ability. Normal dogs usually concentrate to greater than 1.045 when challenged with mild dehydration (5%).

A specific gravity of this magnitude may be associated with abnormal renal function in cats. In one experimental study, cats became azotemic due to renal insufficiency and still concentrated urine to greater than 1.045. A decrease in concentrating ability occurred with the onset of renal failure but was minimal

Essential Components of a Routine Urine Analysis

- Record of method of collection
- Specific gravity
- Dipstick analysis
  - *p*H
  - Protein
  - Ketones
  - Glucose
  - Bilirubin
  - Occult blood
- Sediment examination
  - Red blood cells
  - White blood cells
  - Bacteria
  - Casts
  - Crystals
  - Epithelial cells
  - Miscellaneous

and variable even with mild azotemia. Thus, renal failure is ruled out in dogs, but not in cats, when urine specific gravity is greater than 1.045. To rule out renal failure in cats, blood urea nitrogen (BUN), serum creatinine, or both should be measured. If the cat is not azotemic and urine specific gravity is in this range, renal failure is ruled out (renal disease may still be present but is undetectable by routine laboratory tests).

Specific Gravity >1.030–1.045

In dogs and cats with no internal medical problems and with normal BUN, serum creatinine, and hydration, urine specific gravity in this range is considered normal. With dehydration or azotemia, values in this range are abnormal in cats. In dogs with dehydration, azotemia, or both, this range is more difficult to interpret and may indicate normal concentrating ability or a mild loss of concentrating ability. In general, no further diagnostics are indicated in relation to renal function for urine specific gravities in this range in animals that are otherwise normal.

Specific Gravity 1.013–1.029

Urine specific gravity in this range indicates some ability to concentrate urine. Values in this range may be normal if no stimulus for urine concentration exists; however, values in this range are abnormal if the animal is dehydrated or azotemic due to a prerenal or renal insult. (See chapter 5 [polyuria] to review the causes of the inability to concentrate urine.)

Even if the animal appears normal and other laboratory work is normal, urine specific gravities in this range may warrant further diagnostic work to rule out conditions such as chronic renal failure. The tests indicated (besides complete blood count [CBC], blood chemistry profile, and complete urine analysis, which should be done first) are a water deprivation test and antidiuretic hormone (ADH) response test (see chapter 5).

Specific Gravity 1.008–1.012

Urine with a specific gravity in this range is isosthenuric, meaning that no urine concentration has occurred (its specific gravity equal to that of plasma). This value may be normal if no stimulus to concentrate is present. If a stimulus to concentrate such as dehydration or azotemia of prerenal or renal origin is present, values in this range are definitely abnormal. Routine laboratory work including CBC, blood chemistry profile, and complete urine analysis should be performed. Even if routine laboratory work is normal and the animal is not dehydrated, urine specific gravities in this range may warrant further evaluation. Diagnostic tests to consider include repeat urine specific gravities, water deprivation test, and ADH response test. Refer to chapter 5 to review the causes of inability to concentrate urine.

Specific Gravity <1.008

Urine specific gravities in this range are hyposthenuric, indicating normal renal ability to dilute urine. Values in this range can be normal if the animal has a need to excrete extra water, but they are abnormal in animals with a need to retain water due to dehydration. Urine specific gravities in this range may be produced by a primary polydipsia, lack of ADH, or inability of the kidney to respond to ADH (refer to chapter 5). Urine specific gravities in this range usually warrant further diagnostic testing because they are associated with profound polyuria and polydipsia. A CBC, complete blood chemistry profile, and complete urine analysis are indicated. If these are normal, water deprivation and ADH response tests should be performed.

Urine *p*H

Urine *p*H varies as the kidney maintains electrolyte and acid–base balances in relation to varying dietary intake; therefore, no specific urine *p*H is abnormal. Evaluation of urine *p*H is useful only as it relates to other findings from the urine analysis and in relationship to acid–base and electrolyte balances as a whole.

Urine pH <7.1

Urine *p*H in this range is acidic or neutral. Dogs and cats, as carnivores that eat relatively infrequently, generally have a urine *p*H in this range. If the *p*H is markedly acidic (<6.0), one might suspect a systemic tendency to acidemia. An acidic urine *p*H does not rule out urinary tract infection, as most urinary tract pathogens do not affect urine *p*H *in vivo.*

Urine pH *>7.0*

Alkaline urine is produced for several hours postprandially. The most common disease condition that produces constantly alkaline urine is urinary infection with *Staphylococcus* or *Proteus.* These organisms produce the enzyme urease, which degrades urea to ammonia, causing alkalinity. Thus, when alkaline urine is identified, the rest of the urine analysis (especially the urine sediment) should be examined for evidence of bacterial infection. Consistently alkaline urine in the dog and cat can result in development of struvite uroliths. Monitoring urine *p*H for alkalinity is one method used to prevent recurrence of struvite uroliths.

Another cause of persistently alkaline urine is renal tubular acidosis. In this condition, metabolic acidemia results from the inability of the kidney to reabsorb bicarbonate (proximal renal tubular acidosis, type I) or secrete hydrogen ions (distal renal tubular acidosis, type II). Renal tubular acidosis is apparently rare in dogs and cats. Proximal renal tubular acidosis can be a component of Fanconi syndrome in the dog, in which there is generalized proximal tubular dysfunction. Associated abnormalities in the urine analysis are mild proteinuria and glycosuria.

Proteinuria

Proteinuria is usually assessed by a dipstick analysis. This test is qualitative, not quantitative, and should be recorded as such (trace to 4+). Some dipsticks incorporate milligrams per deciliter on their scale, but these numbers are not sufficiently accurate to quantitate the amount of protein present. Various evaluations of laboratory technicians have indicated that the color change for protein on the dipstick is the most difficult color change to read consistently. This is another good reason for interpreting the result as relative and not absolute. Because of these problems with the dipstick plus its inability to detect Bence Jones proteins associated with plasma cell myelomas, many laboratories utilize a precipitation test such as sulfosalicylic acid, trichloroacetic acid, or Robert's reagent (nitric acid). These tests are also evaluated subjectively on a trace to 4+ basis.

To accurately interpret the significance of proteinuria, the urine specific gravity must be known. A small amount of protein might read as negative in dilute urine at 1.010 but positive (1+) in urine concentrated to 1.040.

A small amount of protein in urine is normal. This protein is derived from small molecular weight proteins, which pass through the glomerulus and are largely but not completely reabsorbed in the proximal tubule, and from proteins produced within the urinary tract (e.g., Tamm Horsfall protein). This amount of protein may register as negative at a specific gravity less than 1.035 or trace to 1+ at a specific gravity greater than 1.035.

A protein of 2+ or greater at a specific gravity greater than 1.035 or any amount of protein at a specific gravity less than 1.035 *may* be abnormal. As specific gravity decreases and urine protein levels increase, the evidence that the proteinuria is abnormal becomes more convincing. Marginal changes may be abnormal or normal because of the subjectivity of the tests involved. The next step in evaluating the proteinuria is to examine the rest of the urine analysis. First, evidence of hemorrhage should be sought. Bleeding into the urinary tract introduces RBCs and serum proteins as well as the other constituents of blood. Since proteins are present in blood in large quantities (g/dl) compared with the amount of protein in normal urine (mg/dl) and since the tests for proteinuria are designed for the small amount of protein in urine, blood in urine results in detectable proteinuria. One should also look for evidence of inflammation (pyuria), since inflammatory exudates also contain sufficient protein to result in significant proteinuria.

When proteinuria is the only abnormality in the urine analysis, one should evaluate renal function by BUN, serum creatinine concentrations, and urine specific gravity. Serum albumin should be measured to determine whether the proteinuria is of sufficient magnitude to cause hypoalbuminemia.

The best method for determining the magnitude and clinical importance of proteinuria in urine with a normal sediment is protein quantitation. One method is to collect all urine produced for a known period (usually 24 hours). The amount of protein in an aliquot of urine is quantitated (mg/dl). The amount of protein in the aliquot is then multiplied by the total urine volume to determine the amount of protein lost per day. Normal values in the dog and cat are less than 200 mg in our laboratory, although others have reported as much as 500 mg per day. Another test that can be used is the urine protein/urine creatinine ratio, in which protein and creatinine are measured in a single random urine sample. This ratio corrects for urine concentration changes. A normal ratio is less than 0.2 and an abnormal ratio is greater than 1.0. Values between 0.2 and 1.0 are indeterminate, and a timed collection should be performed. Quantitative urine protein determinations are only useful when there is no hemorrhage or inflammation.

If there is no evidence of hematuria or pyuria, then the cause of the proteinuria is usually either increased loss of serum proteins through the glomerulus as a result of glomerular disease or a change in glomerular dynamics, a decrease in renal tubular reabsorption of proteins, or excretion of increased quantities of a protein in the glomerular filtrate. An example of the latter is Bence Jones protein (light chain of an immunoglobulin molecule) formed by malignant plasma cells (plasma cell myeloma). This cause of proteinuria can be identified by markedly elevated serum protein concentrations and confirmed by serum and urine electrophoresis. Dipstick analysis for protein may not detect Bence Jones protein: turbidity tests are required.

A change in glomerular dynamics that can cause proteinuria is increased glomerular hydrostatic pressure. This can result from right-sided congestive heart failure or increased intra-abdominal pressure, as might be associated with ascites or a large neoplasm that partially obstructs the caudal vena cava. The degree of proteinuria is usually mild to moderate.

Tubular diseases do not result in severe proteinuria, because protein loss is due to failure of proximal tubular reabsorption of the small amount of small molecular weight proteins in glomerular filtrate. Tubular diseases do not cause hypoalbuminemia. Thus, if the protein loss is large and hypoalbuminemia is present, the cause is probably a glomerular disease, but if the loss is more moderate, further testing may be necessary to determine the cause as a tubular or glomerular disease. With failure of proximal tubular reabsorption, the proteinuria may be associated with glucosuria with a normal blood glucose. An example is Fanconi syndrome in basenji dogs. With chronic renal failure in general (chronic interstitial nephritis), mild proteinuria without glucosuria is characteristic.

Glomerular diseases are characterized by moderate to severe proteinuria. A renal biopsy is required to differentiate the two most common types of glomerular diseases in dogs: amyloidosis and glomerulonephritis. In cats, renal amyloidosis occurs but involves the medullary interstitium more than the glomerulus, so protein loss is less marked. Glomerulonephritis in the cat is frequently associated with feline leukemia virus infection.

Ketonuria

Ketonuria is abnormal. False-positive reactions are uncommon but may occur in highly pigmented urine. The renal tubular reabsorptive mechanism for ketones is rapidly saturated, so ketonuria precedes detectable ketonemia. The most common cause of ketonuria is diabetes mellitus, in which ketonuria is associated with glucosuria and hyperglycemia. Other potential causes are starvation, chronic catabolic diseases, persistent fever, impaired liver function, and hypoglycemic syndromes. Young animals and those of very small body size apparently tend to develop ketonuria faster with anorexia than older, larger animals.

Glycosuria

Normal urine does not contain glucose, so any degree of glycosuria is abnormal. False-positive reactions can occur with dipsticks if urine contains an oxidizing agent such as H_2O_2 or chlorine. The most common cause of glycosuria is a blood glucose (>180 mg/dl) that exceeds the renal threshold for glucose reabsorption. The most common cause is diabetes mellitus. If blood glucose is normal, renal proximal tubular dysfunction should be considered. An associated finding is mild proteinuria. Renal proximal tubular dysfunction (Fanconi's syndrome) can be congenital, as in basenji dogs, or acquired, as with nephrotoxicity due to aminoglycoside antibiotics.

Bilirubinuria

Bilirubinuria can be normal in dogs but is always considered abnormal in cats. In dogs, the degree of bilirubinuria should be compared with the urine specific gravity. A trace to 1+ bilirubin in concentrated urine (>1.035) is normal in dogs. More marked bilirubinuria is abnormal.

Abnormal bilirubinuria indicates increased serum concentrations of conjugated bilirubin, since unconjugated bilirubin does not filter through the glomerulus. Increased concentrations of conjugated bilirubin may be the result of biliary obstruction (hepatic or posthepatic), cholestasis, or increased production secondary to accelerated hemolysis. Bilirubinuria will precede bilirubinemia in these conditions (see chapter 37, Icterus).

Positive Occult Blood

The occult blood reaction will become positive in the presence of hemoglobin, myoglobin, or intact red blood cells. To determine which is present, the rest of the urine analysis should be examined and the serum color should be determined. Hemoglobinuria can result from hemoglobinemia or release of hemoglobin from RBC breakdown in urine. RBCs in the urine sediment plus a positive occult blood reaction indicates hematuria. If there are no RBCs in the urine, serum color should be examined for hemolysis. If the serum is not red, the positive occult blood reaction is unlikely to be the result of hemoglobinuria from hemoglobinemia. Other possibilities are the presence of hemoglobin in contaminants of urine (*e.g.*, flea dirt in voided samples), complete RBC breakdown in urine (uncommon in a fresh sample), or myoglobin. Myoglobinuria is uncommon in dogs and cats and should be accompanied by clear serum and evidence of severe muscle disease. An ammonium sulfate precipitation test can be used to help differentiate hemoglobin from myoglobin.

Urine Sediment Results

Red Blood Cells

An occasional RBC per high power field (hpf) is normal. Greater numbers are either iatrogenic or abnormal, except in a voided sample from a proestral bitch. To evaluate the RBCs, two determinations must be made: the site of bleeding and the cause. One must know the method of urine collection to determine the site. If the sample was voided, the external genitalia and reproductive system as well as the entire urinary tract must be considered. If the sample was collected by cystocentesis or bladder catheterization, the bladder, kidneys, ureters, or prostate may be the origin. If the sample was collected by cystocentesis or catheterization, an iatrogenic injury during collection must also be considered. For this reason, if an animal is presented for the problem of hematuria, a voided sample should be collected first to confirm the hematuria. Causes of hematuria include trauma, uroliths, infection, inflammation, neoplasia, infarction, prostatic hyperplasia, parasites, toxins, and coagulopathies (see chapter 39, Discolored Urine).

Pyuria

A few white blood cells (WBCs) in urine (<5/hpf) is normal. A greater number of WBCs indicates inflammation at or in advance of the sampling site. One exception is the prostate gland in the male dog, since prostatic fluid refluxes back into the bladder. If WBCs are found in a voided sample, they may be the result of contamination from the reproductive tract or external genitalia or they may indicate inflammation in the urinary tract. A sample collected directly from the bladder, preferably by cystocentesis, is *essential* to differentiate these possibilities. A conclusion that these cells are from contamination without examining urine from the bladder is *incorrect.*

Causes of inflammation within the urinary tract include infection, urolithiasis, neoplasia, trauma, toxins (including drugs such as cyclophosphamide [Cytoxan]), and idiopathic granulomatous diseases. Diagnostic tests, including urine culture and survey and contrast radiographs, may be necessary in addition to the history, physical examination, and urine analysis to differentiate these possibilities.

Bacteruria

As with pyuria, knowing the method of sample collection is essential for accurate interpretation of bacteruria. Urine from the bladder is normally sterile, but the distal urethra, vagina, and prepuce have resident bacterial populations. Thus, bacteruria is abnormal in urine collected by cystocentesis as long as contamination does not occur during or after collection and as long as sterile urine containers are used. Bacteruria in samples collected by voiding or catheterization may be normal or abnormal, depending on the degree of contamination from the urethra, vagina, or prepuce. If a voided sample is bacteruric, a sample should be collected by cystocentesis to determine if the bacteria are contaminants. If a catheterized sample is bacteruric, either a quantitative culture of the sample or a cystocentesis can be performed. More than 100,000 bacteria per milliliter in a catheterized sample usually indicates infection. Lesser numbers may be significant in male dogs and in cats (>10,000/ml). In female dogs, contamination may cause greater than 100,000/ml. This fact plus the possibility of inducing infection with catheterization in female dogs reinforces the importance of cystocentesis.

Estimation of numbers of bacteria on urine analysis often does not correlate with actual numbers. Some bacteria, especially cocci, are difficult to differentiate from amorphous debris with brownian movement. Bacteria are not reliably seen until numbers exceed 100,000/ml (cocci) or 10,000/ml (rods); therefore, absence of bacteruria does not rule out infection. A culture of bladder urine is the best method to establish the presence or absence of infection.

Occasionally bacteria are seen, but a urine culture is negative. The possibilities are that the bacteria died or were killed prior to or during culturing or that the bacteria had unusual growth requirements (*e.g.*, anaerobes). Urinary tract infections are usually caused by common aerobic bacteria (*Escherichia coli*, staphylococci, streptococci, *Proteus*), so only aerobic cultures using common media are routinely done.

Cylindruria

A few granular casts are normally present in urine from turnover of renal epithelial cells. Larger numbers of granular casts and other types of casts are abnormal.

Increased numbers of granular casts indicate active renal tubular cell injury. The type of injury may be ischemic, toxic, infectious, immune-mediated, or traumatic. WBC casts indicate renal inflammation. RBC casts indicate renal bleeding. Absence of WBC or RBC casts does not rule out renal inflammation or hemorrhage. Hyaline casts are composed of Tamm-Horsfall protein, which precipitates in the presence of increased quantities of albumin; thus, hyaline casts are usually associated with glomerular proteinuria. Hyaline casts are more apparent in very concentrated or very acidic urine. They dissolve in alkaline urine. Waxy and broad casts are thought to be degenerate granular casts that form in collecting ducts and indicate current or previous slow urine flow rates (oliguria).

Crystalluria

Crystalluria may be normal or abnormal and primarily indicates the presence of the composing minerals in the urine. Struvite crystals are common in the urine of normal dogs and cats. However, in the presence of radiodense uroliths, urinary tract infection with staphylococci or *Proteus,* and alkaline urine, struvite crystals suggest that the uroliths are also struvite.

Biurate crystals are normal in dalmation dog urine because of the reduced capacity of the liver of dalmatians to convert uric acid to urea. In the presence of uroliths in the dalmatian dog with acid urine, no infection, and minimal radiodensity, the finding of biurate crystals suggests that the uroliths are uric acid. In dogs other than dalmatians, the presence of biurate crystals suggests hepatic insufficiency. Tyrosine crystals also may indicate hepatic insufficiency.

Hippurate and oxalate crystals suggest ethylene glycol toxicity, especially when present in large numbers. Absence of these crystals does not rule out the diagnosis, since slow urine flow rates may keep the crystals in the kidney. Oxalate crystals are occasionally found in normal canine or feline urine.

Bilirubin crystals can be normal in concentrated canine urine. Cystine crystals suggest poor renal tubular ability to reabsorb cystine. Cystinosis predisposes the dog to cystine calculi.

Epithelial Cells

Squamous epithelial cells usually enter urine as it is voided through the vagina or prepuce. Other epithelial cells found in urine are transitional and renal, which are normally present in low numbers. Renal epithelial cells are small, just slightly larger than WBCs. The size of transitional cells varies markedly. It is difficult to differentiate small transitional cells from renal epithelial cells. Caudate cells are small transitional cells with a tail-like appendage. Large numbers of transitional epithelial cells are present with infection, inflammation, injury, and neoplasia. If one suspects lower urinary tract neoplasia, the transitional cells should be examined closely for evidence of malignancy (mitoses, number of nucleoli). This may be a difficult determination to make with the normal size and shape variability of urine transitional cells.

Miscellaneous

Urobilinogen

So many problems exist in the dipstick measurement of urobilinogen that evaluation is not recommended. False-negative and false-positive results are common.

Parasites

The eggs of *Dioctophyma renale* (dog) and *Capillaria plica* (dog, cat) may be found in urine. Intestinal parasite ova may be found if the colon is inadvertently aspirated during cystocentesis.

Spermatozoa

Spermatozoa are often found in the urine of male dogs. Sperm migrate up the deferent ducts and enter the urethra at the prostate gland and then reflux back into bladder urine.

Fat

Lipid can be found in urine of normal cats.

Fungi

Fungi or yeasts are usually contaminants during collection, in transport containers, or in stain. Fungal urinary tract infection can occur but is rare. Some coliforms will assume a markedly filamentous morphology in urine and may be mistaken for fungal hyphae.

SUGGESTED READINGS

Barsanti JA, Finco DR: Protein concentration in urine of normal dogs. Am J Vet Res 40:1583, 1979

Biertuempfel PH, Ling GV, Ling GA: Urinary tract infection resulting from catheterization in healthy adult dogs. J Am Vet Med Assoc 178:989, 1981

Bovee KC, Joyce T, Blazer-Yost B, et al: Characterization of renal defects in dogs with a syndrome similar to the Fanconi-syndrome in man. J Am Vet Med Assoc 174:1094, 1979

Carter JM, Klausner JS, Osborne CA, et al: Comparison of collection techniques for quantitative urine culture in dogs. J Am Vet Med Assoc 173:296, 1978

Chew DJ: Urinalysis: In Bovee KC (ed): Canine Nephrology, pp 235–274. Philadelphia, Harwal Publishing, 1984

Comer KM, Ling GV: Results of urinalysis and bacterial culture of canine urine obtained by antepubic cystocentesis, catheterization, and midstream voided methods. J Am Vet Med Assoc 179:891, 1981

Hardy RM, Osborne CA: Water deprivation in the dogs: Maximal normal values. J Am Vet Med Assoc 174:479, 1979

Ihrke PJ, Norton AL, Ling GV, et al: Urinary tract infection associated with long-term corticosteroid administration in dogs with chronic skin diseases. J Am Vet Med Assoc 186:43, 1985

Lees GE, Simpson RB, Green RA: Results of analyses and bacterial cultures of urine specimens obtained from clinically normal cats by three methods. J Am Vet Med Assoc 184:449, 1984

Ling GV, Ruby AL: Aerobic bacterial flora of the prepuce, urethra, and vagina of normal adult dogs. Am J Vet Res 39:695, 1978

Osborne CA, Low DG, Finco DR: Canine and Feline Urology. Philadelphia, WB Saunders, 1972

Padilla J, Osborne CA, Ward GE: Effect of storage time and temperature on quantitative culture of canine urine. J Am Vet Med Assoc 18:1077, 1981

Ross LA, Finco DR: Relationship of selected clinical renal function tests to glomerular filtration rate and renal blood flow in cats. Am J Vet Res 42:1704, 1981

63

Abnormal Blood Gases, *p*H, and Anion Gap

LARRY M. CORNELIUS

BLOOD GASES AND *p*H

Definition

The acidity of body fluids is expressed in terms of hydrogen ion (H^+) concentration or, more conveniently, as *p*H. The suffix "emia" refers to *p*H of blood. Acidemia (increased H^+ concentration) is defined as an acidic blood *p*H (<7.39), and alkalemia is an alkaline blood *p*H (>7.51). The terms *acidosis* and *alkalosis* refer to processes that cause acid and alkali to accumulate and that, if not halted, will cause a change in blood *p*H.[10]

Pathophysiology

Body fluid pH is normally maintained within narrow limits despite the continuous addition of large quantities of metabolic acids synthesized via intermediary metabolism from dietary precursors and the addition of carbon dioxide (CO_2) from complete cellular oxidation of carbohydrates, fats, and proteins. Three different types of mechanisms defend against large changes in the pH of body fluids:

1. *Chemical buffers* include proteins and phosphates (mostly intracellular), hemoglobin (erythrocytes) and HCO_3- (mostly extracellular). Buffers are compounds that can absorb or donate H^+ ions and thereby minimize changes in *p*H. Since all blood buffers act as if they were in functional contact with a common pool of H^+ ions, the assay of both members of any blood buffer should reflect blood *p*H. The HCO_3^-/H_2CO_3 buffer system is especially important to the clinician and will be discussed later.
2. *Ionic shifts* between extracellular and intracellular fluid help protect extracellular pH. When acid or base is added to extracellular fluid, approximately half of the added ions eventually difuse into cells, where they are buffered chemically.[9] In order for electroneutrality of extracellular and intracellular

fluid to be maintained, other ions of the same charge diffuse in the opposite direction or ions of opposite charge accompany the diffusing ions.

3. *Organ-mediated compensatory responses* include renal and respiratory mechanisms. The kidney can either retain or excrete acids and bases. Respiratory regulation of acid-base balance is through the retention or excretion of CO_2 via changes in the rate and depth of respiration. Disturbances of acid–base homeostasis may be simple or mixed.

Classification of Simple Acid–Base Disturbances[3]

Disease states that initially alter blood PCO_2 are termed *respiratory acidosis or alkalosis,* whereas those initially affecting plasma HCO_3^- concentration are termed *metabolic acidosis or alkalosis.* Changes in blood *p*H are determined by changes in the ratio of plasma HCO_3^-/H_2CO_3.* This ratio (and therefore *p*H) is stabilized by the ability of primary respiratory disorders to initiate offsetting metabolic changes and the ability of primary metabolic disorders to effect counterveiling respiratory changes. Thus, the secondary increase in HCO_3^- induced by primary respiratory acidosis and the secondary decrease in HCO_3^- caused by primary respiratory alkalosis tend to return the HCO_3^-/H_2CO_3 ratio toward normal. Generally, the compensatory processes do not completely normalize *p*H, since to do so would remove the stimulus to compensation. These counterveiling responses are physiologic consequences of the primary or initiating disturbance and are termed *secondary or metabolic compensation* for primary disturbances. The terms *acidosis* and *alkalosis* should not be used to describe compensatory changes in HCO_3^- and PCO_2 but should be reserved for primary pathologic processes.[10]

Respiratory Acidosis

Whenever CO_2 production in body tissues exceeds the rate of its removal by the lungs, blood PCO_2 increases and the patient is said to have respiratory acidosis. Based on clinical experience, primary respiratory acidosis is less common than primary respiratory alkalosis in unanesthetized animals. Depression of the medullary respiratory center by anesthetic agents, when accompanied by inadequate assisted ventilation, frequently causes respiratory acidosis and acidemia (Table 63-1). CO_2 rapidly diffuses across the blood–brain barrier and combines with water to form H_2CO_3, thus lowering cerebrospinal fluid (CSF) *p*H. CSF acidosis causes central nervous system depression and even coma in human patients.[9] Lower airway disorders such as pneumonia and pulmonary edema are more commonly associated with either respiratory alkalosis or normal PCO_2 values; however, severe pneumonia or pulmonary edema may cause respiratory acidosis. Two other causes of respiratory acidosis are laryngeal or tracheal ob-

* HCO_3^- and H_2CO_3 are used as representatives of all body fluid buffers. The kidneys regulate HCO_3^- concentration and the lungs regulate PCO_2 (and therefore H_2CO_3) concentration.

struction and diaphragmatic paralysis. Increased PCO_2 (hypercapnia, hypercarbia) may also occur as a compensatory response to metabolic alkalosis (Table 63-1).

Defense mechanisms against acidemia due to CO_2 retention include chemical buffering by blood and cellular proteins (limited magnitude) and renal compensation (retention of HCO_3^-, excretion of H^+ ions).

Respiratory Alkalosis

Whenever CO_2 removal by the lungs exceeds its production by body tissues, decreased PCO_2 (hypocapnia, hypocarbia) results. Decreased PCO_2 due to a primary disease process is termed *respiratory alkalosis.* As previously stated, respiratory alkalosis is relatively common in lower respiratory disorders such as pneumonia and pulmonary edema. It is theorized that lowered arterial PO_2 in these disorders becomes the driving force for respiration, resulting in hyperventilation and excessive exhalation of CO_2. Respiratory alkalosis frequently results from hyperventilation caused by use of a mechanical ventilator. Hypocarbia is also observed as a compensatory response to metabolic acidosis.

Defense against alkalemia due to hypocarbia consists of chemical buffering by hemoglobin and other blood proteins (acute respiratory alkalosis), renal excretion of HCO_3^-, and renal retention of H^+ ions. Chronic respiratory alkalosis appears to be unique among the simple acid–base disorders in its ability to

Table 63-1. Causes of Abnormal Arterial PCO_2

INCREASED PCO_2	DECREASED PCO_2
Compensation for metabolic alkalosis	Compensation for metabolic acidosis
Respiratory acidosis	Respiratory alkalosis
CNS depression	Mild or moderate lung disease
Sedation or anesthesia	Pneumonia
Damage to respiratory center	Pulmonary edema
Airway obstruction	Mild or moderate restrictive airway disease
Foreign body	Pleural effusion
Laryngospasm	Pneumothorax
Severe tracheal collapse	Diaphragmatic hernia
Enlarged left atrium with left heart failure	Anxiety/panting
Severe lung disease	Mechanical ventilation
Pneumonia	Fever/sepsis/endotoxemia
Pulmonary edema	Hepatic encephalopathy
Restrictive airway disease	
Pleural effusion	
Pneumothorax	
Diaphragmatic hernia	
Thoracic cage limitation/flail chest	
Neuromuscular disorder	
Phrenic nerve paralysis	
Botulism	
Coonhound paralysis	

induce compensatory responses that return blood *p*H completely to normal.[10] The cause of enhanced buffering in chronic respiratory alakalosis is unexplained.

Metabolic Acidosis

Reduction in plasma HCO_3^- due to accumulation of H^+ ions from acids other than H_2CO_3 or from actual loss of HCO_3^- ions from the body is termed *metabolic acidosis*. Whether or not blood *p*H is actually decreased (acidemia) will depend upon the severity of the primary disturbance, the buffering capacity of blood and tissues, and the efficiency of respiratory compensation. Metabolic acidosis is the most common acid–base disturbance in dogs and cats. Various causes include diarrhea (loss of HCO_3^-), severe azotemia (renal H^+ ion retention), diabetic ketoacidosis (ketones are acids), and circulatory collapse (shock) (Table 63-2).

Compensation for metabolic acidosis occurs as the chemoreceptors in the respiratory center of the medulla respond to increased H^+ ion concentration and cause increased ventilation and loss of CO_2 from the lungs. This respiratory response to metabolic acidosis is apparently sluggish, often requiring 12 to 24 hours for maximal response to develop.[10]

Metabolic Alkalosis

Increase in plasma HCO_3^- due to loss of H^+ ions from noncarbonic acids or from excessive alkali therapy is defined as metabolic alkalosis. As is true for each acid–base disorder, whether or not blood *p*H is changed will depend upon the severity of the primary disturbance and the efficiency of body defense mechanisms. Causes of metabolic alkalosis include profuse vomiting, accumulation of gastric juice in the stomach (gastric atony, pyloric obstruction), and overzealous alkali administration (Table 63-2). Metabolic alkalosis is usually more severe when vomiting is caused by a lesion near the pylorus, resulting in loss of mostly gastric juice with its high content of hydrochloric acid (HCl).

Body defense against *p*H increase (alkalemia) due to metabolic alkalosis is principally respiratory. Hypoventilation and retention of CO_2 in response to

Table 63-2. Causes of Abnormal Plasma HCO_3^-

INCREASED HCO_3^-	DECREASED HCO_3^-
Compensation for respiratory acidosis	Compensation for respiratory alkalosis
Metabolic alkalosis	Metabolic acidosis
Vomiting of mostly gastric contents (see chapter 32)	Diarrhea
Sequestration of fluid in stomach	Renal failure
Gastric atony	Diabetic ketoacidosis
Gastric volvulus	Lactic acidosis
Fluid or drug therapy: HCO_3^-, lactate, citrate	Drugs or toxins
	Ammonium chloride
	Ethylene glycol

metabolic alkalosis occur but are reportedly somewhat erratic.[10] The kidney would be expected to maximize H^+ ion retention and HCO_3^- excretion, resulting in an alkaline urine; however, in metabolic alkalosis due to profuse vomiting, acidic urine is frequently observed. The precise mechanism of paradoxical aciduria during severe vomiting is not fully understood, but it may be a consequence of the necessity by the body to retain equivalent quantities of cations and anions.[7] Since large amounts of chloride are lost in gastric juice, HCO_3^- is required to match quantities of sodium reabsorbed in the renal tubules. The result is an acid urine nearly devoid of HCO_3^-.[7] An additional factor that can impair body defenses against alkalemia during metabolic alkalosis is potassium depletion.[15] Hypokalemia causes relatively more H^+ ions to be available for secretion into the urine, thus enhancing paradoxical aciduria and worsening metabolic alkalosis. Furthermore, hypokalemia causes potassium to diffuse out of cells into extracellular fluid in exchange for H^+ ions, which move into cells. This exchange further enhances metabolic alkalosis (see chapter 61).

Mixed Acid–Base Disorders

Recalling the definition of acidosis and alkalosis given earlier—processes that cause acid and alkali to accumulate in the body—it should be clear that mixed acid-base disturbances are common in clinical disorders. For example, a patient with pyloric outlet obstruction resulting in vomiting will probably have metabolic alkalosis due to loss of HCl in gastric juice. The expected compensatory response would be hypoventilation and resultant secondary increase in PCO_2. If this patient develops aspiration pneumonia, hypoxemia may result in hyperventilation and subsequent respiratory alkalosis. This would be an example of mixed metabolic alkalosis and respiratory alkalosis. It is entirely possible that metabolic acidosis may develop in this animal also. Metabolic acidosis could be a result of (1) hypoxemia (from aspiration pneumonia) severe enough to cause increased cellular anaerobic metabolism and lactic acid production, (2) dehydration severe enough to cause prerenal azotemia and retention of inorganic acids, and (3) enhancement of glycolysis by alkalosis with increased lactic acid production.[10] This is an example of a so-called triple acid–base disorder[10] (metabolic alkalosis, metabolic acidosis, and respiratory alkalosis). In this clinical example, blood *p*H and plasma HCO_3^- may be increased, decreased, or normal, depending upon the relative severity of the opposing processes causing accumulation of acid and alkali. Despite a normal or near normal arterial *p*H, recognition of mixed disturbances is very important because each process requires appropriate corrective therapy. The treatment of only one process without attention to the other can result in severe acidemia or alkalemia. Although mixtures of metabolic disturbances may occur, it should be apparent that mixed respiratory acid–base disorders are impossible, because CO_2 cannot concurrently be overexcreted and underexcreted by the lungs. An in-depth discussion of mixed acid-base disorders is beyond the scope of this chapter.

Diagnostic Plan

History and Physical Examination

The history may provide information concerning the type of acid-base disturbance present in a patient. By considering the severity of the signs of the primary disorder, it may be possible to predict whether the acid–base disorder is mild or severe. Physical examination is notoriously unreliable in predicting the type and severity of acid–base disturbances.

Laboratory Evaluation

The most reliable information about acid–base status is gained from laboratory data. All that is necessary for initial acid–base evaluation is a routine set of serum electrolytes (sodium, potassium, chloride, and calculated HCO_3^-) and blood *p*H and PCO_2. Calculation of the anion gap from serum electrolyte values is also helpful in the assessment of acid–base balance (see the section on anion gap in this chapter). A hemogram, serum biochemistry profile, and urine analysis are also helpful in evaluation of the patient. Ideally, arterial blood should be collected for acid–base evaluation. Most instruments that are used to measure *p*H and PCO_2 also determine PO_2, which can provide additional information related to the respiratory component of acid–base balance. Procurement of blood from the femoral artery of most dogs is not difficult. Whenever it is not practical to obtain arterial blood, free-flowing jugular venous samples will usually provide reliable information.

If blood for acid–base evaluation is contaminated with air, falsely decreased PCO_2 and falsely increased PO_2 and *p*H values will result. Carefully filling the dead space of a syringe with heparin will usually avoid contamination with air bubbles. It is best to do the analyses immediately. If the procedure must be delayed for more than 15 to 20 minutes, satisfactory results can still be obtained for up to 2 to 3 hours by placing the stoppered syringe into an ice water bath.

Total CO_2 (TCO_2) concentration is included in many serum biochemical profiles. Since about 97% of TCO_2 is bicarbonate, the clinician should interpret TCO_2 as bicarbonate in the evaluation of acid–base disorders.

Symptomatic Therapy[4]

Symptomatic treatment of acid–base disturbances depends on the cause, type, and severity of the primary disorder.

Respiratory Acidosis

The treatment of respiratory acidosis should be directed at the cause of the CO_2 retention. Ventilatory assistance may also be needed.

Respiratory Alkalosis

Symptomatic therapy of respiratory alkalosis is not indicated. Treatment of the cause of the disorder should be undertaken.

Metabolic Acidosis

Whenever the primary disorder that has resulted in mild metabolic acidosis can be quickly resolved, it may not be necessary to treat the metabolic acidosis. In mild to moderate acidemia (*p*H 7.20–7.39), lactated Ringer's solution is generally the fluid of choice. Solutions containing acetate instead of lactate are also available and are acceptable in most instances. Lactate and acetate are metabolized by the liver to HCO_3^- (1 mEq of lactate or acetate = 1 mEq of HCO_3^-), thus providing buffer base to body fluids. For life-threatening metabolic acidemia, the use of sodium bicarbonate solution, usually as an additive to 0.45% saline or 5% glucose solutions, may be justified.

If the patient's plasma HCO_3^- concentration is known, the approximate quantity of lactate, acetate, or HCO_3^- required to correct the bicarbonate deficit can be estimated from the following formula:[6,8]

$$\begin{aligned} HCO_3^- \text{ required} &= 0.5 \times \text{body weight (kg)} \\ &\quad \times HCO_3^- \text{ deficit in plasma (normal } HCO_3^- - \text{ patient } HCO_3^-) \end{aligned}$$

For example, the HCO_3^- requirements of a 10-kg dog with a plasma HCO_3^- of 8 mEq/liter can be estimated as follows:

$$\begin{aligned} &= 0.5 \times 10 \text{ kg} \times (20 \text{ mEq/liter [normal]} - 8 \text{ mEq/liter [patient]}) \\ &= 60 \text{ mEq of } HCO_3^- \text{ required} \end{aligned}$$

In general, estimated HCO_3^- requirements should be administered slowly over a 24- to 48-hour period; half of the calculated HCO_3^- needs can be administered during the first 4 to 6 hours if necessary. Because of sluggish penetration of HCO_3^- across the blood–brain barrier, parenteral therapy with HCO_3^- alkalinizes blood faster than CSF. The persistent CSF acidity perpetuates compensatory hyperventilation and loss of CO_2 (respiratory alkalosis), which adds to the alkalinizing effect of HCO_3^- on blood. The HCO_3^-/H_2CO_3 ratio may increase enough to cause alkalemia. Sustained lowering of arterial PCO_2 for 12 to 36 hours may be present during the correction of metabolic acidosis.

Paradoxical CSF acidosis and coma have been documented in acidotic human diabetics[12] and following experimental cardiac arrest and resuscitation in acidotic dogs[1,2] as a result of excessively rapid intravenous administration of sodium bicarbonate solution. This apparently happens because the administered HCO_3^- combines with H^+ ions in the extracellular fluid to form H_2CO_3, which dissociates to CO_2 and H_2O. Bicarbonate penetrates the blood–brain barrier slowly, but CO_2 enters the CSF rapidly. Once in the CSF, CO_2 combines with H_2O to form H_2CO_3, resulting in a progressive fall in CSF *p*H at the same time the blood *p*H is increasing. Neither the incidence nor the consequences of paradoxical CSF acidosis caused by rapid sodium bicarbonate administration to dogs and cats are known.

This complication is most likely whenever relatively large quantities (>2–4 mEq/kg) of sodium bicarbonate solution are being repeatedly administered intravenously during a short period (<24 hours). Resulting central nervous system depression or coma could be serious consequences or even fatal in critically ill patients.

Other reported side effects of excessive sodium bicarbonate administration include a decrease in ionized serum calcium concentration of extracellular fluid (shifts to protein-bound form), hypokalemia (potassium ions enter cells in exchange for H^+ ions), left shifting of the oxyhemoglobin dissociation curve (increased affinity of hemoglobin for oxygen, resulting in less oxygen release to tissues), and plasma hyperosmolality with hyperosmolal coma.

HCO_3^- may be given by the oral route if vomiting is not present and if the need is not immediate. Sodium bicarbonate tablets, either 5-grain or 10-grain, are available. To convert grains to milliequivalents, it should be remembered that 4 grains of sodium bicarbonate are equal to about 3 mEq each of sodium and bicarbonate.

Regardless of the compound and route used in the treatment of metabolic acidosis, it is best to monitor plasma HCO_3^- (or TCO_2) periodically to assess results of therapy. Increasing urine *p*H is generally associated with correction of metabolic acidosis but is only a rough guideline at best.

In considering the usual efficiency of body defense mechanisms against blood pH change, and the number of potentially hazardous consequences of excessive alkali administration, it is best to be conservative when treating metabolic acidosis.

Metabolic Alkalosis

The treatment of metabolic alkalosis depends on the cause. If excessive alkali administration caused the disorder, discontinuance of the alkali should lead to a prompt restoration of acid–base balance. Metabolic alkalosis due to vomiting is associated with chloride depletion and sometimes potassium deficit. It can be effectively treated by administration of solutions containing high chloride concentration and enough potassium to repair potassium deficit, if present. It is generally unnecessary to administer strong acid solutions to correct H^+ ion deficit, because acids are continually being produced endogenously as waste products of cellular metabolism. Ringer's solution contains sufficient chloride to replenish chloride deficits but is low in potassium. Once hydration has been reestablished and adequate urine output documented, extra potassium (as potassium chloride) should probably be added to the Ringer's solution (see chapter 61).

ANION GAP

Definition

The anion gap (AG) is a major tool used in evaluating acid-base disorders in humans, and its usefulness in veterinary medicine has been reported.[5,13,14] The formula most commonly used to estimate AG is

$$AG\ (\text{mEq/liter}) = (Na^+ + K^+) - (Cl^- + HCO_3^-)$$

With the common use of biochemical profiling, more veterinarians routinely determine serum Na^+, K^+, Cl^-, and TCO_2 (which can be substituted for HCO_3^- in the above formula) on clinical patients and can estimate AG. Normal AG for dogs is about 15 to 25 mEq/liter and it is probably similar for cats.

Pathophysiology[4]

The term *AG* is a misnomer, because it implies that there is a gap between, or a difference in, plasma anion and cation concentration. This is certainly not the case, because total plasma cation concentration must always be equal to total plasma anion concentration to maintain electroneutrality in body fluids.

It is helpful in understanding AG to derive another formula that more clearly states the true meaning of AG *in vivo*.[10] Since total serum cations equals total serum anions,

$$(Na^+ + K^+) + UC = (Cl^- + HCO_3^-) + UA$$
$$(Na^+ + K^+) - (Cl^- + HCO_3^-) = UA - UC$$
$$AG\ (\textit{in vivo}) = UA - UC$$

where UC is unmeasured cations in plasma and UA is unmeasured anions in plasma. Thus, whereas the AG is *estimated* from the concentrations of Na^+, K^+, Cl^-, and HCO_3, AG is actually *determined in vivo* by the concentrations of UA and UC in plasma.[11] Since plasma UA and UC in the patient do not change in the same direction in equal quantities simultaneously, "true" changes in plasma UA and UC can be accurately predicted by the following formula:

$$AG = (Na^+ + K^+) - (Cl^- + HCO_3^-)$$

Changes in AG can occur as a consequence of only three basic processes:

1. A change in plasma UA or UC in the patient
2. A gain or loss of water from plasma in the patient
3. Laboratory error in Na^+, K^+, Cl^-, or HCO_3^- measurement

Common causes of increased and decreased AG are shown in Table 63-3.

The most common change in AG is an increase and, except for a few unusual situations, an increased AG is synonymous with accumulation of acids, other than HCl, in the body (metabolic acidosis). It should be understood, however, that anions, measured or unmeasured, are not acids. Only when anions are

Table 63-3. Causes of Abnormal Anion Gap*

INCREASED ANION GAP	DECREASED ANION GAP
Increased unmeasured anions	Decreased unmeasured anions
Diabetic ketoacidosis	Decreased plasma albumin
Lactic acidosis	Acidosis, decreasing negative charge on albumin
Azotemia	Dilution of extracellular fluid
Increased plasma albumin	Increased unmeasured cations
Dehydration	Hypercalcemia
Alkalosis, increasing negative charge on albumin	Hypermagnesemia
Exogenous anions: penicillin, carbenicillin, salicylate	Cationic proteins in multiple myeloma
Ethylene glycol toxicity	
Dehydration	
Decreased unmeasured cations	
Hypocalcemia	
Hypomagnesemia	

* Laboratory error in the measurement of sodium, potassium, chloride, or bicarbonate will cause an erroneous anion gap.
(Cornelius LM: Principles of fluid therapy [small animal]. In Anderson NV [ed]: Veterinary Gastroenterology. Philadelphia, Lea & Febiger [in press])

accompanied by H^+ ions that dissociate from the anion and titrate buffers (*e.g.*, HCO_3^-), thus lowering the HCO_3^-/H_2CO_3 ratio, is acidosis observed.

Shown below are illustrations of the effects on AG of the accumulation of two different types of acids in the body:

1. $H^+ \text{ lactate}^- + Na^+HCO_3^- \rightarrow Na^+ \text{ lactate}^- + H_2CO_3 \rightarrow CO_2 + H_2O$
2. $H^+Cl^- + Na^+HCO_3^- \rightarrow Na^+Cl^- + H_2CO_3 \rightarrow CO_2 + H_2O$

In example 1, the accumulation of lactic acid lowers the measured anion, HCO_3^-, and replaces it with the unmeasured anion, lactate. Therefore, AG increases in this example of metabolic acidosis. In example 2, the accumulation of HCl also lowers the measured anion, HCO_3^-, but replaces it with another measured anion, chloride. Therefore, AG does not change in this example of hyperchloremic metabolic acidosis. Causes of metabolic acidosis with elevated and normal AG are shown in Table 63-4. An increased AG may be the only laboratory evidence of acidosis in some patients with mixed metabolic acidosis and metabolic alkalosis.[10]

Diagnostic Plan

Anion gap is estimated from serum sodium, potassium, chloride, and HCO_3^- (or TCO_2) and is used in the interpretation of acid–base balance.

Table 63-4. Selected Causes of Metabolic Acidosis

INCREASED ANION GAP	NORMAL ANION GAP (HYPERCHLOREMIC ACIDOSIS)
Diabetic ketoacidosis	Diarrhea
Azotemia	Renal tubular acidosis
Lactic acid accumulation (hypoxic tissues)	Addition of HCl
Toxins	Ammonium chloride therapy
Ethylene glycol (antifreeze)	Methionine sulfate therapy
Salicylates	
Paraldehyde	

(Cornelius LM: Principles of fluid therapy [small animal]. In Anderson NV [ed]: Veterinary Gastroenterology. Philadelphia, Lea & Febiger [in press])

Symptomatic Therapy

Symptomatic treatment of abnormal anion gap is not required. The primary disorder should be corrected. If acid–base abnormalities are present, they should be treated appropriately.

REFERENCES

1. Berenyi KJ, et al: Cerebrospinal fluid acidosis complicating therapy of experimental cardiopulmonary arrest. Circulation 52:319, 1975
2. Bishop RL, Weisfeldt ML: Sodium bicarbonate administration during cardiac arrest. JAMA 235:506, 1976
3. Cornelius LM: Fluid, electrolyte, acid-base, and nutritional management. In Bojrab MH (ed): Pathophysiology in Surgery, pp 12–32. Philadelphia, Lea & Febiger, 1981
4. Cornelius LM: Principles of fluid therapy (small animal). In Anderson NV (ed): Veterinary Gastroenterology. Philadelphia, Lea & Febiger (in press)
5. Feldman BF, Rosenberg DP: Clinical use of anion and osmolal gaps in veterinary medicine. J Am Vet Med Assoc 178:396–398, 1981
6. Finco DR: General guidelines for fluid therapy. J Am Anim Hosp Assoc 8:166, 1972
7. Finco DR: Fluid therapy for profuse vomiting. J Am Anim Hosp Assoc 8:200, 1972
8. Garella S, et al: Severity of metabolic acidosis as a determinant of bicarbonate requirements. N Engl J Med 289:121, 1973
9. Makoff DL: Acid-base metabolism. In Maxwell MH, Kleeman CR (eds): Clinical Disorders of Fluid and Electrolyte Metabolism, pp 297–346. New York, McGraw-Hill, 1972
10. Narins RG, Emmett M: Simple and mixed acid-base disorders: A practical approach. Medicine (Baltimore) 59:161–187, 1980
11. Oh MS, Carroll HJ: Current concepts: The anion gap. N Engl J Med 297:814–817, 1977
12. Posner JB, Plum F: Spinal fluid pH and neurologic systems in systemic acidosis. N Engl J Med 277:605, 1967
13. Polzin DJ, Stevens JB, Osborne CA: Clinical application of the anion gap in evaluation of acid-base disorders in dogs. Comp Cont Ed 4(12):1021–1032, 1982
14. Shull RM: The value of anion gap and osmolal gap determination in veterinary medicine. Vet Clin Pathol 7:12–14, 1978
15. Welt LG: Agents affecting the volume and composition of body fluids. In Goodman LS, Gilman A (eds): The Pharmacological Basis of Therapeutics, pp 773–804. London, Macmillan, 1970

Index

The letter *f* after a page number indicates a figure; *t* following a page number indicates tabular material.